MATERNAL AND CHILD HEALTH NURSING

Special contributions

CHAPTER 15

Intensive care of the newborn

John E. Wimmer, Jr., M.D.
Assistant Professor,
Department of Pediatrics, Neonatology Section,
School of Medicine,
East Carolina University,
Greenville, North Carolina

Linda Jean Cramer, R.N., B.S.
Neonatal Staff Educator,
Good Samaritan Hospital and Medical Center,
Portland, Oregon

CHAPTER 20

Rehabilitation of the long-term pediatric patient

Helen Linn, R.N., B.S.N.
Resource Nurse,
Donald N. Sharp Rehabilitation Center,
San Diego, California

Carol D. Heylman, R.N.
Head Nurse,
Special Care Unit,
Children's Hospital and Health Center,
San Diego, California

MATERNAL

AND CHILD HEALTH

NURSING

A. JOY INGALLS, R.N., M.S.

Instructor, Maternal and Child Health Nursing, Grossmont Vocational
Nursing Program, Grossmont Health Careers Center, La Mesa, California

M. CONSTANCE SALERNO, R.N., M.S., S.N.P.

Professor of Child Health Nursing,
San Diego State University, San Diego, California

FIFTH EDITION
with 640 illustrations

The C. V. Mosby Company

St. Louis • Toronto • London   1983

A TRADITION OF PUBLISHING EXCELLENCE

Editor: Alison Miller

Assistant editor: Susan R. Epstein

Manuscript editor: Suzanne Harrawood

Design: Nancy Steinmeyer

Production: Carol O'Leary, Mary Stueck, Jeanne A. Gulledge

Conversion chart on back endpaper from
Chinn, P.L.: Child health maintenance:
concepts in family-centered care, ed. 2, St. Louis, 1979,
The C. V. Mosby Company

FIFTH EDITION

Previous editions copyrighted 1967, 1971, 1975, 1979

Printed in the United States of America

The C. V. Mosby Company
11830 Westline Industrial Drive, St. Louis, Missouri 63141

Library of Congress Cataloging in Publication Data

Ingalls, A. Joy.
  Maternal and child health nursing.

  Bibliography: p.
  Includes index.
  1. Obstetrical nursing. 2. Pediatric nursing.
I. Salerno, M. Constance. II. Title. [DNLM:
1. Obstetrical nursing. 2. Pediatric nursing.
WY 157 I44m]
RG951.I5   1983   610.73'62   82-14160
ISBN 0-8016-2324-3

TS/VH/VH 9 8 7 6 5 4 3 2   03/B/312

To
The bedside nurse
whatever her title

CONTRIBUTORS

JULIE COWAN NOVAK, R.N., M.A., P.N.P.

Coordinator, Child-Health Nurse Practitioner Program,
University of California, San Diego,
San Diego, California

JUDITH MILLER PETERS, R.N., M.S.

Assistant Professor of Parent-Child Nursing,
Loma Linda University,
Loma Linda, California

JANET MEIER CETTI, R.N., M.S.

Educational Consultant, Donald N. Sharp Memorial Community Hospital,
San Diego, California

PREFACE

The dynamic, revolving sphere that is our world vividly displays the seasonal cycles of birth, growth, maturation, aging, and death reflected in generations of nature and mankind. The person engaged in nursing is in a privileged position to observe and participate in particularly significant events and periods in the calender of human life. This book continues to be an introductory text for the bedside nurse who, as a student or staff member, is serving in the setting of maternity and pediatrics where the processes of birth and growth are most obvious and the life cycle begins anew.

This fifth edition incorporates numerous changes in content, while retaining its basic structure. Almost every page has undergone alteration. Considerable new material has been added, and obsolete subject matter has been deleted. Significant additions to the maternity section are: new discussions and charts concerning high-risk pregnancy, preeclampsia-eclampsia (pregnancy-induced hypertension), and teratogens; a section on the Friedman Labor Curve for evaluating the progress of labor; and a brief discussion of cultural effects on maternal care and individual patient compliance. The subjects of obstetric complications and pain relief during labor and birth have been almost completely rewritten. The pediatric sections have been revised to include problems related to vision and hearing (including assessment and treatment). The chapters devoted to contagious diseases and isolation procedures, nursing aspects of pediatric urology, the young burned patient, and the terminally ill child have been extensively revised. The sections dealing with genetics, childhood diabetes, and cystic fibrosis have also been rewritten.

Several new teaching illustrations increase the usefulness of the text. Noteworthy additions are an expanded CPR reminder chart, a series of drawings and photographs designed to assist the nurse's understanding of chest therapy, and diagrams depicting the positioning and care of the rehabilitation patient.

We are fully aware of the contribution men are making to the nursing profession, and we have made every effort to eliminate all sexism from this text. For clarity and simplicity, however, the feminine pronoun has been used to refer to the nurse. For the same reasons, the masculine pronoun has been used to refer to the infant and child.

A textbook of this scope, though representing beginning levels of understanding, incorporates the work of many minds and hands. Writers are fortunate indeed who have the help and support of such contributors as: John E. Wimmer, Jr., M.D., who carefully revised the chapter treating intensive care of the newborn, first prepared by Linda J. Cramer, R.N., B.S., and himself; and Helen Linn, R.N., B.S.N., and Carol Heylman, R.N., who rewrote portions of the chapter entitled "Rehabilitation of the Long-Term Pediatric Patient," which was initially prepared in previous editions by Larry Christenson, R.N., M.A. We also continue to recognize the work of Julie Cowan Novak, R.N., M.A., and Janet Meier Cetti, R.N., M.S., who helped strengthen the previous revision, and we are delighted to recognize the continuing contribution of Judith M. Peters, R.N., M.S., who graciously helped update the chapter on prenatal care. The expertise and literary abilities of these professionals have contributed significantly to the usefulness and readability of this text.

We cannot adequately express our appreciation for the generous assistance of the following physicians, nurses, and other professionals who reviewed and critiqued various chapters or sections of the manuscript: Helen Brophy, R.N., M.S., William H. Browning, M.D., Carolyn Colwell, R.N., M.A., Thomas Cullison, M.D., Douglas Dechario, M.D., Stephan Drosman, M.D., Hugh

A. Frank, M.D., Emanuel A. Friedman, M.D., William F. Friedman, M.D., William R. Griswold, M.D., Barry H. Gruer, D.D.S., Charles B. Hargrove, M.D., Mary Ingalls, M.T.M.A., Kenneth Lee Jones, M.D., Jon Lischke, M.D., William M. McGuigan, M.S., J.D., Daniel J. Marnell, M.D., David G. Martin, M.D., James Mascarello, Ph.D., Eli O. Meltzer, M.D., Robert E. Novak, Ph.D., Sung Min Park, M.D., Alex F. Pue, M.D., Teri L. Richards, R.N., M.S., Katherine Sheehan, M.D., Rayburn R. Skoglund, M.D., John J. Spinetta, Ph.D., F. Bruder Stapleton, M.D., and William J. Thomas, M.D. We are pleased and honored to be associated with all those who have shared their knowledge and expertise to make this edition possible.

As authors, we are indebted to several accomplished artists and photographers. The talents of Sue Seif, medical illustrator, MCV, Virginia Commonwealth University; Carol Land, Graphic Arts Department, San Diego State University; and Phyllis Stookey of Medigraphix are recognized with gratitude. Photographers Karla Barber, Chris McGirr, and Ed Keenan also added a visual aspect to learning not conveyed by the printed word. The fine artistic work of Martha B. Lackey and Mary Fritchoff continues to offer meaningful clarification. We are particularly appreciative of the time and effort of James Mascarello, Ph.D., Director of Genetic Services, Children's Hospital and Health Center, San Diego, California, for contributing the new karyotype, and Eveline Buchanan, C.R.T.T., who graciously demonstrated the position in the photos of chest physiotherapy.

We also wish to express our thanks to our faithful typists, Pat Summers and Jimmy Nichols, two very valued persons who often performed above and beyond the call of duty. We thank Jan and Robert Brown, who came willingly when a call for assistance was sounded. As always, we express our appreciation for the encouragement of Ellen M. Abbott, the Director of the Health Careers Center Grossmont Adult School, Grossmont Union High School District, whose early and continuing support helped make the text first possible.

Most of all, as teachers and students, we wish to recognize the contributions that our patients, large and small, young or old, solemn or smiling, have made to our nursing experience. They have enriched our personal and professional lives and have taught us much regarding the seasons of life.

A. Joy Ingalls
M. Constance Salerno

CONTENTS

xii   Contents

Current perspectives in maternal-child care

Nurses engaged in maternal and child care must be aware of current developments and goals in these fields, both locally and nationally, if they are to function meaningfully in hospitals and clinics. This brief introduction contains some definitions, important statistics, and a short historic review designed to increase the student's appreciation of the progress that has been made and the problems that still remain.

That progress has been made cannot be denied. Great reductions have been realized in the number of illnesses and deaths involving both mothers and children. The overlapping disciplines of *obstetrics*, the art and science of maternal-fetal and newborn care, and *pediatrics*, the art and science of the care of children and youth, have made tremendous, almost miraculous advances in the last 60 years. Indeed, it is out of these twin concerns that the new discipline of *perinatology*, or the study and support of the fetus and neonate, has developed.

To help the student understand the extent of this improvement, it will be necessary to introduce some statistics; however, they need not be complicated or lengthy to tell an important story.

Maternal mortality

Among health statistics the term "mortality" often is encountered, meaning the number of persons per given population who died in a given period of time. Maternal mortality refers to the number of mothers who die per 100,000 live births for a

certain period. In 1915 maternal mortality in the United States equaled 608 per 100,000; by 1978 maternal mortality had fallen to 9.6 per 100,000.

Year	Maternal Mortality
1980 (Est.)	6.9
1979 (Est.)	7.8
1978	9.6
1977	11.2
1976	12.3

A gradual reduction in maternal mortality has continued steadily as revealed by the 1979 and 1980 estimated statistics.*

Although these figures represent a splendid reduction in the maternal death rate, it should be much lower. The national statistics for 1978 continue to demonstrate a great but narrowing difference between the maternal death rate among nonwhite mothers (23.0 per 100,000) and white mothers (6.4 per 100,000), reflecting a significant inequality in the availability or use of maternity services. Shifting centers of population, lack of education, strained and understaffed public facilities, maldistribution of services, and ineffectual health delivery systems all help contribute to a higher maternal death rate than should occur in the United States.

Leading causes. The final maternal mortality statistics for 1978 cite "toxemias of pregnancy," infec-

---

*U.S. Department of Health and Human Services, Public Health Service, NCHS. Monthly Vital Statistics Report **29**(6):37, supplement 2, Sept. 1980.

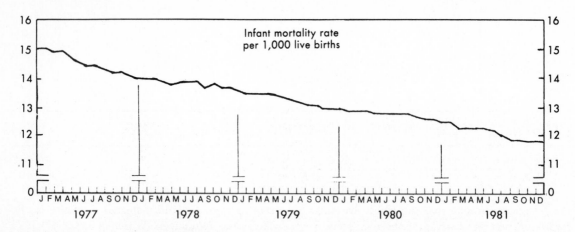

FIG. 1.A   United States infant mortality rate Jan. 1977-Dec. 1981.

Data from U.S. Dept. of Health and Human Services, Public Health Service, NCHS Monthly Vital Statistics Report, Vol. **30**:3, March 18, 1982.

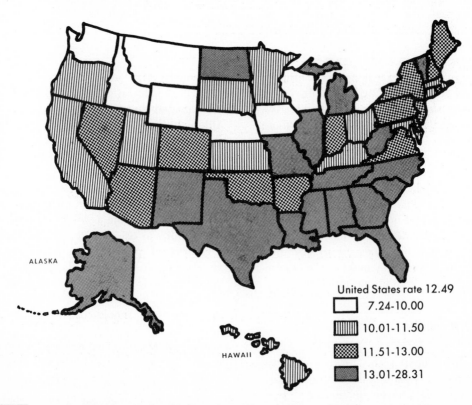

FIG. 1.B   United States infant mortality, per 1,000 live births, January to June, 1981.

Data from Monthly Vital Statistics Report, U.S. Dept. of Health and Human Services, Public Health Service, Office of Health Research, Statistics and Technology, Publication No. HE20.6217, vol. 30: Sept. 15, 1981.

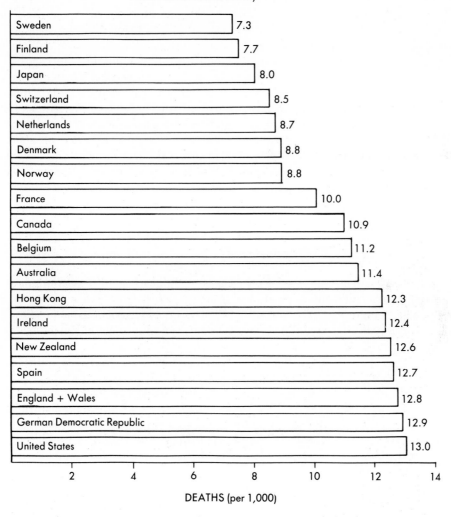

International Infant Mortality

Country	Deaths (per 1,000)
Sweden	7.3
Finland	7.7
Japan	8.0
Switzerland	8.5
Netherlands	8.7
Denmark	8.8
Norway	8.8
France	10.0
Canada	10.9
Belgium	11.2
Australia	11.4
Hong Kong	12.3
Ireland	12.4
New Zealand	12.6
Spain	12.7
England + Wales	12.8
German Democratic Republic	12.9
United States	13.0

DEATHS (per 1,000)

FIG. 2 International infant mortality, 1979, of lowest eighteen countries with a population of 2 million or more.

Data from Statistical Papers: Population and Vital Statistics Reports, New York, United Nations, 1980, Series A, vol. 32; Demographic Year Book, 1979. New York, 1980, United Nations.

tion, ectopic pregnancy, and hemorrhage as the four leading causes of maternal death in their order of incidence.

The statistical category labeled toxemias of pregnancy includes several associated signs and symptoms such as elevated blood pressure (hypertension), albumin in the urine (albuminuria), and an abnormal amount of fluid in the tissues (edema). Edema reveals itself by swelling and rapid weight gain, headache, and, in extreme cases, convulsions. At this time there is no agreement among clinicians regarding the cause of toxemic complications. Newer terminology used to describe these signs and symptoms includes preeclampsia-eclampsia and pregnancy-induced hypertension. Ectopic pregnancy refers to those pregnancies that develop in places other than the normal location within the uterus. Ectopic pregnancies are often associated with significant blood loss early in gestation.

Hemorrhage is by far the most common major maternal complication. It should be appreciated that many times hemorrhage may predispose a mother to fall victim to other difficulties, such as infection. The greatest progress in the overall reduction of maternal mortality through the years has been in the prevention of infection.

Infant mortality

Infant mortality statistics concern the number of children per 1,000 live births who die before their first birthday. In 1900 the average rate in those states reporting was 200 per 1,000; in 1980 the rate had dropped to 12.6 per 1,000 live births (provisional figures).* But lest health professionals become too self-congratulatory, they should be aware that this figure is not consistent throughout the United States and still ranks approximately eighteenth among the nations recording such sta-

*U.S. Department of Health and Human Services, Public Health Service, NCHS Monthly Vital Statistic Report, **30:**6, Sept. 1981.

tistics (Figs. 1 and 2). Reduced to more shocking proportions, United States infant mortality statistics mean that 1 out of every 79 babies born dies before his first birthday. The national lag in lowering infant mortality is related to the reasons cited for the rate of maternal mortality. It is no doubt caused by the many different economic, cultural, and educational backgrounds and levels found in the United States and the failure of the health care delivery system to meet the needs of these diversified groups. The country's international standing may also be influenced slightly by the different ways in which statistics are formulated in various countries, despite attempts at standardization. However, the fact remains that, compared to the records of other nations, performance in infant mortality in the United States leaves much to be desired.

About 65% of infant deaths occur in the first 28 days of life, the *neonatal* period. Estimated data for 1980 reported by the U.S. Department of Health and Human Services (formerly the Department of Health, Education and Welfare) indicates that the leading causes of *infant* death were, in the order of their frequency, congenital anomalies, respiratory distress syndrome, sudden infant death syndrome, and disorders related to short gestation and low birth weight. Prematurity is a leading cause of neonatal death.

It will readily be seen that any method that decreases the incidence of prematurity or improves medical-nursing management of premature infants would profoundly affect infant mortality statistics. In the past the most commonly used definition of prematurity was a birth weight of less than 5½ pounds (2,500 g), although it is recognized that not all infants of low birth weight are born before term. The current definition, birth before the end of 37 weeks' intrauterine development, is more logical but not always verifiable.

Another statistical category is that of *perinatal mortality*. This figure includes recorded deaths of fetuses of more than 20 weeks' gestation added to those of the first 4 weeks of life (the neonatal period).

CHANGE AND PROGRESS IN MATERNITY CARE

Although maternity care could be improved a great deal, clearly conditions have changed radically for the better. It would be worthwhile for us to discuss the major reasons that this great progress has been made.

Acceptance of the germ theory

First, the acceptance of the germ theory led to a greater understanding of the causes of infection. Less than a hundred years ago, infection was such a common companion of childbirth in some communities, notably among hospital patients, that its symptoms were termed childbed, or puerperal, fever (referring to the puerperium, the approximate 6-week period after birth). Standards of cleanliness in most nineteenth century hospitals were nonexistent, and the suggestion that illness might be spread by the contaminated hands of physicians and medical students met with much opposition and scorn. Nevertheless, despite much difficulty and even persecution, certain individuals began to persuade the medical world that puerperal fever was really a contagion borne by many hands and common objects.

Chief among these medical pioneers was a Hungarian, Ignaz Philipp Semmelweis (1818-1865), whose sad but fascinating biography should be read by every maternity nurse. The American poet-physician, Oliver Wendell Holmes (1809-1894), is probably best remembered for his "Chambered Nautilus," but medical historians record his concern with maternal mortality and his widely criticized paper entitled "The Contagiousness of Puerperal Fever." The famed French chemist, Louis Pasteur, confirmed that childbed fever was indeed caused by bacteria and was contagious in character.

Improvement of techniques and teaching

Second, obstetric techniques and teaching have vastly improved. With the acceptance of the germ theory, new concepts of care evolved. Britain's Joseph Lister, the Father of Antisepsis, began to combat infection by chemical means and new wound-dressing techniques. Students of obstetrics were given more clinical instruction at the bedside, and their "experience" was less confined to the printed page or the dissecting table. New tools, such as improved obstetric forceps, sutures, and syringes; antibiotic medications; laboratory clinical tests; transfusions; and anesthesia were developed. Hospitalization of the childbearing woman and her child became an asset.

More recently there has been the development of new laboratory methods of assessing fetal maturity and health, the wide use of ultrasonic and electronic fetal monitoring, and more aggressive techniques in treating the immature or sick newborn. Greater technologic aid is available to the mother facing high-risk pregnancy and labor. These advances along with the regionalization of maternal and infant intensive care centers have further reduced mortality and morbidity.

Development and extension of prenatal care

Third, and probably most significant, has been the development of *prenatal care* and extended obstetric services by private and governmental public health facilities. Nurses relate proudly that prenatal care began as a nursing contribution instigated by the Instructive Nursing Association of the Boston Lying-In Hospital in 1901. From one visit before childbirth, prenatal care has now developed into close supervision of the expectant mother from the time her pregnancy is confirmed. Prenatal care has been extended to more and more Americans through the services of public health departments, visiting nurses, nurse practitioners, and nurse-midwives, as well as private clinics and individual physicians. However, despite these efforts, many women in the United States still do not obtain adequate prenatal care. Much analysis of health delivery systems, funding, promotional expertise, and education is still needed.

Today the entire nation as never before is experiencing the stresses of structural change and modification. These changes are reflected in numerous patterns of family organization, divisions of labor, and sexual relationships. Women who need maternity care in the United States are representatives of a mobile, pluralistic, multicultural society. They face the experience of childbearing with differing concerns, expectations, goals, and resources. Maternity nurses must increasingly be aware of the wide variety of backgrounds their patients represent, their differing needs, and the individualized care they may require.

One of the major developments of this decade has been the increasing assertiveness of consumers of health services. A growing number of expectant parents are demanding to participate as a family more actively in the process of pregnancy and childbirth, relatively free of medical intervention. To fulfill this desire, some couples have sought alternatives to so-called traditional hospitalization such as home birth or, where available, a birth center.

The declaration that childbirth is a normal rather than a pathologic event has much to commend it. Also praiseworthy is a childbearing woman's willingness to accept responsibility for the birth process and the parents' commitment to the promotion of normal childbirth. Difficulty may arise, however, when differences between normal and abnormal are not adequately appreciated in time to allow successful treatment of complications. It is extremely interesting that as more technical and mechanical methods of detecting complications are being introduced and perfected, emphasis on humanistic values increases. The two are not necessarily incompatible; they are complementary. Indeed, maternal and child care has been described as both a science and an art.

CHANGE AND PROGRESS IN CHILD CARE

Naturally, the same factors that improved maternity care have helped to enhance the lives of children of all ages. However, pediatrics is a more recent specialty than obstetrics. Until the 1800s there was little formalized recognition of the special needs of children, the medical and surgical problems peculiar to childhood, or the different ways in which infants and children, in contrast to adults, respond to the presence of disease.

Development of pediatrics

In 1802 the first children's hospital was founded in Paris, France. In 1855 the first children's hospital in the United States was established in Philadelphia. But in most regions sick, hospitalized children were often quartered with ill adults, sometimes in the same bed! Gradually, the consideration of pediatrics as a separate study was initiated. As medical schools recognized the unique qualities of the childhood period, nursing schools followed their lead and offered special classes in pediatric nursing. General hospitals established pediatric departments, and more separate treatment centers for children were inaugurated. An early leader in the recognition of the special needs of children was Abraham Jacobi, first president of the American Pediatric Society and founder of the first clinic operated exclusively for children.

Responses of a changing society to children's needs

Change in itself does not automatically guarantee progress, and certainly the vast technologic changes of the late nineteenth and early twentieth centuries did little to improve the immediate outlook of a great number of the world's growing children. The new demands of the rapidly accelerating industrial revolution, often untempered by regard for the individual, child or adult, caused sudden urban congestion, and although standards of living rose for some, often the industrial laborer suffered from deprivation and exploitation. Some of those laborers working in the mills, factories, and mines were children. Two early major events, the inauguration of the White House Conferences and the establishment of the Children's Bureau, reflected a definite improvement and promotion of a better life for all children.

White House Conferences. From 1909 through 1971, close to the beginning of each decade, the very important national White House Conferences were held. These focused attention on the current prominent needs of children and youth. Delegates of private and governmental agencies at local, state, and federal levels concerned with maternal and child care as well as selected youth representatives convened for evaluation of these needs and ways in which they could be met. One of the most significant documents in the history of child care was prepared at the 1930 White House Conference on Child Health and Protection. Entitled "The Rights of the Child as an Individual in the State," it has been called the "Children's Charter." The theme of the midcentury White House Conference was "A Fair Chance to Achieve a Healthy Personality." At this conference the "Pledge to Children" was adopted. (See p. 8.) The 1970-71 White House Conference focused on children and youth in the changing social scene. The White House Conferences on children scheduled for the 1980s were terminated by presidential order.

Children's Bureau. Principally because of the problem of child labor, the Children's Bureau was founded in 1912 as a result of the support of the first White House Conference on Children and Youth; it was initially placed under the jurisdiction of the Department of Labor. When the Department of Health, Education, and Welfare (DHEW) was created in 1953, it became part of the responsibility of this cabinet post. In its founding legislation, as amended, the Children's Bureau was charged with the responsibility "to investigate and report on all matters pertaining to the welfare of children and child life among all classes of our people"; to carry out research, demonstration, and training func-

tions; to help coordinate the programs for children and parents throughout the Department of Health, Education, and Welfare (today known as the Department of Health and Human Services); to promote programs for youth; and to identify areas requiring the development of new projects. In 1969 the Children's Bureau was transferred to the newly created Office of Child Development, where it continued to provide a wide range of technical assistance services to children and families. In 1977 the Office of Child Development was replaced by the Administration for Children, Youth and Families. The Children's Bureau now administers the National Center on Child Abuse and Neglect, established in 1974, under the Child Abuse Prevention and Treatment Act. Through this act, funds have been made available for 3-year demonstration projects that provide preventive, social, and medical services, as well as treatment services, to families and children at risk.

Social Security legislation. The Social Security Act, passed in 1935, provided for a federal-state partnership to promote maternal and child health. Title V of this legislation (Child Health Act of 1967) is the basis for extensive programs including nutrition, family planning, prenatal, and other services for mothers and children. It reinforced the principle that all people in the United States, through the federal government, share responsibility with the state and local governments for helping to provide essential community services for children. To back up this principle, the Social Security Act authorizes Congress to appropriate funds each year to be given to the states to help them extend and improve their maternal and child health, crippled children's, and child welfare services. Under Title XIX of the Social Security Act, Medicaid was authorized. With matching funds states may receive federal aid to pay for comprehensive health care for children. Whether a child is eligible for such aid depends on his problem or diagnosis and the financial position of his family. In 1972 an extension of Title XIX provided that preventive child health services would be made available to all Medicaid recipients under age 21 years through the Early and Periodic Screening, Diagnosis, and

PLEDGE TO CHILDREN

To you, our children, who hold within you our most cherished hopes, we, the members of the Midcentury White House Conference on Children and Youth, relying on your full response, make this pledge:

From your earliest infancy we give you our love, so that you may grow with trust in yourself and in others.

We will recognize your worth as a person and we will help you to strengthen your sense of belonging.

We will respect your right to be yourself and at the same time help you to understand the rights of others, so that you may experience cooperative living.

We will help you develop initiative and imagination, so that you may have the opportunity freely to create.

We will encourage your curiosity and your pride in workmanship, so that you may have the satisfaction that comes from achievement.

We will provide the conditions for wholesome play that will add to your learning, to your social experience, and to your happiness.

We will illustrate by precept and example the value of integrity and the importance of moral courage.

We will encourage you always to seek the truth.

We will provide you with all opportunities possible to develop your own faith in God.

We will open the way for you to enjoy the arts and to use them for deepening your understanding of life.

We will work to rid ourselves of prejudice and discrimination, so that together we may achieve a truly democratic society.

We will work to lift the standard of living and to improve our economic practices, so that you may have the material basis for a full life.

We will provide you with rewarding educational opportunities, so that you may develop your talents and contribute to a better world.

We will protect you against exploitation and undue hazards and help you grow in health and strength.

We will work to conserve and improve family life and, as needed, to provide foster care according to your inherent rights.

We will intensify our search for new knowledge in order to guide you more effectively as you develop your potentialities.

As you grow from child to youth to adult, establishing a family life of your own and accepting larger social responsibilities, we will work with you to improve conditions for all children and youth.

Aware that these promises to you cannot be fully met in a world at war, we ask you to join us in a firm dedication to the building of a world society based on freedom, justice, and mutual respect.

So may you grow in joy, in faith in God and in man, and in those qualities of vision and of the spirit that will sustain us all and give us new hope for the future.

Treatment (EPSDT) program. The EPSDT program directs its efforts toward reaching children of low-income families with preventive and case-finding health services while they are in school in an attempt to correct or reduce health problems before severe handicaps develop. In 1975 a wide variety of social services was authorized under Title XX of the Social Security Act. Funds were allocated to each state to provide family planning and child care services, including foster care for needy children.

Project Head Start. Continued organized public concern for the health and welfare of children has resulted in great progress in society's efforts to protect their rights and promote their well-being.

Project Head Start is a comprehensive program launched by the Office of Economic Opportunity in the summer of 1965 and delegated to the Department of Health, Education, and Welfare (now the Department of Health and Human Services) in July, 1969. It is designed particularly for preschool children from disadvantaged backgrounds to help them develop their full potential and promote individual social competence. It provides for a daily program of learning activities, nutritious meals, medical and dental care, and psychological, social, and economic services for these children and their families. Parental participation is a vital requirement of the program.

The Parent and Child Center Program was established to meet the needs of poor children who enter Head Start with physical, mental, or language problems. The project provides a full range of services to disadvantaged families. It provides practical encouragement and assistance to parents in overcoming economic and personal problems and in learning the importance of their role in child development. Head Start has proved helpful in preparing culturally disadvantaged children for their public school experience. Its effectiveness is prolonged and enhanced by continuing educational enrichment of parents and elementary school programs.

Administration for Children, Youth and Families (ACYF). This new agency will administer all programs formerly in the Office of Child Development, which it replaces. The Administration for Children, Youth and Families includes three major divisions: the Head Start Bureau, the Children's Bureau, and the new Youth Development Bureau, which will have responsibility for the runaway youth program and other youth activities. ACYF coordinates and serves as an advocate for all children's programs throughout the federal government in an attempt to improve the wide range of services for children, youth, and their families. Numerous other programs concerned with the health of mothers and children are located within the Department of Health and Human Services. However, at this writing many of the services supported by federal and state funds are being reevaluated and reorganized.

American Academy of Pediatrics. An important analysis of health status goals for children has been conducted by the executive Board of the American Academy of Pediatrics (AAP). The academy, now composed of a membership of over 17,000 pediatricians, has assumed a leadership role in establishing standards of child health care. It approved 10 health status goals for children that outline the basic requirements for good child health.

1. All children should be wanted and born to healthy mothers.
2. All children should be born well.
3. All children should be immunized against the preventable infectious diseases for which there are recommended immunization procedures.
4. All children should have good nutrition.
5. All children should be educated about health and the health care system.
6. All children should live in a safe environment.
7. All children with chronic handicaps should be able to function at their optimal level.
8. All children should live in a family setting with an adequate income to provide basic needs to insure physical and intellectual health.
9. All children should live in an environment that is as free as possible from contaminants.
10. All adolescents and young people should live in a societal setting that recognizes their special health, personal, and social needs.

Private volunteer programs. Numerous private voluntary organizations are interested in certain specific diseases or conditions and provide considerable funds for research, diagnosis, and treatment. The National Foundation is particularly interested in birth defects. The Cystic Fibrosis Research Foundation, the American Cancer Society, the Muscular Dystrophy Association, The American Heart Association, the Epilepsy Association of America, and the National Association for Retarded Children are all examples of such private voluntary groups. Other private social agencies help by providing essential community services, such as adoption, care of unwed mothers, counseling and psychiatric services, homemaking, and recreational facilities.

International organizations. On an international scale two organizations under the auspices of the United Nations immediately come to mind. Perhaps the first is the United Nations International Children's Emergency Fund, called the United Nations Children's Fund since 1950, although the former initials, UNICEF, have been retained. This worthy organization, supported entirely by voluntary contributions, was established in 1946 to meet the distress of children caused by war. It has now greatly expanded its scope. It currently includes not only distribution of food, clothing, and medicine, but also provision for education and training of needed national workers in the health field. It is the world's largest international agency devoted to children and has received the Nobel Peace Prize for its efforts in behalf of children.

In 1956 the General Assembly of the United Nations, showing international concern for a popular topic, approved another important statement in the history of child care, "The Declaration of the Rights of the Child." Representative of UNICEF activity was its role in promoting the International Year of the Child (IYC), proclaimed by the United Nations for 1979.

The second United Nations–sponsored agency is the World Health Organization (WHO), formed in 1948. It helps coordinate efforts for disease control, provides a method of sharing new information in the fight against disease, and cooperates with UNICEF in promoting maternal and child health.

The continuing challenge

In spite of significant progress during the past decade, much remains to be done. Although the United States is ranked as the most affluent country in the world, many Americans continue to be burdened with poverty, hunger, illness, and despair. The concentrated urbanized and dispersed rural poor, changing population patterns, increasing health costs, an unevenly distributed medical care have necessitated alterations in health care delivery.

An increased number of extended nursing roles involving advanced preparation has been and is now being defined. Some of these roles would include family, pediatric, and school nurse practitioners, geriatric practitioners, and nurse-midwives.

To meet the desires of consumers for more control over health care decisions and more emphasis on the promotion of health rather than the treatment of disease, new types of health insurance and prepaid medical care are being formulated. Nursing in the combined maternal-child or family care settings of the future may change in form, but its basic intent, to promote health and to cope with the threat and discomfort of disease, remains constant.

These are some of the many challenges still to be met that profoundly affect the quality of the basic unit—the family and the child it produces. Continued effort must be exerted in order to strengthen the family unit and lend stability, depth, and purpose to the daily lives of all persons so that individually and collectively they and coming generations may enjoy creatively the best that life can offer.

The present-day maternal-child nurse works in an area that demands increasing knowledge, skill, and sensitivity. Responsibilities embrace an understanding of the reproductive process, its possible complications, care of the mother and her growing child in health and illness, an ability in health teaching, an appreciation of the role of the family, and a knowledge of community resources. Each patient is an individual with particular needs. For the alert nurse there is abundant opportunity for real challenge and achievement.

SUGGESTED SELECTED READINGS AND REFERENCES

Brodie, B.: Children: a glance at the past, Am. J. Mat. Child Nurs. **7**:219+, July-Aug. 1982.

Claiborn, S., and Walton, W.: Pediatricians' acceptance of pediatric nurse practitioners, Am. J. Nurs. **79**:300, Feb. 1979.

Dixon, M.S.: United States government health programs for children, Pediatr. Clin. North Am. **28**:689-701, Aug. 1981.

Dunlop, R.: Abraham Jacobi, the children's physician, Today's Health **48**:58+, Apr., 1970.

Dzik, R.S.: Childbirth: two approaches, introduction, JOGN Nurs. **5**:19-21, Mar.-Apr. 1976.

Edmundson, M.A., Jennings, B.J., and Kowalski, K.: A nurse practitioner program for women's health care, Am. J. Nurs. **80**:1784-1785, Oct. 1980.

Ford, K.: Child advocacy: ideas for action, Pediatr. Nurs. **5**:18-19, Jan.-Feb. 1979.

Haire, D.B.: The pregnant patient's bill of rights, J. Nurse-Midwifery **20**:29, Winter 1975.

Holaday, B. Changing views of infant care 1914-1980, Pediatr. Nurs. **7**:21-25, Jan.-Feb. 1981.

Lieberman, J.J.: Childbirth practices: from darkness into light, JOGN Nurs. **5**:41-45, May-June 1976.

Lourie, I.S., et al: Adolescent abuse and neglect: the role of runaway youth programs, Child. Today **8**:27-29, Nov.-Dec. 1979.

Marlow, D.R.: Textbook of pediatric nursing, ed. 5, Philadelphia, 1977, W.B. Saunders Co.

McAtee, P.R.: School nurse practitioner, Pediatr. Nurs. **4**:44-49, Mar.-Apr. 1978.

McGrellis, N.M.: Labor and delivery 120 years ago, JOGN Nurs. **5**(3):56-58, May-June 1976.

McGrellis, N.M.: Prenatal care 120 years ago, JOGN Nurs. **5**(2):56-58, Mar.-Apr. 1976.

Miller, M.A., and Brooten, D.A.: The childbearing family: a nursing perspective, Boston, 1977, Little, Brown & Co.

NAACOG statement on the role of the OB/GYN nurse practitioner, JOGN Nurs. **1**:56, June 1972.

Quinn, N.K., and Somers, A.R.: The patient's bill of rights: a significant aspect of the consumer revolution, Nurs. Outlook **22**:240-244, Apr. 1974.

Reed, J.: The child in America, Child. Today **8**:20-22, Nov.-Dec. 1979.

Reed, J.: Childhood in America: a folk artist's record, Child. Today **9**:18-23, Nov.-Dec. 1980.

Rubenfeld, M.G., et al: The nurse training act: yesterday, today, and . . ., Am. J. Nurs. **81**:1201-1204, June 1981.

Schweitzer, B. and Griffith, H.D.: The new federalism and health care, Pediatr. Nurs. **7**:35-36, 52, Nov.-Dec. 1981.

Smith, F.T.: Florence Nightingale: early feminist, Am. J. Nurs. **81**:1020-1024, May 1981.

Steinman, M.E., and Farr, J.D.: Nurse practitioner acceptance in private OB/GYN practice, JOGN Nurs. **9**:240-242, Jul.-Aug. 1980.

The story of the White House Conferences on Children and Youth, Washington, D.C., 1967, U.S. Department of Health, Education and Welfare, pp. 20-21.

Waserman, M.: An overview of child health care in America, Children **5**:24-29, 44, May-June 1976.

Wegman, M.E.: Annual summary of vital statistics, 1980, Pediatrics **68**:755-762, Dec. 1981.

Youmans, P.M.: The developmental pediatric nurse practitioner, Nurs. '79 **9**:113-116, Nov. 1979.

REPRODUCTIVE ANATOMY AND PHYSIOLOGY

CHAPTER **1**   Female reproductive anatomy

THE PELVIS, THE BONY PASSAGEWAY

To understand the events of labor and birth, the nurse must be acquainted with the first journey the fetus takes—the all-important journey of a few inches through the mother's birth canal. Since this canal is shaped largely by the bones of the pelvis, we will begin with a discussion of its formation and contours.

The word "pelvis" means basin. It is used to describe the cavity in the kidneys into which the urine drains before flowing down the ureter. It is also used to describe the bony ring located between the trunk and thighs, joining the spine above and the femurs below. This is the pelvis to which we refer now.

Anatomy

The pelvis is formed by the two innominate bones and the sacrum and coccyx (Fig. 1-1). Each innominate bone, however, is the end result of the fusion of three distinct bones: ilium, ischium, and pubis.

LANDMARKS AND JOINTS

The names of these three bones often recur in the descriptions of the following pelvic landmarks:

anterosuperior iliac spines The lower front end of the iliac crest line.

iliac crests The hip bones. Convenient for book or baby balancing.

iliopectineal line (**linea terminalis, brim**) Divides the upper, or false, pelvis and the lower, or true, pelvis.

ischial spines Two important landmarks in determining the depth of the fetus in the passageway. The location of the presenting part of the fetus in the pelvic canal in relation to the ischial spines is termed its "station." If the presenting part is at the level of the ischial spines, its station is said to be 0, or zero. If it is above the ischial spines, it is termed minus so many centimeters (for example, −1 or −2 cm). If the presenting part is below the ischial spines, its location is termed plus so many centimeters (for example, +1 or +2 cm). Naturally, it is important for the nurse to be able to interpret this information. When a woman in labor nears full cervical dilatation and has a station of +2 cm, the nurse must realize that if the mechanism of labor is normal, it will probably be only a relatively short time before the infant will be born.

ischial tuberosities Major bony sitting support; important in measuring a transverse diameter of the pelvis.

pubic arch Formed by the lower border of the symphysis pubis and the ischial bones.

sacral promontory The internal junction of the last lumbar vertebra and the sacrum; important in obtaining an internal obstetric measurement, known as the true conjugate, conjugata vera, or C.V.

sacrococcygeal joint Located between the sacrum and coccyx, retains limited mobility, which may offer additional room for the passage of the fetus by bending the coccyx slightly backward. Some authorities say that as much as 1 inch (2.54 cm) is occasionally gained in this way at the outlet.

sacroiliac joints Found at either side of the sacrum joining with the iliac bones.

symphysis pubis Junction of the pubic bones.

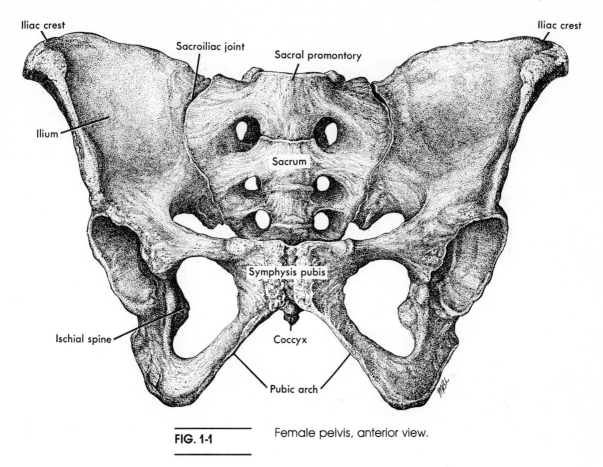

Iliac crest

Sacroiliac joint

Sacral promontory

Iliac crest

Ilium

Sacrum

Symphysis pubis

Ischial spine

Coccyx

Pubic arch

FIG. 1-1   Female pelvis, anterior view.

TRUE AND FALSE PELVIS

The *false pelvis*, formed chiefly by flaring wings of the iliac portions of the innominate bones, helps guide the fetus into the true obstetric canal. Its measurement may at times indicate possible difficulties in the structure of the true pelvis just below, but other methods utilizing x-ray pelvimetry are much more reliable. The *true pelvis* is the real concern of the obstetrician. In its journey the fetus must adapt to its different diameters and shapes to reach the outside world successfully.

INLET AND OUTLET

The entrance to the true pelvis is termed the "inlet" (Fig. 1-2). Its shape is traced, in part, by the iliopectineal line. It is wider from side to side than from front to back. Therefore the head usually enters the true pelvis with its longest diameter (which is from front to back) pointed from side to side or in transverse position. Mechanically, it is either easier or absolutely necessary.

The exit of the true pelvis is termed the "outlet" (Fig. 1-3). The outlet is wider from front to back than from side to side. To pass through the outlet, the head, in most cases, must turn to accommodate its longest diameter to the longest diameter of the exit. This turning is called *internal rotation*. The canal formed by the true pelvis forms a slight curve near the outlet and has been likened in shape to the letter J.

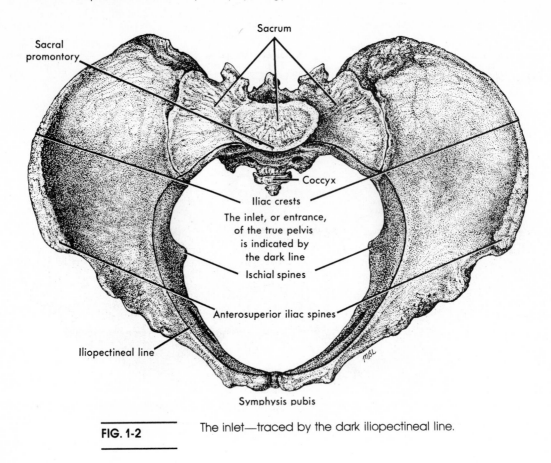

Sacrum

Sacral
promontory

Coccyx

Iliac crests

The inlet, or entrance,
of the true pelvis
is indicated by
the dark line

Ischial spines

Anterosuperior iliac spines

Iliopectineal line

Symphysis pubis

FIG. 1-2   The inlet—traced by the dark iliopectineal line.

PELVIC DIFFERENCES

Classifications. No two pelves are exactly alike although they may be classified according to their measurements. The most common classification concerns the shape and dimensions of the inlet (Fig. 1-4). The typical female pelvic inlet is labeled *gynecoid*. The typical male inlet is *android*. Unfortunately, some women have android-type pelves. A look at a male pelvis offers at least one reason why the human male could not bear children. The inlet is heart shaped and angular. The whole pelvic structure is heavier and more confining than that of the female. The pubic arch, under which every fetus should pass, is steep and narrow. In contrast, a typical woman's pelvis is relatively light and com-

modious, and the pubic arch is shallow and wide. Occasionally, a woman's pelvic inlet will be abnormally flat, or *platypelloid*, with a decreased anteroposterior diameter or it may have an *anthropoid* or apelike configuration with an enlarged anteroposterior measurement and a restricted transverse diameter. These problems may necessitate a cesarean section (abdominal delivery). But whether a birth will terminate abdominally or vaginally will depend on several factors, including the type of passageway; the size; position, and well-being of the fetus; the strength of the uterine contractions; and the condition of the laboring mother.

Causes of abnormalities. A history of certain conditions may alert the physician to expect trou-

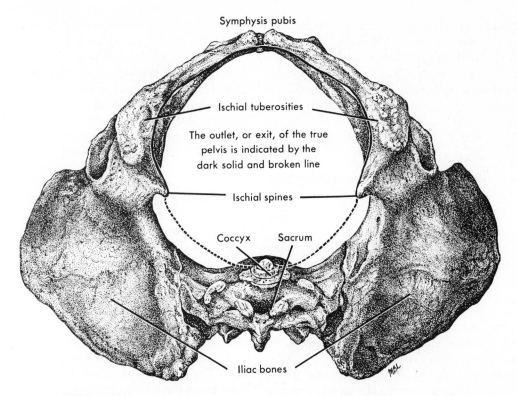

Symphysis pubis

Ischial tuberosities

The outlet, or exit, of the true pelvis is indicated by the dark solid and broken line

Ischial spines

Coccyx   Sacrum

Iliac bones

FIG. 1-3   The outlet—traced by the solid and broken dark lines.

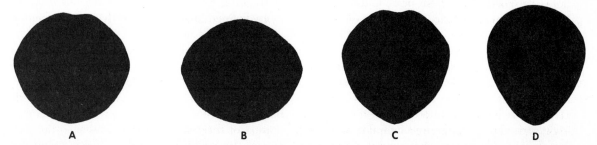

A   B   C   D

FIG. 1-4   Types of pelves. A, Normal female pelvic inlet (gynecoid); B, flattened female pelvic inlet (platypelloid); C, typical male pelvic inlet (android); D, ape-type (anthropoid).

ble because of pelvic abnormalities. The six main causes of abnormal pelvic measurements are (1) heredity (characteristic familial problems, dwarfism); (2) infections (poliomyelitis, osteomyelitis, tuberculosis of the bone); (3) poor nutrition (rickets); (4) accidents (fractured pelves); (5) paralysis of one or both extremities; and (6) poor posture and exercise habits.

Four methods of pelvic measurement

The pelvis may be measured by the following methods:

1. *External palpation* with instruments called pelvimeters (Fig. 1-5). The most important external measurement that may be determined is the distance between the ischial tuberosities (Bi. Isch. or T.I., averaging 10 to 11 cm). This measurement may indicate the distance between the ischial spines, a critical transverse measurement that is possible only with x-ray pelvimetry.

2. *Internal palpation* with a lubricated gloved finger. The distance between the sacral promontory and the outer inferior border of the pubis, known as the *diagonal conjugate* (C.D., averaging 12.5 cm), may be sought. From this measurement a closer estimate of the anteroposterior diameter of the inlet, referred to as the *true conjugate*, conjugata vera, or C.V., may be made. To do this, one subtracts 1.5 to 2 cm from the diagonal conjugate to compensate for the thickness and tilt of the pubic bone. The true conjugate usually averages 11 cm (Fig. 1-6). The shortest distance between the posterior surface of the symphysis pubis and the sacral promontory, the *obstetrical conjugate*, like the true conjugate, is only estimated clinically, but may be measured by x-ray pelvimetry.

3. *X-ray pelvimetry* (Fig. 1-7), generally involving two views. One is made with the woman in a semirecumbent position, her pelvic inlet parallel with the x-ray plate, and another with the woman upright and sideways to secure a lateral view of the pelvis. This method is most accurate and allows evaluation of additional crucial obstetric diameters as well as the relationship of the size and posture of the fetus to the passageway. But this procedure should be scheduled only near term or during labor for significant reasons: to reduce the exposure of the young developing fetus to radiation and to avoid possible damage to fetal structures during early gestation, the most vulnerable period for the fetus.

4. *Ultrasonography*, the use of ultrasound to detect differences in tissue density by directing high-frequency sound waves into tissue and electrically measuring the reflected echoes from internal structures. This technique is now of clinical importance in obstetrics. Although it has seemingly not been used to determine relative pelvic and fetal size as has x-ray pelvimetry, with perfection of technique and experience it may be. It offers no known hazards to the mother or fetus. It has been employed to detect single or multiple pregnancy and abnormal fetal or placental positions or conditions. It also supplies helpful estimates of fetal age and growth through determination of the biparietal diameter of the infant skull, comparisons of the size of the amniotic sac to the size of the uterine cavity, indications of the length of the fetus, and the amount of fetal bone formation observed (Fig. 1-8). It is increasingly used to help detect fetal abnormality. (See also pp. 41, 50, 51.)

Physicians working in areas well supplied with adequate hospital facilities have discontinued the determination of external pelvic measurements except perhaps an evaluation of the pubic arch. In fact, some believe that if cephalopelvic disproportion becomes a practical problem, it can be evaluated and faced best at the time of labor using the more refined diagnostic and treatment facilities available in the hospital.

A knowledge of the structure of the obstetric passageway is basic to an understanding of the mechanism of labor and the problems that will be faced by the physician. So far we have discussed only the bony pelvis. We shall continue now with a consideration of the soft structures involved—the muscles of the pelvic floor and the organs they support.

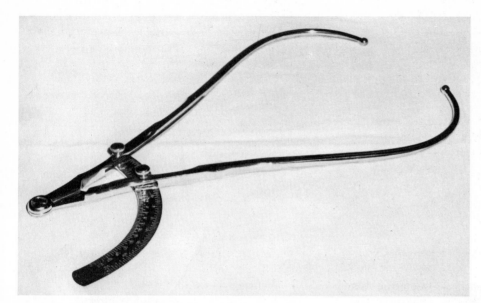

FIG. 1-5

One type of pelvimeter.

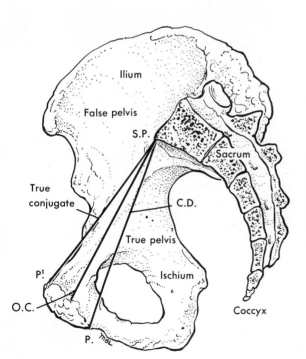

FIG. 1-6

Female pelvis, sagittal section. C.D., Diagonal conjugate; P, inner superior border of the pubis; P., outer inferior border of the pubis; S.P., sacral promontory; O.C., obstetrical conjugate.

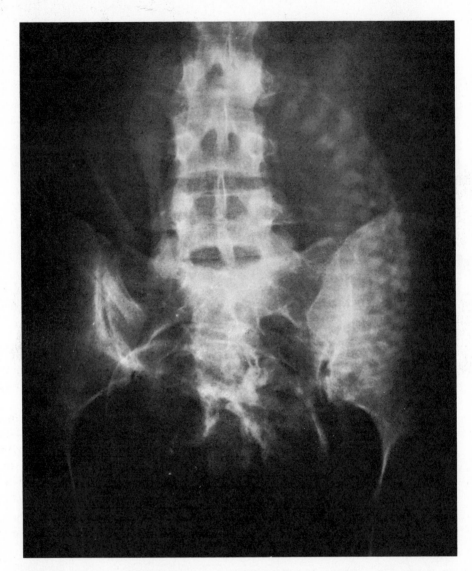

FIG. 1-7   Photograph of x-ray film. Pelvimetry showing a cephalic presentation.

Courtesy Grossmont Hospital, La Mesa, Calif.

Amniotic   Abdominal
fluid   wall   Heart   Head

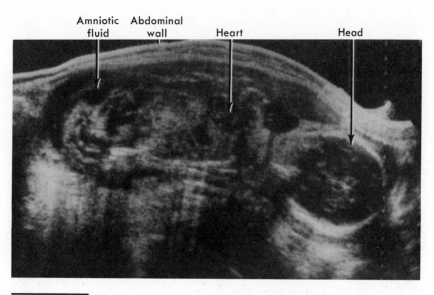

FIG. 1-8   Longitudinal view of a fetus taken using ultrasound.

Courtesy George R. Leopold, M.D., University Hospital, San Diego, Calif.

PELVIC CONTENTS AND SUPPORT

The pelvis, through which the fetus must pass, contains many soft tissue structures vital to normal body function. These structures are supported by layers of muscle, fibrous coverings called *fascia*, and various ligaments and tendons. They help to cushion the passage of the fetus through the hard, bony canal, help direct its descent, occasionally impede its progress, and may sustain damage at the time of birth.

Soft tissues of the vulva

Looking at the external female genitalia when the woman is on her back with her knees flexed, one observes the superficial relationships of many of these vital soft tissue organs (Fig. 1-9). The vulva, or external genital area, includes the following structures.

1. *Mons veneris* (Mount of Venus—mons pubis).

This is a fatty pad over the symphysis pubis that after puberty becomes covered with curly hair in the form of an inverted triangle extending between the legs.

2. *Labia majora* (larger lips, singular, *labium majus*). These are two fleshy, hair-covered folds, extending on each side of the midline from the mons veneris almost to the anus. In a child or a woman who has not borne a child, these folds almost completely cover the structures between. They correspond to the two halves of the scrotum in the man. Their inner surfaces are rich in oil and sweat glands.

3. *Labia minora* (small lips, singular, *labium minus*). These are two smaller, more delicate folds of tissue, located just under the labia majora. These small folds are somewhat erectile and are also supplied with oil and sweat glands.

4. *Clitoris*. This is a small, sensitive, erectile structure located at the anterior junction of the labia minora. Actually, folds of the small labia surround the clitoris; the top fold forms a fleshy hood,

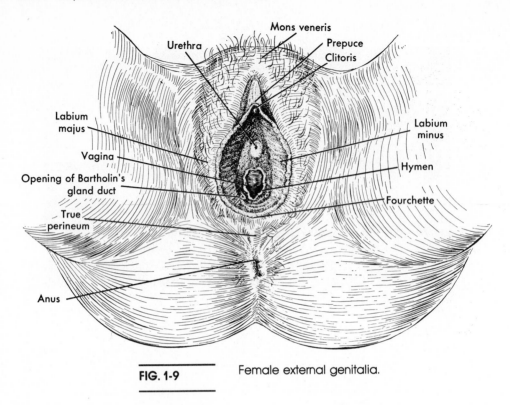

Urethra

Mons veneris

Prepuce

Clitoris

Labium majus

Labium minus

Vagina

Hymen

Opening of Bartholin's gland duct

Fourchette

True perineum

Anus

FIG. 1-9   Female external genitalia.

or *prepuce*, and the lower fold, the *frenulum*. The clitoris corresponds to the penis in the man as the primary anatomic center of sexual arousal.

5. *Vestibule*. This is the triangular space between the labia minora in which are the openings of the urethra, the vagina, and the *Bartholin glands*.

6. *Urethral opening*. The urethra, a tissue tube about 1-1½ inches (2.5-3.5 cm) in length leading from the urinary bladder to the exterior, opens in the midline between the clitoris and vagina. This opening usually appears as a dimple or slit and after childbirth may be slightly displaced or more difficult to locate because of local swelling. On the floor of the urethra open two ducts that lead to *Skene's glands*, structures that have no known purpose but unfortunately may become infected rather easily.

7. *Vaginal opening*. The vagina, a large distensible tube or sheath, leads down and back to the uterine cervix. It serves as the exit point for menstrual flow, the female organ of intercourse, or coitus, and the soft tissue birth canal in labor and birth. In virgins it usually is partially covered by a membrane called the *hymen*, or maidenhead. However, absence of a hymenal membrane does not preclude virginity, since this tissue may be accidentally torn during childhood. On the other hand, the presence of the hymen is no proof of virginity, since it may be elastic and fail to tear during intercourse. Rarely, the hymen completely covers the vaginal opening. This condition is termed "imperforate hymen" and is relieved by a hymenectomy.

8. *Bartholin's glands*. The two Bartholin's glands produce a mucoid substance that drains into the vestibule on either side of the vagina by way of two ducts during sexual stimulation. This drainage, in addition to mucoid secretion from the vaginal walls

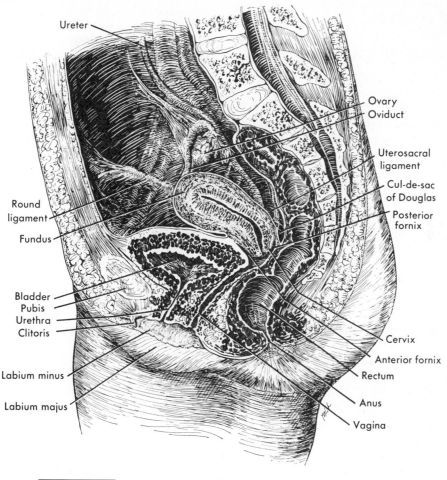

Ureter

Ovary
Oviduct

Uterosacral
ligament

Cul-de-sac
of Douglas

Posterior
fornix

Round
ligament

Fundus

Bladder
Pubis
Urethra
Clitoris

Cervix

Anterior fornix

Rectum

Labium minus

Labium majus

Anus

Vagina

FIG. 1-10   Female reproductive system, midsagittal section.

themselves, provides lubrication for intercourse. Occasionally these glands become infected, and painful abscesses may form.

9. *Fourchette*. This is a tissue fold below the vaginal opening, formed by the fusion of the posterior edges of the labia minora, and often lacerated by childbirth.

10. *Perineum*. This sometimes is considered to be the entire body area between a woman's legs. However, when we speak of the *true* or *obstetrical perineum*, we mean that tissue block found between the posterior edge of the vagina and the anus or rectal opening. It contains the *perineal body*, a mass of connective tissue that forms the point of attachment for the muscles and fascia of the pelvic floor. It is this area that is most frequently injured during childbirth. The true perineum is a critical area of pelvic support. Pelvic organs such as the vagina, uterus, bladder, and rectum may be affected by its injury or inadequate repair. Fig. 1-10 shows these internal pelvic organs and will clarify their relationships and need for support.

Uterus and adnexa

UTERUS AND FALLOPIAN TUBES

An adult, nonpregnant *uterus*, or womb, is a pear-shaped, hollow muscular organ about 3 inches (7.6 cm) long, 2 inches (5 cm) wide, and 1 inch (2.5 cm) thick. It serves as a protector and nourisher of the developing fetus and aids in its birth. Attached to either side of the uterus are the *fallopian tubes*, also called the oviducts or uterine tubes, which help conduct the female sex cell to the uterus.

The uterus is composed of three layers. The vascular mucus-producing endometrium, or inner lining, alters periodically in depth and character, demonstrating the uterine changes of the menstrual cycle. The middle layer, or myometrium, made up of muscular fibers that run in circular, lengthwise, and figure-eight patterns, provides forceful, efficient contraction of the uterine wall during and after birth. The outermost covering layer of the uterus is formed by the enfolding pelvic peritoneum and the parametrium, both strong connective tissues.

The uterus may also be divided into three main parts: the neck portion, or cervix; the main or central portion, called the body, or corpus; and the area above the oviducts, the fundus. Normally the uterus is tipped toward the front of the body, resting on the urinary bladder just below. The cervix dips down into the posterior portion of the vagina from above. Vaginal and cervical tissue ultimately join, forming two pouches, referred to as the anterior and posterior fornices (singular fornix). The posterior fornix is adjacent to a fold in the peritoneal lining of the pelvic cavity, termed the pouch, or cul-de-sac, of Douglas. Occasionally, because of infection or bleeding in the pelvis or abdomen, pus or blood drains into this cul-de-sac and may be aspirated vaginally or rectally by the physician. (See Fig. 1-10.)

UTERINE SUPPORT

Ligaments. The uterus is not only indirectly supported by the true perineum but also, along with portions of the oviducts and ovaries, is enfolded in layers of the so-called *broad ligaments*, portions of the abdominal peritoneal lining. The lower portions of the broad ligaments are thicker and are sometimes called the *cardinal ligaments*. They connect the upper portion of the cervix to the lateral pelvic walls. The uterus is also positioned and stabilized by other fibrous attachments, such as the *round ligaments* leading from the uterine walls toward the front, just below the fallopian tubes, down the inguinal canals, and to the labia majora. The round ligaments hold the uterus in its forward position. The *uterosacral ligaments* connect the posterior cervical portion of the uterus to the sacrum. The oviducts and ovaries and such soft tissue attachments are often referred to as the *adnexa*, or adjacent parts. The ovaries, two almond-shaped glands that produce female hormones and the female sex cells, or ova, are held one on each side of the uterus principally by the ovarian and broad ligaments. (See Fig. 1-11.)

Muscles. The deep muscles of the pelvic floor are arranged in such a way that they form a type of hammock pierced only by the urethra, vagina, and rectum. This muscle grouping, often termed the pelvic diaphragm, is formed by the branches of the large *levator ani* muscles and the *coccygeus* muscles. More muscles converge at the point of the previously described true perineum, reinforcing the levator ani. These are the *bulbocavernosus* muscles, the *transverse* muscles, and the *anal sphincter*. (See Fig. 1-12.)

BLOOD SUPPLY AND NERVES

The blood supply for the uterus is derived mainly from the paired uterine and ovarian arteries. The former branch off the hypogastric (internal iliac) arteries while the latter sprout from the aorta. Together they form an elaborate and rich vascular network over the cervix and body of the uterus. Muscular contractions of the uterus are involuntary, guided by hormonal controls rather than motor nerves. Painful sensations that accompany contractions of the uterus and dilatation of the cervix during labor and childbirth are transmitted by

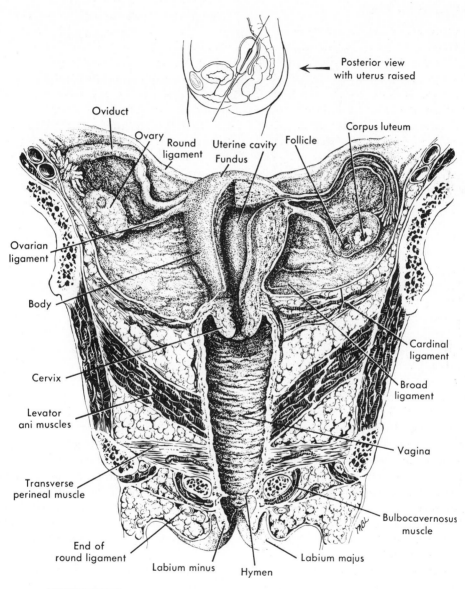

Posterior view
with uterus raised

Oviduct

Ovary

Round
ligament

Uterine cavity
Fundus

Follicle

Corpus luteum

Ovarian
ligament

Body

Cervix

Levator
ani muscles

Transverse
perineal muscle

End of
round ligament

Labium minus

Hymen

Labium majus

Bulbocavernosus
muscle

Vagina

Broad
ligament

Cardinal
ligament

FIG. 1-11   Female reproductive system, inclined posterior view.

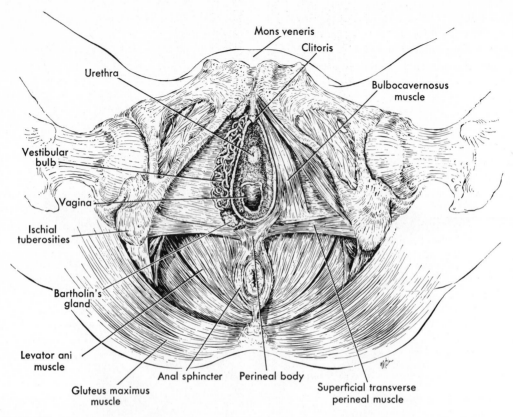

Mons veneris

Clitoris

Urethra

Bulbocavernosus
muscle

Vestibular
bulb

Vagina

Ischial
tuberosities

Bartholin's
gland

Levator ani
muscle

Anal sphincter   Perineal body

Gluteus maximus
muscle

Superficial transverse
perineal muscle

FIG. 1-12   Female pelvic floor in dissection from below. The coccygeus muscle is obscured by the gluteus maximus muscle.

sympathetic nerve fibers passing through the 10th, 11th, and 12th thoracic and possibly the first lumbar spinal nerves. As labor progresses and the baby descends in the birth canal, discomfort is also caused by pressure on pelvic and perineal structures outside the uterus. These sensations are transmitted by nerve fibers leading to sacral nerve pathways.

Protection of the perineum

Various efforts are made to preserve or protect the muscles of the true perineum from tears (lacerations) at the time of birth. The head of the infant is slowly extended by external, manual pressure to force the presentation of the smallest cephalic diameter. It is delivered slowly between contractions. Many physicians, particularly in the United States, perform a prophylactic perineal incision called an *episiotomy* in an attempt to avoid an uncontrolled, jagged tear, reduce possible prolonged pressure on the baby's head and maternal pelvic structures, and speed delivery. Episiotomies may be performed in several ways. The midline, or median, episiotomy extends from the vagina straight down to the anus. It is said to be easier to repair and more comfortable for the mother in the healing period; however, occasionally it may extend by tearing into the anal sphincter. Many physicians now use a combination episiotomy known as a mediolateral, which starts at the midline but then angles from the center, missing the sphincter. Because of its angle, it is more difficult to repair and more painful during the postpartum period, since the suturing is done "on the bias." Episiotomies are so common now that most delivery room setups routinely include the instruments and supplies needed for their execution and repair. However, the use of *routine* episiotomies is increasingly questionable. Reevaluation of birth positions, extended manual support of the perineum, and more patience during the birth process could effectively prevent many lacerations. Low or outlet forceps are frequently used to speed delivery and lessen the pounding of the presenting part on the perineum. Obvious damage to the perineal floor does not always occur as a result of childbirth. Perineal lacerations and other problems related to possible delivery trauma are discussed in greater detail in the chapters on labor and birth and obstetric complications. (See p. 136.)

It is well to note, however, that despite the difficulties that can occur during this first journey taken by human beings through the pelvic passageway, with proper care and management relatively few major problems actually materialize. It is probably true that the first journey from internal to external space, although demanding for mother and child, is far less dangerous than the freeway trip one negotiates every afternoon going home from work.

CHAPTER 2   The menstrual cycle

We have reviewed the anatomy of the pelvis. However, to study the physiology or function of the pelvic organs, we must discuss more than the contents of the pelvis itself.

ROLE OF THE PITUITARY GLAND

Proper functioning of the ovaries and uterus also depends on a gland located a considerable distance from the pelvic cavity but which empties its powerful products directly into the bloodstream. It exerts an influence on the body far beyond that expected, considering its size and position. Remember, glands that empty their manufactured products directly into the blood circulation are called *endocrine* glands. Their products are termed "hormones." The gland outside the pelvis that is so important in ovarian and uterine function is the *pituitary*, located at the base of the brain. It, in part, is regulated by that portion of the brain called the hypothalamus. Some of the pituitary hormones help to regulate a physiologic event universal among women, that of *menstruation*.

MENSTRUATION

Menstruation may be defined as the monthly elimination, through a bloody vaginal discharge, of a portion of the lining of the uterus that had been prepared to protect and nurture the fertilized egg in the event of pregnancy. Menstruation is also properly called menses, catamenia, or, more commonly, a period, or monthly flow. Terminology that implies an undesirable condition or illness should be avoided because menstruation is not an illness but an expected and necessary part of healthy mature womanhood. It may at times be individually inconvenient and troublesome, but it is the way all normal women function, and it declares the possibility for a type of growth filled with meaning and wonder.

Menarche

The advent of menstruation in a girl is a signal of impending physical maturity. This first menses is called *menarche*. It is one of the signs of "growing up." Menstruation occurs periodically throughout the childbearing years, except during pregnancy and lactation, or breast feeding. The age of onset and termination differs from person to person but seems to be affected by heredity, racial background, nutrition, and perhaps climate. On the average, menarche occurs between 10 and 14 years of age. It is preceeded by other body changes, such as the development of breasts, a rounding off of the many angles characteristic of the body of the preadolescent, and the appearance of axillary and pubic hair. Psychologically, a girl's interest turns toward members of the opposite sex.

The cycle

Menstruation occurs approximately every 28 days in most women and lasts about 5 days. The time between the beginning of one period and the

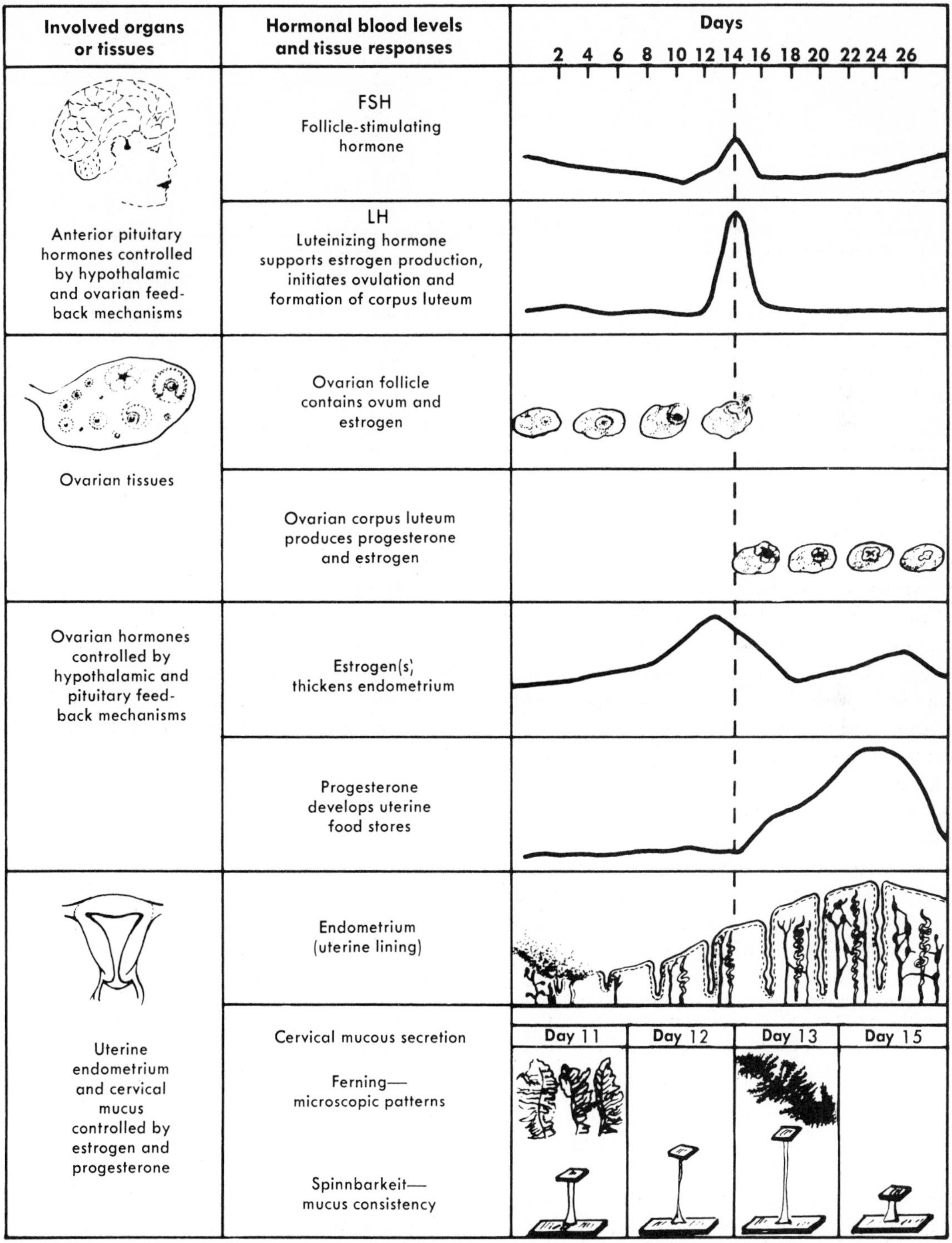

Involved organs or tissues	Hormonal blood levels and tissue responses	Days
		2 4 6 8 10 12 14 16 18 20 22 24 26
Anterior pituitary hormones controlled by hypothalamic and ovarian feed-back mechanisms	**FSH** Follicle-stimulating hormone	
	LH Luteinizing hormone supports estrogen production, initiates ovulation and formation of corpus luteum	
Ovarian tissues	Ovarian follicle contains ovum and estrogen	
	Ovarian corpus luteum produces progesterone and estrogen	
Ovarian hormones controlled by hypothalamic and pituitary feed-back mechanisms	Estrogen(s) thickens endometrium	
	Progesterone develops uterine food stores	
Uterine endometrium and cervical mucus controlled by estrogen and progesterone	Endometrium (uterine lining)	
	Cervical mucous secretion	Day 11 Day 12 Day 13 Day 15
	Ferning— microscopic patterns	
	Spinnbarkeit— mucus consistency	

FIG. 2-1 Normal menstrual cycle schematically depicted to highlight hormone production, ovulation, endometrial response, and changes in cervical mucus.

beginning of the next is called the menstrual cycle. It generally repeats itself about every 4 weeks (Fig. 2-1), although variations of several days in the cycles of different women or even in the cycles of the same woman are normal. Day 1 is distinguished by the appearance of the menstrual flow.

ANATOMY AND PHYSIOLOGY

The physiology of menstruation is complex. However, a basic understanding of some of the relationships involved will increase an appreciation of the human body and its potential. Three organs are primarily involved: the pituitary gland, the ovaries, and the uterus. The ability to analyze the roles and interactions of these three organs and their hormonal controls has greatly improved in the last few years because of the availability of more sensitive, sophisticated research techniques and equipment. However, it should be noted that many unknowns are still encountered in the continued investigation of female reproductive physiology.

In the last decade considerable interest has developed in a special group of fatty acids in the body now classified as hormones called prostaglandins. These substances are produced by many organs of the body in both sexes. However, the endometrium, is especially rich in prostaglandins. These particular prostaglandins are thought to be involved in such diverse reproductive activities as ovulation, the reception and transport of ova and sperm, and the onset of menstruation. They appear to be associated with episodes of uterine hyperirritability or contraction and may be a triggering factor in the onset of labor. The far-reaching functions of this group of hormones are now undergoing extensive study.

There appears to be a wide variation in normal hormonal patterns among women. Disturbances of endocrine glands such as the thyroid and adrenals or nutritional and psychological factors may also influence menstrual function. We will begin our explanation of menstruation with a description of the ovaries.

Ovaries

The ovaries have two basic functions—first, the production of hormones (*estrogen* and *progesterone*), which help regulate the activities of the uterus and pituitary gland and thus bring about the obvious changes that make a little girl a woman, and, second, the formation of the microscopic eggs, or ova, that carry the hereditary characteristics of her family. United with a male sex cell, or sperm, the fertilized egg grows to become a new human being. These eggs are stored in varying degrees of immaturity in the underlying tissues of the ovary. Each month one egg develops to maturity within a protective tissue envelope called a follicle. This follicle and other ovarian tissue are filled with estrogenic fluid, which is secreted in large amounts into the blood to thicken the lining of the uterus. As the follicle develops, it pushes to the surface of the ovary to create a blisterlike bulge that may be clearly seen if the ovary is observed directly. Growth of the follicle in the ovary and development of the egg, or ovum, it contains are not primarily the results of ovarian activity but those of the far-away master gland, the pituitary, which directs ovarian function.

Pituitary gland

It is now believed that two anterior pituitary hormones, the follicle-stimulating hormone (FSH) and the luteinizing hormone (LH), help govern the ovarian and, more indirectly, the uterine cycles. Previously, a luteotrophic hormone (LTH), or prolactin, also had been thought to be involved in maintaining the production of progesterone by the ovary. Prolactin is now considered not to carry out this function during the human menstrual cycle. However, it is a hormonal stimulus in the production of maternal milk after the birth of an infant and may inhibit but not totally stop ovulation during breast feeding.

A look at the blood levels of FSH during the normal cycle discloses a moderate, early elevation followed by a slight decline until the peak observed at midcycle. This peak is followed by a gradual decrease until just prior to the next menses. FSH, as its name implies, is responsible for the initiation of the ovarian follicle's growth. However, it works in conjunction with LH to continue the follicle's maturation and produce the characteristic increase in estrogen production. The blood level of LH is observed to peak at midcycle, and this surge of LH is responsible for ovulation, or the expulsion of the mature egg from the ruptured follicle, and the beginning production of progesterone. At times fleeting lower abdominal pain (Mittelschmerz) is noted at the time of ovulation. It is thought to be related to peritoneal irritation caused by minor bleeding from the follicle. After ovulation the mature egg is normally swept up into the fallopian tube to begin its journey to the uterus. After ovulation the empty follicle changes its name and alters its function. The walls of the follicle begin to thicken and form a yellow deposit about the size of a lima bean. This deposit is called the corpus luteum (yellow body). The name "follicle" is no longer used. The corpus luteum continues to produce estrogen but, in addition, manufactures the hormone progesterone, initiated by LH.

Pituitary and ovarian hormonal levels inhibit and stimulate each other's hormonal secretions, using rather elaborate negative and positive feedback systems.

Uterus

The effect of estrogen in building up the uterine endometrium has often caused the interval between menses and ovulation to be labeled the *proliferative phase*. The second half of the cycle is frequently called the *secretory phase* because of the secretion or storage of nutrients, glycogen, and mucin in the thickening uterine wall in response to the formation of progesterone produced by the corpus luteum.

Progesterone, which means "a hormone de-

signed to promote pregnancy," helps maintain the soft nutritious wall long enough to receive any fertilized egg and to nourish it until the developing fetus is able to establish its lifeline of placenta and umbilical cord.

In addition to these changes in the uterine lining, there are alterations in the amount and type of mucus formed by the glands of the cervix. During the proliferative phase of the menstrual cycle, cervical mucus becomes typically profuse and thin. It can be pulled into long strands, suspended, for example, between two glass slides. This distensible quality is called spinnbarkheit. When spinnbarkheit is increased, the entry of sperm into the cervix is enhanced. Microscopic changes also are seen when the mucus is placed on a slide and dried. As the time of ovulation nears under the influence of estrogen, special ferning patterns may be detected (Fig. 2-1). When progesterone is secreted in the latter part of the menstrual cycle, these ferning, or arborization, patterns disappear. If ovulation does not occur with subsequent progesterone production, ferning persists. Knowledge of spinnbarkheit and ferning have been used in treating infertility and have been incorporated into so-called natural family planning techniques. On about the twenty-sixth day of the menstrual cycle, if pregnancy has not occurred, the corpus luteum begins to degenerate. Approximately 2 days later the thickened lining of the uterus starts to disintegrate, having lost its progesterone and estrogen support.

CYCLE CONTROL

Pregnancy

If pregnancy does occur, hormones released by the developing fertilized egg interrupt the normal menstrual cycle by maintaining the level of estrogen and progesterone and inhibiting ovulation. Secreted early in the pregnancy is *human chorionic gonadotropin* (HCG). Identification of this substance in the woman's urine forms the basis of some pregnancy tests.

Artificial hormonal control

In recent years oral estrogen- and progesterone-like compounds, which simulate to some degree the changes in the uterine lining and the regulation of ovarian and pituitary activity occurring during pregnancy, have been used to control ovulation and aid in planned parenthood. (See discussion of contraception, Chapter 11.)

Ovulation and menses

The menstrual flow usually consists of less than 60 ml of cellular debris, mucus, and blood. Its appearance signals the advent of another cycle. It is interesting to note that ovulation may not occur each time the menstrual cycle repeats and is not dependent on menstruation. The occurrence of ovulation can be detected by the careful recording of rectal temperatures taken before arising in the absence of temperature-causing disease. Just before ovulation, the temperature drops to the lowest level found in the first half of the cycle. This drop is followed by an abrupt rise of perhaps 1° F, indicating that ovulation has occurred. This information has also been used in trying to plan pregnancies, since the most fertile period is during this temperature change (Fig. 11-1).

PROBLEMS

Dysmenorrhea

The most common menstrual disturbance is dysmenorrhea, or painful menstruation. Although most women observe some discomfort (for example, pelvic congestion, fatigue, or irritability), severe cramping and incapacitation should not be the rule. Repeated experiences of dysmenorrhea should be evaluated by a physician. Occasionally, a physical cause may be found, such as endometriosis (the colonization of endometrial tissue outside the uterus), pelvic inflammatory disease, adhesions, genital tract obstruction, poor uterine positioning, the presence of pelvic tumors, or possible glandular imbalance. Dysmenorrhea may be caused or aggravated by constipation. Its possibility is also greatly increased by fatigue and emotional upset. The maintenance of meticulous hygiene, proper diet, and good mental health is of prime importance to the body's total response during menstruation. Excellent teaching aids dealing with the anatomy, physiology, and hygiene of menstruation are now available through public health departments and private commercial outlets.

Treatment of dysmenorrhea depends on the cause, of course, but moderate exercise, fresh air, a serene philosophy, prevention or relief of constipation, possible application of heat to the pelvis, and mild sedatives or muscle relaxants usually help greatly. Because it has been found that many times dysmenorrhea is not experienced if a menstrual cycle does not include ovulation, contraceptive preparations containing estrogen or estrogen-progesterone combinations are occasionally prescribed with good effect. However, if the contraceptive action of the medication or possible side effects present problems, this method of treatment may not be appropriate. Another method of treating painful menstruation for which no physical cause has been determined is the prescription of one of several drugs that may inhibit the activity of body prostaglandins and, therefore, reduce uterine contraction. Ibuprofen (Motrin), mefenamic acid (Ponstel), and naproxen sodium (Anaprox) have been used.

Disturbances in flow

Other types of menstrual disorders should at least be defined. *Amenorrhea* means the abnormal absence of menses. *Menorrhagia* refers to excessive flow. *Metrorrhagia* identifies the presence of bloody vaginal discharge between periods. All these conditions should be investigated by a physician.

CHAPTER 3

The male parent: his contribution

The role of the mother in the creation of new life has often been emphasized, but the role of the responsible father is also very important. Truly, for an emotionally, socially, and physically healthy child both parents must make considerable contributions of time and effort. This does not mean that if these contributions are absent the child will never achieve a happy, productive life, but if he does, he does so "in spite of" instead of "because of" his early family life. The amount and type of nurturing behavior (by vocal and visual stimulation, touch, and direct participation in child care activities) exhibited by fathers has grown significantly within modern Western society. But great variation is seen within families, influenced by occupational demands, cultural heritage, family structure, personality differences, and the role identification of the mother as well as that of the father. For the mature adult who is capable of giving as well as receiving, parenthood is a demanding responsibility but one that offers a deserved sense of fulfillment and pride.

The male role in the initial creation of his offspring is relatively brief but no less miraculous because of its brevity. The male reproductive system is an intricate mechanism.

ANATOMY AND PHYSIOLOGY

Puberty

Puberty, or the maturation of the reproductive system, usually occurs late in the male (average age 14 years) when compared with the female. The development of the male sex organs and secondary sex characteristics takes place, on the average, 2 years later. It involves changes such as the enlargement of the larynx and the deepening of the voice, the appearance of axillary, pubic, and facial hair, the development of increased musculature, the production of semen, and the normal occurrence of nocturnal emissions, or "wet dreams." Finally, there is a psychological change, and the boy who could not tolerate girls rather suddenly finds them attractive.

Male organs of reproduction
(Figs. 3-1 and 3-2)

The male sex glands, or gonads, are two oval endocrine organs called *testes* (singular, testis), or *testicles,* located in a fleshy pouch suspended from the abdomen called the *scrotum.* The testes (which correspond to ovaries in the female) perform two main functions: the manufacture of male sex cells (gametes), or spermatozoa, and the production of several steroid hormones, chief of which is *testosterone.* This hormone is responsible for the appearance of male characteristics just as estrogen in the woman controls female characteristics. The male pituitary and nearby hypothalamus help regulate events of male reproductive physiology, even as these organs in women assist in the control of female function. The male pituitary also secretes follicle-stimulating hormone (FSH) and luteinizing hormone (LH), but these hormones in the man

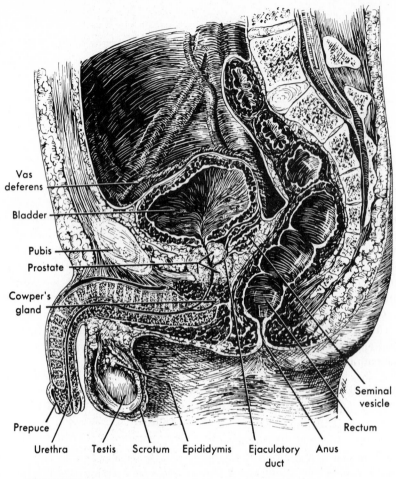

Vas deferens

Bladder

Pubis

Prostate

Cowper's gland

Prepuce

Urethra   Testis   Scrotum   Epididymis   Ejaculatory duct   Anus

Seminal vesicle

Rectum

FIG. 3-1   Male reproductive system, midsagittal view.

perform different tasks. FSH is responsible for promoting the maturation of spermatozoa, whereas LH is involved in the production of testosterone.

The testes are found in the abdominal cavity proper during part of fetal development, but before birth they usually migrate to the scrotal sac by way of the inguinal canal. Occasionally, this migration does not occur, and a condition known as undescended testicles, or cryptorchidism, may exist. If this persists, sterility may occur, since the higher temperature of the abdominal cavity seems to interfere with the manufacture of sperm. If the

condition continues, malignant changes are occasionally diagnosed.

Attached to the top of each testis is a coiled structure called an *epididymis*, which is actually an extension of the tubules of the testis where sperm are formed. In the epididymides (plural of epididymis) the male sex cells mature. Each epididymis is, in turn, attached to a long tube called the *ductus deferens*, or *vas deferens*, which with associated nerves and blood vessels travels up the inguinal canal as the *spermatic cord*. The ductus deferens eventually loops downward in back of the urinary

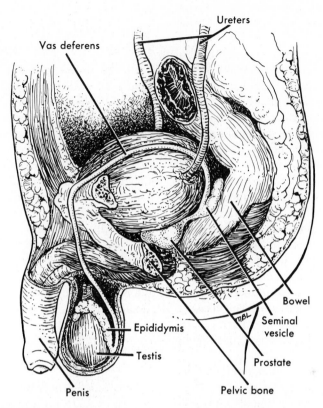

FIG. 3-2   Male reproductive system, sagittal view with partial dissection.

bladder. Attached to the ductus in this area is the *seminal vesicle*. This small pouch secretes a fluid that is added to the spermatozoa and aids the motility of the sex cell. The tube leading forward from the point of attachment of the seminal vesicle is called the *ejaculatory duct*. It joins the long urethra after passing through tissue of the *prostate gland*. Three paired glands add secretions to the spermatozoa traveling from the testes to the exterior to form *semen*, or *seminal fluid*. These glands are the seminal vesicle, the prostate, and the bulbourethral or Cowper's gland, which opens into the urethra proper. These secretions regulate the acidity of the semen and influence the sperm's motility and life-span. As a result of sexual excitement and subsequent ejaculation of 2 to 6 ml of semen,

approximately 250 to 500 million sperm are released at a time from the *penis*, the male organ of intercourse, through the urethral meatus.

When not sexually stimulated, the penis serves as the excretory organ of the male urinary system. The urethra opens at the tip of the penis in a sensitive portion called the *glans*. The glans is hooded by a fold of skin called the *prepuce*, or *foreskin*, which is slit or at least partially removed if a circumcision is performed.

Genetic considerations

The primary function of the reproductive systems of both sexes is the formation of a new developing human being to assure continuation of the species. All cells that compose living things, animal or plant, have within their nuclei the potential of inheritance not only for the species but also for the individualized representatives of that species. Each living thing has a certain number of thread-like strands, or chromosomes, of transmitable characteristics, or genes, within the nuclei of its tissue cells. This chromosome number is constant for each species. For example, human beings have forty-six chromosomes in each body tissue cell. However, because the child necessarily inherits qualities from both parents and the body tissue chromosome count must be unaltered for the species, the sex cells (gametes) of the male and female are unlike the rest of the cells found in the body. Through a special process called *meiosis*, the chromosome count in these cells is reduced by half. When male and female sex cells unite, fertilization, or conception, takes place, and the species' chromosome count is restored in the new developing representative of the race.

In the 1970s another proposed method of reproduction that would duplicate the genetic inheritance of an individual by substituting the nucleus of a donor's tissue cell for the nucleus of an ovum and provide an appropriate environment for growth of the developing embryo and fetus received considerable publicity. This technique, called *cloning*, has been used experimentally in the reproduction of genetically duplicate frogs but has not been demonstrated, although it has been claimed, in the development of a human being. Certainly, perfection and use of such a technique would be accompanied by startling scientific, social, and ethical implications.

SEX DETERMINATION

Because there has been considerable consternation in the past concerning the sex of certain heirs, perhaps it should be pointed out that the potential sex of the child is determined by the type of sex cell contributed by the man that penetrates the ovum, or egg. Only the male sex cells, the spermatozoa, may carry the Y chromosome, and when the sperm that unites with an ovum carries the Y chromosome, a boy will result; but if the sperm that fertilizes the egg carries an X chromosome, a girl will result. Although research continues regarding possible ways to preselect the sex of one's offspring, such as controlling the acidity or alkalinity of the vagina or using certain techniques and timing for intercourse, the results have been highly controversial.

"OUR HUMANITY"

Although few people would deny that a baby is a human being, it must be agreed that the true process of reproduction of the human race does not end at conception or at birth. It only enters another phase. Just how "human," in the best sense of the word, the child becomes depends on the humanity he observes and feels about him within his own family circle—what he finds within the lives of his mother and father that he values as true and lasting.

SUGGESTED SELECTED READINGS AND REFERENCES

Anthony, C.P., and Thibodeau, G.A.: Textbook of anatomy and physiology, ed. 10, St. Louis, 1979, The C.V. Mosby Co.

Cath, S.H., Gurwitt, A., and Ross, J.M.: Fathers, 1982, Boston, Little, Brown & Co.

Chaffee, E.E., and Lytle, I.M.: Basic physiology and anatomy, Philadelphia, 1980, J.B. Lippincott Co.

Comerci, G.D., Symptoms associated with menstruation, Pediatr. Clin. North Am. **29:**177-200, Feb. 1982.

Crouch, J.E.: Functional human anatomy, ed. 3, Philadelphia, 1978, Lea & Febiger.

Gantt, P.A., and McDonough, P.G.: Adolescent dysmenorrhea, Pediatr. Clin. North Am. **28:**389-396, May 1981.

Haughey, C.W.: Understanding ultrasonography, Nursing '81 **11:**100-104, Apr. 1981.

Jensen, M.D., Benson, R.C., and Bobak, I.M.: Maternity care: the nurse and the family, ed. 2, St. Louis, 1981, The C.V. Mosby Co.

Kohn, C.L., Nelson, A., and Weiner, S.: Gravidas' responses to realtime ultrasound fetal image, JOGN Nurs. **9:**77-80, Mar.-Apr. 1980.

Macvicar, M.G., Harlan, J.D., and Ouellette, M.: What do we know about the effects of sports training on the menstrual cycle? Am. J. Mat. Child Nurs. **7:**55-58, Jan.-Feb. 1982.

Masters, W., and Johnson, V.: Human sexual response, Boston, 1966, Little, Brown & Co.

Moore, M.L.: Realities in childbearing, Philadelphia, 1978, W.B. Saunders Co.

Netter, F.H., and Oppenheimer, E., editors: The Ciba collection of medical illustrations. Vol. 2, The reproductive system, Summit, N.J., 1954, Ciba Pharmaceutical Products, Inc.

Patient assessment: examination of the male genitalia: programmed medical instruction, Am. J. Nurs. **79:**689-712, Apr. 1979.

Phillips, C.R., and Anzalone, J.T.: Fathering: participation in labor and birth, ed. 2, St. Louis, 1982, The C.V. Mosby Co.

Reiber, V.D.: Is the nurturing role natural to fathers? Am. J. Mat. Child Nurs. **1:**366-367, Nov.-Dec. 1976.

Roberts, S.J.: Dysmenorrhea, Nurse Pract. **5:**9-10, Jul.-Aug. 1980.

Shettles, L.B., and Vande Weile, R.L.: Can parents choose the sex of their baby? Birth Fam. J. **1:**3-5, Spring 1974.

Tortora, G.J., and Anagnostakos: Principles of anatomy and physiology, ed. 2, New York, 1978, Harper & Row, Publishers, Inc.

PERIOD OF GESTATION

CHAPTER **4**   Embryology, fetal development,
and signs and symptoms of pregnancy

The event of *conception* (Fig. 4-1), the union of the male sex cell (sperm) and the female sex cell (ovum), sets into motion a period of growth unequaled at any other time in the life of the individual.

Just after *fertilization*, or conception, the ovum is not quite as large as the dot used to complete a sentence, but within approximately 9 calendar or 10 lunar months (266 days) that particle of life will increase in size approximately 200 billion times and become the highly complex structure and personality known as a baby.

EMBRYOLOGY (Table 4-1)

Early beginnings

Conception normally takes place in the fallopian, or uterine, tube. The single cell soon becomes two, then four, then eight, multiplying until keeping count would be impossible. The fertilized egg, or zygote, assumes the bumpy appearance of a mulberry, and, for that reason, is called a *morula* as it journeys down the tube in search of a warm, safe place to grow. The journey from ovary to uterine cavity, where nesting, or *implantation*, takes place, involves about 7 days. At the end of this time the zygote, now a hollow, fluid-filled blastocyst, burrows into the soft uterine lining. Its outer surface becomes covered by fingerlike tissue projections called *chorionic villi*, which aid in the process of implantation into the endometrium (known as the

decidua during pregnancy.) These villi also manufacture the human chorionic gonadotropin (HCG) that initially signals the corpus luteum in the ovary to continue to manufacture progesterone and estrogen to prevent menstruation and additional ovulation. The aggregation of cells begins to form a definite pattern. The microscopic embryonic disc develops, and primitive beginnings of the child and his basic support system appear.

Of course, the possibility of a purposeful alteration in the initiation and early development of selected pregnancies now exists. In 1978 an ovum obtained from a woman's ovary, fertilized by her husband's sperm in a laboratory and placed in her uterus as a blastocyst, resulted in the birth of an apparently normal, healthy infant girl. At this writing, more than a dozen infants, both girls and boys, including twins, have been born as the result of this complex process of *in vitro fertilization*, allowing couples who previously were denied biological parenthood because of blocked fallopian tubes to have children.

Placental development and role

Fairly soon a supply and disposal system across the uterine wall is initiated through a special intermediary organ called the *placenta*, or *afterbirth*. The placenta, a miraculous structure, forms from part of the chorionic villi that extended from the outside of the egg. Attached to the uterine wall, it manufactures estrogen, progesterone, chorionic

Text continued on p. 46.

THE MENSTRUAL CYCLE
- Menstruation
- Ovulation

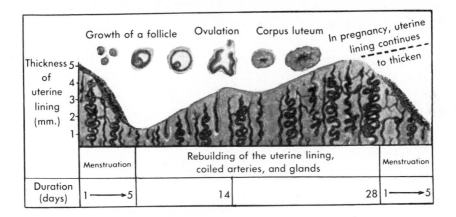

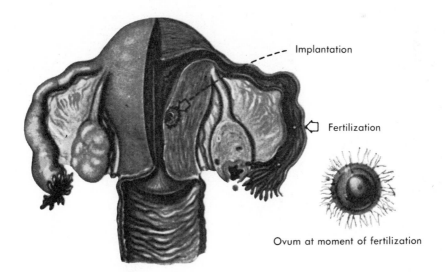

Ovum at moment of fertilization

FIG. 4-1   The event of pregnancy.
Courtesy Carnation Co., Los Angeles, Calif.

TABLE 4-1   PRENATAL CALENDAR (USING FERTILIZATION AGE)

General developmental characteristics (schematically pictured)	Average weight and size	Possible maternal findings and diagnostic aids
GERMINAL STAGE (1 TO 10 DAYS)		
First week		
Zygote forms: ovum fertilized in fallopian tube undergoes cell divisions (cleavage) on way to uterus 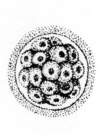 Ovum — Fertilizing sperm	Just visible to eye	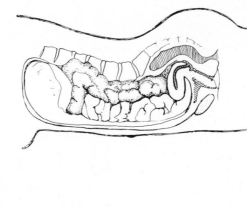
Morula forms: solid mass of about 16 microscopic cells resembling mulberry; enters uterus on third day		
Blastocyst: morula develops fluid-filled cavity; *trophoblast:* outer wall of blastocyst; *embryoblast:* inner cell mass from which embryo eventually forms 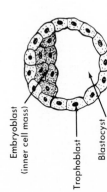 Embryoblast (inner cell mass) — Trophoblast — Blastocyst cavity		Normal female pelvis before implantation (sagittal section)

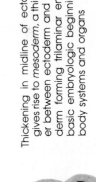

From Hertig, A. T., and Rock, J.: Contr. Embryol. Carneg. Instn., Wash. **25**:127, 1941.

Implantation site of human embryo at about 12 days (see arrow)

Endometrium covers blastocyst, producing elevation or wartlike bulge on uterine surface

Amenorrhea

Human chorionic gonadotropin (HCG) in urine beginning 10 days after conception, but tests not always sensitive

Ultrasonogram may reveal pregnancy as early as 3 to 4 weeks postconception

2 to 3 mm (1/10 inch)

Continued.

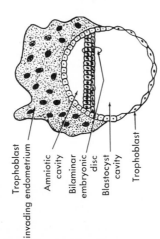

Beginning implantation of blastocyst in endometrium by invading trophoblastic tissue ±7 days

Trophoblastic tissue

Endometrium

Inner cell mass

EMBRYONIC STAGE (10 DAYS TO 8 WEEKS)

Second week

Implantation deepens and completes; primitive uteroplacental circulation originates from enlarging trophoblast and maternal endometrial tissues

Amniotic cavity appears as opening between inner cell mass and invading trophoblast; a thin lining becomes amnion

Two-layered (bilaminar) embryo called *embryonic disc* develops, formed by ectoderm and endoderm

Yolk sac present

Trophoblast invading endometrium

Amniotic cavity

Bilaminar embryonic disc

Blastocyst cavity

Trophoblast

Third week

Thickening in midline of ectoderm gives rise to *mesoderm*, a third layer between ectoderm and endoderm forming trilaminar embryo; basic embryologic beginnings of body systems and organs

Embryonic disc

Connecting stalk

Yolk sac

Embryonic ectoderm

Intraembryonic mesoderm

Embryonic endoderm

Trilaminar embryonic disc

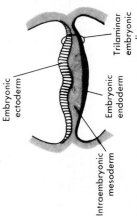

TABLE 4-1   PRENATAL CALENDAR—cont'd

	General developmental characteristics (schematically pictured)	Average weight and size	Possible maternal findings and diagnostic aids
	Three basic embryonic layers form:		
	1. *Endoderm:* forerunner of lining of gastrointestinal tract from pharynx to rectum; epithelial parts of trachea, bronchi, lungs, liver, pancreas, and urinary bladder		
	2. *Ectoderm:* forerunner of mucous membrane, enamel, hair, nails, mammary glands, and nervous system		
	3. *Mesoderm:* forerunner of heart and blood vessels, spleen, blood and lymph cells, bones, and muscles		
	Neural tube, beginning of central nervous system, forms in midline of cranial portion of ectoderm		
Fourth week	Cells group in mesoderm to form primitive blood vessels and blood cells; heart tube forms and contracts to circulate blood by end of third week; umbilical vessels pass through connecting stalk to placenta	5 mm (³⁄₁₆ in)	Nausea and vomiting(?) Urinary frequency Breast tenderness, tingling, swelling Montgomery's tubercles visible Uterine enlargement Increased cervical secretion
	Flat, disclike embryo folds to form typical C-shaped cylinder		
	Rapid development of forebrain portion of neural tube		
	Heart prominence seen		
	Arm and leg buds; forerunners of ears and eyes appear		
	Primitive gut formed with incorporation of dorsal yolk sac		
	Rudimentary lungs, kidneys		

Otic pit (primitive ear)

Forebrain

Primitive eye

Heart prominence

Arm bud

Leg bud

Softening of cervix (Goodell's sign)
Softening of uterine isthmus (Hegar's sign)
Violet coloration of cervix and vagina (Chadwick's sign)

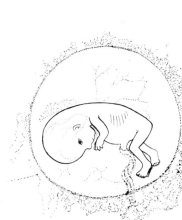

Abdominal wall
Bladder
Embryo
Gestational sac
Cervix
Vagina

Sonogram of 6 weeks' gestational sac containing embryo (Courtesy George R. Leopold, M.D., University Hospital, San Diego, Calif.)

Fifth to seventh weeks

Rapid brain development
Retina of eye forms
Heart becomes chambered
Fingers, toes, and eyes are becoming visible
Palate and upper lip forming
Gastrointestinal tract develops; part of intestine still in umbilical cord
Rapid formation of urogenital systems

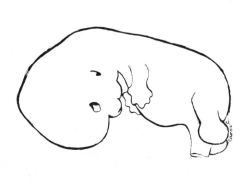

By end of seventh week all essential systems present

FETAL STAGE (EIGHTH WEEK TO BIRTH)
Eighth to tenth weeks

3 cm (1⅛ inches)
2 gm (⅕ oz)

Development mainly involves growth and maturation of structures begun in embryo; fetus less vulnerable to effects of drugs, most infections, and radiation
Head almost half fetal length at 8 weeks (illustration shows fetus within amniotic sac)

8 weeks

Continued.

TABLE 4-1 PRENATAL CALENDAR—cont'd

General developmental characteristics (schematically pictured)	Average weight and size	Possible maternal findings and diagnostic aids
Eleventh to twelfth weeks		
Facial features forming Eyelids present and fused Intestine retracted from umbilical cord into abdomen Palate fusion complete External sex identification possible Well-defined neck Nail beds beginning Tooth buds forming	Crown-heel length: 11.5 cm (4½ inches) 20 g (⅔ oz)	Frequent urination and nausea have usually disappeared Fetal heart tone may be detected with Doppler techniques 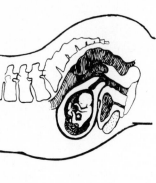 Fundus of uterus rises above pubic bone between 12 and 16 weeks
Thirteenth to sixteenth weeks		
Rapid growth of limbs and trunk; head less prominent Active fetus Skeleton calcified on x-ray examination by sixteenth week Increasing respiratory movement detected by sonogram Approximately 150 to 280 ml amniotic fluid present Placenta distinct	19 cm (7½ inches) 100 g (3⅓ oz)	Debut of maternity clothing(?) Usual time of amniocentesis between fourteenth and sixteenth weeks Quickening felt at 16 weeks by some mothers 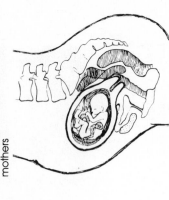 Fundus half distance between pubis and umbilicus at 16 weeks(?)

12 weeks

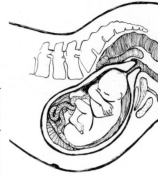

Quickening at 16 to 18 weeks
Fetal heart tone detected by standard fetoscope (18 to 20 weeks)
Secondary areola prominent
Linea nigra identified

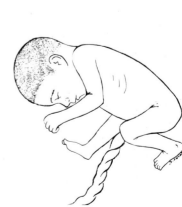

Fundus at umbilicus or slightly above
Chloasma (mask of pregnancy)
Striae may develop

Continued.

22 cm (8¾ inches)
300 g (10 oz)

Eyebrows, lanugo, and vernix appear
Nipples barely visible (illustration shows placental relationship)
Scalp hair visible

32 cm (12½ inches)
600 g (1¼ lb)

External ear soft, flat, shapeless
Skin wrinkled, translucent, appears pink; blood in capillaries shows
Lanugo covers body

Seventeenth to twentieth weeks

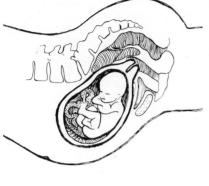

Twenty-fourth week

Currently accepted lower level of viability(?)
Only rare survivals

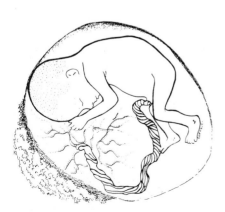

TABLE 4-1 PRENATAL CALENDAR—cont'd

General developmental characteristics (schematically pictured)	Average weight and size	Possible maternal finding and diagnostic aids
Twenty-eighth week 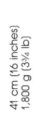 Subcutaneous fat appears; finger-nails and toenails Testes at internal inguinal ring or below Eyes open Scalp hair well developed	36 cm (14 inches) 1,100 g (2¼ lb)	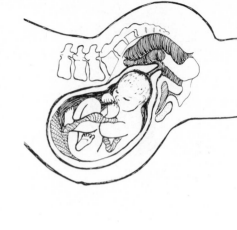
Thirty-second week Hair fine and woolly Nails to fingertips Prominent clitoris; labia majora small and separated Skin pink and smooth 1 or 2 creases on anterior portion of soles Breast areolae visible but flat	41 cm (16 inches) 1,800 g (3¾ lb)	

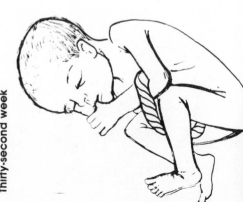

Thirty-sixth week

Body, limbs more rounded
Skin thicker, whiter; lanugo disappearing
Breast tissue develops under nipples
Scrotal rugae few
Testes in inguinal canal
Sole creases involve anterior two thirds of sole

46 cm (18 inches)
2,200 g (4½ lb)

Dyspnea due to pressure on diaphragm
Lightening in primigravidae about 38 weeks
Urinary frequency returns
Increasing prominence of Braxton Hicks contractions
Milk may appear in breasts
In primigravidae, characteristic effacement may be noted by pelvic exam

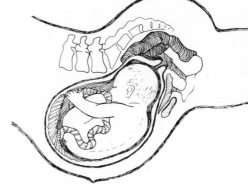

TERM
Thirty-seventh to forty-second weeks

Skin whitish pink
Lanugo gone from face
Hair in single strands
Vernix decreasing
Areola 5 to 6 mm with 7 to 10 mm breast tissue
Ear well defined by outer incurving to lobe, erect from head
Testes in scrotum
Labia majora meet in midline; cover labia minora and clitoris

51 cm (20 inches)
3,200+ g (6.6+ lb)

At term

Newborn

gonadotropin, and various other hormones and enzymes that apparently influence the growth and maintenance of the pregnancy and maternal preparation for birth and lactation. It also transports from the mother's blood the food and oxygen necessary for fetal growth. In addition, through the process of osmosis, hormones and protective substances called antibodies cross over the placental link to the fetus by way of the umbilical cord. Then, too, the placenta handles waste products brought to its tissues from the fetus: it allows carbon dioxide and other metabolic wastes to pass from the fetal circulation to the maternal bloodstream. The mother and fetus do not share a common bloodstream; the fetus manufactures its own blood. Normally the whole blood of the mother and that of the fetus stay within their separate, although closely related, channels. Blood flows from the placenta to the fetus by means of a large umbilical vein in the cord. The two arteries in the cord, wound about the umbilical vein, carry the waste to the placenta.

"Bag of waters"

As the embryo develops, the chorionic villi that face the interior of the uterus and are not involved in the formation of the placenta fall off the spherical covering, leaving a transparent sac made up of two membranous layers called the *chorion* and *amnion*. The inner layer, the amnion, contains a salty liquid known as *amniotic fluid,* in which the fetus may be said to float. It helps to control the environmental temperature of the fetus and shield it from trauma and infection. Perhaps weightlessness is not such an extraordinary condition for mankind after all! This amniotic sac is commonly known as the "bag of waters," or the membranes. Normally, it persists intact until the time of labor and birth.

THE FETUS

At about the end of 8 weeks of growth, the embryo is recognizable as a small, unfinished human, and its name is changed to fetus, meaning "young one." It is less than 2 inches (about 3 cm) long and weighs a fraction of an ounce. Although rudimentary, body systems are formed and working. The calcified skeleton has even begun to be established. (See Fig. 4-2.)

At 12 weeks. By the close of the third lunar month, the sex of the fetus may be clearly discerned if it is directly inspected. Needless to say, there is always considerable curiosity regarding the sex of the developing fetus. However, no *completely* safe way exists yet to discover its sex before birth. Nevertheless, a technique called amniocentesis now makes possible sex identification before birth if it is genetically important. Amniotic fluid is aspirated from the bag of waters and examined for cellular content and chromosome determination later in the pregnancy (see Fig. 4-3).

The fetus is most susceptible to malformation from the effects of maternal drug ingestion, radiation, or infection in the first trimester, when basic organs and systems are being formed. It is even possible for certain drugs to distort fetal development within 11 days of conception, before the woman realizes that she may be pregnant. Such an "assault" at that early period usually causes fetal death. Drugs or conditions that produce fetal structural defects are termed *teratogenic.* They are currently the object of much concern and study. (See also p. 69.)

At 16 weeks. At 16 weeks' *gestation,* or pregnancy, the fetus has increased considerably in size. It is approximately 7½ inches (19 cm) long and weighs about 3⅓ ounces (100 g). The uterus will be correspondingly larger, and the expectant mother's maternity clothes may make their debut. At about 16 to 18 weeks, expectant mothers usually report feelings of life, or *quickening.* Elbows, feet, and hands punch and twitch as the fetus attempts more vigorous exercise in its confining temporary home.

At 20 weeks. The fetus is about 8¾ inches (22 cm) long and weighs approximately 10 ounces (300 g) at this time. The examining physician may begin to listen for the fetal heart tone, which, although

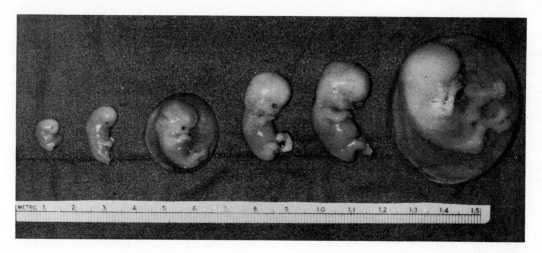

FIG. 4-2　Progressive growth of the human fetus (measured in centimeters). Two amniotic sacs are pictured still intact.

Courtesy Jeanne I. Miller, M.D., Modesto, Calif.

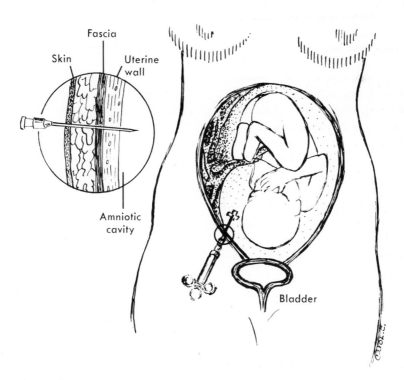

FIG. 4-3　Amniocentesis—a diagnostic tool. To help lessen risk of fetal or placental trauma, ultrasound is used to localize intrauterine structures before insertion of the needle. A full or partially filled bladder is now desired by some physicians during amniocentesis to push the uterus out of the pelvis and to aid visualization. Check your local procedure. Amniocentesis is usually performed for genetic analysis between 14 and 16 weeks' gestation.

present before, was too faint to be heard using a standard fetoscope.

Some state laws declare that the legal threshold of viability is 24 weeks' gestation; others use 20 weeks as the lower limit. However, the true length of a pregnancy may be difficult to determine and can lead to moral-ethical dilemmas involving the rights and responsibilities of the parents and the community, as well as consideration for the life and well-being of the developing fetus. Infants diagnosed as less than 24 weeks' gestation have made postnatal respiratory efforts. Special neonatal care units employing exceptional techniques supporting or monitoring body warmth, ventilation, cardiac function, and nutrition have been able to save fetuses of increasingly shorter gestations. Nevertheless, when all births are evaluated, such survivals still must be considered a rare occurrence. (See a brief discussion of premature care on pp. 253 to 258.)

The characteristics of the premature infant and his so-called grip on life depend on his genetic endowment, the length and quality of his prenatal environment, and his immediate postnatal care. Assuming his prenatal environment and personal condition is satisfactory, each additional day the fetus is able to remain in the uterus until maturity is reached at a little less than 40 weeks of gestation is of benefit. Each day increases his ability to withstand the demands of extrauterine life and to adjust to the tremendous circulatory, respiratory, and digestive alterations that must take place at birth. (See Table 4-1.)

Fetal circulation

A diagram of fetal circulation is shown in Fig. 4-4 to give a better understanding of the circulorespiratory changes. The umbilical vein extends from the placenta to the fetus, entering the body at the umbilicus. It travels upward, branching through the liver eventually to join the inferior vena cava. There its richly oxygenated blood mixes with the oxygen-poor blood flowing from the lower extremities and abdominal cavity toward the heart. The blood enters the heart by way of the right atrium, as in postnatal circulation, but because the pulmonary circulation is unnecessary to oxygenation, much of the blood entering the heart from the inferior vena cava crosses directly to the left atrium through the fetal shunt, or interatrial opening, called the *foramen ovale*. This blood then is guided into the usual circulation pattern, left atrium → left ventricle → aorta.

Blood entering the right atrium from the superior vena cava, draining the head and upper extremities, flows for the most part into the right ventricle and is eventually pushed into the pulmonary artery. However, the trip to the lungs is superfluous at this time, and another shunt, the *ductus arteriosus*, is employed. This short duct leads from the pulmonary artery to the aorta. Relatively little blood flows to the lung fields and back to the left heart by way of the pulmonary veins.

The blood flow down the aorta is eventually channeled into the iliac arteries to the hypogastric arteries that join with the umbilical arteries leading to the umbilical cord and placenta.

The pulmonary circulation becomes established within a relatively short time after birth. The umbilical cord is cut and clamped, and the blood vessels it contains become occluded. Because of the changes in thoracic pressures initiated by postnatal expansion of the lungs, the foramen ovale begins to close, and the ductus arteriosus collapses and becomes a ligament within a period of days or weeks.

Methods of evaluating the fetus

Because the maturity of an infant is so important to his survival outside the uterus, improved techniques to determine the state of his intrauterine growth, as well as his general health in utero, have been very welcome. Before labor, types of tests that help assess fetal age, size, and maturity (not necessarily synonymous) have included (1) an examination of amniotic fluid aspirated with sterile

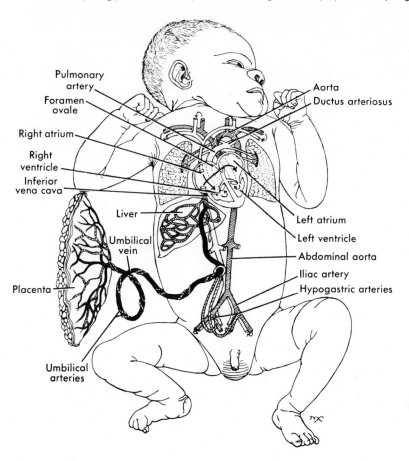

Pulmonary artery
Foramen ovale
Right atrium
Right ventricle
Inferior vena cava
Liver
Umbilical vein
Placenta
Umbilical arteries

Aorta
Ductus arteriosus
Left atrium
Left ventricle
Abdominal aorta
Iliac artery
Hypogastric arteries

FIG. 4-4   Fetal circulation. The darker the blood in the vessels, the greater its oxygen content will be. (See text for blood flow patterns.) The size of the placenta has been reduced to save space. Normally, it would be about twice the pictured size in relation to the size of the infant at term. At birth the normal placenta equals about one sixth the weight of the newborn.

precautions, transabdominally, from the amniotic sac, called amniocentesis (Fig. 4-3); (2) ultrasonography, which, unlike x-ray examination, *appears* to be a safe technique for the fetus and mother at any stage in the pregnancy; and (3) maternal blood and urine analysis. These tests are highlighted in Table 4-2. During labor the immediate status of the baby may be evaluated through simultaneous monitoring of the fetal heart rate and contraction patterns and, in certain cases, by fetal blood sampling. (See pp. 109 to 113.)

Knowledge about the fetus has grown tremendously in the last decade. The intensive study of the fetus and newborn has developed into the rapidly expanding clinical specialty of perinatology, which crosses the ill-defined borders of maternity and pediatric practice. Scattered reports of successful medical and surgical interventions that have been used to treat the unborn have caused this small representative of the human race to gain in many minds much more status as a person and a patient.

•   •   •

TABLE 4-2   EVALUATION OF THE UNBORN INFANT

AGE

Important for medical-legal considerations, e.g., dating of prospective abortion (or elective cesarean birth)
 	
An indirect, unreliable assessment of maturity
	1. Based on date of first day of last normal menstrual period (Nägele's rule: count back 3 months, add 7 days to determine delivery date)
	2. Based on fundal height (assumes normal fetal growth) (Fig. 4-7)
	3. Based on appearance of fetal heart tone at 18 to 20 weeks using standard fetoscope
	4. Ultrasound measurements
	  a. Size of amniotic sac/uterine cavity
	  b. Fetal crown to rump length
	  c. Biparietal diameters, abdominal or thoracic circumferences at approximately 20 to 24 weeks for greatest accuracy
	5. Amniotic fluid analysis (amniocentesis)
	  a. Bilirubin levels during pregnancy uncomplicated by maternal-fetal blood incompatibilities usually reach peak at 16 to 30 weeks, then fall, disappearing by 36 weeks
	  b. Creatinine levels rise as fetal urine increases; unreliable if maternal-fetal complications occur
	  c. L/S ratio usually 2 at 35 weeks, but appearance of normal levels may be accelerated or retarded by maternal-fetal disorders

---

MATURITY

Various body system development may be monitored, but overall fetal maturity difficult to ascertain	1. Amniotic fluid analysis (amniocentesis)
	  a. L/S ratio usually rises to 2 or more when lungs have matured; other biochemical tests (e.g., amount of saturated fats) increase reliability of lung maturation evaluation in complex obstetric cases
	  b. Positive foam or shake test usually rules out lung immaturity
	  c. Fatty cell recovery percentage—low reliability
	  d. Creatinine levels may assist in assessment of renal maturity

---

WELL-BEING

Indications of some specific defects as well as clues of general fetal well-being possible, but not all problems identifiable	1. Ultrasound measurements
	  a. Evaluation of fetal presentation; multiple pregnancy
	  b. Detection of some structural abnormalities, e.g., hydrocephalus
	  c. Localization of placenta; diagnosis of placenta previa
	  d. Motion picture (real-time techniques) may confirm fetal death
	2. Amniotic fluid analysis (amniocentesis)
	  a. Chromosomal studies may reveal the following:
	    (1) Fetal abnormalities in chromosome number and gross structure (e.g., Down syndrome)
	    (2) Sex of infant to help evaluate probability of sex-linked genetic disorders (e.g., Duchenne's muscular dystrophy, classic hemophilia)
	  b. Biochemical studies may reveal the following:
	    (1) Anencephaly-myelomeningocele, based on presence of alpha fetoprotein
	    (2) A number of metabolic and blood diseases (e.g., thalassemia)

TABLE 4-2   EVALUATION OF THE UNBORN INFANT—cont'd

WELL-BEING—cont'd

	3. Meconium-stained amniotic fluid; possible fetal oxygen lack (hypoxia)
	4. Fetal movement—usually reassuring if not exaggerated
	5. Fetal heart rate and contraction monitoring—external or internal
	a. Helps identify episodes of hypoxia resulting from uteroplacental insufficiency or cord compression during labor (pp. 109 to 113)
	b. Positive oxytocin challenge test may reveal in "trial labor" fetal jeopardy in event of true labor (p. 488)
	c. Fetal heart rate changes in response to fetal movement without uterine contractions before labor are consistent with fetal health and form basis of *nonstress* test
	6. Fetal blood sampling (microsamples drawn from presenting part, usually scalp)
	a. Helps identify fetal hypoxia, retention of CO_2, and developing acidosis
	b. Serial samples are more meaningful
	c. pH Values of below 7.2 in two or more samples usually indicates need for assistance
	d. Maternal acidosis may cause misleading interpretations of fetal status
	7. X-ray examination (used only late in pregnancy because of radiation risk; less common where ultrasound available)
	a. Fetal presentation; multiple pregnancy
	b. Fetopelvic disproportion
	8. Maternal urine or serum analysis to detect serial estriol levels to evaluate functioning of placenta and fetal adrenal glands

SIGNS AND SYMPTOMS OF PREGNANCY

All the activity initiated within the uterus with the onset of pregnancy cannot be kept a secret for long. Widespread changes take place in the body, creating various signs and symptoms that possess varying degrees of importance in the diagnosis of pregnancy.

Although these signs and symptoms are usually arranged according to their accuracy into three groups comprising the presumptive, probable, and positive signs of pregnancy, there is no universal agreement regarding the contents of these categories.

Presumptive signs and symptoms

The presumptive signs and symptoms of pregnancy are those that taken by themselves could easily be an indication of other conditions. They usually include the following.

Amenorrhea. Although absence of menses may be an early sign of developing pregnancy, it certainly is not always. Amenorrhea may occur as a result of sudden changes in environment or occupation, emotional upset, malnutrition, fatigue, hormonal disorders, and the menopause.

Nausea and vomiting (particularly in the morning). Nausea and vomiting, presumably the results of changes in hormone levels in the body in the first weeks of pregnancy, are obviously not confined to this cause, since they are a common accompaniment of gastrointestinal tract irritation and emotional stress.

Frequent urination. Frequent voidings, usually of small amounts, are common during the first and last weeks of pregnancy because of pelvic congestion and the particular pressure of the uterus on the bladder. But frequency may also be present because of excitement, large fluid intakes, or irritation of the urinary tract.

Breast changes. Tingling, swelling, and tenderness involving the breasts are also found rather early in pregnancy. But a minimal number of such symptoms may be experienced during each menstrual cycle just before menses. Color changes causing a deepening of pigmentation in the breast or production of breast secretion (colostrum) are considered to be probable signs of pregnancy in a woman who has not been pregnant previously, but have little value in a woman who has had children recently or has been nursing. Tiny nodules on the nipple and areola, which are enlarged lubricating glands called tubercles of Montgomery, are often seen.

Color changes in the skin and mucous membranes. Another pigmentation characteristic of pregnancy is a bronze-type of facial coloration called *chloasma*, or the *mask of pregnancy*, often seen on dark-haired women. Development of a dark line (linea nigra), extending from the sternum to the pubis in the midline, is considered by some to be a probable sign if the woman has not been pregnant before. These changes in coloration are probably related to hormonal alterations. Most references now list the violet coloration of the vagina, cervix, and vulva, which is apparent at about 6 to 10 weeks' gestation (Chadwick's sign), as a presumptive indication of pregnancy. It is caused by increased circulation to the area and may be associated with any cause of pelvic congestion.

Quickening. Quickening, meaning the first time life or fetal movement is felt by the woman, can sometimes be imitated by peristalsis or gas and be wrongly interpreted. By the time quickening is felt (at approximately 16 weeks by mothers who have had previous children and 18 weeks or more by those experiencing their first pregnancy) other more definite signs should be manifest.

Fatigue. Fatigue, often included on the list, is a widespread complaint.

Probable signs and symptoms

The probable signs of pregnancy are more certain, but not infallible. They usually include the following: enlargement of the abdomen, certain other changes in the reproductive anatomy and physiology, and positive pregnancy tests.

Changes in shape of abdomen. Increases in abdominal size may be accompanied by pink to purplish "stretch marks," known technically as *striae gravidarum* (Fig. 4-5). It is now thought that their presence is probably more related to increases in the production in or sensitivity to adrenocortical hormones during pregnancy than to gain in weight alone. Such skin changes are also noted in patients with Cushing's disease and, to a lesser degree, with sudden great weight gains not associated with pregnancy. Unfortunately, the contour of one's abdomen may depend on dietary willpower rather than gestation. It may also be influenced by the growth of tumors or hernias.

Changes in reproductive organs. The enlargement of the uterus, rather than an increase in abdominal circumference, is a more definitive sign of pregnancy. Nevertheless, uterine tumors or inflammation may cause an increase in size. At about 6 to 8 weeks' gestation a special softening of the region of the uterus between the body and the cervix, called the *isthmus*, occurs. It is determined by a simultaneous abdominal and vaginal examination, a bimanual maneuver illustrated in Fig. 4-6. This softening is termed "Hegar's sign." Another softening of the uterus, this time affecting the cervix, is detected by the examiner's finger. In the nonpregnant state the cervix feels somewhat like the cartilage at the tip of one's nose. During preg-

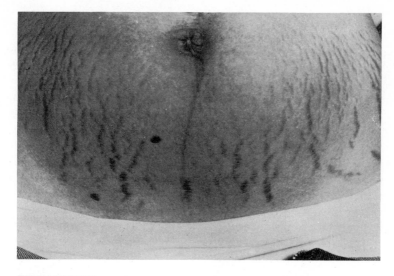

FIG. 4-5 Striae (stretch marks).
Courtesy Mercy Hospital and Medical Center, San Diego, Calif.

FIG. 4-6 Hegar's sign.

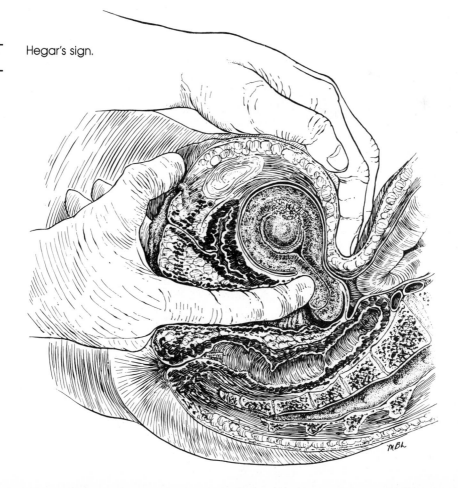

nancy it changes in consistency to resemble the pliability of the ear lobe or lips (Goodell's sign).

Basal body temperature elevation. This is one of the earliest diagnostic observations possible and is considered to have 97% accuracy. However, for this basal or waking temperature to have meaning, the woman must have taken her temperature consistently, using proper technique both before and after ovulation to detect the persistent relative increase in basal readings. (For interpretation of the temperature readings, see p. 208.)

Positive biologic and immunochemical pregnancy tests. Pregnancy tests are based on the fact that the chorionic villi of an implanted ovum or of the developing placenta secrete human chorionic gonadotropic hormone (HCG), which is excreted in small amounts in urine and blood. The first tests were biologic. A concentrated urine sample obtained from a morning specimen, voided after a period of fluid limitation, was injected into a laboratory animal. The animal was then observed for changes in its reproductive cycle. Rabbits, mice, and frogs were used.

Immunochemical tests that no longer require laboratory animals are now employed. Manufacturers of pregnancy tests usually state that HCG may be accurately identified in urine 42 days after the last menstrual period (LMP). Special blood tests known as radioimmunoassays (RIA) may also be used to obtain even earlier confirmation. The RIA for the β (beta) subunit of HCG is said to be capable of diagnosing pregnancy as early as 5 days *before* the first missed period.

Most pregnancy tests are only about 95% to 99% accurate depending on when they are performed, the method used, and the presence of factors that may cause both false negatives or positives. For these reasons "positive" results are still considered probable and not positive signs of pregnancy. Although a firm diagnosis of pregnancy can usually be made after the eighth week without any special chemical tests, there is a growing tendency to use the tests to help detect pregnancy as soon as possible. The earlier pregnancy can be documented, the sooner prenatal care can be initiated and a more

accurate estimated date of birth be established. In those instances when a pregnancy outside the uterine cavity (ectopic pregnancy) or an abnormal growth of the fertilized ovum (hydatidiform mole) is suspected, when surgery involving anesthesia, diagnostic or therapeutic radiation, or prescription of medications potentially toxic to a developing pregnancy is planned, or when abortion may be contemplated, the results of such tests continue to be especially significant.

Positive signs

Three positive signs of pregnancy are usually cited.

1. Presence of a fetal heart tone, usually heard after 18 to 20 weeks by conventional auscultation with a standard fetoscope. (Up to the 20th week the fetal heart is best heard at the center of the pubic hair line. Fetal heart tones are usually detected by 10 to 12 weeks after conception using ultrasonic or Doppler effect techniques. The presence of the so-called uterine souffle is not diagnostic. This swish-like tone, which is at the same rate as the maternal pulse, originates from the pulsating uterine arteries and not from the placenta itself and may also be heard in the presence of large vascular pelvic tumors.)
2. Fetal movement detected by a trained examiner.
3. Visualization of the fetus during ultrasonography or x-ray studies.

Some references also include bouncing of the fetus against the examiner's fingers during a vaginal examination (ballottement) and palpation of fetal parts by a physician.

PROGRESSIVE FETAL GROWTH

With the growth of the embryo and fetus, as shown in Table 4-1 and Fig. 4-7, the contours and silhouette of the expectant mother change progres-

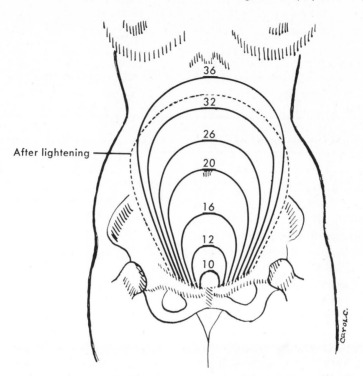

After lightening

FIG. 4-7   Progressive growth of fundus during pregnancy, measured in weeks. Note that the fundus is lower at term than at 36 weeks' gestation.

sively. The fundus, or top of the uterus, is felt about halfway between the top of the pubic bone and the umbilicus at approximately 16 weeks. It is found almost at the umbilicus at about 20 weeks. Near term it is almost at the level of the tip of the sternum. A woman expecting her first baby usually experiences a sudden relief from shortness of breath about 2 weeks before her delivery when the fetus "drops" and *lightening* occurs, taking pressure off the diaphragm.

The increasing size of her temporary boarder puts greater demands on her respiratory, circulatory, and urinary systems. Her intestines and stomach experience crowding and compression. Increasing size necessitates changes in wardrobe, creates a typical posture of pregnancy, and finally makes the heretofore simple process of tying shoes almost impossible. The onset of labor terminating her long period of waiting is usually a welcome event.

When she suspects she is pregnant, a woman should consult a physician to gain optimum care even during the early months of pregnancy. Since women are not certain that they will become pregnant and often are not aware of the fact of pregnancy until several weeks of gestation have elapsed, the earliest prenatal care is always the responsibility of the woman herself. Her general health habits and physical condition before a physician is ever consulted are of considerable importance. When pregnancy is established, provision for regular medical supervision and suitable plans for the baby's arrival must be made.

In the physician's office and in the hospital, an expectant mother is given certain professional labels by the staff to help in anticipating her needs and to briefly describe her obstetric history. This terminology, with certain modifications, is used throughout her care. It consists of a series of prefixes and base words to help describe the number of times the woman has been pregnant and the number of times she has carried a child to a viable age. The word elements are as follows:

gravida Means the number of pregnancies a woman has had regardless of outcome.
para Means the number of infants a woman has delivered weighing 500 g or more or, if weight is unknown, the number having an estimated gestational age of 20 completed weeks or more, whether born living or dead. In most areas the birth of twins or triplets would only be considered as one delivery. Both abdominal and vaginal deliveries are recorded in "para" counts. A *parturient* is a woman in labor.

nul (a prefix) Means none. A *nulligravida* has never been pregnant. A *nullipara* has never delivered a viable child.
prim (a prefix) From primary, or first. Combined with gravida, it reads *primigravida* and means a woman who is having or has had one pregnancy. Combined with para, it reads *primipara* and technically means a woman who has had one delivery of a viable child. However, once she is admitted into the labor-delivery suite, attending nurses usually refer to a woman who is carrying her first child but is not yet delivered as a primipara, or "primip," to differentiate her from a woman who has been through the birth process.
mult (a prefix) Meaning many, or at least more than one. Combined with gravida it reads *multigravida* and means a woman who has had more than one pregnancy. Combined with para it reads *multipara*, or "multip," and technically means a woman who has borne two or more viable infants. Actually, in the labor-delivery suite the term is applied to a woman who has delivered one viable child or more, to differentiate her from a "first timer." Sometimes women who have had six or more viable births are called "grandmultips."

GOALS AND IMPORTANCE OF PRENATAL CARE

The term "antepartal or prenatal care" as used by physicians and nurses refers to the planned examination, observation, and guidance of an expectant mother. It is well to remember that the extension of prenatal care is probably the primary factor in the improvement of maternal morbidity and mortality statistics. Society needs to appreciate its importance. The goals are as follows:

1. A pregnancy with a minimum of mental and physical discomfort and a maximum of gratification
2. A birth under the best circumstances possible
3. A normal, well baby
4. The establishment of good health habits benefiting all the family
5. A smooth, guided postpartum adjustment

For many years the overall goals of prenatal care have probably remained much the same, but interpretation of these goals and the methods for accomplishing them are undergoing continual change and accelerated expansion. During the late 1800s and early 1900s, the focus of the attending physician and nurse was on the physical needs of the parturient. Later, the psychological aspects of her needs drew deserved attention. More recently, the physical and psychosocial needs of the entire family unit, as well as the needs of the childbearing woman, have been emphasized as health professionals concern themselves with the concept of "family-centered maternity care."*

For example, goals 1 and 2 above underline the need for better health care delivery systems that would encourage socioeconomically disadvantaged urban and rural clients to receive needed care and vital health instruction. Because of financial strain, transportation difficulties, child care problems, or fear and distrust of established depersonalized and fragmented institutional management, they may not have sufficiently obtained or used these facilities. These goals also imply for many parents more knowledge of the processes of pregnancy of childbirth and more participation in the control over these processes than were requested by recent previous generations.† For some expectant parents, these goals have encouraged childbirth in settings

other than the traditional hospital maternity unit. Primarily, psychological factors have prompted their consideration of more flexible family-centered maternity care programs, alternative birth centers, or possible home birth.* (See pp. 139-141.) Goal 3 now allows more legally permitted decision making than ever before as genetic counseling and abortion services become increasingly accessible. Goal 4 may encompass not only physical health but emotional well-being, knowledge and appreciation of life processes, and a sense of responsible personhood that considers individual differences as well as the common good. Future parents, consumers of maternity care, today do not wish to be treated all alike. They wish to have comprehensive care that will allow them certain choices, variations of expression, and informed consent. "A smooth, guided postpartum adjustment" entails more knowledge of childcraft and parenting skills and more premeditated control of family composition.

THE FIRST VISIT

Usually prenatal care is formally begun shortly after the second menstrual period is missed. But in a broader and very real sense, prenatal care, negative or positive, has gone on in the life of a young woman long before she becomes pregnant. Her basic physique was determined by her parents before her birth. Her environment has left its physical and emotional imprint. Her own family circle and close friends have greatly influenced her attitude toward pregnancy and the challenges and responsibilities of motherhood. Today much controversy exists regarding the need for sex education, what should be taught by whom, and at what age level. Sex education and preparation for marriage and parenthood are taught—sometimes negatively, by default. Children and young people do not live in a vacuum.

---

*Ryan, G.M.: Prenatal care and pregnancy outcome, Am. J. Obstet. Gynecol. **137**:876-881, August 15, 1980. Joint position statement on the development of family-centered maternity/newborn care in hospitals, Chicago, June, 1978, Interprofessional Task Force on Health Care of Women and Children.
†Elkins, V.H.: The rights of the pregnant parent, Ottawa, 1976, Waxwing Productions.

*Kramer, R.: Giving birth: childbearing in America. Chicago, 1978, Contemporary Books, Inc. Olds, S.B.: Obstetric nursing. Menlo Park, Calif., 1980, Addison-Wesley Publishing Co., Inc., p. 15.

What, in more detail, does formal prenatal care entail? Perhaps it would be easiest to describe the visits of the future mother to the physician's office or clinic. Usually the most lengthy visit she makes is her first.

The first prenatal visit is usually a particular time of stress. Some women are concerned because they want very much to be pregnant. Some are anxious about the nature of the examination and the tests to be made. Others may be concerned because they had not planned to have a child. Family financial problems may be mounting. A number of small children may already be part of the family. Health problems at home may cause worry. Previous unfortunate obstetric experiences and half-believed gossip about pregnancy and childbirth may concern her. The marriage or relationship may be undergoing a period of instability or even dissolution. All these possible situations tend to heighten the emotional content of the visit.

Setting and "climate"

The "climate" of the first as well as subsequent visits to the physician or, in some settings, nurse-midwife is all important. A nurse who has the responsibility of greeting and caring for these women has a key position. A cordial, respectful environment in which the woman feels personally important to the office or clinic staff and physician is a goal to be sought.

Preparation for the visit is usually made by a telephone call. At this time it is customary for a new patient to be asked to bring a sample of the first voided urine on the day of the appointment if her visit will be made early in the morning. When the time of the appointment arrives, it is hoped that the prospective patient will not have to wait too long, but because of the very nature of a physician's practice, which deals with the unscheduled arrivals of babies, some waiting is almost unavoidable. However, some of this time can often be put to excellent use. The nurse or receptionist can start to make contact with the patient and make her feel welcome. Brief information cards for office use may

be completed. Frequently changed, attractive bulletin boards may emphasize nutrition and meal planning, mental health practices, good grooming, maternity wardrobe styles, and approved courses in preparation for childbirth and child care. Up-to-date pamphlets on maternal and child care and breastfeeding literature may also be available. Not all reading material should be pregnancy oriented, however. Just because a woman is pregnant does not mean that is all she wants to think about! When waits are protracted, an offer of coffee or fruit juice may be appreciated. The way to the public rest room should be clearly indicated, since frequent urination is an often encountered annoyance, and general nervousness will usually exaggerate this symptom. Just before the pelvic examination, the patient should have an opportunity to empty her bladder to ease the examination and to allow a more accurate measurement of the height of the fundus.

Vital signs and history

Before actually seeing the physician the woman is usually weighed and her temperature, pulse, and respiration are checked by the nurse. In some clinics, nurses may also take the blood pressures and medical and obstetric histories of new patients, but many practitioners prefer to complete the blood pressures and the histories themselves. A carefully secured history is very important in helping to determine any special care of the patient. Early detection of reproductive risk is essential to help prevent maternal or fetal problems. What previous medical or surgical difficulties has she had? Any problems involving mental or emotional instability? Any family problems that may affect her toleration of the stress of pregnancy? A record of previous pregnancies and their outcome is extremely important in indicating the need for special emphasis in prenatal care. One method of coding the results of previous pregnancies involves the use of four consecutive digits. The first refers to the number of full-term deliveries, the second to the number of premature births, the third to abortions, and

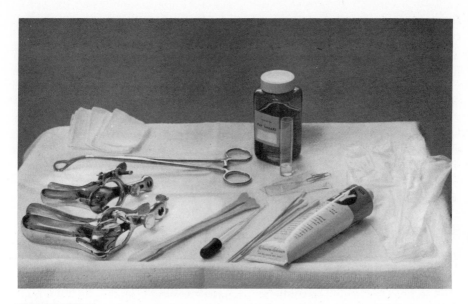

FIG. 5-1   Typical pelvic tray (sterile gloves are not shown). The small test tube contains physiologic saline solution for wet mount of vaginal discharge.

the fourth to children now living. Using this code, what would 3215 mean? Many physicians believe that the time spent in recording the historic data is more than repaid by the greater opportunity to evaluate the childbearing woman and her child and establish rapport.

Pelvic examination

The visit usually continues with the determination of the presence of pregnancy. Physicians have individual routines, but it is our opinion that the pelvic examination should be done first in the schedule of the physical examination to alleviate the additional anxiety of waiting and to avoid a filling bladder! The nurse, by her manner and efficiency, can help the patient immensely.

Preparation. An adequate gown, which gives reassuring coverage but opens in such a way to facilitate a physical examination, is desirable. A drape that makes the patient feel covered, even if

she is not, is a real aid. The hips should extend about 1 inch over the edge of the table with the feet supported in stirrups. Various drapes may be used. A nurse should always be present during the examination to give reassurance to the patient and to protect the physician from criticism. Necessary instruments should be ready (Fig. 5-1): warmed speculum, spatula or applicator, or vaginal pipette with rubber bulb, slides and preservative for cervical cancer detection; long swabs or cotton balls, sponge sticks, both sterile and clean rubber gloves, lubricant, and paper tissue wipes. A good light and a convenient stool must be provided. If the woman is able to let her knees fall outward and relax, the examination will be less difficult. Having her breathe through her open mouth usually helps promote relaxation, although there is some danger of hyperventilation in very tense patients.

Progression. The pelvic examination yields considerable information. The physician first inspects the external genitalia. Next, if a Papanicolaou smear for cancer detection is desired (and it is almost always part of the routine), a warmed but unlubricated bivalve speculum is inserted to reveal the cervix. Specimens of secretion may be aspirated from the posterior fornix with the pipette or secured with the applicator or spatula from the cervix and placed thinly and evenly on one or two slides. These slides must not be allowed to dry out but should immediately be placed in a fixative (usually equal parts of 95% alcohol and ether). The physician will then observe the cervix and vaginal mucosa for any abnormalities or unusual discharge; specimens of any discharge can be obtained for future study. Fungous infection caused by *Candida albicans* or infection initiated by microscopic animals, or protozoa, called *Trichomonas vaginalis*, is fairly common. Routine culture of cervical mucus for *Neisseria gonorrhoeae*, the cause of gonorrhea, has been helpful in detecting significant numbers of so-called silent infections within certain high-risk populations. The mucosa will be checked for Chadwick's sign—a violet tinge caused by increased circulatory congestion in the area.

After general inspection of the vulva, cervix, and vagina, the speculum will be gently removed and a digital examination will be made with the lubricated gloved hand. At this time the physician will feel the size and position of the uterus, the consistency of the cervix, and perhaps try to elicit Hegar's sign, the softening of the uterine isthmus, through vaginoabdominal pressure. The pelvic contents will be palpated to try to identify any abnormal masses or tumors. Usually before completing the examination, the physician will attempt to measure the *diagonal conjugate* to estimate the size of the pelvic canal and will evaluate the position of the ischial spines and tuberosities. At the end of the vaginal examination a rectal examination is usually carried out. Generally the physician can report at the end of the pelvic examination whether or not the woman is actually pregnant.

Determination of delivery date

The most common method of determining the date of delivery involves a record of the menstrual cycle. The woman is asked to name the *first* day of her last *normal* menstrual period. The physician then counts back 3 months and adds 7 days to calculate the estimated date of confinement (EDC). (Confinement is a rather old term used to indicate the period of labor and birth.) For example, if a woman said that her last normal menstrual period occurred between May 7 and May 12, her EDC would be February 14 of the following year. This method of calculation is called Nägele's rule. Of course, if the patient cannot remember the necessary vital statistics, calculation may be more difficult. Then the size of the uterus may be interpreted, or the time of the intercourse that preceded conception may be known. Ultrasound evaluation may be used if it is important to know the age of the fetus. Occasionally *quickening* may be used as a measurable landmark, but it is not too reliable. However, even Nägele's rule offers only an estimation. It is said that only 4% of all babies arrive "on time" using this schedule, whereas 60% appear 1 to 7 days early or late.

Complete examination

The first prenatal visit may continue with a complete physical examination, or the physician may only talk with the patient, giving appropriate guidance and information and making arrangements for a more detailed physical examination during the following visit.

In addition to the pelvic examination, the physician checks the woman's blood pressure; listens to her heart and lungs; examines her mouth, eyes, ears, nose, and throat; observes and palpates her breasts for any abnormalities; and inquires about her preference for feeding the infant. The breast examination should be conducted to determine whether normal breast changes are occurring and whether infection or even malignancy is present. The abdomen is palpated with the knees flexed for greater relaxation of the abdominal wall, and the extremities are checked for bruises, swelling, and enlarged veins.

Usually at the conclusion of the physical examination, arrangements are made for the necessary laboratory tests. A sample of venous blood is drawn. A complete blood cell count may be ordered or perhaps a hemoglobin alone or a hematocrit to determine the amount of hemoglobin present in the blood in relation to its volume. Any pregnant woman may be or may become anemic. Dietary deficiencies of iron are common. Although hemoglobin and hematocrit levels in nonpregnant women would be considered suspiciously low if less than 12 g/100 ml and 36%, respectively, the standards of possible anemia used during pregnancy are usually less than 11 g/100 ml and less than 33%. The differences are the result of the increased fluid content in the blood during gestation. Prenatal testing for sickle cell anemia in previously unscreened black patients is becoming more common.

A serology test for the detection of syphilis (STS) is a routine screening procedure of prenatal care. A determination of main blood group and Rh status is made to assist in maternal care in the event of hemorrhage and to detect the possibility of blood protein incompatibility, which could threaten the life of the developing fetus or infant. If the patient is found to be Rh negative, the Rh status of the baby's father should be ascertained.

Another potential threat that can now be identified by the laboratory is rubella, or German measles. A history of the disease in childhood is not always reliable, since other conditions may have been incorrectly called rubella and since the disease does not always manifest a rash. The measurement of rubella antibody level in a woman's blood has become a premarital or prenatal legal requirement in some states. The presence of antibodies in a 1:10 or greater dilution of serum is said to indicate immunity. Some physicians in practice consider the 1:10 dilution reaction evidence of only "borderline" protection and consider the mother still at risk unless a weaker dilution (more than 1:10) demonstrates antibody levels. Pregnant women are *not* given the available immunization against rubella. There is a real possibility that the fetus could contract the deforming contagion whether or not the mother shows clinical signs of the disease. However, if immunity is considered absent, the antibody titer obtained can be used as a base line to help determine subsequent contact with the disease and the need for possible immune serum globulin or consideration of an abortion. New mothers at risk are immunized during the postpartum period only after reliable contraception techniques have been instituted. See discussion of rubella, pp. 293-294.

The urine specimen brought in the same morning or secured later at the office is tested for albumin and glucose. Many physicians order a complete urinalysis initially.

In many patients, chest x-ray examination for detection of tuberculosis is being avoided through the use of Mantoux or Tine skin testing. If the skin test is positive, a full-sized, conventional chest x-ray examination is recommended to rule out possible pathology more easily and to avoid the higher amount of x-ray exposure involved in the use of photofluorographs or miniature films. Screening for tuberculosis, hepatitis, and malaria is becoming more important as the refugee population increases.

Guidance

After all these procedures have been completed, if they take place during one visit, the patient is usually tired. Lengthy instructions and explanations are not properly assimilated. Perhaps the best method of imparting needed information is through the use of some kind of prenatal instruction booklet that has been approved by or perhaps even written by the patient's physician. Some practices program a series of teaching films that individuals or groups can view while they are waiting to see the physician. Such guidance is absolutely necessary, but all of it need not be provided on the first visit. However, some time should be spent answering questions, discussing patient expectations for the childbirth, and giving some general instructions regarding dietary requirements, risks of self-medication, excessive smoking and alcohol consumption, and the situations that should be reported to the physician.

Reportable signs and symptoms

The physician should indicate the signs and symptoms that must be reported in a manner that will not be too alarming to the pregnant woman. They may or may not be significant, but only qualified personnel are capable of deciding their importance and must be notified of their presence. They include the following:

1. Bleeding from the vagina at any time
2. Uncontrollable leaking of fluid from the vagina
3. Unusual abdominal pain or cramps
4. Persistent nausea or vomiting, especially in the second or third trimester
5. Persistent headache or any blurring of vision
6. Marked swelling of the ankles and especially of the hands and face
7. Painful or burning urination
8. Chills or fever

Then, armed with information, the woman may make an appointment for her next visit. Before her return she can jot down questions that come up about which she needs to be reassured.

SUBSEQUENT VISITS

During the first half of the pregnancy, expectant mothers most often visit their physician every 3 or 4 weeks unless special needs become apparent. After 5 months, visits are usually scheduled every 2 or 3 weeks, and in the last month, checkups may be made every 1 or 2 weeks or more often.

Examination

The subsequent visits are not as long or involved. The woman is weighed by the nurse, and the blood pressure is recorded. A urine specimen is checked for albumin and glucose. The urine examination for glucose, of course, is made to detect dia-

betes mellitus. All of the other above determinations are done to reveal the beginnings of preeclampsia. (Remember that the major signs of preeclampsia are elevated blood pressure, edema, excessive weight gain, and albuminuria. See p. 171.) The physician measures the height of the uterus to see if the pregnancy is progressing at the expected rate and may repeat the pelvic examination during the first return visit. The Doptone may be used in early pregnancy to evaluate the fetal heart rate. After about 4½ calendar months' gestation the physician may hear the fetal heart tone with a nonelectronic fetoscope. After 8 months' gestation the physician can palpate the abdomen to determine the presentation of the fetus. Hemoglobin or hematocrit levels should be repeated for all pregnant women at least once late in pregnancy (at about 32 to 36 weeks). Women who earlier had been found to have iron or folic acid deficiency anemias or other causes of hemoglobin reduction should be checked more frequently to determine their response to therapy.

If Rh incompatibility is a possibility, antibody titers should be done not only at the initial prenatal visit but also at 24, 28, 32, and 36 weeks' gestation, even if the woman received Rh immune globulin, such as RhoGAM, after previous pregnancies. Rising titers may indicate whether the baby is Rh positive and will alert the physician to developing erythroblastosis fetalis. A more reliable technique for evaluating fetal jeopardy related to blood factor incompatibility involves the aspiration of amniotic fluid by transabdominal needle insertion (amniocentesis) and its analysis for elevated bilirubin levels (p. 47).

Because maternal syphilitic infection may be acquired *after* a negative prenatal serology result is obtained, the prudence of securing a repeat serology test close to term should be considered. Since initial testing for maternal syphilitic infection will be positive in less than 80% of patients with primary syphilis, it is essential to repeat the test near the end of pregnancy (36 weeks). Follow-up may utilize the fluorescent treponemal antibody absorption (FTA-ABS) test if the VDRL is reactive. In this instance, even though treatment has been instituted, the newborn should be tested using cord and serum VDRL and FTA-ABS tests as well as IgM-specific FTA-ABS testing.*

Genital herpes can be transmitted to the baby as it passes through the birth canal. When suspicious lesions are found, a test for herpes should be performed. It takes a few days for a current, active infection to be detected by laboratory studies, but if the herpes culture is positive, the test should be repeated at 38 weeks. If this repeat culture is negative and no lesions develop, a vaginal delivery may be done. Otherwise, cesarean section would be safer for the baby.† Other laboratory evaluations of fetal and maternal health and gestational maturity are possible but would depend on the specific problems discovered.

Guidance

During the initial and return visits a feeling of trust should be built up between the pregnant woman and the physician, any other maternity team members,‡ and office staff. The physician and nurse should be able to identify areas in which special help is required, whether the woman needs information, reassurance in her own capacity to be a good mother, possible help in organizing her household to achieve more rest and peace of mind, or simply an interested human listener.

NUTRITION

The subject of nutrition has long been considered important in prenatal care. Increasing numbers of health professionals now recognize that nutrition is not only important but crucial in determining the health of the childbearing woman, her offspring, and perhaps even that of ongoing generations. It is imperative that girls and women consider themselves as possible prospective mothers by preparing themselves for the potential responsibility of such nurture long before a mate is selected. Their health, knowledge, and skills will profoundly influence the structure of any future family. A woman who furnishes her body with what it needs nutritionally to enjoy optimum personal health and who augments her diet as needed as a pregnancy progresses gives her child a better opportunity to be both well formed from his earliest days of development and well born as he ends his intrauterine growth period. A well-nourished mother and baby are less often the victims of obstetric and perinatal complications, such as preeclampsia, prematurity, growth retardation (small for dates), or significant residual neurologic damage (for example, cerebral palsy, mental deficiency, or behavior disorders in the child).

Various aids have been devised to try to help Americans eat more nourishing food according to their body build, age, activity, or special physiologic needs. The National Research Council publishes periodically a quantitative list of calories and nutrients needed. In 1980 this list, the Recommended Daily Allowance, or RDA, was newly revised. (Table 5-1 is an abbreviated version.) The council indicates that a normal, healthy, pregnant woman of any age needs *greater amounts of calories* and every *nutrient* listed during the last half of her 40-week pregnancy than she does when not pregnant.

Since 1974 the requirement for ascorbic acid has been increased from 60 mg/day to 80 mg/day for the pregnant woman. Vitamin B_6 recommended daily intake was changed from 2.5 mg to 2.6 mg. The iodine recommendation has been elevated from 125 to 175 μg per day. (Use of iodized salt can meet this requirement.) Zinc has been shown to affect over 70 enzymes in the human body—an important element to consider when planning the dietary intake. It is usually associated with protein foods and nuts.

---

*Syphilis before birth, Emergency Medicine, June 15, 1980, pp. 126, 127. Jones, J.E., and Harris, R.E.: Diagnostic evaluation of syphilis during pregnancy, Obstet. Gynecol. **54**:611-614, Nov., 1979.

†Boehm, F.H., and Estes, W.: Genital herpes simplex during pregnancy, Perinatology/Neonatology **6**(1):21-24, Feb., 1982.

‡Bash, D.B., and Gold, W.A.: The nurse and the childbearing family, New York, 1981, John Wiley & Sons, p. 205.

TABLE 5-1 RECOMMENDED DAILY DIETARY ALLOWANCES (DESIGNED FOR THE MAINTENANCE OF GOOD

		Weight		Height				Fat-soluble vitamins			Water-soluble vitamins		
	Age (years)	kg	lb	cm	in	Energy (kcal)	Protein (g)	Vita- min A (µg RE)[a]	Vita- min D (µg)[b]	Vita- min E (mg α TE)[c]	Vita- min C (mg)	Thiamin (mg)	Ribo- flavin (mg)
Females	11-14	46	101	157	62	2200	46	800	10	8	50	1.1	1.3
	15-18	55	120	163	64	2100	46	800	10	8	60	1.1	1.3
	19-22	55	120	163	64	2000	44	800	7.5	8	60	1.1	1.3
	23-50	55	120	163	64	2000	44	800	5	8	60	1.0	1.2
	51+	55	120	163	64	2000	44	800	5	8	60	1.0	1.2
Pregnant						+300	+30	+200	+5	+2	+20	+0.4	+0.3
Lactating						+500	+20	+400	+5	+3	+40	+0.5	+0.5

From Food and Nutrition Board, National Academy of Sciences–National Research Council, Washington, D.C., 1980.
*The allowances are intended to provide for individual variations among most normal persons as they live in the United States under usual environmental stresses. Diets should be based on a variety of common foods in order to provide other nutrients for which human requirements have been less well defined.
[a]Retinol equivalents 1 Retinol equivalent = 1 µg retinol or 6 µg β carotene.
[b]As cholecalciferol. 10 µg cholecalciferol = 400 IU vitamin D.
[c]α tocopherol equivalents. 1 mg d-α-tocopherol = 1 α TE.

Iron deficiency anemia is the most common anemia of pregnancy. Although the pregnant woman should increase her iron intake during pregnancy, the requirement is usually not met from dietary sources alone. The fetus needs to lay down an iron reserve for hemoglobin formation during the first few months of extrauterine life, when the main source of nutrition will be milk, which is normally iron poor. Therefore, the National Research Council advises that an iron supplement of 30 to 60 mg/day be taken by the pregnant woman. This could be continued for 2 to 3 months after delivery to help replenish the mother's iron store. Excessive vitamin intake can be dangerous as well as wasteful. Routine multivitamin supplementation should not be necessary if a varied nutritious diet is consumed. Folacin or folic acid requirements should be met; a specific megaloblastic anemia does occasionally occur as a result of folacin depletion in pregnancy. It is interesting to note that steroid contraceptives that the expectant mother may have used in the recent past may also inhibit folic acid absorption. Nondietary folic acid is often pre-scribed by clinicians. Prescription of prenatal fluoride has not proved to be an asset. Calcification of the permanent teeth and much of that of the deciduous teeth occurs after birth. The RDAs determined by the council are designed to indicate safe dietary levels of selected nutrients for a wide range of normal healthy persons. Individual differences in the dietary background or obstetric histories of pregnant women may suggest the need for variations in these allowances.

An increasing trend (at least among some physicians) emphasizes the quality of the pregnant woman's diet with less concern about a certain total number of pounds gained. The need for quality intake is present throughout pregnancy. One can see in Fig. 5-3, which indicates the average relative-weight increase curve advocated as a pattern for evaluation by the National Academy of Sciences, Committee on Maternal Nutrition, that approximately two thirds of the weight gain occurs in the last half of pregnancy, paralleling fairly closely the baby's own weight gain curve. Quantitative increases in maternal intake are recommended for

NUTRITION OF PRACTICALLY ALL HEALTHY PEOPLE IN THE UNITED STATES)*

Water-soluble vitamins				Minerals					
Niacin (mg NE)[d]	Vitamin B₆ (mg)	Folacin[e] (μg)	Vitamin B₁₂ (μg)	Calcium (mg)	Phosphorus (mg)	Magnesium (mg)	Iron (mg)	Zinc (mg)	Iodine (μg)
15	1.8	400	3.0	1200	1200	300	18	15	150
14	2.0	400	3.0	1200	1200	300	18	15	150
14	2.0	400	3.0	800	800	300	18	15	150
13	2.0	400	3.0	800	800	300	18	15	150
13	2.0	400	3.0	800	800	300	10	15	150
+2	+0.6	+400	+1.0	+400	+400	+150	f	+5	+25
+5	+0.5	+100	+1.0	+400	+400	+150	f	+10	+50

[d]1 NE (niacin equivalent) is equal to 1 mg of niacin or 60 mg of dietary tryptophan.

[e]The folacin allowances refer to dietary sources as determined by *Lactobacillus casei* assay after treatment with enzymes ("conjugates") to make polyglutamyl forms of the vitamin available for the test organism.

[f]The increased requirement during pregnancy cannot be met by the iron content of habitual American diets nor by the existing iron stores of many women; therefore the use of 30-60 mg of supplemental iron is recommended. Iron needs during lactation are not substantially different from those of nonpregnant women, but continued supplementation of the mother for 2 to 3 months after parturition is advisable in order to replenish stores depleted by pregnancy.

healthy, well-nourished women only in the last half of pregnancy.

Because a pregnant woman cannot (as yet) go to the grocery store to purchase a package labeled "74 grams of protein," and because buying many of the nutrients as pills in a bottle would be expensive, inefficient, and unsatisfying, there needs to be a way to interpret her caloric and nutrient needs in terms of market basket commodities. For a number of years the concept of the Basic Four Food Groups and the suggested number of servings have been helpful in planning balanced family meals (Fig. 5-2). These four groups—milk, meat, vegetables and fruit, and breads and cereals—only contain those foods high in leading nutrients. In the second half of pregnancy many women benefit by including 3 or 4 cups of skim (lowfat 2%) or whole milk in their diets. Using nonfat dairy products reduces the total fat and cholesterol intake. Some fat is necessary in the diet, but it is not a scarce nutrient. Milk (and the calcium and protein it provides) is considered an important constituent of the pregnant woman's diet. However, at times its use must be modified.

The woman who does not care for milk per se is free to use flavoring, make what she does drink more concentrated in value by adding skim milk powders, use it in cooking, or select a milk exchange of approximately equal value for calcium. For example, 1 slice of American cheese or 1 cup of creamed cottage cheese equals approximately ⅔ glass of milk. Some adults, especially blacks and Asians, experience a digestive intolerance to the lactose found in milk and may develop abdominal cramping, intestinal gas, and diarrhea. However, they are often able to eat cheese. The harder or more aged varieties of cheese contain less lactose than processed types. Chilled dairy products, such as yogurt or ice cream, may also produce fewer symptoms. The calcium provided in milk and its products is important. There is a tendency for calcium to be drawn from the maternal skeleton, causing *osteoporosis*, weakening its structure if dietary needs are not met. If a pregnant woman cannot tolerate milk or is having muscle cramps due to phosphorus/calcium imbalance in the blood, calcium pills may be given, but in this case a fine, rel-

A Guide to Good Eating

Use Daily:

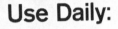

Milk Group

3 or more glasses milk — Children
smaller glasses for some children under 9

4 or more glasses — Teen-agers

2 or more glasses — Adults

Cheese, ice cream and other milk-
made foods can supply part of the milk

2 or more servings

Meats, fish, poultry, eggs, or
cheese — with dry beans,
peas, nuts as alternates

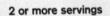

Meat Group

Vegetables and Fruits

4 or more servings

Include dark green or
yellow vegetables;
citrus fruit or tomatoes

4 or more servings

Enriched or whole grain
Added milk improves
nutritional values

Breads and Cereals

This is the foundation for a good diet. Use
more of these and other foods as needed for
growth, for activity, and for desirable weight.

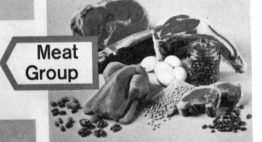

FIG. 5-2   Guide to good eating. Indicates recommended diet for
nonpregnant women and other family members. See
p. 65 for modifications during pregnancy.

Courtesy National Dairy Council, Chicago, Ill.

atively inexpensive source of protein is lost. Milk is also usually fortified with vitamin D, an important consideration in planning meals in climates with little sunshine or for women who receive inadequate exposure to sunlight.

Three servings of the meat group are usually recommended during the latter part of pregnancy. (This generally includes one or two eggs per day in addition to two servings of the other meat group foods listed.) Eggs are recommended particularly for the rich iron source found in the yolk. Meat, eggs, even fish and poultry are expensive, but they are complete proteins, containing all the amino acids necessary for growth, repair, and development. The essential amino acids (eight to ten in number, depending on age requirements) must be available to form new tissue within the mother's body, and they must be supplied in the diet; the body cannot manufacture these protein-building blocks by rearranging molecules within its own cells. Such proteins are critical to the growth of the embryo and fetus as basic body systems are formed early in pregnancy and as different organs, especially the brain, undergo growth spurts in the last weeks of gestation. They are also critical for the pregnant woman if she is to maintain her health and avoid obstetric problems such as toxemia. If legumes such as beans or peas, corn, nuts, and gelatin are used as major protein sources, they must be mixed in such a way that all essential amino acids are represented in a single meal, since none of these protein sources is complete in itself. Mixing certain incomplete proteins conscientiously or serving them with milk provides an adequate diet but is more difficult to plan. Examples of adequate protein mixes using incomplete proteins are combinations of cornmeal and kidney beans or whole wheat, soy beans and sesame seeds. Pure vegetarian, or "vegan," diets without any animal sources, dairy products, or eggs can supply adequate protein with careful planning. But other deficiencies (for example, vitamin B_{12}) may become a problem.

High-grade biologic sources of protein, such as meat, fish, poultry, milk, and eggs, contribute other nutrients as well. For example, liver, although it

may not be everybody's choice, is strongly favored in the diet because of its high iron content.

Whole-grain or enriched breads and cereals provide sources of the B vitamins thiamine and niacin, as well as some iodine and iron and needed cellulose. Four or more servings are indicated. One slice of bread equals one serving. A helpful chart designed to help meet the dietary needs of pregnancy is from Williams' excellent text, *Nutrition and Diet Therapy* (Table 5-2).

Fruits and vegetables are important sources of vitamins, minerals, and fiber (if they are eaten unmodified). Constipation is a real problem for many pregnant women. The increasing pressure exerted on the bowel by the enlarging uterus, diminished intestinal tone, and decreased physical exercise have all been blamed for this trouble. The use of high-fiber foods, mainly whole-grain breads and cereals, and increased fluids usually helps solve the problem. A high vitamin C (ascorbic acid) intake is advised for tissue building; the fruits and vegetables especially helpful are grapefruit, oranges, lemons, limes, tomatoes, strawberries, cantaloupe, green peppers, and cabbage. Two servings a day of fruits in raw, cooked, or juice forms are recommended. Two portions of vegetables, especially dark green and yellow types, are considered optimum.

Items that contribute little or no nutrient value other than calories for energy are called "empty calorie" foods. Examples of these items are candy, cake, pie, soft drinks, spaghetti, doughnuts, and potato chips. They add pounds but contribute nothing that would assist the pregnant woman or developing fetus except potential heat and energy. Remember, carrying this excessive weight requires more energy, and it is infinitely better to obtain energy plus nutrients with one's food.

Sometimes women during pregnancy experience special cravings for unusual foods or food combinations. Generally these desires are trivial and may be humored if they do not threaten good nutrition. However, there is a type of unusual ingestion called "pica" that is characteristic of, but not confined to, lower socioeconomic ethnic groups. Women exhibiting symptoms of pica may eat rela-

TABLE 5-2   DAILY FOOD PLAN FOR PREGNANCY AND LACTATION

Food	Nonpregnant woman or during first half of pregnancy	Second half of pregnancy	Lactation
Milk, cheese, ice cream, skim or buttermilk (food made with milk can supply part of requirement)	2 cups	3 to 4 cups	4 to 5 cups
Meat (lean meat, fish, poultry, cheese, occasional dried beans or peas)	1 serving (3 to 4 oz)	2 servings (6 to 8 oz); include liver frequently	2½ servings (8 oz)
Eggs	1	1 to 2	1 to 2
Vegetable* (dark green or deep yellow)	1 serving	1 serving	1 to 2 servings
Vitamin C-rich food* Good source—citrus fruit, berries, cantaloupe Fair source—tomatoes, cabbage, greens, potatoes in skin	1 good source or 2 fair sources	1 good source and 1 fair source or 2 good sources	1 good source and 1 fair source or 2 good sources
Other vegetables and fruits	1 serving	2 servings	2 servings
Bread† and cereals (enriched or whole grain)	3 servings	4 to 5 servings	5 servings
Butter or fortified margarine	As desired or needed for calories	As desired or needed for calories	As desired or needed for calories

From Williams, S.R.: Nutrition and diet therapy, ed 4, St. Louis, 1981, The C.V. Mosby Co.
*Use some raw daily.
†One slice of bread equals one serving.

tively large amounts of substances such as laundry starch or river clay. Such ingestions interfere with good nutrition and cause anemia.

Anything that depresses good nutritional intake, whether it be nausea and vomiting, food fads, lack of finances, smoking, alcoholism, or other personal or social problems, should be evaluated and relieved or eliminated to achieve good dietary prenatal care.

The restriction of salt or sodium intake has long been considered by many physicians almost part of the prenatal diet. It has been advocated in an attempt to help prevent and treat the symptoms of preeclampsia-eclampsia (toxemia of pregnancy), a serious complication characterized by edema, hypertension, and albuminuria, possibly leading to convulsions and death. Preeclampsia-eclampsia has

been a major cause of fetal, neonatal, and maternal mortality for many years. Considerable controversy continues regarding its cause, prevention, and treatment. In the last 25 years increasing evidence has shown that the type of toxemia that appears in the last trimester of pregnancy is associated with a poor nutritional (particularly low protein) intake. Some clinicians believe that malnutrition is the long-sought cause of toxemia of late pregnancy. Severe weight gain restriction, enforced weight loss through prescription of extreme, low-caloric diets, limitation of sodium intake to below the "season to taste" standards, and the use of diuretics are increasingly considered to be of no therapeutic benefit and to represent even dangerous attempts at symptomatic prevention and control of this disorder. Such efforts deprive both the mother and fetus of essential nutrition and jeopardize their health and development. (See discussion of preeclampsia-eclampsia, also called pregnancy-induced hypertension, pp. 171 to 176.)

Studies have corroborated the assertion that protein or caloric restriction below that needed physiologically for the growth of the fetus and for preparation of the maternal system in meeting the demands of pregnancy and lactation results in a smaller infant and reduction of maternal nutritional stores. Although not all big babies are healthy babies, low birth weight babies make up a disproportionate percentage of infant mortality. Unless the woman's prenatal and postnatal health is threatened by the known strain exerted on body systems by obesity, weight gain in itself is not detrimental and may represent only real nutritional gain or the usual increase in body fluids associated with normal pregnancy. The problem again seems to center on the quality of food intake. One woman can gain excessive weight eating "empty" calories, contributing very poor nutritional resources to herself and her child. Such a woman is a good candidate for complications such as toxemia, low birth weight, and premature birth. Another woman may also gain more than the norm but have a diet rich in nutrients and not suffer the same complications. Currently an average total weight gain of 10 to 12 kg (22 to 27 pounds) is being suggested in the literature.* Some physicians have found no problems with higher gains if nutritional intake was maintained. Recent studies have also indicated that obese patients should not be placed on a diet to reduce weight during pregnancy nor should their weight gains be limited to less than the weight of the fetus and supporting tissues and fluids. Again, a quality diet is the important key. Weight reduction is recommended only in the interpartum period after lactation to protect the fetus from low birth weight as well as acidosis, which may be associated with maternal starvation and its possible effect on

*Weight gain and pregnancy outcome, Briefs 43(9):141-144, Nov., 1979; Naeye, R.L.: Weight gain and the outcome of pregnancy, Am. J. Obstet. Gynecol. **134**:3-9, Sept. 1, 1979.

the baby's intellectual capacity. Approximate physiologic weight gain in pregnancy has been explained in the following way:

	lb	kg
Fetus	7.5	3.4
Placenta	1.0	.5
Amniotic fluid	2.0	.9
Uterine weight increase	2.5	1.1
Breast tissue	3.0	1.4
Blood volume	4.0	1.8
Maternal stores	4 to 8	1.8 to 3.6
Totals	24 to 28 or	10.9 to 12.7

On the average, 3 to 4 pounds are gained in the first trimester. During the remaining weeks, a weight gain of approximately 1 pound or less a week is considered normal (Fig. 5-3). Any sudden weight gain should be suspected as a sign of developing preeclamptic toxemia.

TERATOGENS

A teratogen is defined as an agent or factor that causes the production of physical defects in the developing embryo or fetus. Table 5-3 lists substances and infections proven to be teratogenic. Other factors must be studied further to be proven conclusively teratogenic. However, the pregnant woman should be cautioned not to utilize medications unless she consults her physician. Over-the-counter medicines, such as nose drops, cold remedies, sleep medications, and diuretics, may cause problems. Certain drugs such as methotrexate and phenytoin are known teratogens. Others may cause hemorrhage, jaundice, neurologic symptoms, and abnormal dental pigmentation. Drugs such as heroin and methadone taken during pregnancy may produce addiction in the newborn. The effects that all substances prescribed to treat illness will have on the fetus have not been determined. Then, too, effects of drugs taken during pregnancy may not become obvious in the child until years later (for example, the incidence of vaginal malignancy in young girls or sperm changes causing infertility in men whose mothers had received diethylstilbestrol in early pregnancy to help prevent their miscar-

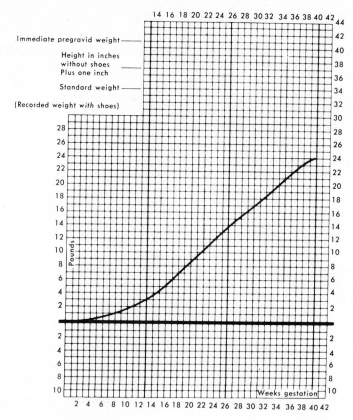

FIG. 5-3 Prenatal gain in weight.

From Maternal nutrition and course of pregnancy, ISBN 0-309-01761-0, Washington, D.C., 1971, Food and Nutrition Board, National Academy of Sciences–National Research Council.

riage). Teratogenic effects take place especially at the beginning of a pregnancy before a woman is certain she is pregnant. The stage of development determines the vulnerability of the embryo or fetus.

Smoking, alcohol, and other drugs. Smoking tobacco decreases the oxygen supply to the unborn fetus by displacing oxygen with variable quantities of carbon monoxide and decreasing intrauterine blood flow. Mothers who smoke frequently (more than 10 cigarettes a day) bear smaller infants than do nonsmoking women. In some studies late fetal and newborn mortality for infants born to cigarette smokers was significantly higher than for those

born to nonsmokers. Utilization of vitamins and minerals and transport of amino acids is compromised in smoking mothers.

It is interesting to note that the smaller babies of women who smoke grow faster during the 6 months after birth than do infants of nonsmokers. This is interpreted as a response to the removal of the infant from an "inhibiting and toxic" influence in utero.* However, evidence also indicates that a

---

*McKay, S.R.: Smoking during the childbearing year, Am. J. Mat. Child Nurs., **5:**46-50, Jan.-Feb. 1980; Diebel, P.: Effects of cigarette smoking on maternal nutrition and the fetus, JOGN Nurs. **9:**333-336, Nov.-Dec. 1980.

TABLE 5-3 POTENTIAL HUMAN TERATOGENIC FACTORS

Substances
    Alcohol
    Aminopterin
    Tobacco smoke
    Diethylstilbestrol
    Dilantin
    Heroin
    Lithium
    Methadone
    Methyl mercury
    Tetracycline
    Thalidomide
    Trimethadione
    Warfarin (Coumadin)

Infections
    Coxsackie B
    Cytomegalovirus (CMV)
    Herpes simplex
    Rubella
    Syphilis
    Toxoplasmosis
    Varicella

Other
    Hyperthermia
    Maternal disease (as diabetes)
    Maternal malnutrition

Adapted from Jones, K.L.: Teratogens: what we know and don't know about them—genetic issues in pediatrics and obstetrical practice, Chicago, 1981, Year Book Medical Publishers, Inc., p. 117.

relationship exists between mothers who smoke excessively at home and the incidence of pneumonia and bronchitis in their babies from 6 to 9 months of age. Of course, from the perspective of general maternal health, smoking is an important factor in respiratory and circulatory disease processes. Pregnant women should be encouraged to decrease or stop the habit.

Intrauterine exposure to alcohol is an important teratogen. Babies born with sufficient intrauterine exposure to alcohol often demonstrate fetal alcohol syndrome (FAS). Chronic, excessive use of alcohol has been identified as a significant cause of fetal growth retardation, impaired intellect, and congenital malformation, particularly microcephaly and facial abnormalities. Both the amount and timing of the alcohol consumption by the mother, as well as her own physical condition, appear to be important. No minimum safe levels of alcohol during pregnancy have been determined. Some pregnant women may need specific suggestions on how to decrease or eliminate their alcohol intake.

The use of methylxanthines (such as caffeine and theobromine found in coffee, tea, chocolate, and colas) by the prospective mother has been questioned. The FDA stated that conclusions about teratogenic effects of the xanthines cannot be made.* However, at normal dosage (less than 600 mg/day), teratogenic effects have not been demonstrated. The pregnant woman should be counseled to limit consumption of foods and drinks containing xanthines. A cup of coffee has 75-155 mg of caffeine (up to 330 mg has been reported). Caffeine does cross the placenta. Research needs to be done on effects of xanthines taken during pregnancy, which may affect the child after birth.†

Bendectin, which is used to combat "morning sickness," has been studied several times; no teratogenic relationship has been demonstrated.

Viruses and parasites. The fetus is particularly vulnerable to viral infections during the early weeks of development. The newborn also may be at special risk. Pregnant women should not knowingly expose themselves unnecessarily to any viral disease to which they have not proved immunity, for example, rubella (German measles), or to cytomegalovirus (CMV) or the herpesvirus. While CMV can have teratogenic effects, it is usually more significant in the neonate as a congenital infection. Another infection—herpes simplex—may also cause fetal damage and/or serious disease

---

*Stephens, C.L.: The fetal alcohol syndrome: cause for concern, Am. J. Mat. Child Nurs., 6:251-256, July-Aug. 1981; National Institute on Alcohol Abuse and Alcoholism: Alcohol and your unborn baby, DHEW Publication No. (ADM) 78-521, 1978, U.S. Government Printing Office.
†Luke, B.: Does caffeine affect reproduction? Am. J. Mat. Child Nurs. 7:240-244, July-Aug. 1982.

in the newborn. This infection is most often contracted at the time of a vaginal delivery. A pregnant woman with diagnosed genital herpesvirus should be delivered by cesarean birth in an effort to avoid contamination of her infant (see p. 165). Influenza is thought by some to be teratogenic in the first few weeks of pregnancy. Another potential danger to the unborn infant is a parasitic disease called toxoplasmosis, transmitted to the pregnant woman chiefly by cat feces. An expectant mother should not handle Tabby's litter box! In addition, she needs to be reminded to wash her hands carefully after handling raw meat, to cook meat well, to wash fruits and vegetables before eating them, and to wear gloves while gardening.

Other items that may cause teratogenic effects in the fetus include environmental pollutants, lead, and excessive use of vitamins A, D, and K. Increase in maternal age is said to be correlated with fetal deformities.

While diagnostic x-ray films should not be taken unless necessary, no conclusive evidence indicates that the levels of exposure associated with these x-rays cause fetal injury. The effects of these x-rays on the life of the child after birth are questionable. Lead aprons and shields should be used when possible.

GENERAL HYGIENE

Good prenatal guidance involves more than the questions of diet, smoking, drugs, and exposure to disease. The pregnant woman will undoubtedly have questions regarding many other subjects. Sometimes she wants information regarding general hygiene—the need for rest, relaxation, and exercise. Pregnant women need to conserve their resources by getting adequate rest. They may not want actually to nap in the morning and afternoon, but at least they can sit down and put their feet up. Because the bulk of the fetus in later pregnancy may compress the inferior vena cava and crowd the diaphragm, resting in a flat supine position may interfere with venous blood return to the heart and placental circulation as well as embarrass respirations. At such a stage in pregnancy, a side-lying position is frequently advised. Walking outdoors is wonderful exercise. Golfing, bowling, dancing, and swimming, when not done to the point of fatigue, are usually endorsed.

More research regarding the effects of exercise during pregnancy is needed. What sports are an asset will probably depend on the health, exercise habits, and obstetric history of the individual. Some exercise is to be encouraged for the normal expectant mother. Curtailing the exercise of a previously active woman may be a negative factor in her physical, emotional, and mental health. Horseback riding and competitive tennis, especially singles, have been generally not recommended for the usual pregnant woman until after her postpartum checkup.

Bathing. A woman is likely to perspire profusely during pregnancy, and frequent baths and showers are needed. Bathing may become a problem in late pregnancy because of the woman's awkwardness, and great care must be taken that she does not fall. Some physicians recommend that tub baths not be taken late in pregnancy and that only sponge baths be used because of the risk of falls. The possibility of infecting the vaginal tract and uterus was another consideration, but most now consider this highly unlikely.

Hair may need special attention because of the increased activity of the oil glands of the scalp. A permanent, if desired, will "take" during pregnancy.

Preparation for nursing. If the woman is planning to nurse her baby, the physician may advise certain routines to prepare her breasts for lactation and identify community groups such as La Leche League who can help breastfeeding mothers. If she has inverted or flat nipples, the physician may prescribe the use of a manual breast pump, teach finger compression of the breast or nipple rolling, or recommend the use of Woolwich plastic breast shields, which are worn for varying intervals inside the bra, to draw out the nipple to make it easier for the newborn infant to grasp. The expression of colostrum, the early breast secretion, may be recommended in the last trimester of pregnancy to encourage milk production, try to prevent engorgement, and toughen the nipples. Advice differs.*

Some pregnant women, especially primigravidas, develop rather prominent pink marks called striae on the abdomen and breasts, probably related to hormonal increases as well as rapid weight gain. Some people think that they are not so prominent if cocoa butter is applied to the skin. Certainly it does not hurt to use it if one does not object to the odor. These lines usually retract appreciably after pregnancy and become less noticeable.

Wardrobe. Never before have expectant mothers had an opportunity for such an attractive, versatile wardrobe as they have today. Since maternity patterns are also available in the fabric stores, attractive clothing need not be expensive. Maternity clothes should be lightweight, nonconstrictive, adjustable, and absorbent and should also provide a boost to the morale.

It is especially important that the pregnant woman have good breast support to prevent fatigue and maintain a good figure. She will not be able to go through her entire pregnancy with the same size brassiere! If she plans to breast-feed her baby, nursing bras are a fine investment. A maternity corset is usually not advised. The tendency in the last few years is to counsel its use only for older multiparas if needed. Primigravidas and younger multiparas are usually told to practice certain exercises during pregnancy (especially the "pelvic rock, or tilt") that will improve posture and strengthen muscles. However, a light maternity girdle may be used with satisfaction. Specially designed garter belts are available. No constrictive round garters should be used because of interference in the blood's circulation from the legs.

If a woman has been accustomed to wearing high-heeled shoes, it will probably be difficult for her to descend suddenly to fairly flat heels. However, as pregnancy progresses and her center of gravity moves forward, she will find lower heels much less awkward and more flattering to her total silhouette. She will want to avoid shoe styles with ties or buckles; toward the end of her 260 plus days of waiting, tying shoes will not be easy.

Dental care. The old saying "for every child a tooth" is not true. But it is a good plan for the pregnant woman to have a dental checkup during the second trimester so that plenty of time is available for any needed repairs. The gums may become swollen and exhibit a tendency to bleed in pregnancy. These symptoms are probably caused by the increase in estrogen in the body and are not necessarily related to a vitamin C deficiency. Symptoms typically recede after the eighth month. The presence of gingivitis previous to pregnancy fostered by plaque formation and malocclusion may cause the condition to become a continuing problem without care. Some women experience an annoying increase in salivation (ptyalism) in pregnancy.

Douching. Some women wonder whether they should douche or not. Normal vaginal secretions are usually intensified during pregnancy. Some physicians believe that douching should be done only for a specific condition with a low-pressure fountain syringe, gently introduced. Others do not recommend the practice at all.* The possible introduction of infection or incidence of air embolism is a real concern (p. 159).

Employment. Many pregnant women are employed. Whether they continue their employment and for how long depends on several factors, one of which is the type of work in which they are engaged (heavy lifting, exposure to potential hazards of radiation or chemicals, or long hours of standing without relief). The employment of pregnant women in certain occupations is often restricted by state law, policies of the individual employer (dependent on insurance coverage, previous experience, etc.),

---

*Whitley, N.: Preparation for breast feeding: a one year follow-up of 34 nursing mothers, JOGN Nurs. **7**:44-48, May-June 1978; Atkinson, L.D.: Prenatal nipple conditioning for breast feeding, Nurs. Res. **28**:267-271, Sept.-Oct. 1979.

*Kuczynski, H.J.: Pros and cons of douching, JOGN Nurs. **9**:90-93, Mar.-Apr. 1980; Pritchard, J.A., and Macdonald, P.C.: Williams obstetrics, ed. 16, New York, 1980, Appleton-Century-Crofts, p. 319.

and the health of the employee (whether she is experiencing any complications).

Recently women have been challenging disability benefit regulations and pregnancy leave rulings that require a working, expectant mother to resign her position because she has reached a certain month in her pregnancy. Numerous changes in policy affecting the working pregnant woman are probably to be seen in the future.

Travel. Sometimes pregnant women ask whether they should restrict travel. If a trip can be so arranged, it is best to travel during the middle trimester, since the pregnant woman is more comfortable, the danger of abortion is not so great, and the threat of premature or unprepared-for births is at a minimum. If trips must be made by car, schedules should allow for adequate rest stops and should be carefully paced. Commercial airline travel in pressurized planes is now considered as safe as other methods of transportation for this traveler. However, last-minute protracted journeys close to term are to be discouraged no matter how they are made.

Sexual relations. Instructions regarding sexual intercourse during pregnancy are now much more liberal than formerly. Many physicians are now allowing most couples to have sexual intercourse until full term is reached, unless the bag of waters has ruptured or discomfort is encountered. Others, believing that orgasm may initiate painful uterine contractions or premature labor, still take a more conventional approach and would limit sexual response in the last few weeks before term. If there has been a previous problem with abortion, premature birth, or bleeding during pregnancy, additional modifications in sexual life would probably be advised. Most couples find such privations stressful and may need counseling regarding alternate modes of mutual sexual gratification and other adjustments that would be helpful.

COMMUNITY EDUCATION RESOURCES

In many communities classes are offered to help expectant parents prepare for the changes pregnancy and parenthood will bring. They may be sponsored by the local childbirth education association, American National Red Cross, YWCA, public health departments, adult education programs, postpartum support groups, hospitals, or groups of physicians. Participation in such approved groups is recommended, especially for primigravidas. Some classes concentrate on imparting an understanding of the basic anatomy and physiology of reproduction, what to expect during the "waiting months," what occurs during labor and birth, how to prepare the baby's nursery and layette, how to bathe the newborn infant, techniques of breast feeding, and how to prepare an artificial formula. Others emphasize exercises in training the body and mind for peak performance during pregnancy, labor, and childbirth and are usually led by a physical therapist or nurse specializing in childbirth education (Fig. 5-4). Preparation for childbirth involving techniques such as those advocated with Lamaze or other methods of instruction may be intensive. Attendance of the expectant parents at a series of classes with assigned practice sessions is strongly recommended. Information and exercises to promote good posture, strengthen key muscles, enhance relaxation, and lessen fear and discomfort during the birth experience are emphasized. (See also pp. 153 to 155.) In our opinion they are helpful to the expectant parents no matter what their preference may be regarding the use of analgesics, anesthetics, or birth procedures.

Such informal group sessions with other couples facing similar experiences, expectations, hopes, and fears guided by competent leaders are especially helpful in assisting new prospective fathers and mothers to gain needed instruction and self-esteem for their changing roles.

Pregnancy and new parenthood are developmental crises for the man as well as the woman, and new self-identities must be clarified and accepted. The crises may be changed or lessened when parenthood is repeated, but the sense of wonder, the expectations, and the strains recur. Adjustments are still to be made whether the child is the first or fourth. The processes of role identification are more obvious perhaps in this culture for the pro-

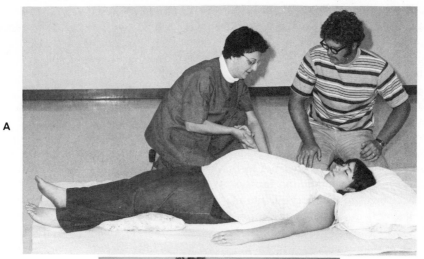

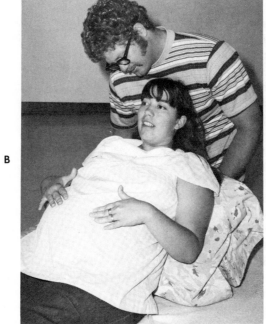

FIG. 5-4   **A,** The childbirth education instructor teaches the father to check for muscular relaxation. **B,** Relaxation and breathing techniques such as "pant-blow" and effleurage (light massage) must be practiced regularly.

spective mother. Indeed, the increasingly manifest changes in her body dramatically declare a changed status in society. Psychologists who are describing the focal changes during a normal woman's pregnancy usually speak of her emotional preoccupation with self, an introversion that occurs and predominates her thinking in early pregnancy. At this time the growing fetus is part of her and is yet to assume a real identity of its own. Consciously—or most often subconsciously—she sorts through her feelings concerning motherhood and her early experiences with her own mother. As the pregnancy continues and her body image changes, her feelings of dependency typically grow and her focus of attention generally changes to that of the father of the child as he represents protection and continuity. Later, in the third trimester, her interest is centered on preparations for the baby, who by this time has become an unknown but acknowledged individual, and on her feelings and expectations concerning labor, birth, and her ability to cope at that time with the demands of her body, her family, and society.

Pregnancy is normally characterized by feelings of ambivalence. One day the mother-to-be may be pleased and proud concerning her condition. The next day she will be fretful and even resentful regarding the disturbance in her life that the coming baby represents. Prospective mothers and fathers need to know that these contradictory feelings are normal. Men need especially to be alerted regarding the sudden mood swings and fantasies that may trouble their mates' emotional and mental equilibrium. Such knowledge will help smooth the many difficult adaptations that need to be made. Pregnancy is a developmental crisis, but it is also an opportunity for real emotional and psychological growth. Having peers and knowledgeable professional people with whom to share some of the experiences of this process is a tremendous asset.

THE LAYETTE

Provided finances are not too strained, preparing the layette for the new baby can be one of the most pleasurable duties of the expectant parents. For first-timers, baby showers may also help in this regard but are not dependable. Contributors at such affairs should be told that the baby will grow, and perhaps half the group could purchase basic clothes for the 1- to 2-year-old child. If the baby is not a "firstborn," infant clothes will probably be left over from the last time. Babies usually do not wear out their clothes, but they do grow out of them quickly.

A basic layette, at least enough to start with, consists of the following items:

1. Six cotton shirts, short or long sleeves, depending on the weather (Stretch shirts cost more but can be worn by the baby longer. Long-sleeved shirts can have a fold-over cuff enclosing the hands. To purchase a 3-month size is a waste of money.)
2. Four dozen cotton gauze, bird's-eye, or flannelette diapers if diaper service is not used; 1 dozen, if it is; or disposable diapers
3. Two or three plastic diaper covers, to be used only if the baby does not have any skin irritation
4. Four or five long gowns, opening down the front with grip fasteners
5. Two or three sweaters with no more than 10% wool content to prevent allergic skin rash
6. Three or four soft, light receiving blankets
7. One square, heavy blanket for use outdoors
8. One cap
9. Booties if it is cold
10. One bunting if in a climate requiring such protection. (The tendency is to overdress rather than underdress infants.)
11. Two or three waterproof squares for protecting surfaces from the baby's urine
12. Two washcloths, just for the baby
13. Six cotton sheets; two crib blankets

Basic furniture includes a bed (a bassinet, although pretty, is unnecessary), a firm mattress, and cover. No pillow should be used because of the danger of suffocation. Some type of chest of drawers for storage, a covered diaper pail, and a large plastic tub or, if preferred, a canvas bathinette (this, too, is a frill) will be needed. A bath tray is a great convenience, but it does not have to be expensive. Any clean tray will do. On it should be a jar of cotton balls, a jar of safety pins, a mild soap and dish, a supply of baby oil or lotion, a box of paper tissues, and perhaps baby powder.

Even if the baby is to be nursed, there should be equipment in the home for preparing artificial feedings, or for storing and feeding breast milk when the mother is away. Approved baby car seats are a necessity, and portable infant seats or baby carriers worn by the infant's caretaker can be helpful (p. 381). Do not forget that mothers can often borrow needed items.

There are many things on the market for babies, but many of those cute eye-catching gadgets and extras require money better spent elsewhere.

WHAT TO TAKE TO THE HOSPITAL

There are other things the mother should have ready before that special date comes due. She should consider what she will take to the hospital with her. Usually, the following list suffices:

Recommended articles to assist with Lamaze-type labor techniques (extra pillows, Chap-Stick, focal point, etc.)

Two nightgowns (the short type)

Robe, slippers

Two brassieres (nursing-type if breast feeding), one sanitary belt

Toothbrush, dentifrice, brush, comb, cosmetics

Deodorant, shower cap

Writing materials, stamps, birth announcements, checkbook or cash for deposit at hospital, insurance identification if applicable, and a good book

Cross-cultural components influencing maternity care

When caring for a pregnant woman from another culture or ethnic group, the nurse must understand the variations in this mother's attitudes and behaviors that may result from cultural influences. Perceptions of health and illness are culturally derived. Culture definitely influences her reactions and behaviors concerning pregnancy. The care given should fit in with the prospective mother's cultural life style when possible. Failure in maternity care may result from not taking into account the patient's customs and belief system. The concepts of transcultural nursing need to be applied to the planned care. For example, nutritional guidance must consider food practices and the symbolic significance of food. In some cultures certain foods are not to be eaten (taboo) during pregnancy. Certain groups do not assign any active role to the father regarding prenatal care or labor and delivery.

While individuals must not be stereotyped, it is helpful to look even briefly at a few of the ethnic groups the nurse may encounter. However, practices and views associated with childbearing will also vary with the individual. Discussing cultural influences with the mother herself will help the nurse better plan for her special needs.

Black cultural practices. Many black families from lower socioeconomic groups are headed by women. Other relatives may form an extended family; grandmothers may be responsible for raising the children. Nurses teaching child care should find out who is going to give the care. The cultural patterns of blacks in the middle and upper socioeconomic groups may more closely resemble the patterns of the majority of members of these groups.

Black Muslim women often follow meat-restricted diets. Their prenatal nutrition, as well as that of the breast-feeding mother, should be examined. They characteristically wear long garments and cover their hair.

Hispanic cultural practices. This is the largest ethnic group in the United States. They have come from many different Spanish-speaking regions of the world. Some of these families have also adopted the middle-American culture, while others have retained the concepts and life styles of their Hispanic heritages. Again, extended families are very common and important. The advice given by a family member may be accepted by the mother in preference to that given by a member of the health team. The "hot-cold theory" of disease and health may influence the mother's diet and compliance. Certain foods are considered hot or cold, though these concepts may have no relationship to their actual temperatures. A balance of certain foods based on this classification may be sought. Since pregnancy is viewed as normal, going to the physician may be delayed. This group is characterized by male-dominant relationships. Large families are often desired.

Asiatic cultural practices. Asian families in the United States currently represent particularly diverse cultures and socioeconomic levels. The extended family is dominant. While some taboos govern food and activity during pregnancy, pregnancy is seen as a normal, healthy process in which family members should have the major role. When caring for patients from the Asian culture, nurses should particularly protect the modesty of the patient. Male participation in the direct care of the mother is usually minimal, but does not represent a noncaring attitude. The concepts of *yin* and *yang* (in some ways similar to the hot-cold theory of disease and health) and the need to balance these contrary forces in an individual's life can affect diet, hygiene, and activity, particularly in the postpartum period.

Arab cultural practices. Arab families feel strong family unity among extended family members and rely on them for help before going outside the family. The experience of pregnancy and birth is usually seen as an exclusively female affair. Having children, especially sons, is the important function of women. Arab women feel a special need for modesty. Often families from the Arab culture are oriented to the present; planning ahead for the care of the coming baby is not part of the culture. This should not be viewed as showing less concern for the baby, but as an aspect of the culture perhaps prompted by ancient high infant mortality rates. This emphasis on the present rather than the future should also be remembered if contraception is to be taught. Including other adult family members in health teaching is helpful. Having both the husband and wife together during such discussions may increase compliance.

Perhaps socioeconomic constraints have as big a place in the outcome of the pregnancy as do the cultural and ethnic variations, because nutrition plays such a vital role in the pregnancy and is affected so greatly by socioeconomic factors.

PERSPECTIVE

The period of pregnancy is a creative, productive period in a woman's life from many points of view. It should be a happy, truly expectant interval. But how a woman reacts to the challenge of pregnancy will be, in the main, determined by her basic emotional maturity or lack of it. The physician, the nurses, the clergy, and members of the community health agencies have an opportunity to help a pregnant woman and her partner mature in the understanding of themselves and their role in life at this crucial time. If these care-givers help the expectant parents, they are also helping the generation to come.

UNIT 2

SUGGESTED SELECTED READINGS AND REFERENCES

GENERAL

Antle, K.: Psychologic involvement in pregnancy by expectant fathers, JOGN Nurs. 4:40-42, July-Aug. 1975.

Bash, D.B., and Gold, W.A.: The nurse and the childbearing family, New York, 1981, John Wiley & Sons.

Butnarescu, G.F., et al: Perinatal nursing, vol. 2: reproductive risk, New York, 1980, John Wiley & Sons.

Carter-Jessop, L.: Promoting maternal attachment through prenatal intervention, Am. J. Mat. Child Nurs. 6:107-112, Mar.-Apr. 1981.

Colman, A.D., and Colman, L.L.: Pregnancy: the psychological experience, New York, 1971, Herder & Herder, Inc.

Colman, A.D., and Colman, L.L.: Pregnancy as an altered state of consciousness, Birth Fam. J. 1:7-11, Winter 1973-74.

Dodendorf, D.M.: Expectant fatherhood and first pregnancy, J. Fam. Pract. 13:744,751, Oct. 1981.

Ellis, D.J.: Sexual needs and concerns of expectant parents, JOGN Nurs. 9:306-308, Sept.-Oct. 1980.

Friederich, M.A.: Psychological changes during pregnancy, Contemp. OB/GYN 9:27-34, June 1977.

Greenhalf, J.O.: Constipation during pregnancy, Contemp. OB/GYN 2:29-31, Aug. 1973.

Hogan, L.R.: Pregnant again—at 41, Am. J. Mat. Child Nurs. 4:174-176, May-June 1979.

Lamb, G.S., and Lipkin, M.: Somatic symptoms of expectant fathers, Am. J. Mat. Child Nurs. 7:110-115, Mar.-Apr. 1982.

Marquart, R.K.: Expectant fathers: what are their needs?, Am. J. Mat. Child Nurs. 1:32-36, Jan.-Feb. 1976.

Moore, M.L.: Realities in childbearing, Philadelphia, 1978, W.B. Saunders Co.

Oakley, G.P., et al: Prenatal diagnosis, Ped. Ann. 10:(entire issue), Feb. 1981.

Queenan, J.T.: The role of ultrasound in high-risk obstetrics, Contemp. OB/GYN 18:44-80, Nov. 1980.

Ryan, G.M.: Prenatal care and pregnancy outcome, Am. J. Obstet. Gynecol. 137(8):876-881, Aug. 1980.

Saxena, B.B.: New methods of pregnancy testing in adolescent girls, Pediatr. Clin. North Am. 28:437-453, May 1981.

Sherwen, L.N.: Fantasies during the third trimester of pregnancy, Am. J. Mat. Child Nurs. 6:398-401, Nov.-Dec. 1981.

Sweet, J.B.: Pregnancy associated dental problems, Contemp. OB/GYN 16:33-38, Aug. 1980.

Williamson, P., and English, E.C.: Stress and coping in first pregnancy: couple-family physician interaction, J. Fam. Pract. 13:629-635, Oct. 1981.

Wanson, J.: The marital sexual relationship during pregnancy, JOGN Nurs. 9:267-270, Sept.-Oct. 1980.

EMBRYOLOGY

Arey, L.: Developmental anatomy, Philadelphia, 1965, W.B. Saunders Co.

Dickinson-Belskie: Birth atlas, ed. 5, New York, 1968, Maternity Center Assoc.

Moore, K.: The developing human: clinically oriented embryology, ed. 2, Philadelphia, 1977, W.B. Saunders Co.

NUTRITION

Kitay, D.F.: Folic acid deficiency, Contemp. OB/GYN 10:30-36, July 1977.

Lemasters, G.K.: Zinc insufficiency during pregnancy: a review, JOGN Nurs. 10:124-125, Mar.-Apr. 1981.

Luke, B.: Lactose intolerance during pregnancy, Am. J. Mat. Child Nurs. 2:92-96, Mar.-Apr. 1977.

Luke, B.: Understanding pica in pregnant women, Am. J. Mat. Child Nurs. 2:97-100, Mar.-Apr. 1977.

Rosso, P.: Prenatal nutrition and fetal growth development, Ped. Ann. 10:21-29,32, Nov. 1981.

Weathersbee, P.S., et al: Weight gain and pregnancy outcome, Briefs 43(9):141-144, Nov. 1979.

Worthington, B.S.: Nutrition during pregnancy, lactation and oral contraception, Nurs. Clin. North Am. 14:269-283, June 1979.

Worthington-Roberts, B.S., Yermeersch, J., and Williams, S.R.: Nutrition in pregnancy and lactation, ed. 2, St. Louis, 1981, The C.V. Mosby Co.

CULTURAL DIFFERENCES

DeGracia, R.T.: Filipino cultural influences, Am. J. Nurs, **79**:1412-1414, Aug. 1979.

Grosso, C., et al: The Vietnamese American family—and grandma makes three, Am. J. Mat. Child Nurs. **6**:177-180, May-June 1981.

Hollingsworth, A.O., Brown, L.P., and Brooten, D.A.: The refugees and childbearing: what to expect, RN **43**:44-48, Nov. 1980.

Johnson, M.: Cultural variations in professional and parenting patterns, JOGN Nurs. **9**:9-13, Jan.-Feb. 1980.

Meleis, A.I.: The Arab American in the health care system, Am. J. Nurs. **81**:1180-1183, June 1981.

Meleis, A.I., and Sorrell, L.: Arab American women and their birth experiences, Am. J. Mat. Child Nurs. **6**:171-176, May-June 1981.

Santopietro, M.S.: How to get through to a refugee patient, RN **44**:42-48, Jan. 1981.

Santopietro, M.S., and Lynch, B.: What's behind the "inscrutable" mask? RN **43**:54-62, Oct. 1980.

EDUCATION FOR CHILDBIRTH

Bing, E.D.: Six practical lessons for an easier childbirth, New York, 1967, Grosset & Dunlap, Inc.

Bonovich, L.: Participation: the key to learning for patients in antepartal clinics, JOGN Nurs. **10**:75-79, Mar.-Apr. 1981.

De La Fleur, T.P., and Payne, J.P.: Role playing in childbirth education classes, Am. J. Mat. Child Nurs. **6**:333-336, Sept.-Oct. 1981.

Dore, S.L., and Davies, B.L.: Catharsis for high-risk antenatal inpatients, Am. J. Mat. Child Nurs. **4**:96-97, Mar.-Apr. 1979.

Dzurec, L.C.: Childbirth educators: are they helpful? Am. J. Mat. Child Nurs. **6**:329-332, Sept.-Oct. 1981.

Ewy, D., and Ewy, R.: Preparation for childbirth, New York, 1972, The New American Library, Inc.

Genest, M.: Preparation for childbirth—evidence for efficacy: a review, JOGN Nurs. **10**:82-85, Mar.-Apr. 1981.

Jimenez, S.L.M.: Education for the childbearing years: comprehensive application of psychoprophylaxis, JOGN Nurs. **9**:97-99, Mar.-Apr. 1980.

Lamaze, F.: Painless childbirth: the Lamaze method, New York, 1972, Pocket Books.

Pridham, K.F., and Schutz, M.E.: Preparation of parents for birthing and infant care, J. Fam. Pract. **13**:181-188, Aug. 1981.

TERATOGENS

Bibbo, M., and Gill, W.B.: Screening of adolescents exposed to diethylstilbestrol in utero, Pediatr. Clin. North Am. **28**:379-388, May 1981.

Burgess, H.A.: When a patient on lithium is pregnant, Am. J. Nurs. **79**:1989-1990, Nov. 1979.

Chernoff, G.F., and Jones, K.L.: Fetal preventive medicine: teratogens and the unborn baby, Ped. Ann. **10**:14-27, June 1981.

Deibel, P.: Effects of cigarette smoking on maternal nutrition and the fetus, JOGN Nurs. **9**:333-336, Nov.-Dec. 1980.

Jones, K.L.: Teratogens: what we know and don't know about them—genetic issues in pediatric and obstetrical practices, Chicago, 1981, Year Book Medical Publishers, Inc.

McKay, S.R.: Smoking during the childbearing year, Am. J. Mat. Child Nurs. **5**:46-50, Jan.-Feb. 1980.

Moore, M.L.: More on smoking and birth weight, Briefs **35**(3):38-39, Mar. 1981.

Soyka, L.: Caffeine ingestion during pregnancy: in utero exposure and possible effects, Semin. Perinat. **5**(4):305-308, Oct. 1981.

Stephens, C.J.: The fetal alcohol syndrome: cause for concern, Am. J. Mat. Child Nurs. **6**:251-256, July-Aug. 1981.

Tull, M.W., and Brown, A.L.: Effects of caffeine on pregnancy and lactation, Pediatr. Nurs. **7**(2):51-52, Mar.-Apr. 1981.

INFECTIONS

Amstey, M.S.: Managing herpes in pregnant patients, Contemp. OB/GYN **16**:87-92, Aug. 1980.

Bettoli, E.J.: Herpes: facts and fallacies, Am. J. Nurs. **82**:924-929, June 1982.

Boehm, F.H., and Estes, W.: Genital herpes simplex during pregnancy, Perinatology/Neonatology **6**(1):21-24, Jan.-Feb. 1980.

Felman, Y.M.: Sexually transmitted disease in women: an agenda for action, J. Fam. Pract. **13**:289-290, Aug. 1981.

Mocarski, V.: Asymptomatic bacteriuria: a "silent" problem of pregnant women, Am. J. Mat. Child Nurs. **5**:238-241, July-Aug. 1980.

Olds, S.B., et al: Preventing congenital toxoplasmosis, Briefs **35**(1):12-14, Jan. 1981.

Test yourself: nongonococcal urethritis and related chlamydial infections, Am. J. Nurs. **80**:1097, June 1980.

Wilbanks, G., and Chez, R.: How to diagnose and treat genital herpes, Contemp. OB/GYN **16**:81-85, Aug. 1980.

UNIT **3**

PARTURITION

CHAPTER **6**   Presentations, positions,

and progress

The relationship of the fetus to the obstetric passageway is of great interest to both physician and nurse. It will usually influence the length of labor, preparation of the delivery room, and type of complications possibly encountered.

TERMINOLOGY

Some common words are used in special ways to describe this relationship. For instance, in obstetrics one often refers to the following terms: lie, presentation, attitude, position, station, engagement, effacement, and show.

Lie and presentation

The *lie* of an infant means the relationship of the long axis of the fetus to the long axis of the uterus. If the length of the fetus is parallel to the length of the uterus, the lie may be called "longitudinal." If, instead, the body lies crosswise in the uterus, the term "transverse lie" may be used.

Many times the term *presentation* is used synonymously with the phrase *presenting part*—that part of the baby which is coming through or attempting to come through the pelvic canal first. Headfirst placement is referred to as a cephalic presentation. Feet or buttocks first is termed breech. Approximately 96% of all births are headfirst, or cephalic; about 3.5% are breech. Trans-verse presentations account for the remaining percentage. Presentation may be determined by abdominal palpation and rectal, vaginal, ultrasonic, or x-ray examinations. Today, because of the increased safety of abdominal, or cesarean, birth, few attempts are made to turn a fetus through external or internal manipulation (version) to a cephalic presentation.

Attitude

The *attitude* refers to the degree of flexion of the body, head (Fig. 6-1), and extremities. The normal attitude is complete flexion. A well-flexed head presents the smallest cephalic diameter and fewer mechanical problems in descent and delivery. This "chin-on-chest" posture makes possible the *vertex* delivery so desired.

Position (Figs. 6-2 to 6-5)

The *position* technically is the relationship between a predetermined point of reference or direction on the presenting part of the fetus to the pelvic quadrants *of the mother*. It gives more detailed information about the fetus's progress as the presenting part seeks to adapt to the shape and size of the various parts of the birth canal. The maternal pelvic quadrants are identified as right and left posterior and right and left anterior (Fig.

Complete flexion   Moderate flexion   Poor flexion
(extension)

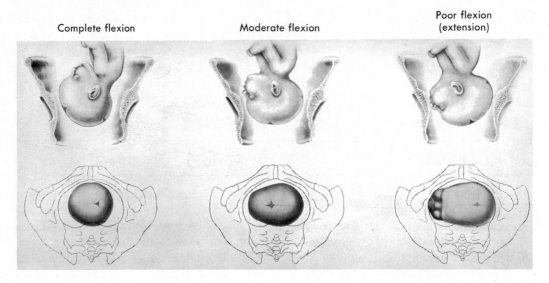

FIG. 6-1   Head diameters in various degrees of flexion.

From Phenomena of normal labor, Columbus, Ohio, 1964, Ross Laboratories.

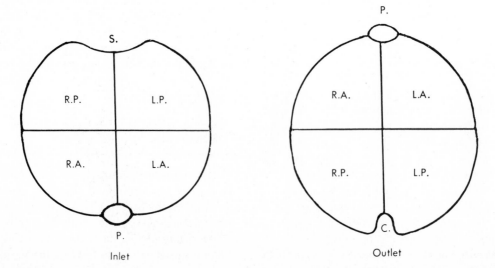

Inlet   Outlet

FIG. 6-2   Maternal pelvic quadrants stay the same; however, the student's perspective may change! *C*, Coccyx; *P*, pubic bone; *S*, sacrum.

6-2). They never change location, although the different perspectives from which they are viewed in illustrations and diagrams can confuse the student. Sometimes the quadrants are seen from "below," that is, as they appear to the physician in front of the delivery table ready to receive the baby. Sometimes they are viewed from "above," from the vantage point of the unborn child entering the true pelvis. In some other diagrams, students miraculously look directly through the abdominal wall to view the fetus within the canal. The point of reference, of course, will vary according to the presenting part discussed and the amount of flexion present. In the event of a well-flexed cephalic or vertex presentation the point of reference employed is the occipital bone, or occiput. It is the most accessible bone to identify in rectal or vaginal examination. The vault of the fetal skull is made up of three paired bones and one single bone separat-

ed by tough but softer membranous seams, or sutures. It is fairly easy to follow these sutures with a gloved finger after sufficient cervical dilation has occurred and to determine the placement of the occiput. The sutures trace a Y, and the occiput is found between the top shafts of the Y just in back of the triangular posterior fontanel (Fig. 6-3).

To simplify reference to the various positions possible, the descriptive phrase usually begins with either right or left (of the mother's pelvis), followed by the point of reference used (on the infant) and the adjectives anterior, posterior, or transverse (referring again to the part of the mother's pelvis toward which a particular point on the baby is directed). Thus one refers to the most common vertex position as "left occiput anterior" or, shortcutting further, L.O.A. Each presenting part has the possibility of eight positions following the same pattern. Only the middle initial or code let-

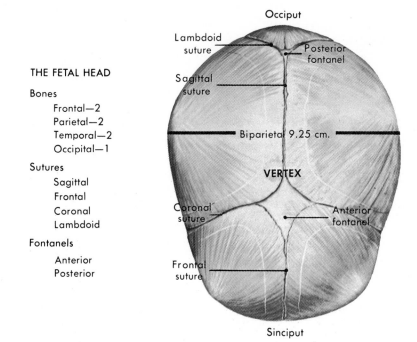

THE FETAL HEAD

Bones
    Frontal—2
    Parietal—2
    Temporal—2
    Occipital—1

Sutures
    Sagittal
    Frontal
    Coronal
    Lambdoid

Fontanels
    Anterior
    Posterior

FIG. 6-3   Fetal head—physician's map.

From Phenomena of normal labor, Columbus, Ohio, 1964, Ross Laboratories.

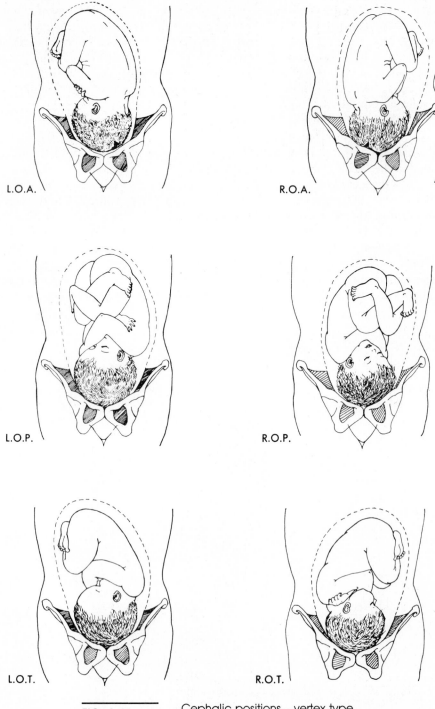

FIG. 6-4   Cephalic positions—vertex type.

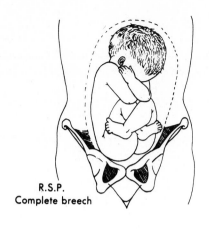

R.S.P.
Complete breech

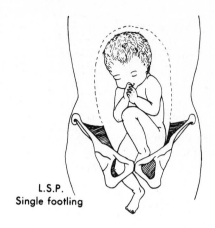

L.S.P.
Single footling

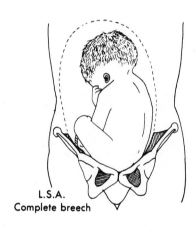

L.S.A.
Complete breech

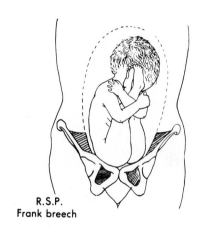

R.S.P.
Frank breech

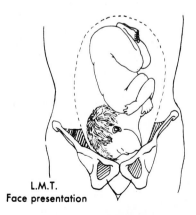

L.M.T.
Face presentation

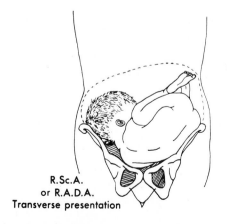

R.Sc.A.
or R.A.D.A.
Transverse presentation

FIG. 6-5   Various presentations and positions.

ters representing the point of reference need be changed. For example:

1. Right occiput* anterior   R.O.A.
2. Left occiput anterior   L.O.A.
3. Right occiput posterior   R.O.P.
4. Left occiput posterior   L.O.P.
5. Right occiput transverse   R.O.T.
6. Left occiput transverse   L.O.T.
7. Occiput at sacrum   O.S.
   Occiput posterior   O.P.
8. Occiput at the pubis ⎫
   Occiput anterior   ⎭   O.A.

Note that a transverse position is *not* the same thing as a transverse presentation, or lie. The letter "O" is usually employed only in the case of well-flexed or median vertex presentations (military). In the rare cases of cephalic presentations demonstrating more deflexion, other points of reference must be sought, since the occiput is no longer available or meaningful to the examiner. In a brow presentation, the letter "F" for fronto is used, referring to the area of the anterior fontanel. Brow presentations are usually slow and difficult because of the increased diameter of the skull trying to force its way through the passageway. A cesarean section may be the procedure of choice. In instances of full extension of the head, resulting in a face presentation, the letter "M" for mentum, or chin, is seen. Face presentations, although slow, usually terminate satisfactorily without intervention. However, the infant's remarkable but temporary facial edema and distortion proclaim to all his unorthodox entry into the world.

Breech presentations employ the sacrum or coccyx as a point of reference and the code letter "S." Characteristically, three types are described. A *complete*, or *full*, breech involves the flexion of the infant's legs usually tailor fashion so that the buttocks and feet appear at the vaginal opening almost simultaneously. A *frank*, or *single*, breech is said to occur when the thighs are flexed on the abdomen with the extended legs against the trunk and the feet against the face (sort of foot-in-mouth posture).

---

*Sometimes the combining form "occipito" is used instead of the noun "occiput."

The term *incomplete* breech may indicate the initial appearance of either the feet or knees. The presentation of one or both feet is labeled a *single* and *double* footling, respectively. Frank breech is the most commonly encountered. Breech birth is associated with a higher perinatal mortality. (See p. 144.)

A transverse lie, sometimes called a shoulder presentation, usually employs the scapula or its upper tip, the acromion, for reference, and "Sc" or "A" is the code. The baby lying crosswise in the uterus may be positioned with its back toward the front or back of its mother. The baby's scapula, posteriorly located, indicates the position of its back. Sometimes the terms "dorsoanterior" or "dorso-posterior" may be used to clarify this. A fetus whose shoulder and head occupy the right side of the mother's pelvis and whose back is toward her front may be said to be in the right acromiodorsoanterior position, or R.A.D.A. This is an impossible presentation for normal birth.

Station and engagement

Another measurement related to the location of the fetus in the passageway is *station*, which may be defined as the relationship of the presenting part to the ischial spines of the pelvis. When the presenting part is at the level of the spines, it is usually considered engaged, and the station is said to be 0. If the presentation is above the spines, it is usually considered high, and the station is said to be -1, -2, etc., an estimate of its location in terms of centimeters above the ischial spines. If the presenting part is below the ischial spines, the station is coded as $+1$, $+2$, etc., again making the estimate in centimeters. (A centimeter is a little less than ½ inch.) A plus station is considered low (Fig. 6-6).

Effacement and dilatation

One should not forget that the power accomplishing the shortening and thinning (effacement) and dilatation of the cervix to an opening approxi-

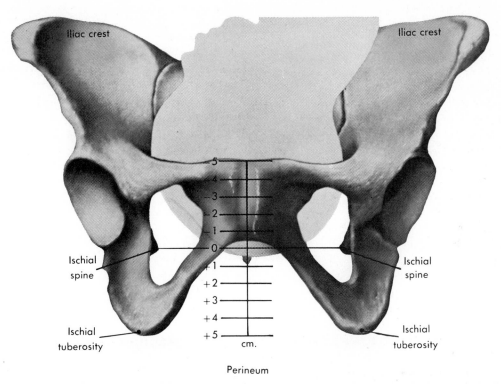

Iliac crest

Iliac crest

Ischial
spine

Ischial
spine

Ischial
tuberosity

Ischial
tuberosity

cm.

Perineum

FIG. 6-6   Stations of presenting part, or degree of engagement. The location of the presenting part in relation to the level of the ischial spines is designated *station* and indicates the degree of advancement of the presenting part through the pelvis. Stations are expressed in centimeters above *(minus)* and below *(plus)* the level of the ischial spines *(zero)*. The head is usually engaged when it reaches the level of the ischial spines.

From Phenomena of normal labor, Columbus, Ohio, 1964, Ross Laboratories.

mately 10 cm (or about 4 inches) in diameter is provided by the intermittent but increasingly frequent and progressively stronger uterine contractions. It should be noted that effacement may occur rather "silently" as the result of unobtrusive contractions before the onset of more definitive, vigorous labor. Limited cervical dilatation (approximately 1 to 3 cm) may also take place before the onset of the "formal" labor period. The disappearance, or effacement, of the cervical canal as its walls move upward to become part of the lower uterine segment is expressed in percent. Primigravidas usually undergo 100% effacement before dilatation (Fig. 6-7). The cervix of a multipara typically undergoes

effacement and dilatation at the same time. For a more detailed discussion of expected rates of dilatation, see pp. 91-95 and 103.

Show

Dilatation of the cervix is usually accompanied by what is called *show*. During pregnancy, the mucus-producing glands of the cervix have formed a mucoid deposit in the cervical canal that helps protect the interior of the uterus from the introduction of infection. When the cervix begins to dilate, this mucous plug is discharged. As the cervix con-

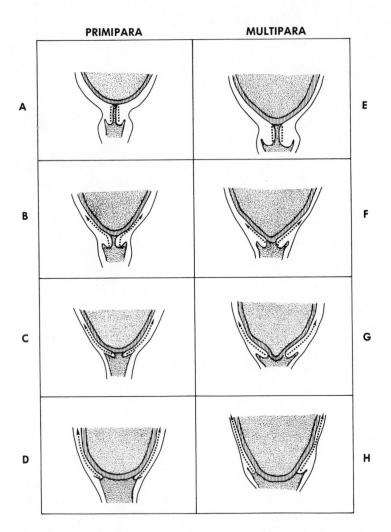

PRIMIPARA   MULTIPARA

A   E

B   F

C   G

D   H

FIG. 6-7   Typical cervical dilatation (first stage labor) primiparas contrasted with multiparas. **A,E,** Cervix long—cervical canal characteristically more "relaxed" in multiparas; **B,F,** Effacement or shortening and thinning of cervix begins; **C,G,** Cervix thins in primiparas but little dilatation occurs. Effacement and dilatation occur simultaneously in multiparas; **D,H,** Effacement and dilatation complete.

tinues to dilate, small capillaries in the cervix break and stain the mucus with blood. The faster the cervix dilates and the closer it is to complete dilatation, the more abundant and red will be the "show." However, it should not assume the proportions or characteristics of frank bleeding or contain clots.

After complete dilatation is accomplished, both abdominal and uterine muscles contract to push the fetus to the exterior. The mother has no control over the contractions of her uterus; they are under involuntary control. However, once dilatation is complete, she may aid immensely by pushing with her abdominal muscles when her uterus contracts to help make the fetus descend in the pelvic canal.

Thus to help determine the progress of the passenger, the physician is interested in the *presentation*, the body part that is trying to come first; the *position*, the relationship of the presenting part to the pelvic quadrants; and the *station*, the depth of the presenting part in the pelvic canal. If these things are known plus the relative size and shape of the pelvis and fetus, the condition of the soft-tissue uterine exit called the cervix, and the quality and frequency of the uterine contractions providing the power, the physician has a good basis for an evaluation of the progress of the labor and the mechanisms involved.

MECHANISM OF LABOR

Textbooks usually speak of the cardinal movements in the mechanism of labor. In the vertex delivery they usually include the following: descent, flexion, engagement, internal rotation, extension, external rotation, and expulsion (Fig. 6-8). The first *four* movements are not necessarily in order, since flexion may be present before descent and may increase thereafter. Descent and internal rotation will also continue after engagement. These mechanisms may occur concurrently and defy a 1-2-3 order.

Descent, flexion, and engagement

In a primipara,* or woman bearing her first baby, *descent* of the fetus into the true pelvis usually occurs about 2 weeks before the actual birth of the child. This descent is referred to as *lightening* and results in *engagement*, or passage of the largest diameter of the presenting part into the true pelvis. Lay people remark about this change in fetal location by the phrase "the baby has dropped." The expectant mother, with less pressure on her diaphragm, happily finds that she can breathe more freely. The increased tilt and lowered location of the fetus produce a characteristic change in the maternal silhouette. In a multipara, descent and engagement may not occur until dilatation of the cervix begins.

Internal rotation

The amount of *internal rotation* necessary will depend on the position of the fetus and the way the head rotates to accommodate itself to the changing diameters of the pelvis. The most common rotation is that which involves the turning of the head to occiput anterior position. If the fetus begins its descent in L.O.A. or L.O.T. position, this rotation represents only a short distance of 45 to 90 degrees. If, however, the internal rotation involves moving from a posterior position, it may mean a turn of 135 degrees. For this reason posterior positions usually entail a longer labor and more lower back discomfort for the mother, who will usually appreciate firm, cool, intermittent sacral support. Occasionally, instead of rotating to an anterior position, the occiput turns to the sacrum, and the child is born in O.S. or O.P. position—a mode of delivery usually slower and more dangerous to the maternal tissues.

---

*The words "primipara" and "multipara" in this section are used from the delivery-labor room perspective. More correct would be the terms "primigravida" or "nullipara" but these are less frequently employed.

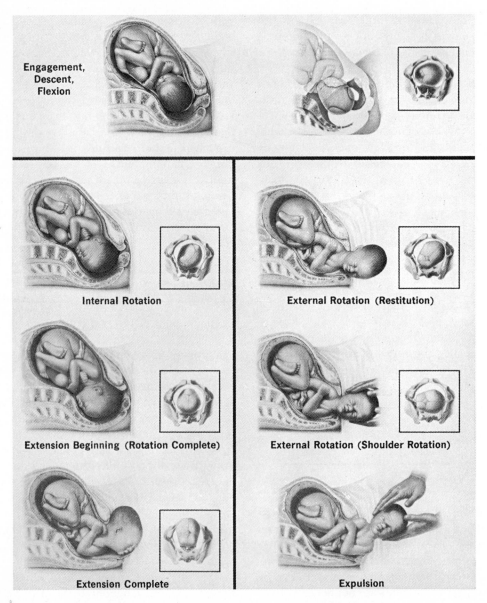

Engagement,
Descent,
Flexion

Internal Rotation

External Rotation (Restitution)

Extension Beginning (Rotation Complete)

External Rotation (Shoulder Rotation)

Extension Complete

Expulsion

FIG. 6-8   Mechanism of normal labor, L.O.A. position showing head rotation in square inserts.

From Nursing education aid, No. 13, Columbus, Ohio, 1964, Ross Laboratories.

Often the occiput will complete the longer rotation from the posterior position to the pubis. Sometimes the occiput lingers unduly in the posterior position or stops its rotation in transverse. The former situation is called "persistent posterior" and the latter a "transverse arrest." This can occur at almost any station or depth in the pelvic canal and may necessitate manual rotation or the use of rotation forceps by the obstetrician.

Extension

In a vertex delivery the head is delivered by *extension*. During descent it is normally forced into a flexed attitude by the pressure of the cervix, pelvic walls, and floor. Once the occiput has rotated to anterior position and occupies the pubic arch, the head cannot make any further progress unless extension is accomplished. Because of this extension plus the natural curve of the lower pelvis, the baby's head is born pushing upward out of the vaginal canal. The rate of extension is gently controlled by the physician. If the bag of waters (membranes) has not previously broken during labor, it must be artificially broken now by the physician to avoid the baby's aspirating amniotic fluid. To try to prevent uncontrolled tearing of the perineum, an *episiotomy*, or surgical incision extending the soft tissue vaginal opening, may be executed by the physician just before the birth of the head. (See also pp. 129-131.)

External rotation (restitution, shoulder rotation) and expulsion

When the perineum slides over the chin of the baby and temporarily only the neck occupies the outlet, more room is available to the infant for head movement. Usually without coaxing by the physician, the back of the baby's head will then turn to line up with his back, revealing the baby's position just before internal rotation of the head took place. This movement is called *restitution*. The turning movement of the head generally continues and influences the location of the back, helping to line up the unborn shoulders just beneath the pubis in anteroposterior position. This process of alignment is called *shoulder rotation*. Usually the top of the anterior shoulder is next seen just under the pubis—generally aided by the physician, who may exert gentle but firm downward traction on the head. Then the head is gently raised to clear the posterior shoulder, and the entire body follows without any particular difficulty. *Expulsion* of the infant is accomplished.

STAGES OF LABOR

Labor has been classically divided into three stages. In recent literature a fourth stage has been identified:

Stage 1—from the onset of regular labor contractions, beginning the effacement and dilatation of the cervix to complete dilatation, 10 cm

Stage 2—from complete dilatation to the birth of the baby

Stage 3—from birth of the baby to the expulsion of the placenta and membranes

Stage 4—normally about a 2-hour period of transition, stabilization, and "initial recovery" from childbirth

The Friedman labor curve

Another more elaborate way of describing labor that includes the classic first and second stages has gained particular prominence in the last decade. It employs what is called the Friedman Labor Curve. Dr. Friedman has emphasized that two measurements, when serially repeated and graphed, reveal whether or not the journey through the pelvic passageway is in preparation or process and whether satisfactory progress is being made. Those two measurements are *cervical dilatation* and *station*.

Changes in cervical dilatation. After statistical study of many thousands of birth histories, two sim-

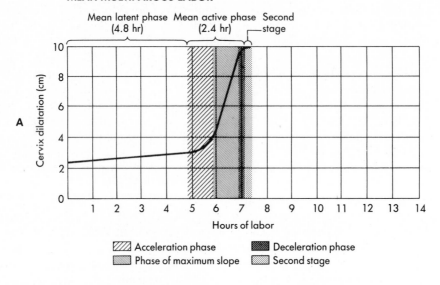

FRIEDMAN LABOR CURVE
MEAN MULTIPAROUS LABOR

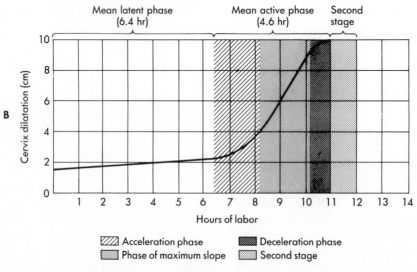

FRIEDMAN LABOR CURVE
MEAN NULLIPAROUS LABOR

FIG. 6-9   The Friedman labor curve formed by plotting the rate of cervical dilatation of the **A,** mean multiparous labor; **B,** mean nulliparous labor ("mean" indicates average).

Based on revised mean labor statistics in Friedman, E.A.: Labor: clinical evaluation and management, ed. 2, New York, 1978, Appleton-Century-Crofts, and personal correspondence.

ilar though not identical S-shaped curves based on the speed of dilatation of multiparas and primiparas (nulliparas) were identified. When the rates of cervical dilatation of individual women in labor are plotted against the appropriate curve, disturbances in progress related to dilatation may be diagnosed more readily. Both curves may be divided into sections describing different phases of the labor process (see Fig. 6-9, *A* and *B*). The veritcal side of the graph indicates the cervical dilation 0 to 10 centimeters; the horizontal side indicates the number of hours in labor. The length of labor is much shorter for the multipara, accounting for the variance in the curves.

Two main phases are described: a relatively slow-moving, flat first section called the *latent phase,* involving cervical softening, effacement, and early dilation (it traces the period extending from onset of labor until more rapid dilatation manifests itself at approximately 2 to 3 cm); and a second section, the *active phase,* which is indicated by the rather sudden upswing and steep ascent of the tracing, ending with a brief rounding at the apex. This active phase of dilatation has in turn been divided into three phases: (1) the obvious curve upward from the latent phase which first identifies that cervical dilation has increased in tempo, called the *acceleration phase;* (2) the steepest part of the tracing called the *phase of maximum slope;* and (3) the rounding at the apex, which represents a slowing of the dilatation just before the patient is completely dilated, called the *deceleration phase.* Existence of this phase has been disputed, and it has often been characterized as short or absent in multiparas.

It may be difficult at times to determine just when the latent phase begins, since effacement and early cervical dilatation may be "silent," or false labor may confuse the issue. The patient's labor graph is usually begun when a nullipara's contractions are experienced at regular 3- to 5-minute intervals or when a multipara attains regular contractions at 5- to 10-minute intervals. The following limited analysis includes some selected findings and conclusions from Dr. Friedman's study that makes the graphed information more meaningful. The abnormalities in dilatation described below are depicted in Fig. 6-10.

I. Length of the *latent phase of dilatation*
   A. Does not predict the length of the active phase
   B. May be quite easily affected by varying conditions or factors
   C. Is considered *prolonged* if it lasts:
      1. 14 hours or more for multiparas
      2. 20 hours or more for nulliparas
   D. Possible causes are:
      1. Long, firm (unripe) cervix
      2. Premature or excessive sedation, analgesia or conduction anesthesia
   E. Possible effects may be:
      1. Maternal dehydration, exhaustion
      2. More risk of infection if bag of waters ruptures early in labor
   F. Possible actions:
      1. Sedation to rest mother
      2. Uterine stimulation by oxytocic medication
II. Length of the *active phase of dilatation*
   A. Protracted active-phase dilatation (slow-slope)
      1. Maximum rate of slope is:
         a. 1.5 cm/hr or less for multiparas
         b. 1.2 cm/hr or less for nulliparas
      2. Possible causes are:
         a. Cephalopelvic disproportion (CPD)
         b. Abnormal presentation and position
         c. Early or excessive sedation, analgesia impairing uterine contractions
         d. Early rupture of the bag of waters
      3. Possible effects are:
         a. Maternal exhaustion, dehydration
         b. Usually no real risk to mother or infant from the labor pattern itself, but longer, more difficult labor and potential risk from the delivery if by forceps
      4. Possible actions:
         a. Expectant observation—intervention may worsen situation
         b. Sedation to rest mother
         c. Possible uterine stimulation by oxytocic medication, but usually no increase in *rate* of progress attained
         d. Possible cesarean birth (if CPD)
   B. Secondary arrest of active phase of dilatation
      1. No progress in maximum rate of slope for 2

hours or more (potentially most damaging dilatation pattern)

2. Possible causes:
   a. Cephalopelvic disproportion (CPD)
   b. Abnormal presentation and position
   c. Early or excessive sedation, analgesia impairing uterine contractions
   d. Multiple pregnancy (twins, etc.)
   e. Prematurity, malformed fetus
3. Possible effects:
   a. Increased risk of fetal distress or damage
   b. Maternal exhaustion and trauma
4. Possible actions:
   a. Reevaluation of infant presentation, position, and maternal pelvis (x-ray examination, ultrasound)
   b. Sedation to rest mother
   c. Uterine stimulation by oxytocic medication
   d. Cesarean birth

Changes in station or descent. Friedman's study of the rate of descent of the fetus through the pelvic canal also produces a curve that can be divided almost the same way as the dilatation curve has been. It is sometimes superimposed on the dilatation graph, showing that the phase of maximum slope for cervical dilatation normally corresponds to the phase of acceleration for descent (see Fig. 6-11).

Abnormalities of descent occur alone or in conjunction with problems in dilatation. Some important deviations are mentioned below.

I. Length of maximum slope of descent extended
   A. Is considered *protracted* if rate of descent is:
      1. 2 cm/hr or less for multiparas
      2. 1 cm/hr or less for nulliparas
   B. Is considered *arrested* if rate of descent is stopped for 1 hour or more
   C. Possible causes of protracted or arrested descent may be:
      1. Cephalopelvic disproportion (CPD)
      2. Abnormal presentation and position
   D. Possible effects of protracted or arrested descent—if unrelieved, increased incidence of maternal and fetal trauma
   E. Possible actions:
      1. Reevaluation of infant presentation, position, and maternal pelvis

2. Uterine stimulation by oxytocic medication
3. Cesarean birth

II. Length of maximum slope of dilatation or descent shortened (precipitate labor)
   A. Not to be confused with precipitate *delivery* which means a birth without adequate preparation and supervision
   B. Often defined as labor lasting less than 3 hours
   C. As defined by Friedman, involves:
      1. Maximum slopes of dilatation or descent of 10 cm/hr or more for multiparas
      2. Maximum slopes of dilatation or descent of 5 cm/hr or more for nulliparas
   D. Is associated with:
      1. Little soft-tissue resistance to cervical dilation or descent
      2. Abnormally strong uterine and abdominal contractions
   E. May be accompanied by:
      1. Maternal uterine and perineal lacerations
      2. Lowered fetal oxygenation and increased infant birth injury (especially cerebral hemorrhage)

The Friedman Curve is not universally employed to monitor labor progression, but it is a useful concept and tool which has added specific terminology to the analysis of childbirth.

A wise nurse or physician makes no specific predictions regarding the length of the stages of labor. However, Table 6-1 may be of some aid in estimating possible time intervals. Labor lengths for both primiparas and multiparas have decreased in the last generation.

Third stage: special considerations

The third stage of labor is characterized by the separation of the placenta and its expulsion.

Placental separation. Separation of the placenta from the uterine wall is accomplished by the contraction of the uterus. The site of the placental attachment suddenly becomes reduced, but the placenta itself remains the same size, causing a separation of the two structures. The placenta slides down into the lower portion of the uterus and vagi-

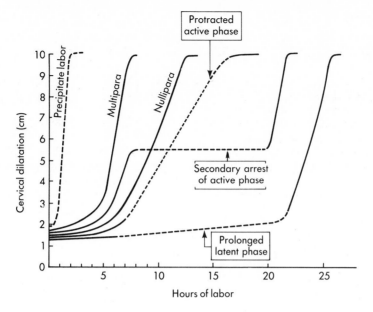

FIG. 6-10   Deviations in rate of cervical dilatation (as described by Friedman).

NULLIPAROUS DILATATION AND DESCENT CURVES

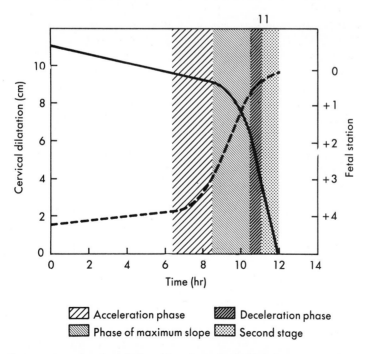

FIG. 6-11   Shows approximate relationship of cervical dilatation rate to fetal descent rate in average nulliparous labor.

Adapted from Friedman, E.A.: Labor: clinical evaluation and management, ed. 2, New York, 1978, Appleton-Century-Crofts.

TABLE 6-1   USUAL DURATION OF THE STAGES OF LABOR

	First stage	Second stage	Third stage
Primi-para	10 to 12 hours	30 minutes to 2 hours	5 to 20 minutes (usually aided by oxytocics or manual pressure)
Multi-para	6 to 8 hours	20 minutes to 1½ hours	5 to 20 minutes (usually aided by oxytocics or manual pressure)

na. The physician watches for signs of placental separation, which include the following:

1. The rise of the uterus to the umbilicus or above—pushed up by the bulky placenta in the vagina
2. The increased firmness and rounded shape of the fundus
3. The lengthening of the exposed umbilical cord at the exterior as the placenta descends
4. The sudden appearance of moderate temporary vaginal bleeding originating from the site of the placental attachment at the time of separation

Placental expulsion. After the placenta is separated it may be pushed out by the mother as uterine contractions resume, and she is again instructed to "bear down". More commonly she is assisted by the physician, who—*after* separation of the placenta—may carefully exert abdominal pressure with one hand just above the pubic bone momentarily pushing the uterus higher to help the placenta slip further down the birth canal, while he gently pulls on the umbilical cord with the other (the Brandt-Andrews maneuver) causing the placenta's expulsion. At times the physician may elect to help deliver the placenta through cautious intravaginal, intrauterine, or abdominal maneuvers. Manual extraction may be a necessity in cases of abnormally retained placenta or excessive uterine bleeding. Most physicians routinely carry out manual palpation of the uterine cavity after the delivery of the placenta in an effort to make sure that it is normal and empty. Visual inspection of the cervix is part of the usual follow-up. The expelled placenta is checked for abnormality and completeness.

The third and fourth stages of labor are probably the most dangerous for the mother because hemorrhages most often occur during this time. In an effort to speed the separation of the placenta and lessen blood loss, *oxytocics*, medications that help contract the uterus, are often employed. The medications used will depend on the time during the delivery sequence that their action is desired, the condition of the patient, the anesthesia used, and the personal preferences of the attending physician.

The satisfactory completion of the mechanisms of labor and birth as seen in all stages is indeed cause for congratulation for all concerned.

The following discussion of the needs of the laboring patient reflects the traditional departmentalized structure of hospital maternity care in the United States (separate labor/delivery, nursery, and postpartum areas). This pattern of care will probably be that most frequently encountered by students using this text. However, it should be emphasized that many maternity services are undergoing changes, and that various nursing roles are being created that overlap and extend those formerly described. Indeed, different birth settings, both within and outside hospital walls, are being sought by some parents, and the reader should be aware of alternatives available. (See p. 139.)

Normally, the onset of labor is the anticipated climax of 9 months of very constructive waiting. Under normal conditions each day has better prepared the fetus to make the transition from intrauterine to extrauterine existence smoothly, without undue strain. As the time of labor and birth approaches, the pregnant woman should be alerted to certain "get set" signs, and she should be instructed when to call the physician and come to the hospital.

SIGNS OF IMPENDING LABOR

Several signs and symptoms usually precede the onset of true labor—the opening of the cervix and expulsion of the baby and placenta. These hints of things to come are usually welcome. At the end of a full-term pregnancy the mother is willing to relinquish her lively and bulky boarder; however, she also has feelings of anxiety as she considers the actual period of labor and birth.

Lightening. In a woman bearing her first infant, usually about 2 weeks before birth a relative change in fetal location may be suddenly apparent. As the fetus "drops" into the true pelvis (a process called *lightening*) and the presenting part "becomes engaged" (the largest diameter of the presenting part passes the pelvic brim), she finds herself able to breathe more freely with less pressure on the diaphragm. Primigravidas are expected to experience lightening and engagement before true labor begins. If it does not occur, the possibility of too small a pelvic inlet or too large a presenting part (fetal-pelvic disproportion) may be considered. Women who have borne children previously may not undergo lightening until just before or during true labor.

Frequent urination. The woman may also find, alas, greater pressure on her bladder and may be troubled with frequent urination.

Energy. Many women experience a phenomenal "burst of energy" just before going into labor and want to clean the whole house. They should be advised to resist the impulse.

Uterine contractions. The uterus contracts and relaxes intermittently all during pregnancy, but its contractions are usually mild and not detected by the mother-to-be. However, in the last few weeks of waiting, these uterine contractions may become annoying and, contrary to what some texts declare, may be painful. The most discouraging aspect about these contractions of late pregnancy is that they are often only a rehearsal for the real thing. They do not serve to dilate the cervix and therefore are called false labor, or Braxton Hicks' contractions, after the British obstetrician who described them. Characteristics of false labor contrasted with true labor contractions include the following:

1. The duration of the contraction remains about the same, not becoming appreciably longer or more intensive as do true contractions.
2. The period between contractions remains long and irregular. True contractions are regular, with a gradually decreasing interval.
3. Pressure or pain is felt primarily in the abdomen rather than in the small of the back.
4. Walking can be tolerated during the contraction. In fact, walking may help relieve discomfort, whereas true labor contractions may be intensified by ambulation.
5. Show, or the appearance of a mucoid vaginal discharge tinged with blood, is absent in false labor but is usually present in true labor.
6. On rectal or vaginal examination the cervix is usually found to be long and closed in false labor but is effacing or dilating in true labor.

An expectant mother should be counseled to contact her physician about the onset of labor if (1) contractions are regular, becoming increasingly frequent and intensive; (2) show is present; or (3) the bag of waters, or membranes, ruptures.

THE TRIP TO THE HOSPITAL

The time at which the woman is instructed to go to the hospital depends on her reported progress, the distance she must travel, how many babies she has had, and the history of her previous labors. Usually, physicians want all their patients to be admitted as soon as the bag of waters ruptures or show appears. If these signs are absent, admission is advised when the contractions of primigravidas are regular at about 7-minute intervals. With mothers who previously have had one baby or more,

physicians usually want them hospitalized when contractions have achieved some regularity, but they do not wait until a certain frequency is reached. Women who have previously experienced a full-term normal birth usually deliver more rapidly than those who have not. They are encouraged not to wait at home too long. If the onset of labor is suspected, the prospective mother should eat nothing and limit her intake of fluids until evaluated by the physician to prevent possible aspiration at the time of birth if general anesthesia is required.

It is hoped that the ride to the hospital will not turn into a race or be complicated with too many obstacles. Certainly it is best to be able to be admitted without rush and confusion. Detailed planning for the journey should be made. The woman should be told by her physician or office nurse before her entry what the admission procedures involve so that she may be more prepared for what will transpire.

HOSPITAL ADMISSION

Admission directly to the labor room unit with a minimum of front office procedure is desirable. Usually only one signature is needed, that of the woman herself, for permission to perform the routine procedures necessary during labor and birth. "Routine procedures" do not include a cesarean section. The husband or chosen companion may help complete any other office admittance procedure needed while the woman is being cared for in the labor room area. Answers to study questionnaires indicate that a number of prospective fathers resent being sent to the admission desk to complete lengthy forms at a time when they feel that they can be supportive to their wives. Preadmission arrangements to obtain as much information as possible regarding the physical, mental, and social status of the patient and the expectations and desires of the parents as they may affect their birth experiences are to be encouraged. If brief information sheets could be filled out before admission by the woman and the clinic or office personnel and forwarded with the current prenatal record close to term, the individual needs and preferences of the woman and her family might be better understood and considered. The so-called assembly-line maternity care of many hospitals has caused some women to feel more like objects than human beings. Some have so resented or feared hospitalization experiences that they seek alternatives to a hospital birth. These expectant parents may plan a home birth or search for a birth center available in their community. These choices are discussed further on pp. 139-141.

All women harbor anxiety regarding their hospital experience, and some are very nervous and fearful. The nursing staff should do everything in its power to alleviate this anxiety and make the woman and her partner or family feel welcome and secure. A gracious welcome makes a lasting impression. Unfortunately, so does a rude, thoughtless, or disorganized admission experience. The expectant mother does not want to hear about the current problems of the maternity service, experiences of former patients, or the personal histories of her attending nurses. Such recitals are indiscreet, impolite, and worrisome to the woman and her family. Her chosen companion or members of the immediate family should be shown a place where they can comfortably wait during the completion of the admission procedures. If it is indicated that the laboring mother wishes to have one person remain with her during the entire admission, this desire should be honored if possible. Once the admission is completed, most hospitals encourage visitation of the woman by her immediate family or companion, one or two persons at a time.

Role of vocational or practical nurse

The prepared vocational nurse, as a part of the maternity staff, can make a real contribution to the well-being of the expectant mother and her family. Under the supervision of an experienced registered nurse, she can render valuable assistance to the department and the patient. We believe that the use of the prepared licensed vocational nurse (LVN or LPN) in nonsupervisory capacities in this department is legitimate and desirable but that it is a misuse of personnel to expect her to assume the role of a charge nurse or, on the other hand, to delegate to her only those duties that can be accomplished by workers with less training.

The vocational nurse can provide valuable assistance in the admittance of the patient to the labor-delivery suite. After the woman arrives at the hospital, she is usually taken by wheelchair to the labor room area. The nurse helps the patient remove her clothes and put on a hospital gown. She makes special note of valuables, such as watches and eyeglasses. If the bag of waters has ruptured, the patient should remain in bed. As soon as possible the patient is properly identified, preferably by use of a careful banding technique. The nurse asks the name of the attending physician and secures the patient's prenatal record if one is present at the hospital. With the supervising registered nurse, she may read the record to determine as much as possible about this patient before continuing with the admission. Important factors to check are (1) the obstetric history—the number of viable births she has had, previous difficulties, the rapidity of former labors, and Rh status; (2) the record of the current pregnancy—the expected date of birth, laboratory results, present physical or psychosocial problems, and any known allergies; (3) plans for the labor and birth—type of anesthesia, if desired, whether she has attended childbirth education classes; (4) accommodations preferred, method selected for feeding the infant, and name of the physician to care for the baby; and (5) marital status.

Some of the necessary admission information will, by its very nature, be absent from the prenatal record. The admitting nurse must inquire when the contractions (if any) began, if any show has been noted, and if the bag of waters is known to have broken. The staff should know if the patient has recently eaten. In some maternity services a voided urine specimen is routinely obtained for urinalysis at the time of admission. In others, a specimen is secured on admission only if prenatal history prompts the physician to order it. A specimen may be obtained by catheterization just prior to the birth. Some maternity services include weighing the patient in their admission procedure. Although most of the time a call will have previously been received from the attending physician regarding the admission, in some situations the nurse may want to know if the patient has contacted and been examined by the physician. She will take the patient's temperature, pulse, and respiration, determine the blood pressure, in the *absence of a contraction*, and time the duration, interval, and intensity of contractions. She will listen for and count the fetal heart rate and note the presence of amniotic fluid drainage and any show. Application of external fetal and contraction monitors is often part of her care. In some settings she may be expected to perform a rectal or vaginal evaluation of the patient's progress in labor (see below).

Role of the registered nurse

The registered nurse, having overall responsibility for the case, greets the patient, noting any special needs. She palpates the abdomen, evaluates contractions, and examines the patient rectally or now more often, vaginally, to determine fetal station and presentation, the dilatation and effacement of the cervix, and the condition of the membranes and position of the fetus. These last two are sometimes difficult or impossible to discern through the rectal-vaginal wall. If the rectum is not empty, the results of the examination may be questionable. The position of the cervix may make the estimation of dilatation difficult. The patient's condition, progress, and reaction to labor are evaluated. The individual orders of the attending physician are consulted regarding types of analgesia and anesthesia and the expected delivery setup. If no previous arrangement is known, the physician is called regarding the arrival of the patient at the

maternity service, and any unusual vital signs and pertinent information gained from the pelvic examination and other evaluations of the patient are relayed.

Unless the presence of true labor is doubted, perineal preparation of some type is usually carried out. Whether an enema is given will depend on the progress, condition, and consent of the patient and her physician's desires. If analgesia is ordered, side rails should be in place. Which staff member carries out the necessary admission procedures depends on the competencies of the personnel and the patient's condition and needs.

Procedures

Principles of the admission procedures should be discussed. It is impossible to describe in detail an admission that fits the needs of every hospital. There are many ways to accomplish similar aims. However, certain principles are followed in every good maternity service no matter where it may be. We will now discuss the admission perineal "prep," the labor room enema, the timing of contractions, and the determination of fetal heart rate.

Perineal preparation

Purpose: To cleanse the external genitalia in preparation for birth. This usually entails a "mini shave" of the true perineum and/or clipping of perineal hair. However, some physicians are now ordering "no prep." No increase in infection has been noted because the patient has not been shaved. However, the perineum should be carefully cleansed before the birth. Cleansing does help prevent infection. Minimal shaving or clipping helps make a possible episiotomy repair and postpartum perineal observation easier.

Setup: Provide individual equipment for each patient or equipment that is used in such a way that no cross infection can take place. Provision should be made for the following:
1. Privacy
2. Adequate lighting
3. A waterproof pad under the patient's hips to protect the bed

4. A supply of clean, warm water
5. A sudsing antiseptic solution
6. A sharp safety razor (if shaving is desired)
7. Two or three clean dry cotton balls or gauze compresses to help pull back on the skin if it is being shaved and to clean the labial folds
8. An irrigation pitcher and/or folded soft paper or cloth towels to help rinse off the soapy solution and dry the area
9. Several paper towels or a plastic sack to receive the waste in a convenient manner and intermittently help to clean off the razor if used
10. Clean disposable gloves for the nurse's use during the procedure
    Procedure:
1. If possible, place light (wall or gooseneck lamp) on opposite side of bed from where you will stand so that no shadows are cast.
2. Screen the patient. The sheet may be over the lower legs and feet; the gown is turned up to just above the perineal hairline giving adequate space to work.
3. Have the patient bend her knees and drop her legs sideways—heels toward one another. Lather the perineal hair. If shaving is ordered, create tension on the skin with a dry compress with one hand, shave with the other, placing your razor approximately at a 30-degree angle to the skin. Cleanse away any collection of smegma (cellular debris found especially in the labial folds). Avoid getting any solution into the vagina. Wipe off prepped area with soft towel dampened with water to remove the solution, which may be irritating. Use a different surface for each stroke (or irrigate the area) and dry with second soft towel, using same technique, never returning to the vulva after passing over the rectal area.
4. Before preparation of the perineal area is complete, you must turn the patient on her side to finish the perianal region. Probably the most important area to clear is between the vagina and anus, the *true* perineum, because this is the area cut during an episotomy. Wipe off any residual solution.
5. Have your first "prep" checked so that you are certain what is expected of you. Even if it is your first "prep," you should not impress the fact on your anxious patient!
6. During the prep, if possible, try to gauge the frequency and quality of any contractions the patient may have, as well as how she is tolerating them. Report any vaginal discharge as to character and amount.

Note: No perineal pads are worn during labor to cut down on the possibility of vulvar contamination resulting from the pad passing from the rectal to the vaginal area. However, the patient may have absorbent, protective bed pads under her hips.

Delivery room enema technique

Purpose: To empty the colon of feces.
1. Help assure a clean delivery and prevent infection
2. Encourage contractions
3. Possibly provide more passageway for the child
4. Facilitate rectal or vaginal examinations during labor

Setup: More and more physicians are prescribing small, prepackaged phosphate enemas. Some are ordering no enema for those patients who have had a recent bowel movement who can be easily examined.

Cautions:
1. Enemas are not usually given to primiparas after a dilatation of 6 to 8 cm or to multiparas above 4 to 5 cm dilatation to avoid expulsion of the enema during birth.
2. Enemas should not be given to a frankly bleeding patient, since this will further encourage bleeding.
3. Enemas are not usually given to patients with a high presentation (unengaged) with ruptured membranes because of the danger of prolapsed cord. Some physicians prefer that no enemas be given when membranes are ruptured even after engagement because of the increased danger of infection.

Timing obstetric contractions

Purpose:
1. To help evaluate the efforts of the uterus to dilate the cervix and expel the baby and to aid in determining the progress of the labor
2. To detect any abnormalities such as lack of uterine relaxation, which may reveal the onset of complications
3. To help detect fetal distress by simultaneous observation of contraction and fetal heart rate patterns when internal or external electronic monitors are used
4. To reassure the patient and her family by your presence and interest and, at the same time, to help her better support her labor by:
   a. Encouraging and listening
   b. Rubbing her back or providing sacral support as desired

c. Helping with relaxation, breathing, or pushing techniques as needed

d. Moistening her lips and offering oral hygiene

e. Changing pillowcases and replacing bed pads

f. Watching for signs of the patient's changing needs (for example, the beginning of the second stage of labor)

Procedure:

1. Before going to the bedside, if possible, learn about each patient individually:

   a. Number of pregnancies and viable births

   b. Her marital status and any special arrangements for the baby

   c. Whether she has attended childbirth education classes

   d. Any special complications or problems anticipated

2. The fact that you are feeling her uterus, as it contracts and relaxes under the abdominal wall, to help measure her progress in labor should be explained unless she has previously had contractions timed.

3. Your hands should be clean and not too cold.

4. The term *contractions* should be used, not "pains." Not all contractions are painful. Use of the word "pain" may interfere with maternal conditioning for childbirth.

5. If the pregnancy is full term, the fundus, where the strongest muscular contraction can be felt, will be located just above the umbilicus. The nurse's hand should rest lightly there to best detect the uterine contractions.

6. When the uterus contracts, it gradually becomes hard. The degree of hardness is called the *intensity* of a contraction. As the uterus contracts and the uterine muscle fibers shorten, the uterus may be seen or felt to rise in the abdominal cavity. It then gradually relaxes. The time that the uterus is dis-

cernibly firm or tight is called the contraction's *duration*. Usually contractions are easier to feel on multiparas than primiparas because of differences in abdominal muscle tone.

7. The term *interval* in the timing of contractions is used a bit differently than sometimes supposed. The nurse times from the beginning of one contraction to the beginning of the following contraction, when using manual assessment.

8. The time between contractions is called the relaxation time—a period equally as important as the interval or duration. If the relaxation time is very short or nonexistent, the baby may suffer from lack of oxygen. A continuously contracted, hard uterus may be a symptom of abruptio placentae. Between contractions the fingers should be able to depress the abdominal wall, a sensation similar to depressing a foam rubber pillow.

9. The contraction and relaxation periods and the interval have often been diagramed as shown in Fig. 7-1. The straight line represents complete relaxation, and the curved line the actual tone of the uterine musculature.

10. Usually a relationship exists between the duration and frequency of uterine contractions and the dilatation of the cervix. It follows *somewhat* the pattern shown in Table 7-1 (1 inch = 2.5 cm).

11. Recording of observations of contractions would include duration, interval, and intensity, as well as possible patient tolerance. For example, "Contractions q 5 minutes for 35 seconds, mild in character. Using abdominal breathing effectively."

12. When electronic monitors are used, instructions for individual models must be consulted. Both external and internal contraction monitors are available. When traced electronically, the frequency of contractions is often stated as the time elapsed between

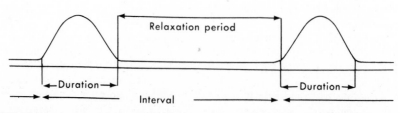

FIG. 7-1   Diagram of the contraction and relaxation of the pregnant uterus.

contraction peaks. Monitor strips are evaluated *at least* every 30 minutes and more frequently during labor induction, active labor, or if possible signs of fetal distress occur. (See Figs. 7-5 to 7-7.)

Fetal heart rate (FHR) evaluation

Purpose:
1. To help detect the presence of fetal life at the time of admission
2. To detect possible fetal distress

Equipment needed: Continuous recorded monitoring of the FHR is probably technically ideal for all laboring women, since research has indicated that intermittent spot checks of the FHR using standard fetoscopes, especially as has been classically taught, are in many instances inadequate for detecting *early* fetal distress. However, such monitors are not always available and their routine use for all labors is controversial. Therefore, the nurse must be familiar with other techniques of intermittent evaluation as well. Indeed, such manually held monitors are sometimes used to verify unusual electronic monitor tracings (for example, doubled beats). The following section discusses the use of "manual" fetoscopes as well as basic principles of simultaneous fetal heart and contraction monitoring.

Manually held monitors—used intermittently:
1. The Leffscope—a stethoscope with a large, heavily weighted bell (Fig. 7-2, *A*)
2. The DeLee-Hollis head scope (Figs. 7-2, *B*; 7-3)
3. An ordinary stethoscope equipped with rubber bands to prevent the sound distortion that results when handling the bell directly
4. Various "lubricated" ultrasonic fetoscopes, which may amplify the FHR (Fig. 7-2, *C* and *D*), held in the examiner's hand against the abdominal wall

Procedure:
1. Explain that you are checking the baby by listening to his heartbeat.
2. Listen to the FHR immediately following a contraction; or better yet, if your patient will allow you, listen during, as well as immediately following, the contraction to hear the heartbeat adequately. This may enable you to detect late deceleration of the heartbeat—a condition thought to be related to fetal distress resulting from uteroplacental insufficiency. (See Fig. 7-5.) However, the pressure exerted on the abdominal wall during a contraction by the manual fetoscope is uncomfortable and annoying to mothers and not easily tolerated by many. For this reason a monitor attached to the mother is superior to manu-

Text continued on p. 108.

TABLE 7-1 COMMON UTERINE CONTRACTION AND DILATATION RELATIONSHIPS AND POSSIBLE DANGER SIGNALS

	Contraction	
Cervical dilatation	**Duration**	**Interval**
1. Fingertip to 2 cm	20-30 seconds	6-8 minutes
2. 2 cm → 4 cm	30-35 seconds	5-6 minutes
3. 4 cm → 6 cm	40-50 seconds	4-5 minutes
4. 6 cm → 8 cm	45-60 seconds	3-4 minutes
5. 8 cm → 10 cm	50-90 seconds	2-3 minutes
(Most difficult period, fatigue, nausea, vomiting, irregular, intensive contractions, "transition")		(Tends to be irregular)

DANGER SIGNALS

Contraction duration more than 90 seconds or tone of more than 75 mm Hg measured by internal monitor
Relaxation period less than 30 seconds
Poor relaxation quality (resting tone more than 15 mm Hg)

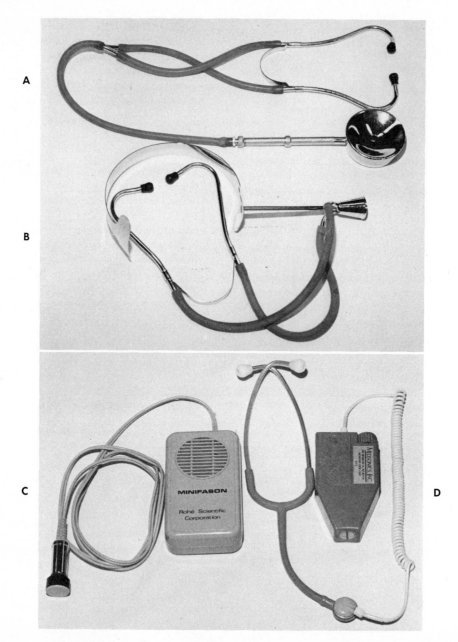

FIG. 7-2   **A,** Leffscope; **B,** DeLee-Hollis head scope; **C,** electronic ultrasound fetoscope, amplifies FHR so that it may be heard by all in area; **D,** electronic ultrasound fetoscope, transmits FHR by means of ear pieces.

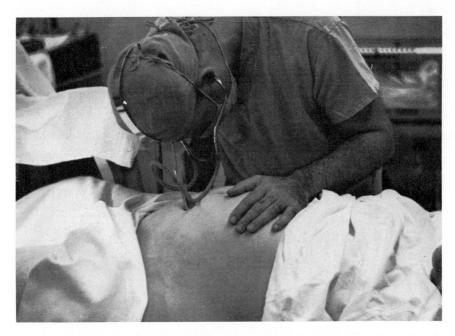

FIG. 7-3

Physician listens to the fetal heart rate (FHR) shortly before the birth. Note the location of the scope on the abdominal wall.

Courtesy Grossmont Hospital and Martin M. Greenberg, M.D., La Mesa, Calif.

FIG. 7-4

Fetal heart tone locations on the abdominal wall indicating possible corresponding fetal positions and the effects of the internal rotation of the fetus.

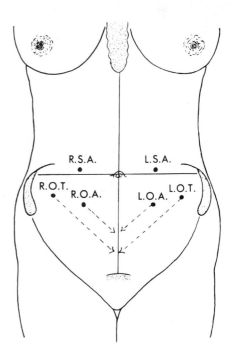

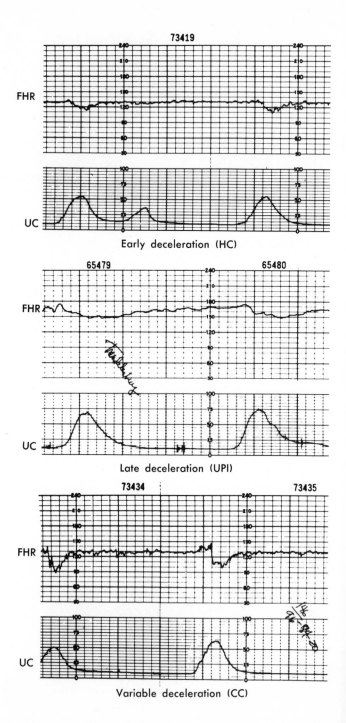

Type I (benign)
"Mirror" coincidental contractions; lowest
point in FHR corresponds to peak of contraction
curve. More common between 4 and 7 cm
dilation and second-stage labor.

Early deceleration (HC)

Type II (ominous)
Mimic somewhat shape of associated contractions,
but onset and lowest point in FHR
occur after peak of contractions. Return to
FHR baseline often exceeds 20 seconds after
end of contractions. Tachycardia, bradycardia
and/or depressed baseline variability
poor signs.

Late deceleration (UPI)

Type III (of varying significance)
Usually V- or U-shaped with abrupt fall and
recovery of FHR. Ominous if below 70 bpm,
last 30 seconds or if recovery sloped or
slow. No consistent relationship to
contraction pattern noted. Tachycardia,
bradycardia, depressed baseline variability
poor signs. More common in advanced labor.

Variable deceleration (CC)

Fig. 7-5   For legend see opposite page.

Intervention

No intervention indicated

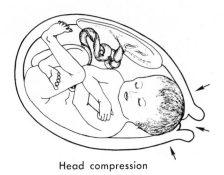

Head compression

Turn patient to either side
Oxygen 6 to 12 liters/min
Stop oxytocin infusion
Elevate legs
Possible fetal blood pH

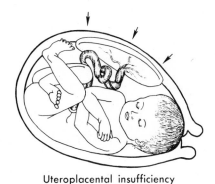

Uteroplacental insufficiency

Turn patient to either side
or place in Trendelenburg's position
Possible vaginal exam to check
for and protect prolapsed cord.
Possible fetal blood pH
Oxygen 6 to 12 liters/min

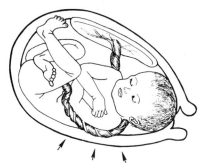

Umbilical cord compression

**FIG. 7-5
cont'd**

Fetal heart rate and contraction patterns have
been found helpful in evaluating maternal-fetal
health during labor.

Courtesy Berkeley Bio-Engineering, San Leandro, Calif.

ally held types, and listening immediately following a contraction will probably be the more frequent observation pattern used. Listen for 30 to 60 seconds if possible. Multiply as necessary to obtain the rate for 1 minute. Every separate beat heard should be counted. It will usually sound like a little watch. At first much concentration will be needed to hear it.

3. Be sure that friction noises from the fingers or the abdominal surface do not distort the sounds. Keep your fingers off the bell. Press firmly on the abdominal wall.

4. The area where the FHR may be heard the best is related to the following (Fig. 7-4):

   a. *Presentation*. In headfirst, or cephalic, presentations the FHR is found in the lower abdominal quadrants, below the umbilicus. In breech presentations the FHR is usually found at the level of the umbilicus or above.

   b. *Position*. If the back of the infant is toward the mother's left (L.O.A. or L.O.P. position), the FHR will probably be heard best on the mother's left. If it points to her right, the FHR will most frequently be heard best on her right. Just because an FHR can be heard in more than one place does not necessarily mean that more than one baby is involved. However, you may want to check by having another nurse listen simultaneously, using a finger-wagging technique to be sure that the rate heard in both areas is the same.

   c. *Station*. As internal rotation and descent occur, the location of the FHR changes, swinging gradually from the right or left quadrants to the midline and dropping until, immediately before birth, it is found just above the pubic bone.

5. It is recommended that the FHR be taken frequently during labor at 15- to 30-minute intervals or less in the first stage of labor. In the event of problems, it would be checked more frequently. The mother should be told at the time of admittance that a frequent check of the FHR is routine. Early in labor she or her partner may enjoy listening once, too.

6. Normal FHR is usually considered to be 120 to 160 beats per minute (bpm). Rates outside this range or a rise or fall of 30 bpm from the usual level of the FHR noted between contractions sustained for 10 minutes or more should be reported to your supervising nurse. Rates determined *between contractions* consistently higher than 160 or showing a 30 bpm baseline increase (fetal tachycardia) may be associated with a variety of problems (for example, maternal fever, fetal hypoxia, or prematurity). Consistent FHR of less than 120 bpm or showing 30 bpm baseline decrease (fetal bradycardia) *not associated with contraction patterns* may signal maternal hypotension. A rate that is too rapid or especially too slow may be a sign of fetal distress. A fetal heart rate under 100 bpm usually signals definite distress. However, even though the heart rate with or without the pressure of a contraction *may* at no time leave the normal range, significant periods of deceleration or slowing may occur undetected unless the labor is continuously monitored. Certain patterns of deceleration may indicate fetal distress. (See Fig. 7-5.) Precise periods of FHR deceleration are difficult to determine with intermittent monitoring techniques, and therefore continuous monitoring technology has developed.

7. Other sounds may be heard in the mother's abdomen as well. *Don't mistake them for the fetal heartbeat.*

   a. The maternal pulse may be heard. You should guard against reporting the maternal pulse as the FHR by feeling the mother's radial pulse at the same time as you are listening with a fetoscope. They should be different rhythms and rates.

   b. The increased sound of the pulsation of the uterine arteries can sometimes be identified. Identification of this "sh" sound with the same rhythm as the maternal pulse does not guarantee that the fetus is alive. Sometimes the FHR can be heard at the same time in the background. Move the fetoscope about 2.5 cm (1 inch), and you will probably hear the FHR better.

   c. Rarely you can hear a sort of soft, whistling sound occurring at the same rate as the fetal heart rate. This has been called the funic souffle, or cord whistle. Some think it is caused by a compression of the cord. Its presence indicates fetal life.

   d. Many expectant mothers are hungry, so you may hear peristalsis!

Monitors attached to mother or fetus for extended or continuous use:

1. External sensors attached to the maternal abdomen to detect the mechanical energy of the fetal heartbeat. These may produce instantaneous visual or audible signals, and when appropriately equipped, they may produce permanent written records. They may be used early in labor before significant cervical dilatation or rupture of the bag of waters. They are simple to use, and there has been no known fetal injury related to their use. However, the position of the sensors

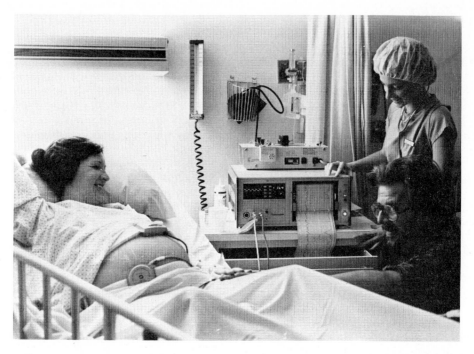

FIG. 7-6   External monitors of FHR and uterine contractions in place. Head of bed elevated to reduce possibility of maternal hypotension.

may need frequent attention as labor becomes more advanced and accuracy of the recording becomes more difficult to obtain. These FHR sensors may be combined with an externally placed diaphragm that is capable of recording the frequency of uterine contractions when held in place with abdominal strapping. (See Fig. 7-6.) Examples are:

a. Small amplifying microphones (phonocardiography) used for antepartum monitoring.

b. Ultrasonic or Doppler-type instruments that produce characteristic reflected sound waves usually more clear

2. Fetal electrocardiography to detect the electrical energy associated with fetal heartbeat.

a. Indirect fetal electrocardiography is possible with electrodes attached to the abdominal wall. It can be used well in early labor, but considerable "electrical noise" may be generated with patient movement during advanced labor, and the recording obtained is inferior to that of direct monitoring.

b. Direct fetal electrocardiography requires ruptured membranes, 1 to 2 cm of cervical dilatation, and a presenting part no higher than −2 station. A physician or specially trained obstetric nurse attaches the electrode vaginally to the presenting part (scalp or buttock), penetrating the epidermis by a tiny metal spiral or clip. Infection and soft tissue injury are possibilities but have not been significant problems.

3. Uterine contraction patterns interpreted by pressure exerted on a catheter inserted cervically into the uterus just beyond the parietal diameter of the fetal head may be viewed and recorded concurrently with the FHR. (See Fig. 7-7.) This arrangement, of course, greatly improves the ability to diagnose correctly early fetal distress.

Basic definitions and concepts regarding monitor strip patterns:

1. *Baseline FHR.* The rate determined either before labor begins or during labor in a 10-minute interval exclusive of any periodic slowdown. Baseline rate is usually 120 to 160 beats per minute. A certain amount of beat-to-beat spacing variation is considered to be an indication of a well-developed, healthy, cardiac

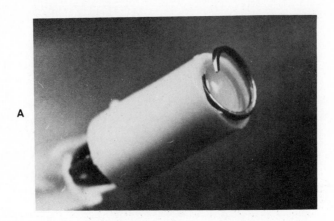

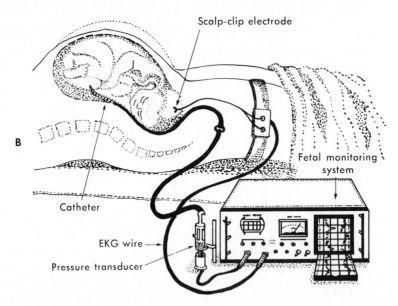

<table>
<tr><td>**FIG. 7-7**</td><td>**A,** Spiral electrode sometimes used to attach FHR monitor to fetal presentation. **B,** Diagram of internal fetal heart and contraction monitoring. Internal monitoring indicates the fetal ECG and the intensity as well as the frequency of uterine contractions. It provides more information but is an intrusive procedure.
A courtesy Corometrics Medical Systems, Inc., Wallingford, Conn.</td></tr>
</table>

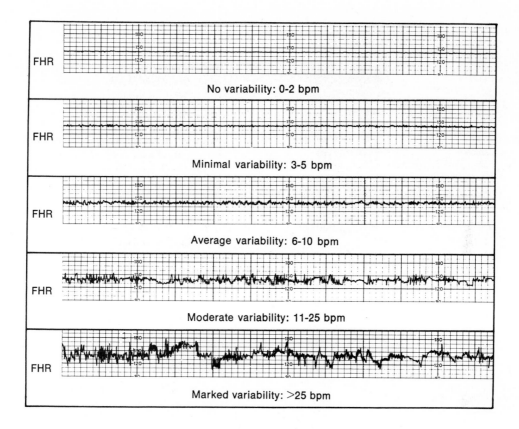

FHR

No variability: 0-2 bpm

FHR

Minimal variability: 3-5 bpm

FHR

Average variability: 6-10 bpm

FHR

Moderate variability: 11-25 bpm

FHR

Marked variability: >25 bpm

FIG. 7-8 Degrees of fetal heart rate variability.

From Tucker, S.M.: Fetal monitoring and fetal assessment in high-risk pregnancy, St. Louis, 1978, The C.V. Mosby Co.

nervous control system. It is best evaluated by internal electrode monitors. Baseline variability of less than 5 beats per minute may be a sign of fetal jeopardy, particularly when lack of variability is found in conjunction with periods of late deceleration of the fetal heart. However, reduced variability may also be produced by the administration of certain analgesic or sedative drugs to the mother. Reduced long-term variability may also be found during 20- to 30-minute intervals of so-called fetal "sleep" or inactivity (Fig. 7-8).

2. *Fetal cardiac deceleration.* Three types of periodic fetal cardiac decelerations, according to their sequential relationships to uterine contractions, have been described and may be detected by continuous moni-

toring devices. (See Fig. 7-5 for tracings, explanations, and possible therapeutic interventions.)

a. Type I. Early fetal cardiac decelerations start at the onset of a contraction and occur only at the same time as the contraction. This pattern is probably due to head compression and increase in the intracranial pressure of the infant. As far as is known, this pattern is harmless. It does not call for an intervention on the part of the obstetric team.

b. Type II. Late deceleration patterns are characterized by a slowing of the fetal heart after the peak, or acme, of the uterine contraction; a delayed return to baseline and a regular waveform reflecting the uterine contraction; they may be found

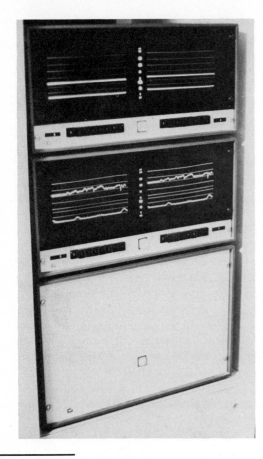

FIG. 7-9

A central monitor, such as might be seen at a nurse's station, displays FHR and contraction patterns of different patients in labor.

Courtesy Corometrics Medical Systems, Inc., Wallingford, Conn.

first within the normal FHR range of 120 to 160 beats per minute. As fetal distress increases, the range and frequency of the FHR deceleration increases. This pattern is frequently associated with uterine hyperactivity caused by oxytocin administration, maternal hypotension, or various high-risk pregnancies. Obstetric interventions to decrease or eliminate fetal distress include stopping any oxytocin administration, providing oxy-

gen by mask or cannula to the mother at 6 to 12 L/min and turning the mother to either side.

c. Type III. Variable deceleration patterns characterized by a periodic, unpredictable slowing of the FHR that show neither a consistent sequential relationship to the uterine contractions nor a regular repetitive range or duration. The deceleration typically traces a steep-sided V or U. This type of pattern is considered to be the result of umbilical cord compression. Changes in maternal posture, to either side or to Trendelenburg's position, oxygen administration to the mother, and possible vaginal exam are recommended interventions.

If either late or variable decelerations persist for 30 minutes after the above interventions have been carried out, operative termination of the labor has been recommended.

3. *Fetal cardiac acceleration.* Periodic accelerations of the FHR are usually considered benign. They are often initiated by fetal movement, uterine contractions, or even maternal abdominal contractions. Indeed, accelerations of the fetal heart rate with fetal movement are an indication of fetal well-being and serve as the basis of the so-called nonstress test (see p. 488). However, occasionally repetitious accelerations associated with contractions may precede the development of progressive late deceleration patterns. For this reason, they should be carefully observed.

Previous comments regarding FHR range also apply with continuous monitoring techniques.*

Other signs of fetal distress: Fetal distress may also manifest itself by the passage of meconium-stained amniotic fluid when the baby is in cephalic presentation; however, this sign is not consistently reliable. Sudden exaggerated fetal movement has at times also been considered a clue of difficulty. Recently in the presence of FHR and contraction patterns that denote possible distress, fetal scalp vein sampling has been used to try to confirm fetal jeopardy. The presence of an acid-base imbalance in the form of pH values below 7.20 in two or more samples usually indicates fetal acidosis requiring prompt delivery by low forceps or cesarean section.

---

*For more detailed discussion of evaluation of FHR patterns, students are referred to Tucker, S.M.: Fetal monitoring and fetal assessment in high-risk pregnancy, St. Louis, 1978, The C.V. Mosby Co.

CONTINUING CARE AND PREPARATION

Once admission is completed, unless birth is imminent, a prolonged period of waiting and observation ensues in which the physical and emotional support of the woman and preparation for the birth are paramount. Usually the presence of her mother, husband, or chosen companion at the bedside is a source of support. Often the husband or companion may have trained to be the woman's labor coach and, as such, is extremely important in sustaining the morale and comfort of the parturient. If such visitation is not supportive or if it appears to antagonize or upset the patient, such observations should be reported to the charge nurse or physician. Sometimes arrangements can be made for the visitor to have a "rest"! Table 7-2 shows some of the relationships between stages of labor, patient behavior and coping techniques, and possible nursing care activities. Table 7-3 provides more details regarding suggested breathing and relaxation techniques. Following is an explanation of terms included:

cleansing breath Deep breath in through nose and out through mouth; used at beginning and end of exercises to ready body for special breathing, to help relaxation, and to restore normal breathing and gas exchange.
focal point Point or object somewhere in room used as center of visual concentration; may be coach's face, picture, furniture, etc.; serves to maintain cerebral input; patient should not close eyes during contraction.
effleurage Light, patterned abdominal massage usually done with tips of fingers.
sacral support Counterpressure exerted to lift sacrum slightly off bed if patient is supine, or firm lower back pressure; may use hands, towels, rolling pins, etc.
pelvic rock Alternately increasing or flattening the lumbar sacral curve of the back.

Early labor

The woman in early labor (usually defined as up to 4 cm dilatation) is characteristically alert, talk-ative, and nervous. She is generally most eager to cooperate with the physician and nursing staff in attendance and responds readily to a calm, cheerful nurse who seems genuinely interested in her welfare. Her contractions, although perhaps uncomfortable, are tolerable. If her membranes are not ruptured, her contractions are not too frequent or intensive, and show is not too remarkable, she will probably appreciate being able to be up and around for a while and not automatically confined to her bed just because she has been admitted to the hospital. It has been found that when she does rest in bed, there is less interference with maternal and fetal circulation, increased urinary function, and greater uterine efficiency if she reclines on her left side. However, it is true that a number of nursing observations and procedures (manual fetal heart rate determination, checking the dilatation or perineum) may be more easily carried out if the patient turns to the supine position intermittently. Later in labor, during transition and while the mother is pushing, the supine position is preferred. If the patient will be supine for an appreciable length of time, the head of the bed should be elevated approximately 30 degrees to prevent circulatory and respiratory disturbances. She should conserve her physical and nervous energy for the more demanding period of labor to come. Her temperature, pulse, and respiration should be taken at least every 4 hours, and more often if individual history or indications warrant it. Many clinicians are advising blood pressure be taken routinely every hour. Fetal heart tones should be checked at approximately 15- to 30-minute intervals or more often during the first stage of labor, with increasing frequency as labor progresses. The amount and character of any show or amniotic drainage, if present, should be noted. At times a question may exist whether or not the bag of waters has broken. It is important to try to determine the time of its rupture, since the possibility of uterine infection after rupture becomes greater as the hours go by before birth. Such a situation may be detrimental to both mother and child. To help find out whether any vaginal leakage is amniotic fluid, the nurse (before

Text continued on p. 118.

TABLE 7-2   THE TYPICAL WOMAN IN NORMAL LABOR

Stages of labor	Physical and psychological characteristics, contraction patterns	Suggested activity, including relaxation and breathing techniques	Recommended nursing care, common physician orders
STAGE I CERVICAL EFFACEMENT AND DILATATION TO 10 CM			
Time range Primipara—10 to 12 hours Multipara—6 to 8 hours Early labor 0 to 4 cm	Cervical dilatation begins; minimal show characteristic; contractions variable, approximately 20 to 35 seconds at 5- to 8-minute intervals; possible backache; intensity of contractions increasingly strong but tolerable Alert, talkative, nervous; may welcome diversion, conversation; coach at bedside	If membranes not ruptured: may prefer to be up and about labor room or unit; when contractions cannot be ignored, slow, deep chest or abdominal breathing, and other relaxation techniques If membranes ruptured: if presenting part not engaged—confined to bed; relaxation techniques as above; if possible, turn to left side, elevate head slightly; should not remain flat on back	*Admission procedures* Welcome, orientation, individual patient assessment Review of prenatal records—TPR, BP, FHR; presentation, cervical dilatation, membranes, station, contractions, show Opportunity to void—urine specimen? enema? perineal preparation? electronic monitor application? *Follow-up nursing duties* TPR and BP at least every 4 hours; BP hourly? FHR, contraction pattern, show, amniotic fluid, labor tolerance every 15 to 30 minutes or less; teach breathing, relaxation IV?—check on need to void every 2 hours or less
Midlabor 4 to 8 cm	Contractions approximately 40 to 60 seconds at 3- to 5-minute intervals; intensity increasing but may still be manageable Becoming less outgoing, more introverted, concentrating on breathing patterns Increased reliance on nurse and coach	Usually confined to bed; more concentration needed; increased emphasis on breathing and relaxation techniques; accelerated shallow panting, effleurage; continued need of encouragement	*Follow-up nursing duties* As above, evaluation of efficacy of breathing, relaxation, teach simple techniques prn; encourage and praise husband/coach and patient; need for medication? Other possible nursing responsibilities: Mouth care, cool cloth, back support, massage, encouragement, aid in maintaining concentration; rectal or vaginal examinations as indicated; prepare delivery room; maintain electronic monitoring, if used
Transition 8 to 10 cm	Most difficult period during labor Fatigued, perhaps nauseated; focus loss of controls, contrac	Switching to more intensive breathing patterns—high chest, pant-blow transition techniques	*Scheduled nursing duties* As above plus increased emotional support, observation for onset of stage II, descent of

...plaints of rectal pressure, desire to push, bulging perineum and caput

Move multipara to delivery room?

STAGE II FROM COMPLETE DILATION (10 cm) TO BIRTH OF BABY

Time range			Scheduled nursing duties
Primipara—30 minutes to 2 hours	Cervix completely dilated; patient desires to push; perineum bulging, anus dilated, contractions long but less frequent; show at maximum of normal	Supine pushing patterns	Check perineum frequently during contractions for signs of progress, FHR every 5 to 10 minutes; stay with patient; move primipara to delivery room when crowning; sterile perineal prep; assist physician
Multipara—20 minutes to 1½ hours	Encouraged by progress made; using all resources for pushing; perhaps drowsing between contractions or intensely aware and alert regarding progress of labor	Rest, doze between contractions—head elevated	Possible anesthesia offered; spinal, epidural, pudendal block, local, or general

STAGE III FROM BIRTH OF BABY TO DELIVERY OF PLACENTA

Time range			
Primipara—5 to 20 minutes	Excited, extremely anxious and curious about infant; reactions vary according to individual and type of birth preparation and anesthesia received	Inspection and touching of newborn, possible breast feeding; may recommence pushing to deliver placenta when separation occurs	Oxytocics as ordered; care for infant, allowing parents to observe; check for abnormality, warmth, eye prophylaxis, identification, cord, Apgar evaluation; assist physician in obtaining cord blood, preparing to suture lacerations or episiotomy as needed; observe mother for relaxed fundus, hemorrhage, problems in delivery of placenta, and interaction with infant
Multipara—5 to 20 minutes (time depends on techniques employed)	Possible resumption of contractions	Resting, visiting with husband or companion and baby	
	Separation and delivery of placenta		

STAGE IV FROM DELIVERY OF PLACENTA TO POSTPARTUM "STABILIZATION"

Time range			
2 to 4 hours	Fundus firm, at or below umbilicus	Quiet, recovery period	Transfer to postpartum recovery area; admission temperature check
	Lochial flow moderate	Visit with husband or companion and baby if possible	Provide period for bonding to continue, if possible
	Relieved that labor has ended	Refreshing bath	BP, P, R, lochial flow and fundus check every 15 minutes for at least 2 hours
	Animated or exhausted; great individual differences seen	Light meal?	Observe for voiding problems
			Observe response to type of analgesia, anesthesia

TABLE 7-3   SUMMARY OF SUGGESTED BREATHING AND RELAXATION TECHNIQUES

Labor phase	Breathing-relaxation techniques, instructions to patient	Suggestions and diagrams
STAGE I		
Early 　0 to 4 cm	Practice distraction When contractions cannot be ignored, use deep chest or abdominal breathing 　1. Cleansing breath 　2. Focal point 　3. 6 to 9 slow breaths/min (in nose, out pursed lips) 　4. Effleurage? 　5. Cleansing breath Possible pelvic rocking, sacral support Relaxation checks	If possible (membranes intact), stay up— walk, play games, plan a vacation, make out the grocery list, etc. 
Midlabor 　4 to 8 cm	Begin when needed: Accelerated-decelerated shallow panting 　1. Cleansing breath 　2. Focal point 　3. Rhythmic slow acceleration-deceleration with contraction 　4. Effleurage 　5. Cleansing breath Sacral support Relaxation checks Increasing coach support	Mouth care Cool cloth 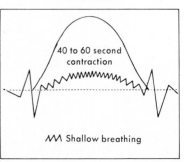

TABLE 7-3 SUMMARY OF SUGGESTED BREATHING AND RELAXATION TECHNIQUES—cont'd

Labor phase	Breathing-relaxation techniques, instructions to patient	Suggestions and diagrams

Transition 8 to 10 cm	Begin when needed:
	Pant-blow breathing
	  1. Cleansing breath
	  2. Focal point
	  3. 4 to 6 shallow breaths, then short blow during length of contraction
	  4. Cleansing breath
	Intensified coach support
		Mouth care
		Cool cloth

STAGE II

From complete dilatation to birth of baby	Begin when completely dilated:
	Pushing technique
	  1. Cleansing breath
	  2. Elevate head and back; second deep breath
	  3. Hold it, trapping air in chest; bend and drop knees to side; pull on thighs, knees, or bed rails while pushing down toward rectum; keep hips motionless on bed
	  4. Quickly take second breath if need more air; avoid short, choppy pushes; push for as long as contraction present to make progress
	  5. Cleansing breath
	Rest; doze between contractions
	Maximum coach support
		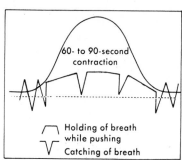

any antiseptic or lubricant other than water is used on the perineal area) may gently insert a sterile applicator or gloved finger into the vaginal canal to be moistened by the fluid present. It is then pressed against a strip of phenaphthazine (Nitrazine paper). If the paper turns blue indicating alkaline drainage, probably the moisture is amniotic fluid—if it is uncontaminated by blood. A yellow or acidic reaction usually indicates urine.

RUPTURE OF THE MEMBRANES (SPONTANEOUS)

If the bag of waters breaks at any time while the patient is in the labor area (if not ruptured before admission), she should be instructed not to get out of bed or sit up completely. The nurse inspects the perineum for signs of a prolapsed cord or, in the case of advanced labor, evaluates signs of the advance of the presenting part (bulging perineum, appearance of the fetal scalp) and the amount and color of the amniotic fluid. Normal fluid is very light yellow. If there is any meconium (infant stool) in the fluid, staining it a brownish-yellow to gray-black, it should be reported immediately. Meconium-stained amniotic fluid during cephalic presentation is considered a sign of fetal distress—the response of the fetus to oxygen lack. Such staining during a breech presentation is usually not considered significant, since the pressure exerted on a breech during its passage through the pelvic canal may cause the discharge of meconium, and no real fetal distress may be involved. The appearance of red-tinged amniotic drainage or old, dark blood, or bright red, frank bleeding at any time during labor should also be reported. Fetal heart tones should be checked immediately after the rupture of the membranes to try to detect possible cord prolapse. The fact that the bag of waters appears to have ruptured should be reported to the head nurse immediately. Contractions should be frequently evaluated, depending on the progress the patient seems to be making.

EVALUATION OF PROGRESS

Rectal or vaginal examinations. Proof of the progress may be gained through rectal or vaginal examinations. Vaginal examinations have been increasingly employed because of the greater accuracy and helpfulness of the information obtained and the lack of infectious complications observed when they are performed properly. Any pelvic examinations should be kept to a minimum because of the discomfort caused to the patient and the possibility of introduction of infection. Student nurses are not routinely taught the techniques of rectal or vaginal examinations. To instruct all students in the techniques would be useless, because unless these techniques are practiced frequently, the ability to interpret what is felt is never learned in the first place or is easily lost. In addition, the patient would have the discomfort of duplicate examinations. In the last few years it has become more common for LVN/LPN staff members assigned regularly to the delivery room area to be taught to perform rectal and vaginal examinations. LVN/LPNs frequently assist the physician and patient during such evaluations.

The patient is usually supine with head elevated slightly for either examination. The attending nurse prepares and assists the patient and helps her to relax during the examinations. If a rectal approach is to be used, only clean gloves and lubricant are needed. If a vaginal examination is desired (and this approach is now much more frequent), preparatory procedures will differ from institution to institution and physician to physician. In some instances the patient is cleansed and draped as for delivery, and the physician may scrub the hands with a brush before putting on sterile gloves. In other hospitals the preparation may not be so elaborate. However, certain principles should always be observed. The vulva should be cleansed. The examiner's hands should be carefully washed. A sterile examining glove should be used. A sterile lubricant and disinfectant should be poured over the gloved fingers and vulva. Care should be taken in inserting the fingers not to touch anything but the actual vaginal canal so that organisms from anal or other areas are not introduced into the canal. Usually it helps if the patient drops her knees toward the outside and breathes deeply through her open mouth during the digital examination. Squeezing the nurse's hand seems to give some patients great comfort, too. After the examinations, the patient's perineal area should be cleansed of any remaining lubricant or antiseptic, and she should be encouraged and reassured. A vaginal examination can reveal information not detected by a rectal examination because the cervix and presenting part are felt directly by the fingers and not through the rectovaginal wall. It may help greatly in the determination of the type of presentation, position, and the condition of the bag of waters. Pelvic evaluations should not be performed routinely if abnormal vaginal bleeding is observed, since such examinations may increase blood loss.

RUPTURE OF THE MEMBRANES (ARTIFICIAL)

At times, in an effort to induce or hasten labor or to apply an internal monitor lead, the physician will artificially rupture the membranes during a vaginal examination. This is done, however, only under certain conditions. The cervix should be effaced, and some dilatation must be present. The head should be engaged. The physician ordinarily uses a sterile instrument with a small clawlike end, such as an Allis or Iowa or special plastic hook. The membranes are ruptured between contractions and the fluid flow is controlled to avoid having the cord swept out of place by a sudden gush of "water." Prolapse of the cord and its subsequent pinching between the presenting part and the bony pelvis is a serious complication that must be watched for. Immediately after the membranes have ruptured, the fetal heart rate should be checked to determine any distress of the fetus. The actual rupture of the bag causes no pain because there are no nerves in the membranes, but the pressure exerted to do the vaginal examination and to position the instrument may cause some discomfort. The patient should be encouraged especially during this period. If rupture of the membranes is anticipated at the time of a vaginal examination, the patient should be placed on several bed-protecting pads to catch the drainage. Some advocate placing the patient on a bedpan; however, the patient's discomfort is usually

increased in such a position. The approximate amount (small, moderate, or large) of fluid expelled and its color should be noted and recorded. Remember, the appearance of meconium in the amniotic fluid during a head presentation is interpreted as a sign of fetal distress. After the examination the patient should be made as comfortable as possible. The excess lubricant should be wiped from the vulva, using good technique (wiping from front to back with no return of a used sponge to the vaginal region). Dry protective bed pads should be in place. The patient should be instructed to stay in bed.

Intensified labor: characteristics and care

As labor progresses, more frequent and intensive contractions are experienced. More and more the woman's attention is focused on meeting the demands of these contractions on her physical and psychological resources. If she has had training in relaxation and breathing techniques, these usually are of great aid. Abdominal and high chest breathing are described in Table 7-3. If a laboring patient has had no previous training in these techniques, she may still benefit from some simple instruction in abdominal breathing. This usually eases the discomfort significantly. Rapid breathing techniques can also be taught; but if the woman is unfamiliar with the method, she is likely to hyperventilate, and the normal proportion of oxygen to carbon dioxide in the blood will be upset. She may feel light-headed, and her fingers may begin to tingle. Such side effects should be avoided. If they appear, it may help if she breathes into a paper bag or places the sheet momentarily over her nose. The patient should be especially encouraged, and signs of her progress and condition should be frequently shared with family members.

Probably the most difficult period of labor is that called "transition" lasting approximately from 8 to 10 cm dilatation. The laboring patient is now fatigued and usually discouraged. She wonders if she is ever going to have her baby and worries about her performance when she does. Her contractions may be irregular, at times seeming to come "one right after another." Nausea and vomiting are common. She is usually most grateful for the presence of the nurse or labor coach, who can help tremendously by offering firm back rubs, sacral support, cool, fresh pillowcases, damp clean gauze sponges to ease the dry mouth, oral hygiene, or a cool cloth on the forehead. The husband or the chosen companion, can often help with these simple methods of relieving distress. The nurse should offer the bedpan at intervals or, if permissible, encourage the mother to ambulate to the toilet to be sure her bladder does not become distended. Distention may delay labor or, rarely, cause laceration of the bladder.

SIGNS OF THE SECOND STAGE OF LABOR

During this period, the patient needs to be evaluated frequently concerning the possibility of the onset of the second stage of labor, the period of expulsion. The physician and other delivery room personnel should be kept informed of the patient's progress. The second stage will ordinarily be heralded by (1) an increase in show, (2) an involuntary urge to push or bear down with each contraction as the presenting part escapes the uterus and descends, (3) the fetal heart tone usually being heard just above the pubic bone in head presentations, and (4) late signs, including the bulging of the perineum, the dilatation of the anus, and the appearance of caput, or the fetal scalp (Fig. 7-10). It is fervently hoped that a multipara will be adequately prepared for the actual birth before these last signs manifest themselves. Usually, multiparas are transferred to the delivery room at about 8 cm dilatation to avoid a last-minute race. However, women bearing their first babies many times are not transferred to the delivery room proper before these last signs appear, since the period between complete dilatation and the birth of the infant may be relatively protracted in a primipara. One of the reasons that the "birthing room" concept is popular is avoidance of patient transfers from one room to

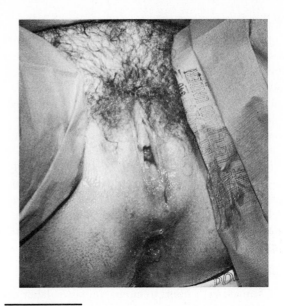

FIG. 7-10

Note bulging of perineum and appearance of fetal head (caput).

Courtesy Grossmont Hospital and Martin M. Greenberg, M.D., La Mesa, Calif.

another for different stages of labor. Such transfers can be quite difficult at times.

Many hospitals in the United States now allow fathers or the expectant mother's chosen companion in the delivery room, especially those who have attended childbirth education classes. The excitement and wonder of the occasion are appropriately shared with these significant persons. The father sits at the head of the delivery table, encouraging the mother in her efforts and watching with her the progress of the birth in an overhead mirror. For most couples, sharing the moment of birth together appears to create a "natural high" that they never forget. However, the father or companion will have previously agreed to leave in the event of problems when his presence is thought to compromise the best interests of the mother. Not all men want to see their children born, but for those who do, it seems to be a memorable, positive experience.

PUSHING

Although she may wish to do so, a laboring woman should not be encouraged by the nurse to bear down or push before complete dilatation of the cervix is determined. To do so could cause greater fatigue for the mother, greater strain on the fetus, and possible swelling and injury to the cervix. After complete dilatation and preparations for the birth are made, pushing is recommended. Unless experienced, the woman must be taught how to push to use her energy most efficiently. Most women are relieved by pushing and cooperate well in following instructions if they are not confused by too many instructors. (See Table 7-3.)

Preparation of the delivery room
(Figs. 7-11 to 7-14)

Before the second stage of labor is reached, the delivery room should be prepared for the actual birth of the baby. The responsibility of its preparation may be that of a trained vocational nurse. Hers is an important responsibility. To execute it correctly, she must have a clear concept of the principles of sterile technique, know where supplies are kept, know the patient's special needs and the attending physician's desires. She should have some idea when the room will be needed so that she can plan her work. The actual preparation of the delivery room will vary in different maternity services, but the basic needs to be met and the principles employed will be the same.

CAPSULE REVIEW OF PRINCIPLES AND PRACTICE OF ASEPTIC TECHNIQUE

The practice of asepsis is not really difficult if the appropriate equipment and supplies are available and if conscientious, knowledgeable persons are involved in their use and care. It is, however, a serious responsibility that involves evaluation of the area environment, including the nurses' dress and personal health problems that may possibly threaten the safety of the patient. Four simple rules sum up aseptic technique:

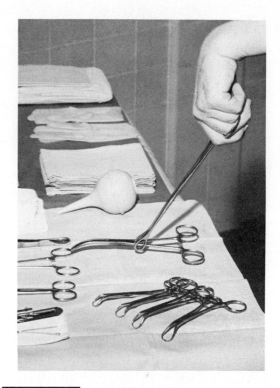

FIG. 7-11

Lifting sterile instruments. For beginners this is a good grip. The instrument is balanced and the hand is far from the surface of the table. Sterile supply tables may also be prepared using sterile gloves instead of sterile transfer forceps.

Courtesy Grossmont Hospital, La Mesa, Calif.

1. Know what is sterile.
2. Know what is not sterile.
3. Keep the two apart.
4. Remedy contamination immediately.*

Using transfer forceps. The use of transfer forceps in the handling of sterile supplies is as safe as the technique employed for their care. The forceps

---

*Hoeller, M.L.: Surgical technology: basis for clinical practice, ed. 3, St. Louis, 1974, The C.V. Mosby Co.

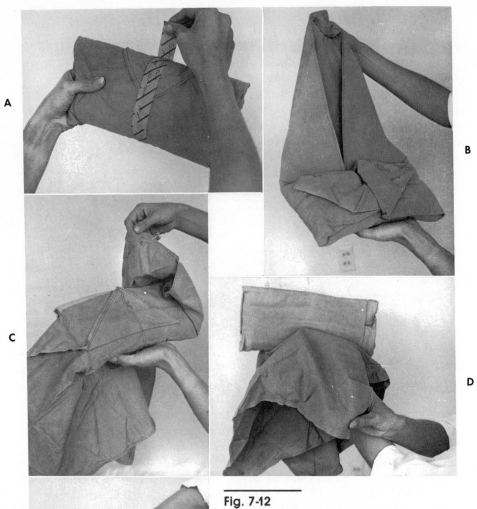

Fig. 7-12

For legend see opposite page.

and their holding canister may be steam sterilized periodically and the holding canister filled with an antiseptic solution between sterilizations to maintain the forceps' sterility, or a new, dry, sterile canister and forceps may be used for each birth. When wet forceps are used, care should be taken not to touch the ends of the instrument on any exposed inner side of the holding canister, since the area above the level of solution cannot be considered sterile because of prolonged exposure to the air. Some specially designed forceps and canister combinations include a lid, which reduces the danger of this complication. Sterile transfer forceps should not be held below the level of the waist or above the shoulder, and the points should always be pointed down. (Keeping the points of the forceps sloped downward is really only critical when wet forceps are used, but it is a good habit to acquire, since both wet and dry "lifts" may be used.) Nurses may also set-up a sterile table using sterile gloves.

General considerations. Review the methods of unwrapping and placing supplies. (Fig. 7-12). When approaching a sterile field to add sterile supplies, take care to avoid accidentally brushing or touching the area. When passing a sterile field, keep a safe distance away and, if possible, face the field. Never turn your back on a sterile area. Avoid turning your back toward an associate who is gowned and masked in a sterile manner.

If contamination of a sterile area does occur, the event must be immediately reported. It is no terrible sin to contaminate, although it is unfortunate. It is dangerous and irresponsible to contaminate a sterile field, know it, and do nothing about it when something could be done. No one at the time may see the lapse of asepsis, but ultimately the patient may suffer from its results. Everyone on the medical-nursing team should be glad to have breaks in technique or inadvertent contamination called to their attention so that they may correct the situation.

Delivery room setup reminder

Purpose: The purpose of this procedure is threefold:
1. To provide an aseptic field for the anticipated birth and subsequent newborn and maternal care.
2. To assure the convenient placement and operation of all necessary articles to promote safety, speed, and confidence on the part of the staff in behalf of the physical and emotional care of the mother and child.

FIG. 7-12   Opening sterile packages. **A,** Remove the heat-sensitive tape closing the package, checking the tape for color change, label and date. Start unwrapping the package with the point of the wrapper facing you. In this way the part of the package next to you will remain covered and protected for the longest period possible. **B,** Pull back the point and let it drop down after assuring yourself that the outside of the dangling wrapper will not contaminate any nearby sterile surface. **C,** Pull back the two side folds by the little turnbacks designed for your use. Uncover the end on the side of the supporting under hand first, then the side next to the active hand. If you are preparing the inner package for a drop onto a sterile surface, stabilizing the pack by bringing your thumb over the top of the wrapper before completely exposing the inner pack is sometimes helpful. **D,** Pull back the last fold covering the inner wrap to expose the sterile surface. The inner pack can now be picked up by a gloved associate or it can be "scooted" onto a sterile table while the ends of the outer wrapper are held back to prevent contamination. **E,** If the hand-thumb grip is used, the pack can be dropped in the manner pictured. Care must be taken not to get too close to a sterile table or field while adding supplies.

Courtesy Grossmont Hospital, La Mesa, Calif.

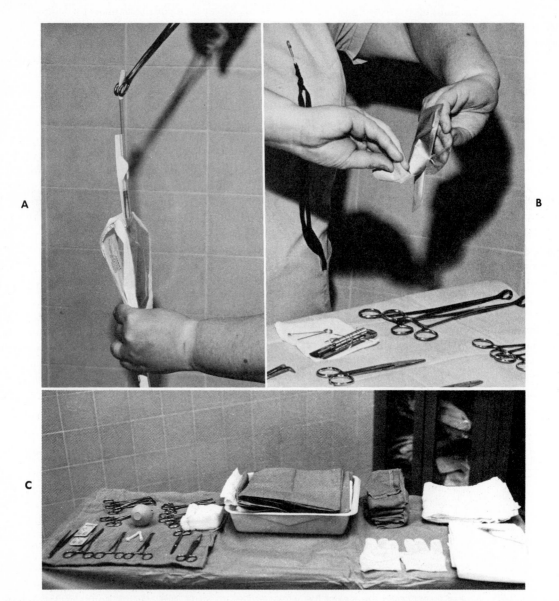

FIG. 7-13   **A,** Extracting a sterile catheter from a commercially prepared peel-back package.
B, Dropping sterile suture from a commercially prepared peel-back package. **C,** One
way to set up a basic delivery room table.

Courtesy Grossmont Hospital, La Mesa, Calif.

3. To aid in the necessary legal and statistical recording of the event.

Setup:

1. Personal preparation.
   a. Secure information.
      (1) Which physician (for glove size, etc.)
      (2) Which delivery room
      (3) Type of anesthesia to be used, if any anticipated
      (4) Special problems involving the patient (Rh-negative, preeclampsia, varicosities of the extremities, etc.)
      (5) Approximate time the room is needed
   b. Put on mask. Be sure all your hair is covered by a cap. Remember, you should not wear clothes worn in areas outside the labor-delivery suite in the delivery room proper.
   c. Wash hands.
   d. Review in your mind the principles of sterile technique.
2. Open necessary sterile packs. Check outside tapes on packs for proof of sterilization if this type of tape is used. Check dates on packs to avoid outdated materials. Usually included are:
   a. The basic delivery pack with drapes and materials used on the patient or to accomplish the delivery.
   b. The instrument pack (unless instruments are taken directly from a sterilizer.)
   c. The basin-set pack, used to provide a sterile basin for the placenta and a sterile basin for lubricating obstetric forceps, rinsing gloved hands, or cleansing the patient.
   d. The perineal preparation tray will usually provide:
      (1) A cleansing solution
      (2) Sterile gauze sponges
      (3) Sterile gloves or sponge sticks
      (4) An antiseptic to be used on the skin after the cleansing of the area
   e. The anesthesia supplies (if appropriate).
   f. Any indicated obstetric forceps are usually placed conveniently (still wrapped) in the room until called for, except Piper forceps used in breech deliveries for the aftercoming head. Piper forceps are usually unwrapped previously and placed on the supply table.
3. Check infant care equipment and supplies (warmer, suction, oxygen and bulb syringe, blankets).

4. At the time of the birth the necessary records are brought into the room for completion, and the identification procedures for mother and child are carried out.

Transfer and immediate predelivery care

The transfer of the patient to the delivery room should be as smooth as possible. If the patient has a strong desire to push and it is not appropriate activity at the time, she should be advised to pant through her open mouth. Care should be taken in the transfer of the patient. She can usually help considerably in the move to the delivery table if the staff is able to wait until a contraction is not present.

While the patient is being prepared in the delivery room, the physician may be dressing and scrubbing for the administration of the spinal anesthesia, if used (analgesia and anesthesia are discussed in Chapter 8), or for the delivery proper. The circulating nurse will uncover the sterile table and basin set and turn on the necessary lights. If no spinal anesthesia is used, the physician generally advises the staff when the patient should be placed in dorsal lithotomy position with her legs in supports, if this position is used.

POSITIONING

It is ideal to have two nurses assist in lithotomy positioning, although it can be accomplished by one. To prevent strain on the patient's back, both legs should be raised or lowered at the same time. Coaching her to bend her knees as her legs are raised helps. Remember, if crutch or stirrup-type leg supports are used, fit the supports to the patient; do not fit the patient to the supports! Often wrist restraints are not used. Most delivery tables have some method of dividing in half, temporarily eliminating the foot portion of the table to allow the buttocks to hang over the end of the upper part of the table and the physician to stand directly in front of the perineum. As soon as the patient's legs are

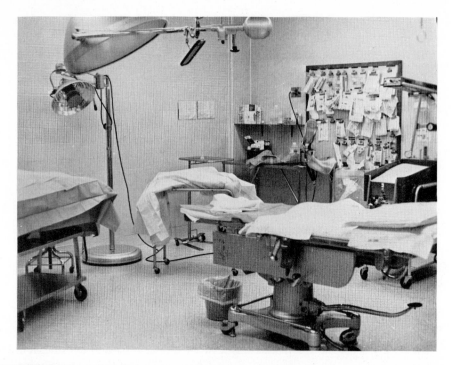

FIG. 7-14   A delivery room in readiness. Not seen are the anesthetic machine and maternal and fetal monitors.

adequately secured in the supports, the table is so adjusted. This is called "dropping," or "breaking the table."

Delivery in lithotomy position is not an anatomic necessity, but it is the position that is associated with the use of spinal or general anesthesia and is most familiar to physicians in the United States. In England a modified side position is often used. In some cultures the mother gives birth in a squatting position. In parts of Europe a modified Fowler's position is typically used with flexion and abduction of the lower extremities. These last two postures allow gravity to aid the mother in her efforts to push the baby to the outside world. Special adjustable combination labor/delivery beds are now available that assist the mother to maintain a more physiologic birth position (Fig. 7-15).

STERILE PERINEAL PREPARATION

As soon as the table is "dropped," the circulating nurse cleanses the abdomen, thighs and complete perineal area with a soap or antiseptic solution. This procedure is the so-called "sterile prep." Again, it is carried out in different ways in different institutions. It may involve sterile gloving or the use of sterile forceps or sponge sticks (Fig. 7-16). The principles are the same: The purpose is to help prevent infection and increase the visibility of the area involved. In performing the prep to prevent contamination of the birth canal, care should be taken to ensure that no sponge is used in the anal-rectal area and then returned to the vulvar region. Usually the first sponge is used to cleanse side to side from the pubic bone to the umbilicus. It is then discarded. The second and third sponges are

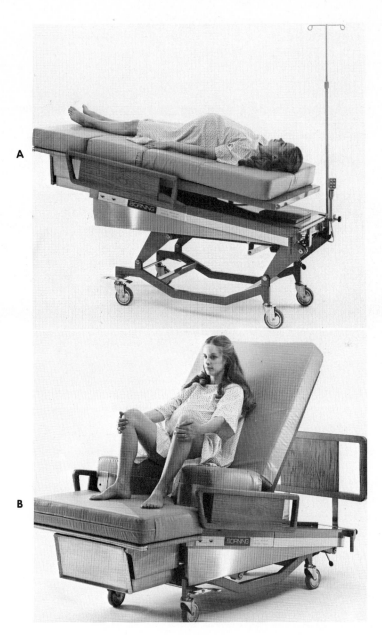

FIG. 7-15 Versatile multiposition maternity beds which may be fitted with stirrups if desired. **A,** The Borning 650 in straight-line Trendelenburg position. **B,** The Borning 650 HR shown in chair configuration.

Courtesy Borning Corporation, Spokane, Washington.

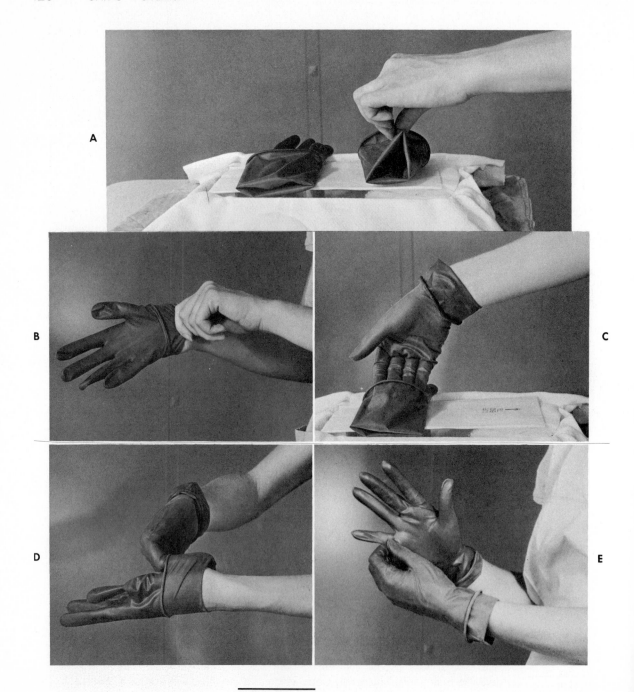

FIG. 7-16

For legend see opposite page.

used to cleanse the thighs with an up-and-down motion from the labia majora to the midthigh. Each is discarded directly after use. The fourth and fifth sponges are used to clean the labia on the right and left of the vagina, avoiding the rectum, and then discarded. The last cleansing sponge passes directly over the vagina and anus. The patient may be rinsed and dried in a similar manner and sprayed or painted with an antiseptic. The purpose of the prep should be kept in mind. The object is not to go through so many prescribed motions but to clean the skin. On the other hand, it must be performed rather swiftly, or the baby may be there before one is through. The gowned physician is usually ready to drape for delivery as soon as the nurse is finished. Care should be taken to see that the physician's hands or gown are not contaminated as the nurse completes the prep.

DRAPING

During the draping procedure, the circulating nurse provides a stool for the physician, pushes the sterile supply table and double basin rack into position, adjusts the light, unwraps the forceps if they are desired, secures any additional supplies if needed, and begins her record of the delivery.

After the patient is draped, no part of the exposed side of the sterile linen (or paper) covering the patient should be touched by anyone not properly gloved or gowned. If pressure must be exerted on the abdomen by a "nonsterile attendant" for any reason, she must reach under the sterile drape, avoiding the exposed perineum to accomplish her task. After the baby is born, if he is placed on his mother's abdomen, the nurse may reach under the covering drape and, using the drape as a hand guard, hold on to an infant arm or leg to help give support while he is aspirated or the cord is tied. Babies can be very slippery.

Delivery

FORCEPS AND EPISIOTOMIES

If the mother is bearing her first infant, many physicians will assist her efforts by employing outlet forceps to lift out the baby's head. This assist may also be given to multiparas. The forceps are applied after an episiotomy or planned incision of the perineum is performed. (See Figs. 7-17 and 7-18.) The bladder may be emptied by catheterization. Many times the episiotomy and judicious use of forceps considerably shorten the second stage of labor, if this is medically necessary and desired by

---

FIG. 7-16   Gloving Procedure. **A,** Sterile gloves usually lie side by side with the thumbs on top at the outside edges, the left glove on the left and the right glove on the right. Pick up the glove by pinching the cuff folded down over the palm of the glove. If right-handed, slide on the right-hand glove first. Your bare fingers may touch any area of the glove that represents the inside of the glove. **B,** Slide your hand in with a rotating motion while pulling on the turned-down cuff. **C,** Pick up the second glove with your gloved hand by sliding your sterile fingers *under* the turned-down cuff. **D,** Place your other hand into the glove, sliding and rotating your hand as you pull out and up against the inside of the cuff with your gloved fingers. Keep your thumb back out of the way. Remember, your arm and the top of the cuff are contaminated and must not be touched with your fingers. When only gloves are worn, it is permissible to retain narrow cuffs at the tops of the gloves, but they, of course, are not sterile and should not be treated as such. **E,** After you are gloved, you may adjust the fingers. Learning to glove takes time, patience, and usually more than one pair of gloves.

Courtesy Grossmont Hospital, La Mesa, Calif.

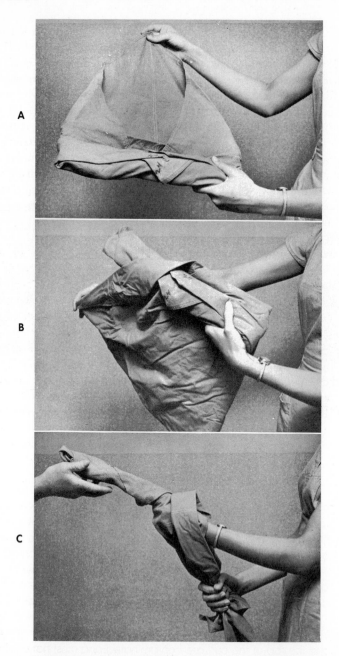

FIG. 7-17   Steps in unwrapping sterile forceps to hand to the physician. **A,** Grasp one end of the package, remove outer tape, and unwind outer wrapper. **B,** Pull back the inner turnback at the top of the package and continue to uncover the inner wrap (rather like peeling a banana!). **C,** Grasp carefully all dangling ends of the outer wrap and pull them out of the way toward your wrist. Do not touch the inner wrap!

Courtesy Grossmont Hospital, La Mesa, Calif.

the physician, especially when the use of general anesthesia makes it difficult or impossible for the patient herself to help push the baby. It also may avoid injury to the maternal perineum and the baby's skull. However, both the *routine* use of forceps and the episiotomy are now being questioned. An episiotomy may be cut from the vaginal opening straight down toward, but not extending into, the rectum (midline). It may be cut at 5 or 7 o'clock position from the vaginal opening to extend sideways away from the anus (lateral). It may originate in the midline just above the anus, but then angle to the left or right (mediolateral). The use of outlet (elective low) forceps is common. A midforceps is occasionally applied. The use of a high forceps is never recommended in modern obstetrics. It is too dangerous to mother and baby. Many babies are born without any previous episiotomy or forceps application.

DELIVERY MECHANISMS (Figs. 7-19 and 7-20)

If forceps are not used for the complete delivery of the head, it may be delivered manually between contractions by slow gentle extension. If the mother is able, she may be asked to bear down between contractions to facilitate the actual passage of the head from the vaginal canal. After the head is delivered, the physician checks to see if the umbilical cord is wound around the baby's neck. If it is, it must be slipped over the baby's head or clamped and cut to avoid strangulation or excessive pulling. Even before the entire body of the baby is delivered, the mouth may be aspirated to clear the airway. To deliver the shoulders, the physician usually turns the baby's head to the side so that the occiput lines up with his back. The physician may then gently but firmly pull down to deliver the top (anterior) shoulder and then gently pull up to deliver the bottom (posterior) shoulder. Scarcely before one realizes it, all of the baby has been born. Further aspiration of the airway may be necessary. Usually the infant cries very soon. His umbilical cord is tied or clamped and cut, and he is handed to the nurse for further care in such a way as to protect the physician's gloves and make a safe transfer. Increasingly the baby is being given to the mother

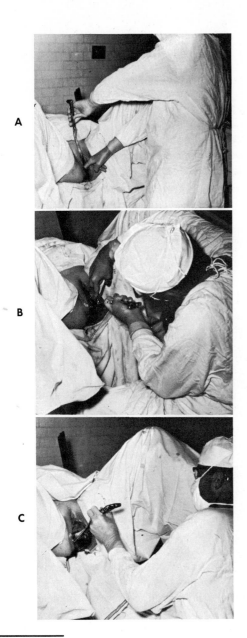

A

B

C

FIG. 7-18

A, Insertion of one forceps blade. **B,** Midline episiotomy (one blade of the forceps has been inserted). **C,** Use of outlet forceps.

Courtesy Wayne B. Henderson, M.D., San Diego, Calif.

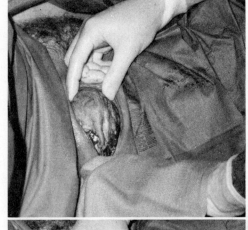

A

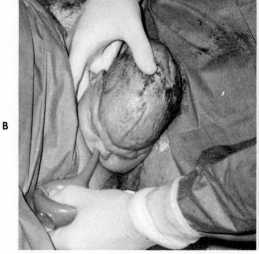

B

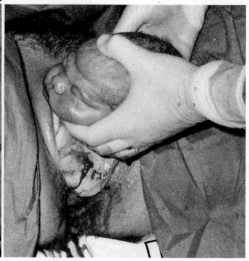

C

FIG. 7-19

Delivery sequence L.O.A.: **A,** Crowning; **B,** delivery of head and clearing of airway, mouth, then nose; **C,** delivery of posterior shoulder.

Courtesy Grossmont Hospital and Mark A. Treger, M.D., La Mesa, Calif.

or father to hold soon after birth. Maternal-infant skin-to-skin contact is believed to promote bonding. Infant heat loss is minimal or nonexistent, particularly if an overhead heat source is available.

THE BABY

Immediate care. The period immediately after birth is hazardous for the baby. Many adjustments must be made in his body to fit him for his new environment. He should be placed on his side and carefully and frequently observed. The nurse caring for the newborn infant should have freshly washed hands and wear a clean overgown. The nurse must provide warmth (usually in the form of an incubator, heated blanket, or a radiant infant warmer), observe his color and breathing pattern, and attach the identification approved by the hospital. During the same period of time, she usually performs the prophylaxis prescribed to prevent gonorrheal infection of the eyes (although some neonatologists state that it may be safely delayed up to an hour after birth to enhance bonding and early breast feeding). The National Society for the Prevention of Blindness and the American Academy of Pediatrics endorse the instillation of 1% silver nitrate ($AgNO_3$) solution into the newborn's

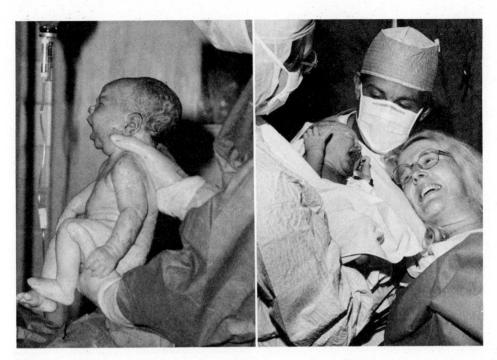

FIG. 7-20   A long-awaited personal introduction! It's good to have Father there for this special moment.

Courtesy Grossmont Hospital, Mark A. Treger, M.D., and Martin M. Greenberg, M.D., La Mesa, Calif.

eyes. They state that the eyes should not be subsequently irrigated with either saline or distilled water since irrigation will not reduce the incidence of chemical conjunctivitis and may curtail the effectiveness of the silver nitrate.* Because of sensitivity problems, penicillin is rarely used.

Apgar evaluation. If the Apgar method of evaluating the newborn infant is used, the infant should also be scored for heart rate, respiratory effort, muscle tone, reflex irritability, and color, 1 and 5 minutes after birth. This scoring may be done by the physician, anesthesiologist, or the nurse; but

the nurse is thought by some to be the more "impartial and available" observer, especially for the 5 minutes' evaluation. The Apgar score is used in follow-up studies of the child and is reviewed in many research inquiries. Infants receiving a score of 7 to 10 are considered vigorous. Scores 4 to 6 are considered to denote mild to moderate depression, while 0 to 3 indicates severe depression. The highest score that can be given is 10. Dr. Apgar believed that few newborn infants conscientiously scored deserve a first rating totaling 10. She believed that few babies are completely pink 1 minute after birth (Table 7-4).

The birth experience and immediate treatment of the newborn have been critiqued provocatively by the French obstetrician, Frederick Leboyer, in his book and film *Birth Without Violence*. His dramatic writings certainly highlight a facet of mater-

---

*Lum, B., Lortz, R., and Barnett, E.: Reappraising newborn eye care, Am. J. Nurs. **80:**1602-1603, Sept. 1980; Silver nitrate prophylaxis for gonococcal ophthalmia neonatorum, Center for Disease Control Morbidity and Mortality Weekly Reports, **27:**107, March 31, 1978.

TABLE 7-4   MODIFIED APGAR SCORING CHART TO EVALUATE NEWBORN STATUS
1 AND 5 MINUTES AFTER BIRTH

New name	Traditional sign	0	1	2
A Appearance	Color	Blue, pale	Body pink Extremities blue	Completely pink
P Pulse	Heart rate	Absent	Slow (below 100)	Over 100
G Grimace	Reflex response (e.g., to catheter in nostril)	No response	Grimace	Cry, cough or sneeze
A Activity	Muscle tone	Flaccid	Some flexion of extremities	Actual motion
R Respiratory effort	Respiratory effort	Absent	Slow, irregular	Good, crying

Total score: 1 min _____

5 min _____

Severely depressed   0 to 3
Moderately depressed   4 to 6
Vigorous   7 to 10

This Apgar scoring chart incorporates a concept first introduced at the University of Kentucky Medical Center, Lexington, Kentucky, by Robert Beargie, M.D. See Campbell, S.J.: New use for the APGAR name, Point of View/Ethicon **17**:6, 1980.

nity care that heretofore has received less attention. His call for more consideration of the sensory needs of the newborn would seem to be legitimate, although his methods have stirred much comment. For normal births he stresses the following: a quiet, dimmed atmosphere; support for the infant's spine; maternal-child skin-to-skin contact; an intact umbilical cord until pulsation has ceased; newborn body massage and a gentle body temperature water bath followed by warm wrapping and breast feeding. Objections most often voiced regarding his techniques involve the dimmed environment and adequate ability to observe, and the additional time and space needed to carry out his recommendations in busy maternity services. An increasing number of couples are seeking out physicians sympathetic to Leboyer's principles.

Third stage of labor

USE OF OXYTOCICS

In most cases some form of oxytocic is ordered after the birth of the baby and/or after the delivery of the placenta. Oxytocin (Pitocin) hastens the delivery of the placenta and is often used in an IV infusion following the birth of the infant. After the delivery of the placenta it is frequently employed to promote uterine contraction.

DELIVERY OF THE PLACENTA (Fig. 7-21)

After it has separated from the uterine wall, the placenta may be delivered through the bearing-down efforts of the mother if she is awake, or it may be expressed by the physician. This must be done

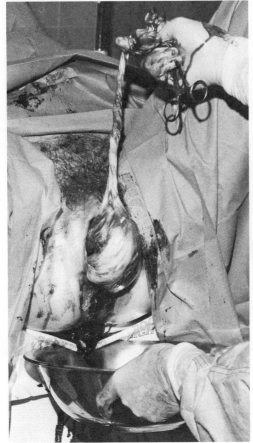

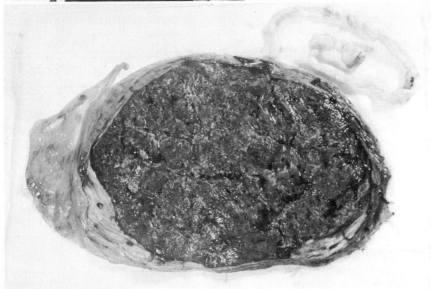

FIG. 7-21

A, Delivery of the placenta, or afterbirth. **B,** Maternal side showing cotyledons and membranes pulled to one side. The cord attaches on the opposite side. If this side appears first at the outlet, the placenta is said to have separated by Duncan's mechanism.

Courtesy Grossmont Hospital and Martin M. Greenberg, M.D., La Mesa, Calif.

Continued.

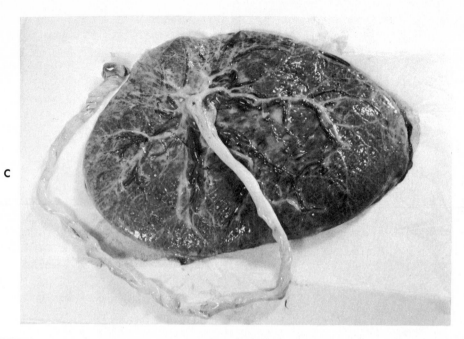

C

**FIG. 7-21,
cont'd**   **C,** Fetal side showing insertion of the cord. If this side appears first at the outlet, the placental separation is by Schultz's mechanism.

very carefully, and only when the placenta has separated and the fundus is firm; otherwise hemorrhage or inversion, a turning inside-out of the uterus, may occur, a grave maternal complication.

Signs of placental separation are (1) the rising of the uterus to or above the umbilicus, (2) the rounding out and firming up of the fundus, (3) the lengthening of the umbilical cord outside the vulva, and (4) a small gush of blood to the exterior. The placenta should be inspected to see if it was delivered in its entirety. Most physicians also perform an internal palpation of the uterus to assure themselves of its condition. In some hospitals, placentas that have not become contaminated with stool or were not born of women whose pregnancies were complicated by infectious disease, fever, or premature rupture of the membranes are saved and later processed by a pharmaceutical concern to extract the immune globulin they contain. The cords of

these placentas have also been especially evaluated and processed to provide vascular grafts to patients with circulation problems.

Immediate postpartum care

LACERATIONS

After the delivery of the placenta, any necessary perineal repair can be made (Fig. 7-22). Generally, if an anesthetic was used for a delivery, the same one can be employed. Sometimes a local anesthetic is administered. If this is used, the physician will need a syringe (usually Pitkin), some infiltration needles, and the local anesthetic of choice as well as the usual materials involved in a perineal repair. A seat and good light should be provided for the physician.

In spite of precautions, lacerations or episiotomy

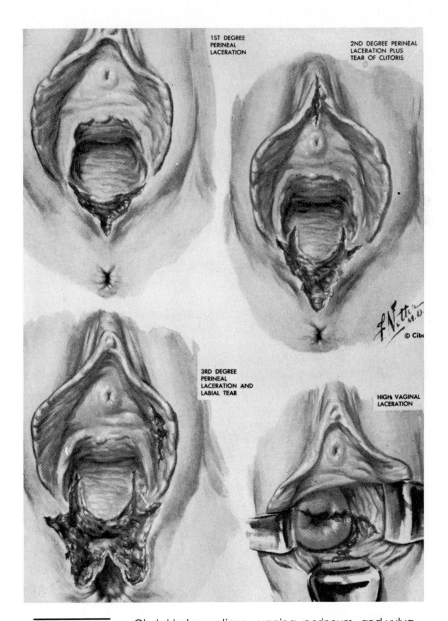

1ST DEGREE
PERINEAL
LACERATION

2ND DEGREE PERINEAL
LACERATION PLUS
TEAR OF CLITORIS

3RD DEGREE
PERINEAL
LACERATION AND
LABIAL TEAR

HIGH VAGINAL
LACERATION

FIG. 7-22   Obstetric lacerations—vagina, perineum, and vulva.

From The CIBA collection of medical illustrations, by Frank H. Netter,
M.D. Copyright CIBA.

extensions will occasionally occur. Some maternal tissues tear more easily than others. Very large babies or unusual positions are a special threat to the perineum. Lacerations of the perineum are described as first, second, or third degree. First-degree lacerations, involving a tear in the mucous membrane and skin only, are fairly common and usually of no permanent consequence. Second-degree lacerations include a tear into the muscles of the perineal block, but exclude the rectal sphincter. Adequately repaired, they usually heal well with little problem. Third-degree lacerations, which by definition involve the circular anal sphincter muscle, however, are more difficult to repair and may result in permanent damage to the perineum and sphincter (review the anatomy of the pelvic floor). To avoid third-degree lacerations or episiotomy extensions that are uncontrolled and more difficult to repair, some physicians are purposely cutting the rectal sphincter (performing an episioproctotomy) when the perineum is endangered. Lacerations may involve areas other than the true perineum. Tears of the labia, interior vaginal wall, and cervix are not uncommon. All these areas should be inspected for such possibilities after a birth.

If repair is nonexistent, inadequate, or improper, the patient is soon a possible candidate for hemorrhage, hematoma, and infection. As weeks and years pass, certain pelvic displacements and malfunctions may show themselves. The woman may be troubled with urinary or fecal incontinence, or she may suffer from a sagging of the pelvic musculature. When the tissue wall between the bladder and the vagina becomes abnormally relaxed, usually because of previous injury, the bladder drops out of place and pushes the anterior vaginal wall backward. The resulting abnormal condition is called a *cystocele*. A similar hernialike abnormality involving the rectovaginal wall and a falling forward of the rectum is what is known as a *rectocele*. Small rectoceles or cystoceles are usually asymptomatic and are not surgically repaired. Large abnormalities of this type, however, may cause complaints such as a "dragging sensation" in the pelvis and conditions such as stress incontinence, urinary retention, and cystitis in the case of cystocele or constipation and hemorrhoids in the case of rectocele. A vaginal repair of these difficulties, or colporrhaphy, may be performed. If both a bladder and a rectal prolapse are surgically treated, the procedure is often called an A and P (anterior-posterior) repair. *Prolapse*, or a falling out of place of the uterus, often accompanies these other displacements. Occasionally abnormal canals or tracts between two body cavities or a body cavity and the exterior develop as a result of obstetric injury. These tracts, most often found between the vagina and the urethra or between the vagina and the rectum, are termed *fistulas* and are difficult to eliminate. An adequate early repair of any obstetric injuries to the birth canal or its supports is very important to continuing good health.

After birth the baby is shown or given to the mother. The infant may remain with her and her husband or companion for a more extended period designed to promote bonding, or he may be taken to the nursery with his birth records after only a short interval. If mother is not alert, definite arrangement should be made for her to see the infant later as soon as she is able.

With the termination of any repair and the cleansing of the perineum, the head and foot of the delivery table are again realigned, and the patient's legs removed from the stirrups or supports. The perineal pads are attached, and a warm, clean hospital gown replaces the one worn by the patient during the birth. She is covered by a warm blanket. In some maternity services any initial preparation of the breasts of nursing mothers is done at this time also. Some mothers nurse their babies while still on the delivery table or in the delivery room if the baby is in good condition and free of excessive mucus and the new mother is alert and so wishes. The nursing of a baby directly following delivery of the placenta has a physiologic basis, since stimulation of the breasts causes the uterus to contract and helps prevent blood loss when other means of control are not available (something to remember in a disaster situation). The early establishment of an intimate mother-child relationship involving touch and nourishment is also considered one way to promote positive maternal emotions or maternal attachment. For some mothers who are not troubled by the relative lack of privacy and are not too tired, this opportunity may be cherished.

OBSERVATION

Throughout this early postpartum period, often called the fourth stage of labor, the patient is being observed for excessive bleeding and signs of shock. The blood pressure and pulse are frequently determined and the respirations observed. The uterus is palpated frequently to discover any relaxation of the fundus. If an intravenous infusion is in place (often used in conjunction with spinal anesthesia), it is carefully watched for rate of administration and possible infiltration. Many of these infusions contain an oxytocic and should not be given rapidly. Great care should be exercised to ensure that the needle is not dislodged during the transfer of the patient from the delivery table. Several hands may be needed for this project if the patient has an intravenous infusion and is temporarily unable to use her legs properly because of the lingering effects of spinal anesthesia, or the staff may be fortunate in having a mechanical aid for the patient transfer. The new mother may remain in the delivery room suite for a specified time for close observation near equipment that may be needed, or she may be transferred to a special postpartum recovery room. At the time of her various changes in location, special attention should be given to the transfer of her personal belongings. Family members should see her as soon after the birth as is appropriate.

Alternative childbirth arrangements

The labor-delivery procedures just described could be called a "modified traditional" hospital maternity experience, although different hospitals incorporate their own variations. Within the last few years a growing number of couples have wished to investigate alternatives to birth in traditional hospital settings. Several reasons are given for their search for other childbirth arrangements. They include a desire for a more relaxed, "personal" atmosphere and more flexibility in the types of care offered with the possible presence of other family members and friends (including, in some instances, sibling observation of the event); a perceived in-hospital attitude that childbirth is an abnormal or pathologic process; a wish for a birth with less medical intervention (for example, obligatory fetal monitoring, administration of drugs, artificial rupture of the bag of waters, routine transfer from the labor area to a "delivery room," episiotomy, and forceps application); an expressed need to have the newborn near at hand; disappointment because of lack of or organization of rooming-in accommodations; concern over possible infant contact with "hospital germs"; lack of rest; and the high cost of hospitalization.

It is important that hospital administrators, physicians, and nurses examine and evaluate these reasons. Consumer discontent may be valid and unnecessary in many instances. The rationale of some hospital routines may be questioned. The alternatives that some families have chosen may not sufficiently recognize that although childbirth is a physiologic process, it can be complicated by unexpected considerations that call for decisions based on professional expertise and experience.

Alternatives to so-called traditional hospital birth vary in availability and safety. Some parents have decided to give birth at home. The birth attendant may be a physician, certified nurse-midwife, lay-midwife, friend, or father. The legality and proficiency of the attendant differs depending on locale and circumstances. Although a minority of physicians will attend home births for selected "low-risk" women, many will not. They contend that although other developed countries such as Great Britain and the Netherlands offer home birth to certain women, the health care system in the United States is not organized to render such care routinely with safety. They cite the small but important percentage (5% to 10%) of mothers and infants

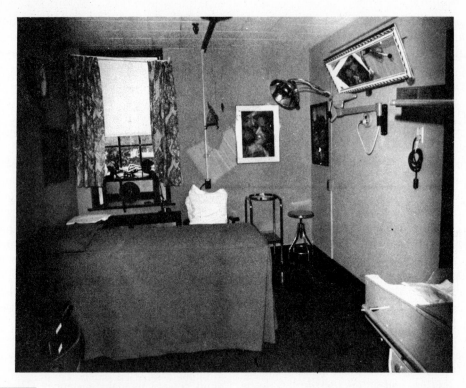

FIG. 7-23   A "birthing room" at Manchester Memorial Hospital in Connecticut. Note overhead mirror and lamp and infant warmer. This simple room is done in warm gold tones.

From Sumner, P.E., and Phillips, C.R.: Birthing rooms: concept and reality, St. Louis, 1981, The C.V. Mosby Co.

who, although not considered high risk, develop problems during the labor-birth period. They are concerned about the possibility of professional backup in the event they cannot attend the birth and the threat of malpractice judgments. They are also influenced by the accessibility of hospital facilities and perinatal centers.

Another method of meeting the objections to traditional childbirth is the use of a birthing room or an alternative birth center (ABC), which is part of or near a hospital or clinic where emergency equipment and staff are available if needed. It is typically designed to care for uncomplicated births in a homelike setting. Such centers have liberal visitation policies and usually discharge the mother and baby several hours after birth. Early follow-up nursing visits are made to the home. Most of these

centers have been in operation a relatively short time. They may use nurse-midwives as well as physicians to monitor the labor and assist at the birth.

While most "alternative birth programs"—to help rule out high-risk situations—require that expectant parents meet rather elaborate criteria before they are approved to participate, the Manchester Memorial Hospital in Connecticut has developed maternity care which includes the "birthing room" concept for *all* women anticipating vaginal childbirth* (Fig. 7-23). Each of its three

---

*Manchester Memorial Hospital established the first modern inhospital birthing room in the United States in 1969. For more details of its experience, you are invited to read: Sumner, P.E., and Phillips, C.R.: Birthing room: concept and reality, St. Louis, 1981, The C.V. Mosby Co.

birthing rooms is designed to handle most obstetrical needs except general or spinal anesthesia, cesarean births, and "difficult obstetric procedures." Mothers who elect to complete their births in these rooms have usually taken childbirth education classes. They may labor with limited or no analgesic drugs and may be given modified paracervical, pudendal or local anesthesia. Traditional delivery rooms are also available as needed or requested. The optional assignment of a nurse-monitrice who usually remains with the parturient until after her labor is ended is also a strong factor in the success of this program. A trained, informed mother attended throughout labor by a skillful nurse-monitrice has valuable supports that speed and enhance her childbirth experience and that of her family and newborn infant.

It will be extremely interesting to observe how maternity care services in the United States will be structured in another 10 years. Certainly they are undergoing a period of intense scrutiny, evaluation, and change. Since families are so diverse in their expectations, desires, and needs, perhaps a "cafeteria of options" (without sacrificing valuable maternal and neonatal safeguards) could be developed to provide true family-centered maternity care.

Special situations

Because questions always develop concerning them, we will now take time to consider some special situations that occasionally arise in the labor-delivery sequence.

PRECIPITATE DELIVERY

First to be considered is what is termed "precipitate delivery." This means a birth that occurs with such speed and in such a situation that proper preparation and medical supervision of the event are lacking. A multipara with a relaxed perineal floor may have an extremely short period of expulsion. Two or three powerful contractions may cause the baby to appear with considerable rapidity. In this instance the nurse may be the only one at the

bedside or delivery table to assist the patient. In no instance should she leave her alone. If it is obvious that the baby would be born before the delivery room is reached (for example, the patient is a para iii and the head is almost delivered), the nurse should do the best she can with what she has at hand. The call light should be turned on. If there is time and it is available, an antiseptic lubricant may be poured over the perineum. The nurse should wash her hands or put on sterile gloves and have a few towels handy.

Birth of the head. The baby's head should not be forcibly held back, since this may cause fetal distress and aspiration, but it should be restrained to prevent a rapid exit from the vaginal canal and greater possibility of perineal laceration or sudden decompression of the infant head with resultant brain damage. This restraint can usually be achieved by allowing the baby to emerge slowly against a guiding hand placed on the top of the advancing head. The fingers of the nurse should not enter the vagina. If the bag of waters is not broken, it must be pinched or torn to release the fluid and protect the baby from aspiration. The actual delivery of the head should be accomplished between contractions, with the mother panting or lightly bearing down as needed to assist. As soon as the head is born, the nurse should wipe off the face and check to determine whether the cord is around the neck. If it is, she should slip it over the head or shoulders to prevent choking. Rarely it may be too tight to slip over with the fingers. If this happens, it is hoped that sterile clamps and scissors are available in the labor room or that a staff member has answered the light and brought the emergency pack containing the clamps and scissors necessary to cut the cord. The mother should be firmly instructed to pant through her open mouth and not push during this interval.

External rotation and expulsion. After the head is delivered, the face wiped, and the location of the cord determined, frequently the rest of the child's body emerges without further assistance. However, if there seems to be no further progress and the back of the head has not already turned toward the mother's thigh, it can be turned in the direction of least resistance to line up with the child's back. There is no need to hurry. Next, the head should gently but firmly be directed downward to deliver the top shoulder. After the top shoulder is expelled, the baby is lifted up toward the pubic bone to release the bottom shoulder. The rest of the child is delivered without any particular problem. Before the birth of the baby, it is sometimes very helpful if the mother's hips can be elevated (or the foot portion of the table lowered a few inches) by another person to give more room for perineal support and the gentle up-and-down maneuvers described and to help keep the baby's face free of vaginal and anal drainage.

Immediate care of the baby. After the complete birth of the baby, care should be exercised that the airway be cleared. The baby should not lie in a puddle of amniotic fluid where aspiration can take place. His body should be supported on the nurse's hand and arm at the level of mother's uterus and tilted to "drain" without any tension being placed on the umbilical cord. After the airway is clear, he may be gently stimulated to cry, if necessary, and placed on his side—head slightly lower than his body—on his mother's abdomen. (Most of these babies cry immediately.) He should be wrapped in a towel or blanket for warmth. There is no haste to cut the cord, or for that matter to deliver the placenta. The cord can wait until proper sterile equipment is available. The nurse should wait for delivery of the placenta unless professional aid is very long in arriving or excessive bleeding occurs. However, if no professional help is forthcoming, if the signs of separation of the placenta have occurred, if the uterus is firm, and if the mother experiences a return of contractions, she may be asked to bear down to deliver the placenta. It should be supported as it is born so that the membranes are not torn. It should be saved for later evaluation by a physician. Usually the physician, who in the meantime has been contacted by the staff, completes the delivery of the placenta and repairs any possible lacerations.

A calm, reassuring manner on the part of the nurse (even if she does not really feel so calm) is very helpful to the mother and all concerned. Usually no great permanent harm results from such an event, but every effort should be made to prevent its occurring. All patients should be evaluated frequently for progress during labor. Signs of the approach of the second stage of labor should not be ignored. In such births the advantages of antisepsis and asepsis are largely lost, there is greater danger of injury to the maternal tissues, danger of aspiration and injury to the baby, and acute embarrassment for the patient, not to mention the nurse.

INDUCTION OF LABOR

At times in the labor suite there may be admitted a pregnant woman who is not in labor. She has come on appointment to have her labor induced.

Reasons for induction. Indications for an induction of labor may include: (1) a problem with erythroblastosis fetalis (isoimmunization), (2) prolonged rupture of the membranes after 37 weeks gestation without spontaneous onset of contractions, (3) increasing symptoms of preeclampsia, (4) postmaturity (baby *definitely* late in arriving), (5) maternal diabetes mellitus, or (6) fetal death without labor onset. Induction planned for the convenience of the patient or the physician is seldom considered a valid reason. Induction to produce abortion is discussed in Chapter 11.

Methods and care. Candidates for induction of labor must be selected carefully, since it is not a procedure totally without risk to the mother and baby. Today, labor is most often induced by intravenous administration of the synthetic pituitary hormone oxytocin (Pitocin or Syntocinon) or the artificial rupture of the membranes. The latter procedure alone is now less frequently performed. Unless the uterus is ready, labor will not occur. The cervix must at least be partially effaced and soft and pliable. If the membranes are artificially ruptured and labor does not begin within 24 hours, the increased possibility of introducing infection must be faced. Posterior pituitary hormone is very powerful and can cause violent uterine contractions which can lead to premature detachment of the placenta, uterine rupture, and fetal hypoxia. For this reason oxytocin (usually 10 units per 1,000 ml of 5% glucose in water) should be given only in small amounts per infusion pump. Another bottle of 5% glucose without oxytocin should be included in the IV setup (piggyback) allowing the nurse to discontinue the uterine stimulation if necessary while still maintaining access to the vein. Ideally, labor of the induction patient should be electronically monitored. A strip showing the FHR pattern before introduction of the oxytocin should be obtained. During induction, it is usually recommended that the FHR, maternal blood pressure and pulse, and the frequency and duration of any contractions as well as the quality of the uterine relaxation period be assessed every 15 minutes. Uterine contractions lasting more than 60 seconds or occurring more than every 2½ to 3 minutes, exaggerated uterine tone and poor relaxation, and signs of FHR abnormalities are usually indications to slow or stop the infusion of oxytocin. Rules regarding use of oxytocin for induction need to be determined and followed. The physician should be readily available in the event of problems.

CESAREAN BIRTH

With the decreasing risk involved in the performance of cesarean birth (the removal of the child through incisions in the abdominal and uterine walls), the operation is used more frequently in modern obstetrics. In fact, in 1980, many hospitals in the United States were reporting that approximately 20% of their births were by cesarean. The rise in cesarean births has been attributed to (1) a more aggressive approach to poor progress in labor, (2) an increased tendency to use cesarean for breech birth delivery, (3) a rise in repeat cesarean patients, and (4) the medical malpractice climate. Although electronic fetal monitoring may be a factor, especially when first introduced to an obstetrical service, with increasing staff experience in its interpretation, it is said to become a less significant consideration.

Reasons for cesarean birth. The most common cause for cesarean birth in the United States has been a previous cesarean birth. Some physicians

now are less reluctant to consider the possibility of a trial labor and vaginal birth if the reasons for the former cesarean birth do not persist. Others think the possibility of uterine rupture is too great.

Needless to say, a mother entering the hospital for a repeat cesarean is usually not enduring the stress of an unexpected surgery hastily arranged because of the appearance of an obstetrical complication. However, sometimes women who are admitted to the labor area will suddenly demonstrate symptoms that will suggest the emergency use of the procedure: conditions such as placentae abruptio, placenta previa, fetal-pelvic disproportion, abnormal presentations, prolapsed cord, uterine inertia (failure of the uterus to contract sufficiently to continue progress in labor), or signs of fetal distress. Conditions that indicate acute fetal distress or maternal jeopardy demand the prompt and rapid preparation of the patient once the condition has been discovered and the course of action determined. A patient scheduled for an emergency cesarean delivery is subjected to many procedures in a very few minutes. Everything should be done with as much calmness and dispatch as possible. The patient's morale should be supported as much as possible, because, if she is alert, she will probably be very frightened.

Preparation. The following procedures are routinely carried out:

1. Signing of the operative permit by the patient or responsible party
2. An abdominal-perineal prep, which starts at the nipple line and includes the entire abdomen from side to side as well as the perineal area visible when the legs are parallel
3. Insertion of an indwelling catheter—sometimes done in surgery after anesthesia
4. Blood type and crossmatch and hemoglobin determination
5. Removal of any hairpins or hard objects from the hair; application of a surgical cap; removal of cosmetics, any extra jewelry, glasses, contact lenses, etc., to be given to the family; taping of wedding and engagement rings to the fingers, but not so as to impede circulation

6. Removal and safekeeping of any dentures
7. Removal of any nail polish from at least two or three fingers of each hand so that the anesthetist can check for cyanosis of the nail beds
8. Preoperative medications as ordered

The patient is given nothing by mouth as soon as cesarean birth is contemplated, if this measure has not been instituted previously. If not already in progress, an intravenous infusion will be started.

Patients may be transferred to the operating room suite for surgery, or a delivery room may be prepared for the procedure. During all the busy preparations, any family members present should not be forgotten, and provision should be made for them to wait in as much mental and physical comfort as possible. Some hospitals are permitting the fathers to stay with the mothers during the section if general anesthesia is not used. Classes are now available to parents anticipating or interested in cesarean birth. (See also p. 201.)

BREECH PRESENTATION

Another situation that is fairly often part of the labor-delivery experience is a breech presentation.

Incidence. You will recall that approximately 3% of all births are breech. In former years, considerable effort was exerted in trying to turn these babies to a cephalic presentation before the onset of labor. Many were turned without too much difficulty only to revert to a breech before the time of labor. Many practitioners now believe that if a baby is found to be a breech, it is because of a valid anatomic or physiologic reason, and there are fewer attempts to turn the child (a process called version).

Complications. Although a breech presentation would probably not be considered an abnormality, it involves more risk to the infant than a cephalic birth, and the mother is likely to have a longer and more tiring labor. As a rule there is greater possibility of prolapse of the umbilical cord during breech labor, and during the delivery of the body of the baby it may be compressed against the pelvic outlet. The baby may try to take a breath before his

head has been born and aspirate tenacious vaginal secretions. Occasionally trouble is encountered in the extraction of the arms. Sometimes an unexpectedly large head may cause concern, and cerebral damage may occur. Although few maternity services today routinely provide a sterile scrub nurse in the delivery room, many physicians appreciate and request the help of such a nurse at the time of breech birth. Such an attendant usually helps support the baby's body or may, when instructed, apply fundal pressure when it comes time for the delivery of the head. A special type of forceps called Piper's forceps applied to the aftercoming head may be used at the time of a breech birth. They should always be on the sterile supply table when a breech birth is anticipated. The delivery of the head is often accomplished in such a way that the baby almost seems to do a guided half somersault over the mother's abdomen. A rather deep episiotomy is customary in breech births. The baby may have edematous or bruised genitalia. Today the physician often elects to perform a cesarean birth because of the increased fetal mortality/morbidity (10% to 15%) of a vaginally delivered breech. However, many of these breech births involve premature infants—another factor to consider when evaluating the statistics.

TWINS OR MULTIPLE BIRTHS

Twins are another interesting occurrence in an obstetric department. Twins occur about once in every ninety pregnancies. There are two types of twins—fraternal and identical (Fig. 7-24). Fraternal twins are the result of two simultaneous pregnancies developing from the fertilization of two separate ova by two distinct spermatozoa. They do not resemble one another any more than siblings resemble one another. They may be of the same sex or of opposite sexes. The placental circulation of each fetus is separate, although the adjoining placentas may be fused. Each fetus develops within its own amniotic and chorionic sac.

Identical twins result from the division of one fertilized ovum into two identical halves that develop into two similar individuals of the same sex. The

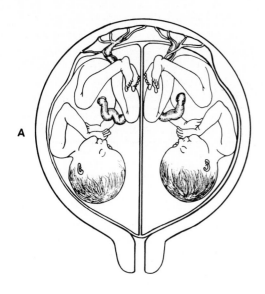

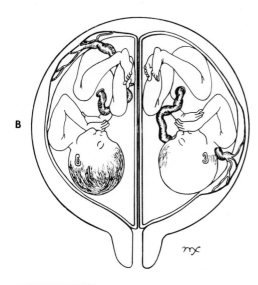

FIG. 7-24

A, Identical twins. **B,** Fraternal twins. Note differences in construction of amniotic sacs.

placental circulation is shared by the attachment of two umbilical cords. Each infant is encased in a separate amniotic sac but shares the chorionic sac with his twin. Fraternal twins are more common than those classified as identical. Approximately 54% of twins are premature, and the risk of intracranial hemorrhage, developmental respiratory distress syndrome, and other neonatal difficulties is high. Mortality for a second-born twin is about three times higher than it is for the sibling, probably because of a greater incidence of malpresentations. Thus the nursery should be alerted when a twin birth is anticipated. Occasionally, such an event is not anticipated, and the family, physician, and nurse are surprised to receive a "bonus baby."

Preparations and complications. When twinning is expected, two sets of identifications should be ready with double newborn record sheets. Two sterile baby receiving blankets, two cord clamps, and two aspirator bulbs should be available. In almost one half of all twin births, both infants are cephalic presentations, but any combination of presentations and positions may exist. Occasionally, the babies' relative positions may cause problems in their birth. Mothers of twins are more likely to suffer from preeclampsia and placenta previa and, because of the greater distention of the uterus, are more often victims of postpartum hemorrhage.

• • •

The nurse's experience in the labor-delivery room area can be a highly satisfying, rewarding type of nursing. If skilled in human relations and the observations and procedural techniques necessary to care for her patients, she can play an indispensable, gratifying role in a very crucial period in a family's life. The alert student in this area can learn much and gain an appreciation of and reverence for life that she will never forget.

CHAPTER 8 Pain relief during labor and birth

METHODS OF PAIN RELIEF

One should not leave the subject of modern childbirth without at least discussing briefly the most common methods being used to make the experience of labor and birth easier and more comfortable for the mother. The physiologic origin of labor pain has not been adequately explained. It results partly from intermittent muscular contractions of the fundus and stretching of muscle fibers of the cervix, lower uterine segment, and vagina. (Review the involved sensory nerve pathways on p. 22.) The amount of painful stimuli produced is also influenced by the individual patient's pelvic anatomy, the size of her baby's head, the strength, duration and frequency of her uterine contractions, and the presence or absence of certain obstetrical deviations or complications.

Within the last few years it has been found that a person's pain threshold also may be significantly altered by the level of available morphinelike hormonal substances in the body called endorphins. These special proteins appear to interfere with the transmission of pain-producing impulses to the brain or the brain's sensitivity to those impulses. The endorphin level falls in the presence of anxiety, tension, fatigue, or extended negative stimuli. This phenomenon may offer a physiologic basis for the observation that a woman's perception of pain and her resulting individual behavior is greatly influenced by her interpretation of what is occurring, the training she has received, her cultural background, and the emotional support she gains from those about her.

Therefore, methods of pain relief employed during labor and birth will involve more than the administration of drugs; they also include ways available to help the patient understand the process of childbirth better and to cooperate consciously with what her body is trying to accomplish. Usually a clean, calm, quiet, attractive environment, attention to techniques of relaxation, application of counterpressure to the mother's back, close supervision and encouragement from a concerned nursing staff and attending physician, and the companionship of those she loves will greatly decrease the need for administration of analgesic and anesthetic medications. Just what methods of relief will be used will depend on the patient's special needs and wishes, the availability of desired agents or equipment, and the expertise and willingness to utilize them.

Key vocabulary

Five words perhaps should be defined for use before a discussion of pain-relieving drugs or procedures is attempted.

amnesic A technique or medication that causes memory loss of varying degrees.

analgesic A technique or medication that reduces or eliminates pain.

anesthetic A technique or medication that partially or completely eliminates sensation or feeling. It may be a nerve-blocking type (local or regional anesthesia) or a sleep-producing type (general anesthesia).

hypnotic A technique or medication that causes sleep.

sedative or tranquilizer A technique or medication that relieves anxiety and quiets the patient.

Obstetric analgesia (first and second stages of labor)

The prescription and administration of analgesic drugs during the first stage of labor must be carefully considered and performed, but may be highly rewarding. The physician actually is caring for two patients. It must be realized that all analgesics may have a hypnotic effect not only on the mother but also on her unborn baby. Dosage and time of administration must be calculated so that the baby will not be "sleepy" at the time of his birth and too drowsy to want to breathe on his own. Before birth, sleepiness of the fetus is not so crucial because he does not have to breathe; he gets all his oxygen from his mother. But after birth, this oxygen supply is no longer available. Failure to breathe, or respiratory depression, results in a condition known as asphyxia neonatorum. If a premature birth is expected, the mother will be encouraged to carry through her labor with a minimum amount of analgesia because the premature infant does not detoxify drugs well and may exhibit respiratory depression at birth. Some antagonistic medications (for example, naloxone hydrochloride [Narcan]) are now available to counteract the depressant action on the newborn infant's respiratory system of drugs containing narcotics. Naloxone is very effective, though its dose may need to be repeated. It has no known detrimental action except when used to treat narcotic addicts or their newborns. Then it may precipitate acute withdrawal symptoms.

Another consideration in the administration of drugs during the first stage of labor is the possible effect of the medication on the progress of the labor. Given too soon during the latent phase, many analgesics may unnecessarily slow down or even stop contractions. Most physicians do not wish to give any drug before active labor has been established or approximately 4 cm of cervical dilatation has been achieved. Many patients will not need medication prior to or even after this dilatation has been reached.

ANALGESICS, HYPNOTICS, AND AMNESICS: EFFECTS AND SIDE EFFECTS

Frequently more than one drug will be used to gain the desired result. For example, the analgesic meperidine hydrochloride (Demerol) and the tranquilizer hydroxyzine (Atarax or Vistaril) are often given together with excellent results. Promethazine (Phenergan) and meperidine is another popular prescription. These combinations are more effective because they increase the analgesic effect and counteract the nausea often associated with the narcotic.

If an amnesic or hypnotic drug is given without an analgesic in the presence of pain, extreme restlessness can be produced in the patient. Amnesics, such as scopolamine, are occasionally ordered, accompanied by pain-relieving drugs such as meperidine. Scopolamine reduces anxiety and promotes amnesia for the period of labor. Scopolamine and morphine combinations formed the basis of the once-popular "twilight sleep." Many patients so medicated did not remember their labors, but their nurses usually did. Often the patients were so restless that it was difficult to minister to their needs. For this reason, this type of pain relief is not common today.

Intermittent inhalation analgesia used in the latter portion of the first and during most of the second stage of labor has had considerable popularity in certain areas of the world. The patient breathes anesthetic gases through a mask. When these gases are properly administered in low concentrations, the patient does not become unconscious but benefits from a real reduction in discomfort. Agents used (for example, methoxyflurane [Penthrane], nitrous oxide) may be self-administered by the patient using a specially designed dispenser, or they may be administered by an anesthesiologist or nurse-anesthetist using an anesthesia machine. It is important that such analgesia not become anesthetic in depth, since regurgitation and aspiration can become a real and deadly complication. Instructions for the use of various types of gases and equipment must be carefully followed. Inhalation analgesia usually does not provide sufficient relief for the entire second stage of labor. Often its analgesic effects are augmented by a pudendal block or infiltration of the perineum with a local anesthetic.

Obstetric anesthesia (first, second, and third stages of labor)

Anesthesia is the province of a trained physician, anesthesiologist, or nurse-anesthetist. Nurses should not attempt to function in this area without skilled advanced training. Administration of anesthesia is not a nursing function.

GENERAL ANESTHESIA

In obstetrics a general anesthetic may be inhaled or administered intravenously. Currently, general anesthesia is used in obstetrics much less than formerly for normal births. This is because of emphasis on parental participation and possible problems with the mother and baby previously mentioned and discussed below.

Special considerations. When a general anesthetic is planned, it is very important to know when the labor started and how recently the patient has eaten, because there is a real danger of aspiration, obstruction of the airway (asphyxiation), and pneumonia. The patient should be given nothing by mouth unless it is ordered, because during labor digestion stops and recent meals may remain in the stomach. Even if a woman in labor has not eaten recently, her highly acidic gastric secretions may pose the threat of acid aspiration pneumonitis (Mendelson's syndrome). To counteract this possibility, some physicians will order oral administra-

tion of 15 ml of an antacid every 3 hours during labor, and most order one dose an hour before a scheduled cesarean birth. Chilling the liquid antacid may increase its acceptance. In case of vomiting, the patient's head should be turned to the side or, if possible, she should be placed on her side. Chewing gum or dentures must be removed from the mouth before administration of anesthetic.

Some anesthetic gases used in the past were either flammable (ether, chloroform) or explosive (cyclopropane). Since other effective gases are now available that do not present these safety hazards, these older products have been essentially phased out or banned. This has largely eliminated the need to be concerned regarding the buildup of static electricity in personnel and other safeguards against explosion, and has facilitated the use of the cautery during abdominal deliveries.

Other considerations are also important when using general anesthetics. During the period when a patient is being put to sleep (the period of induction), the delivery room should be as quiet as possible to make the induction smooth without patient distraction. Undue confusion and noise should also be avoided at the time of emergence.

Because all anesthetics will cross the placenta, and, if given in sufficient concentration, will produce symptoms in the child, they should not be started too far in advance of the expected birth. When the condition of the fetus requires emergency cesarean birth or when rapid uterine relaxation is needed for various obstetrical maneuvers, general anesthetic may be favored. It does not cause the maternal hypotension that sometimes accompanies regional conductive anesthetics and may be administered rapidly with good results. Usually general anesthesia will be induced by an intravenous injection of a sleep dose of thiopental (Pentothal) and a paralyzing dose of succinylcholine (Anectine). This is followed by a rapid placement of a cuffed endotracheal tube into the trachea. The nurse may be asked to help at this time by pushing on the cricoid cartilage of the larynx (just below the "Adam's apple"). This helps close off the esophagus. Both cricoid pressure and endotracheal intubation help prevent aspiration. The anesthesia is then main-

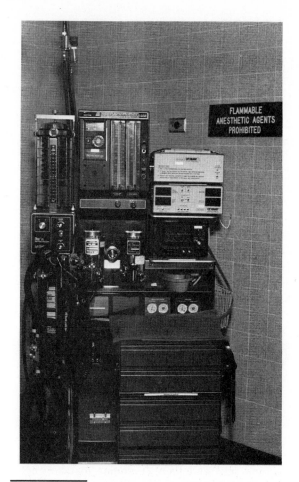

FIG. 8-1

General anesthesia machine capable of providing a number of gas anesthetics. Most hospitals no longer use flammable gases.

Courtesy Alex Pue, M.D., and Donald N. Sharp Memorial Community Hospital, San Diego, Calif.

tained with nitrous oxide, oxygen, perhaps halothane, and a muscle relaxant. Once the baby is delivered, a narcotic and a tranquilizer are usually given intravenously to complete the anesthetic. Oxygen must always be mixed with gas anesthetics to supply the body needs of the mother and her unborn child (Fig. 8-1).

Thiopental (Pentothal) produces a rapid induction by intravenous injection. If thiopental is given for only brief periods, the brain of the fetus is bypassed and little neonatal depression is seen.

Nitrous oxide (laughing gas) is often given for analgesic effect in the period of expulsion during contractions. Administered in low percentages, it relieves the mother's pain but still allows her to bear down with her contractions. When nitrous oxide is used as an anesthetic, care is needed to prevent maternal respiratory and neonatal depression. Nitrous oxide may support combustion but is nonexplosive.

Methoxyflurane (Penthrane) is a nonexplosive, nonflammable, fluorinated anesthetic that has a pleasant odor and produces good analgesia and relaxation. It requires a long period for induction and recovery. Methoxyflurane may be toxic to the kidneys in large doses. For this reason, it is used only in limited doses in obstetrics and is contraindicated in patients with renal problems.

Halothane (Fluothane) is a useful gas producing rapid uterine relaxation. It has been associated with uterine hemorrhage and hypotension if concentrations become too high.

Ketamine hydrochloride (Ketaject), given by intravenous injection, produces rapid anesthesia. It is useful when blood pressure tends to be low. It should not be used with hypertensive patients. It may be associated with dreamlike episodes and hallucinations. Reduced stimulation during emergence is recommended. Its use for obstetrical anesthesia is not widespread but increasing.

Cyclopropane was a useful, fast-acting gas that produced a fairly good muscular relaxation. It allowed a high oxygen concentration and a wide margin of safety for the mother and child. However, it was extremely explosive and could produce laryngospasm and heart irregularities. It is not being manufactured in the United States at the present time.

REGIONAL (CONDUCTIVE) ANESTHESIA

Regional or conductive anesthetics have become considerably popular in recent years.

Saddle block. The use of low spinal, or "saddle," anesthesia has been particularly successful. The patient is supported on the edge of the delivery

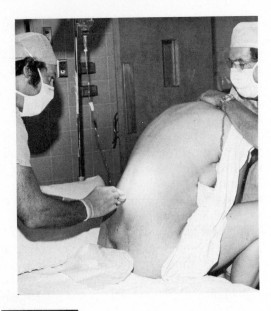

FIG. 8-2

Administration of a low spinal anesthetic.

Courtesy Grossmont Hospital, and Martin M. Greenberg, M.D., La Mesa, Calif.

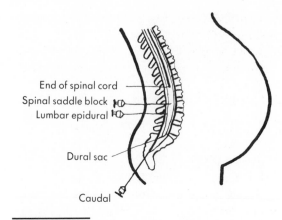

End of spinal cord
Spinal saddle block
Lumbar epidural

Dural sac

Caudal

FIG. 8-3

Types of regional anesthetics. The external sites for the needle insertions for the spinal approach and lumbar epidural may vary slightly depending on the individual patient and the extent of anesthesia desired. The main difference in the two approaches is the depth of the needle placement. An epidural injection does not enter the dural sac; a spinal does.

table in a sitting position or lies on her side with her back bent forward. The physician, using sterile technique, inserts a thin spinal needle between the vertebrae at about the level of the iliac crests. The needle tip is placed in the subarachnoid space below the spinal cord proper. Its position is identified by the appearance of cerebrospinal fluid dripping from the needle's hub. Between contractions, an anesthetic that is heavier than the cerebrospinal fluid such as lidocaine (Xylocaine) is injected into the subarachnoid space. The patient is then positioned on her back with left uterine displacement with only her head and shoulders elevated. Her legs are then placed in stirrups. Such positioning helps localize the anesthetic at the correct level in the spinal canal (Fig. 8-2).

Classically, a saddle block is only supposed to affect those areas of the body that would be touched by a saddle if a person were riding horseback. In practice the anesthesia is usually more

extensive. Low spinal anesthesia as usually used numbs the abdominal and pelvic areas below the umbilicus. It usually affects the abdomen, perineum, and legs and feet. It begins to take effect immediately and gains maximum potency in about 3 to 5 minutes. How long it lasts depends on the medication used (1 to 3 hours). Because of vertebral abnormalities, not all women can have spinal anesthetics. Very few are allergic to the type of medications usually injected. Sometimes lack of time or qualified medical personnel precludes the use of a spinal anesthetic.

Much has been said about the aftereffects of spinal anesthesia. The so-called spinal headache is a complication often feared by patients. Actually the incidence of postdelivery spinal headache has been estimated at less than 5%, and it is decreasing. The use of an intravenous infusion to promote better hydration of the patient and the use of only small-bore needles to cut down on the possibility of cerebrospinal fluid leakage helps prevent spinal headaches. It is debatable whether keeping the patient flat during the postdelivery period is helpful. Spinal anesthesia does entail certain other inconveniences, however. The mother must sit quietly while the procedure is carried out. This is difficult to do during the second stage of labor, even with the support of an understanding nurse. Saddle anesthesia does not stop contractions, but the patient does not feel them. She finds it difficult to push properly, and often outlet forceps are used. Occasionally a patient's blood pressure may drop, possibly affecting the baby's oxygen supply, or the patient may suffer from respiratory problems because of a high level of anesthesia. In the postpartum period the patient may find it more difficult to void spontaneously.

In the minds of many practitioners the negative aspects of this type of anesthesia are outweighed by its positive aspects. The baby is not in danger of being put to sleep by the anesthetic and of having a difficult time breathing at birth because of its action. The mother is awake. She may see her baby born. She can hear his first cry—a real thrill. The regional anesthetics are safer than "gas" for obstetrical patients who have recently eaten, since nausea and vomiting during and after their use are minimal and the patient is awake.

Caudal and lumbar epidural anesthesia techniques. Other types of regional anesthetics are available (Fig. 8-3). In considerable vogue for a time was *continuous caudal anesthesia,* or *one-shot caudal,* which introduces anesthetic agents into the sacral canal, where significant nerves travel outside the meninges or spinal cord coverings. Another kind of regional anesthesia, less difficult to administer than caudal, is called a lumbar epidural block. The drug is injected into the epidural space, usually between the second and third or third and fourth lumbar vertebrae, while the mother lies on her side or is supported in a sitting position. Following careful identification of the desired location, a vinyl plastic catheter is threaded through the needle at the insertion site and the needle is removed. The catheter is conscientiously secured in position with

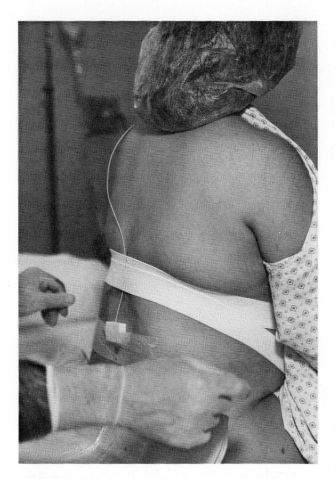

FIG. 8-4

The epidural catheter has just been inserted and is being securely taped in place. The white belts of the fetal heart and contraction monitors also help maintain the position of the catheter.

Courtesy Alex Pue, M.D., and Donald N. Sharp Memorial Community Hospital, San Diego, Calif.

tape. After a small "test dose," cautious instillation of the anesthetic is begun. Currently bupivacaine (Marcaine) and 2-chloroprocaine (Nesacaine) appear to be most frequently employed.

The patient should be alerted regarding what she may experience during the initiation of the epidural. She may detect a burning or stinging sensation at the site of the injection of the local anesthesia given before the insertion of the needle and cannula, local pressure during the insertion, and a "crazy bone" feeling in her leg, hip, or back if the flexible catheter touches a nerve as it is advanced in the epidural space. During the 5-minute period just after the test dose she should be especially observed for the appearance of hypotension and questioned regarding lower extremity sensory changes and loss of ability to move her legs. Such differences may indicate unwanted penetration of the dura mater. Such penetration is to be avoided since the larger amounts of anesthetic routinely used during epidural techniques, if introduced directly into the subarachnoid space, could cause dangerously high spinal anesthesia, compromising respirations and oxygen supply. Such a puncture could also predispose the mother to spinal headache. (See preceding discussion of saddle block.)

Another type of complication that can occur would be the rare unintentional injection of the anesthetic into a blood vessel. Such an occurrence may be first indicated by patient reports of ringing in the ears, light-headedness, circumoral tingling or numbness, and the sudden recognition of a "metallic taste." Convulsions may follow, at which time a side position, preservation of the airway, and oxygenation are necessary. Diazepam (Valium) or thiopental sodium (Pentothal) may be administered to stop the seizure.

When epidural dosage is administered during labor, the patient may remain on her side with her head slightly raised, or she may be placed in a modified supine position with a firm wedge-shaped pillow upon her right hip so that her uterus is tilted to the left. These postures are assumed to help control the level of anesthesia obtained and aid in preventing the weight of the uterus from compressing the maternal aorta and vena cava. This latter compression, which interferes with the circulation of the blood in the mother and eventually deprives the fetus of oxygen, has been called the aortocaval or supine hypotensive syndrome. (See also page 113.) Since maternal hypotension is already one of the looked-for complications of this method of pain control as a result of possible peripheral vasodilation caused by the block of certain sympathetic nerve fibers in the epidural space, it is particularly important to avoid all possible sources of the difficulty. The anesthetic may be infused through the catheter in small continuous amounts using an infusion pump or given intermittently when the analgesic action lessens.

Usually pain relief begins within 3 to 5 minutes after injection, and full effect is obtained in 8 to 15 minutes. According to one study* about 85% of the women receiving epidurals are free of pain, 12% experience partial relief, and a remaining 3% do not benefit at all. Many women will still confirm sensations of abdominal or perineal pressure and note weakness or numbness in their legs. Because of the loss of normal pelvic sensation coupled with routine intravenous hydration, many are prone to urinary distention. They should be asked to empty their bladders before the epidural is begun and should be watched carefully for difficulty in voiding.

Contraindications to this method of pain relief include current anticoagulant therapy, a history of or presence of hemorrhage or shock, septicemia or local infection in the area of the proposed injection, and various spinal problems.

Epidural techniques can be used to good advantage in the latter part of the first stage of labor and continued into the second and third stages. The patient is typically alert and comfortable. Those women wishing medication during their labors are usually enthusiastic regarding the method. However, epidural anesthesia requires the constant supervision of an anesthesiologist, special apparatus, and continuous or at least frequent maternal-fetal monitoring and support by the nurse. It is very important to detect signs of maternal hypotension and to evaluate the duration and quality of uterine contractions, progress in labor, and fetal heart rate response. The mother's urge and ability

---

*Crawford, J.S., Continuous lumbar epidural analgesia for labor and delivery, Br. Med. J. 1:72, 1979.

to push may be impaired, and forcep delivery is fairly common. Today this method of pain relief seems to be growing within certain groups in the United States.

Considerable research is now in progress regarding the subarachnoid (spinal) and epidural infusion of narcotics for pain management during labor and delivery and after cesarean section. These techniques hold promise for the future.*

LOCAL ANESTHESIA AND NERVE BLOCKS

Local anesthesia by direct infiltration of the perineal tissues or infiltration of those nerve centers which serve to relay sensation initiated in the perineal area to the brain is probably the safest anesthesia for both mother and baby available today. A popular technique called *pudendal block* stops sensory impulses from the pudendal nerve by infiltration of a medication into specific areas with a long needle. With its use, an episiotomy may be performed or outlet forceps applied. It may be used in conjunction with nitrous oxide satisfactorily. However, some women do not experience the relief they desire. Some pudendal techniques may cause temporary bruising of the perineum.

Paracervical block. Another type of nerve block that is being used much less frequently but is favored in certain circumstances by individual physicians is the paracervical block. Approximately 10 ml of local anesthetic is injected into the lateral fornices of the vagina at the junctions of the vaginal wall and the cervix that usually correspond to the 3 and 9 o'clock positions on the face of a watch. These injections, usually performed with a special needle guard to prevent unintentional deep infiltration, interrupts the sensory impulses traveling in the paracervical area from the uterus to the spinal cord. Anesthesia relieving the discomfort of uterine contractions develops in 3 to 5 minutes and may last approximately 1 to 2 hours. However, the procedure does not anesthetize perineal tissue and in most instances is not considered sufficient in itself to meet the total needs of the patient during the second and third stages of labor.

Paracervical blocks may be performed in the delivery or labor room when the patient has completed a cervical dilatation of more than 4 cm and less than 8 cm. Most patients report considerable benefit. (When properly done, the technique, barring personal idiosyncratic responses to the anesthetic employed, should have no adverse effect on the mother.) However, reports have associated fetal bradycardia with 10% or more of those labors where the technique was used, and there have even been some fetal deaths associated with paracervical blocks. The cause of this complication has not been completely identified. It is probably related to spasm of the uterine arteries or to high blood levels of the local anesthetic in the fetus. Bradycardia is more frequent when injections are repeated. A modified paracervical approach that features shallow submucosal injections of reduced dosage placed "well lateral to the cervix" seems to reduce the incidence of bradycardia.* Fetal heart tone should be checked frequently.

EDUCATION FOR CHILDBIRTH

Modern trends in obstetrics favor a more alert patient during labor who is able to participate with dignity in her experience of childbirth. To this end greater efforts have been made to educate the woman for her role, both psychologically and physically. Courses have been instituted to teach helpful techniques in posture, breathing, and relaxation, as well as to impart basic information about labor and birth to the expectant mother. Husbands or chosen companions are encouraged to attend the sessions to better understand and aid their partners.

The late English obstetrician Dr. Grantly Dick-Read probably popularized the term "natural childbirth" in his book *Childbirth Without Fear*. In his

---

*Downing, J.N., and Williams, V.: Spinal opiate analgesia for labor and delivery—a new era? Obstetric Anesthesia Digest **1:**121-123, Dec. 1981.

*Sumner, P.E., and Phillips, C.R.: Birthing rooms: concept and reality, St. Louis, 1981, The C.V. Mosby Co., pp. 130-133.

writings and lectures he stressed that much of the fear felt by pregnant women was caused by a lack of knowledge of what was really happening and an ensuing feeling of helplessness. He declared that fear builds tension and that tension eventually produces pain. Because of this, much of his effort was spent in educating the future mother and prescribing exercises to better fit her body for labor and birth.

In 1952 the French obstetrician Fernand Lamaze became intrigued with the labor and delivery techniques based on Pavlov's theories of conditioned response that he had observed during a visit to the Soviet Union. When he returned to Paris, he introduced "psychoprophylactic" concepts into his practice to better prepare his patients for their maternity experiences and to assist them in a conscious, rewarding participation in the birth of their children. Much of what he emphasized was also stressed by Dr. Read. However, the relaxation taught by Dr. Lamaze is based on the principle that a high level of concentrated cerebral activity can inhibit the reception of other stimuli. That is, the mind (psycho) could be induced to prevent (prophylaxis) the reception of unpleasant and painful sensations. Using the Lamaze techniques, the patient is educated (conditioned) to respond neuromuscularly to specific verbal cues. Intense preoccupation with certain muscular tension and release patterns, respiratory movements, and massage helps to attain these goals. A specially prepared labor coach, or monitrice, may be assigned to assist and support the patient in her efforts to utilize her training, or more often her husband or chosen companion fills the role.

The monitrice, if present, the patient's partner, and the entire labor-delivery room staff should work as a team for the realization of a constructive, dignified, aware, satisfying parturition. The attending nurses should be calm, cheerful, and knowledgeable concerning the aims of the techniques employed. The details of the exercises used may differ, but it is helpful if the delivery room nurses acquaint themselves with the psychoprophylactic programs that may be available in their communi-

ties and how the women have been taught. The women so trained for labor need nursing support and encouragement from a nurse who will enhance, not disturb, their concentration during contractions; help evaluate and aid relaxation; render sacral support or pressure as directed; share information regarding progress in labor; and be sincerely complimentary of the idealism and efforts manifested by the patients and their partners.

In addition, the nurse should render the other nursing care services and watchful observation that all laboring women require. Occasionally symptoms of hyperventilation may be associated with some of the rapid-breathing techniques used. The patient may complain of tingling the hands and feet, which causes her annoyance and loss of concentration. Slowing respirations or breathing into a paper bag helps relieve these problems. Symptoms related to hyperventilation have not been as frequent since rapid-breathing patterns have been modified to include slower acceleration and deceleration periods and shallower respirations. The absence of all forms of drug-induced analgesia or anesthesia is not a prerequisite of either the Read or Lamaze method, although this interpretation has been made. However, many women do not use any drugs.

Those who have evaluated psychoprophylactic techniques (cared for patients who were prepared as recommended or used them themselves) generally believe they are of real value. The breathing and relaxation exercises, patterned light massage (effleurage), visual focal point, and the mental and physical conditioning that such team efforts involve represent helpful tools that many mothers can profitably employ as they face the task of childbirth. If a laboring woman decides to use other "tools" (such as analgesia, tranquilizers, or anesthetics), in addition, she should not feel herself to be a failure or guilty of "betraying a concept." She is not a competitor in a contest. She is a participant in an experience.

The main problem in using these techniques seems to be in securing enough time and personnel to prepare the woman adequately. She may find it difficult to attend instruction classes. Many people do not agree that these methods of caring for the childbearing woman are truly "natural childbirth." They look on them as "intensive education and preparation for childbirth." Some women respond very well to the conditioning offered; others have personal histories or personality structures that make constructive participation in labor and birth such as Read and Lamaze recommended very difficult or impossible. Both methods are advised only for those undergoing a normal labor and birth. For those qualified candidates able to seek out a sympathetic practitioner and to undertake the intensive preparation involved, such a management of labor and birth can bring many enduring rewards, not the least of which is a characteristically noisy, vigorous new member of the family.

More information regarding childbirth education can be obtained from the American Society of Psychoprophylaxis in Obstetrics (ASPO), 1411 K St., N.W., Suite 200, Washington, D.C., 20005, or the International Childbirth Education Association, P.O. Box 20852, Milwaukee, Wisconsin, 53220.

HYPNOSIS AND ACUPUNCTURE

No discussion of obstetric analgesia and anesthesia can be undertaken without mentioning hypnosis and acupuncture. Hypnosis, an intense altered state of receptive concentration, is greatly enhanced by high motivation. The psychoprophylactic method of preparation for childbirth incorporates certain aspects of this technique. The ability to attain a trancelike state can be measured by use of the Hypnotic Induction Profile.* Such a trance may be induced by another person or self-induced. Training for this type of pain relief has been typically time consuming and expensive. However, with the use of group sessions, hypnosis is becoming a more accessible method. With its wider availability, more evaluation of its worth for maternity patients will be possible.

The use of acupuncture for vaginal deliveries has received mixed reviews. In a preliminary study, Cosmi and Vellay found that acupuncture associated with electric stimulation (electro-acupuncture) in the dorsolumbar and lumbosacral areas may eliminate painful sensation during labor. It also has been proposed that acupuncture releases endorphins (morphinelike compounds) from the pituitary and midbrain. Surely these forms of pain relief and control are worthy of more study and research.†

No perfect means of pain relief applicable to all women and situations has been found. But physicians have at their disposal many agents of worth, which, when used judiciously and backed up by good nursing care, will assist the patient tremendously.

---

*Spiegel, H.: Obstetrics, pain and hypnosis. In Cosmi, E., editor: Obstetric anesthesia and perinatalogy, New York, 1981, Appleton-Century-Crofts.
†Day, R.L.: Acupunctural anesthesia, a psychological study, Anesthesiology 43:507-517, Nov. 1975.

MINOR PROBLEMS OF PREGNANCY

A French obstetrician named Mauriceau once declared that pregnancy was a disease of 9 months' duration. Today health professionals and prospective parents do not like the term "disease" applied to normal pregnancy, but it is conceded that a number of minor discomforts may be associated with this period of waiting. Some were mentioned in Chapters 4 and 5. Now let us take a more detailed look at those discomforts and others not previously discussed.

Digestive difficulties

Nausea and vomiting. Probably the first discomfort noted by many pregnant women is nausea and vomiting—particularly in the morning, although it may occur at any time. Remember that it is a presumptive signal of pregnancy. This temporary condition is experienced by approximately 50% of pregnant women in the first trimester. It is said to be linked with the great hormonal changes in the body at the onset of pregnancy or a decreased blood glucose or glycogen reserve. Emotional factors may also enter into the cause-and-effect relationship. The most successful preventative seems to be eating more frequent, small meals instead of three rather large meals as is customery. Liquids

are tolerated better if taken between, instead of with, meals. Eating something dry and high in carbohydrate value like a few crackers or a piece of toast 15 minutes before getting up also seems to help. Some physicians may prescribe certain sedatives or antiemetics. Of course, any use of medication by a pregnant woman must be carefully evaluated and closely supervised. If the nausea persists and becomes severe, threatening the nutrition of the mother, it is considered a rather serious complication called *hyperemesis gravidarum*. It may necessitate hospitalization, administration of intravenous feedings, and, in some instances, psychiatric counseling.

Heartburn. Heartburn, or *pyrosis,* an uncomfortable burning sensation felt behind the sternum often accompanied by gas and acid regurgitation into the esophagus, has nothing to do with the heart. It only feels that way. Heartburn becomes more common as pregnancy advances and is thought to be related to decreased peristalsis and the pressure of the growing fetus, which cause stomach acid reflux and secondary esophagitis. For this reason, lying flat directly after eating is not recommended. Since the ingestion of fat inhibits the secretion of stomach acid, a small amount of milk or cream taken about 20 minutes *before* eating might merit some consideration. It can also be prevented or lessened if gas-forming foods, such as cabbage, cauliflower, brussels sprouts, onions, cucumbers, radishes, turnips, and dried beans, are avoided. More frequent, smaller, leisurely meals are also recommended. With the physician's approval, an antacid such as Maalox (a mixture of magnesium and aluminum hydroxides) may be used, especially before bedtime. Sodium bicarbonate or Alka-Seltzer should not be recommended because of their high sodium content.

Constipation. Constipation may also be a problem, especially if the woman has had such difficulty before pregnancy. Four things may help: a diet that includes plenty of roughage, abundant fluids, regular exercise, and a consistent time of day set aside for evacuation when she does not have to hurry. Mild laxatives may also be used, but an expectant mother should check with her physician regarding the type and frequency of such medication. Taking a laxative is one way that labor might be initiated.

Circulatory difficulties (Fig. 9-1)

Varicosities. Many pregnant women suffer from *varicosities*, also called varices, or varicose veins. They most often occur in the lower extremities and rectal area but occasionally may also involve the vulva and groin. These are surface veins, the walls of which are thin and greatly enlarged. Their prominence during pregnancy is especially common because of the increased blood volume, edema, and obstruction in venous return from the lower extremities that accompany gestation. Increased hormonal levels may also cause relaxation of the smooth muscles in the walls of veins. They may appear as a swollen, purple, knotted network just under the skin. The affected lower extremities tire easily. The swollen veins may be more than a cosmetic problem, since occasionally they may be injured, rupture, and bleed or become the point of origin for a blood clot, or thrombus. Most patients find relief with the use of support hose or the application of bandages that stimulate return circulation to the heart. If elastic bandages are used, they should be applied from the foot up, with an even

tension so that they will not become in themselves obstructions to circulation. Ideally support hose or bandages are used after the patient has had her legs elevated several minutes to drain the swollen veins. Swelling and fatigue will be less if the pregnant woman can avoid standing for protracted periods and especially if she can lie down at intervals and elevate her feet above the level of her head. Round garters or knee- or calf-length elastic-topped hose should never be worn. Pooling of the blood in the lower part of the body plus dilatation of the surface blood vessels may be one cause of the faintness experienced by many pregnant women.

Hemorrhoids. Rectal varicosities are termed "hemorrhoids." They may be external or internal and are produced or aggravated by the pressure of the developing fetus or constipation. They can be painful and occasionally become thrombosed or bleed. Most of the time surgical treatment is not contemplated during pregnancy because the condition usually disappears or vastly improves after childbirth. Attention should be paid to the prevention of constipation. Witch hazel compresses, analgesic ointments such as dibucaine (Nupercainal) special suppositories, and sitz baths may help.

Muscle cramps

Muscle cramps are often experienced during pregnancy; they usually involve the calf muscle and can be agonizing. They are said to result from an imbalance in calcium and phosphorus in the body, causing a form of *tetany*. Immediate treatment consists of straightening the leg by pushing down on the knee and pushing the ball of the foot up toward the knee. Preventive therapy for muscle cramps includes increased calcium intake in the form of calcium lactate or gluconate with increased vitamin D intake. Some physicians using this regimen may limit the woman's intake of milk because of its high phosphorus content. Others will continue to recommend a quart of milk a day but prescribe small quantities of aluminum hydroxide gel (Amphojel) in the diet to prevent the assimilation of excess

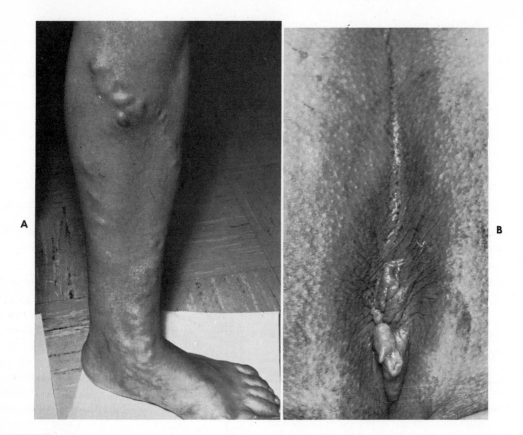

FIG. 9-1 **A,** Varicose veins of the lower extremity. **B,** Varicosities of the rectal area (hemorrhoids).
Courtesy Mercy Hospital and Medical Center, San Diego, Calif.

---

phosphorus. The patient should be advised to avoid fatigue and cold legs, avoid pointing the toes when stretching, and to lead with the heels when walking.

Leukorrhea

The term leukorrhea is used to describe normal increases of whitish mucoid vaginal drainage commonly experienced by women at the time of ovulation, preceding and following menstruation and during pregnancy. This discharge is sometimes labeled physiologic leukorrhea. Confusingly, the word has also been used to indicate profuse, white, cream-colored or yellowish, frequently foul-smell-

ing vaginal drainage, which is often accompanied by vulvar itching or burning. Such secretions may be associated with poor hygiene, lack of perineal ventilation (occlusive underwear), infections by several types of organisms, the presence of cervical polyps (fleshy growths), malignant tissue changes, and vaginal foreign bodies. Descriptions of common vaginal infections follow.

Trichomoniasis. *Trichomonas vaginalis*, a microscopic protozoon, is a common cause of leukorrhea (Fig. 9-2, *B*). This organism may inhabit the vaginal canal without causing noticeable symptoms. However, during pregnancy the increase in alkalinity of the vagina may cause *T. vaginalis* to multiply rapidly and create annoying signs and symptoms. Typically these are an irritating, pro-

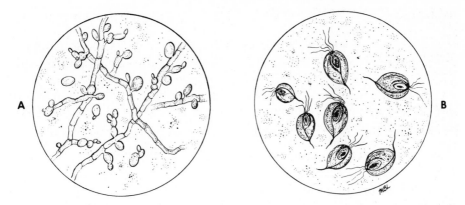

FIG. 9-2   Microscopic views. **A,** *Candida (Monilia) albicans,* a fungus. **B,** *Trichomonas vaginalis,* a protozoon, or microscopic animal.

fuse, foamy yellow vaginal discharge, and vulvar itching or burning. The motile organism may be identified under the microscope in a hanging drop slide or occasionally by culture methods. *Trichomonas* is difficult to combat locally because of the structure of the vaginal folds, and many types of treatment have been attempted. Oral metronidazole (Flagyl) has been successfully prescribed, but its use during the first trimester of pregnancy is contraindicated. It has been identified as a possible cause of fetal abnormality. Sexual partners should be treated to help prevent recurrence. Topical Betadine gel has been advised.

Candidiasis vulvovaginitis. Candidiasis is an infection caused by a yeast or fungus called *Candida albicans,* or *Monilia albicans*. It is easily diagnosed by direct microscopic examination of the discharge or by culture techniques (Fig. 9-2,A). A *Candida* vaginal infection produces a cheesy, whitish discharge and beefy red vulvar irritation. Like *Trichomonas, C. albicans* can inhabit the body without producing any apparent signs or symptoms, or it may spread tremendously and be quite notable. Candidiasis is seen frequently in pregnant women, diabetics (treated and untreated), women using broad-spectrum antibiotics (for example, penicillin, tetracycline, and erythromycin), and women living under stressful conditions. Stress is thought to affect the acid-base balance of the vaginal mucosa. An old remedy consists of locally

applying 1% gentian violet. Miconazole nitrate 2% (MicaTin cream or lotion 2%) applied locally has also been reported to be an effective treatment for external use. The antibiotic nystatin in the form of vaginal tablets and creams has proved to be helpful. Nystatin is given by mouth to prevent monilial overgrowth when broad-spectrum antibiotics are prescribed or to treat an oral infection. *C. albicans* in the oral cavity produces thrush, discussed on p. 224. Intermittent cool tap water compresses applied to the vulva may prove soothing to the patient.

Other causes. Gonorrhea, unfortunately a very common infection that may produce vaginal or urethral discharge, will be discussed under "major problems," p. 164. Most often gonorrhea is asymptomatic in women. Mixed infections of the vaginal tract may be encountered that are especially difficult to treat. Many physicians do not advise douching during pregnancy. Even in the nonpregnant state, evidence indicates that douching usually should not be done; bacteria may be forced in a retrograde fashion through the cervix, uterus, and tubes, causing endometritis and salpingitis. Besides causing an increase in pelvic infections, douching washes away the normal vaginal flora, leading to an overgrowth of hostile bacteria. As an alternative to douching, sitting in a warm tub of water and allowing the water to gently rinse the vaginal vault is recommended.

MAJOR PROBLEMS OF PREGNANCY AND CHILDBIRTH

High-risk pregnancies

Certain characteristics or conditions of the prospective mother or her child cause situations of jeopardy. Some of these can be detected at the onset or shortly after the beginning of a gestation. Such pregnancies are termed *high risk*. For examples of high-risk pregnancies, see the box below. Some of these patients are being referred to regional obstetric intensive care centers, or perinatal centers, where specialists and sophisticated equipment are available. These centers are commonly associated with high-risk or special care nurseries, capable of caring for the endangered newborn in the best manner possible. The maternal, fetal, and infant mortalities for many of these conditions have decreased with the use of these facilities.

DIABETES MELLITUS

Diabetes complicates at least one in three hundred pregnancies in the United States. It represents a significant percentage of maternal and peri-

---

SOME CONDITIONS OR CHARACTERISTICS CONSIDERED TO CONSTITUTE HIGH RISK FOR A MOTHER AND HER UNBORN CHILD

---

1. Low socioeconomic, educational status (influencing especially nutrition, prenatal care supervision, and compliance)
2. Little or no prenatal care
3. Maternal age less than 18 or more than 35 years old
4. More than 4 pregnancies (especially if more than 35 years old)
5. Conception within 2 months of last delivery
6. The presence of coincidental maternal disease or significant health problems involving:
   a. Cardiovascular disease
   b. Renal disease
   c. Diabetes mellitus
   d. Tuberculosis or other pulmonary disease
   e. Herpes simplex type 2, syphilis
   f. Hereditary anomaly or possible carrier state (for example, sickle-cell anemia, myelomeningocele, cystic fibrosis, osteogenesis imperfecta)
   g. Alcoholism or other drug addiction
   h. Ingestion of fetotoxic medication, exposure to radiation or toxic chemicals
   i. Obesity (more than 20% greater than standard weight for height)
7. Previous obstetrical complications that may recur, such as:
   a. Preeclampsia-eclampsia
   b. Severe anemia, clotting problems, intra- or postpartum hemorrhage
   c. Cephalopelvic disproportion
8. Previous poor fetal outcome (repetitive fetal loss, stillbirth)
9. Deviations in the current pregnancy such as:
   a. Twinning or other multiple pregnancies
   b. Premature or small-for-date fetus
   c. Postmature fetus (more than 42 weeks)
   d. Breech presentation
   e. Polyhydramnios or oligohydramnios
   f. Prolonged rupture of the bag of waters
   g. Any of the complications noted in Section 7 above

natal morbidity and fetal mortality. The most common cause of fetal death associated with diabetes is maternal acidosis.

Women who have difficulty metabolizing glucose represent varying degrees of obstetric risk. The potential difficulty facing any diabetic woman and her unborn infant usually can be initially estimated and classified by assessing results of glucose tolerance tests, age at onset and duration of the disease, the extent of control indicated, and the presence or absence of general vascular pathology including urinary and visual complications.

Some pregnant women may develop diabetes without realizing it. They may or may not have a family history of the disease. Clues pointing to the possible presence of the disorder are birth of an infant weighing over 4 kg (approximately 9 pounds), repetitive spontaneous abortions, unexplained stillbirth, infant abnormalities, repeated preeclampsia, excessive amniotic fluid (polyhydramnios), monilial vaginal infection, and, of course, the onset of glucosuria. Any of these factors may cause a physician to seek special identification of the disease process.

Glucose in the urine during pregnancy is not always a symptom of diabetes, but it should always be evaluated. The renal glucose threshold changes during pregnancy, allowing periodic spillage in the nondiabetic pregnant women. Clinistix or Tes-Tape should be used for the original identification of urinary glucose. Clinitest tablets may show a positive response because of other sugars present in a pregnant or nursing woman's urine. If diabetes is present only during pregnancy and needs no continuous therapy after childbirth, the patient is said to have *gestational diabetes*. She must be advised that she carries a higher risk of diabetes in later life and that the onset of the disease often accompanies periods of stress. Maintaining normal weight and following a good nutritional diet will be to her advantage.

Those patients who have taken oral hypoglycemic medications will usually be given insulin, since oral therapy may be inadequate, and the sulfonylureas cross the placenta to the fetus with possible toxic or teratogenic results. Insulin requirements during pregnancy often fluctuate. In early pregnancy the need for insulin may decrease slightly; later, more insulin is usually needed. Immediately after delivery insulin requirements briefly decrease. Periodic fasting and 2-hour postprandial (following a meal) blood glucose level examinations help monitor control. To meet the needs of the developing pregnancy without causing the improper metabolic burning of fats, or developing ketosis and increased acidosis, a more liberal calorie intake is usually endorsed. Considerable patient teaching regarding the needs of the pregnant diabetic must be carried out during office and clinic visits and during the periodic hospitalizations that often take place to maintain proper control of the disease and check on fetal well-being.

Women with diabetes are more likely to have large babies and mechanical problems in childbirth, because the large amounts of insulin produced by most of these infants acts as a growth hormone. Infants of *severe* diabetics, however, may not demonstrate this excessive weight gain. Placental insufficiency, perhaps related to degenerative vascular changes associated with diabetes, may cause the increase in births of stillborn fetuses and premature infants by these patients.

A large percentage of diabetic pregnant women develop preeclampsia. Bed rest in the left lateral–recumbent position is often recommended after the thirty-fourth week to improve intrauterine blood flow. Fetal well-being should be monitored closely, especially during the latter half of the third trimester, by performing biweekly nonstress tests. Response of the fetal heart to the trial adminstration of oxytocin (oxytocin stress test) can also be of help in deciding if termination of the pregnancy should be planned (see p. 488). Diminished placental function may be detected during pregnancy through periodic serial evaluations of the amount of estriol in blood samples or 24-hour urine specimens. If tests of fetal lung maturity (L/S ratio and phospholipid assay) and other growth indices are favorable, the physician may elect to initiate labor before term or perform a cesarean birth, depending on the individual involved. Children of diabetic mothers are more likely to suffer from RDS, because, despite their relatively heavy birth weights, they are often immature. After birth these infants frequently show symptoms of lowered blood glucose (hypoglycemia), probably resulting from overactive pancreatic function initiated in utero because of a high-glucose environment. They often demonstrate hypocalcemia and hyperbilirubinemia. It has been reported that congenital defects are three times more common in children of diabetic mothers than in the population at large. Overt diabetes has been found in approximately 5% of the offspring of pregnancies complicated by maternal diabetes. For a more detailed discussion of diabetes, see p. 295.

CARDIAC PROBLEMS

Patients with cardiac disease are also individually evaluated to determine their capacity to tolerate the increased stresses of pregnancy or a vaginal or abdominal delivery. They should be watched for any signs of possible heart failure, such as increasing shortness of breath, cough, rapid, irregular pulse, progressive generalized edema, and sounds of chest congestion on auscultation. Those patients who have experienced prepregnant incapacity resulting from their cardiac status are particularly at risk. The postpartum period, involving considerable readjustment of vascular volume, is especially hazardous.

URINARY PROBLEMS

The pregnant patient with urinary tract disease is a real challenge to medical management, especially when kidney function is impaired. Pregnancy in itself puts a strain on the urinary system. The developing uterus may pinch or kink the ureters (particularly the one on the right because of the usual location of the uterus). Stoppage of normal urinary flow predisposes the system to infection (pyelonephritis). Infections are often caused by colon bacilli, but other organisms may also be responsible. If the kidneys are already damaged by a previous pathologic condition, the added load imposed by the excretion of fetal waste may be significant. Infection of the kidney and urinary tract may manifest itself in several ways: chills and fever; lower back pain; pain on voiding; and a urinalysis of a clean-catch specimen characterized by the presence of numerous white blood cells, bacteria (100+ colonies per ml), and in more severe cases, perhaps red blood cells and albumin. Recurrent infection may necessitate urologic tests to rule out urinary tract obstruction or other nonpregnancy-related causes. Untreated infection may prompt premature labor and delivery.

Infection of the kidney usually responds well to measures such as bed rest, forced fluids, urinary sedatives or analgesics, and some type of antibiotic therapy based on sensitivity studies. When hospitalized, these patients are routinely on intake and output measurement and have frequent blood pressure and daily weight determinations. Daily urinalysis is often ordered. Renal disease may be inflammatory or degenerative. It is closely connected with the condition of the blood supply to the kidneys, and any continuous process that interferes with this supply will present symptoms in time. Conversely, any significant damage to the kidney will reflect itself in a change in the circulatory system, particularly an elevation of the blood pressure, as more and more pressure is exerted in an attempt to maintain adequate filtration. The onset of significant hypertension is related to a worsening prognosis for both the fetus and mother. Patients whose renal disease is not caused by a current infection (for example, those suffering from glomerulonephritis) receive much the same nursing care as those with a diagnosed bacterial invasion, and antibiotics are often given prophylactically. Chronic or advanced renal disease should be frequently evaluated by renal function tests. It may pose a real threat to both the mother and her unborn child.

SYPHILIS

A complete prenatal examination should always include at least one serologic test for detection of syphilis (STS) (see p. 62). In the 1950s it was believed that the problem of syphilis had been largely solved because of these prenatal precautions and the successful introduction of antibiotics in its treatment. Many "L clinics," so-named for lues, another word for syphilis, were closed. Education of the public and the related necessary casework regarding venereal diseases or conditions that are primarily sexually transmitted (at that time principally syphilis and gonorrhea), which were responding so well to penicillin therapy, were not continued with the same diligence. Health workers were then greatly concerned to find later that national morbidity for syphilis had risen sharply. The reported cases of gonorrhea had also increased alarmingly. These increases were caused in part by the ill-founded sense of security regarding these diseases and by the cutbacks in federal, state, and local budgets helping in its control. These increased rates were also symptoms of the growing restlessness, lack of purpose, family breakdown, and increase in sexual activity that have become major problems of twentieth century society. Syphilis is most common in urban areas in the sexually active population aged 15 to 29.

Transmission. The infectious agent, a corkscrew-like organism, or spirochete, called *Treponema pallidum*, invades the mucous membranes or skin, or both. Syphilis may be acquired through accidental inoculation by contaminated needles or exposure to infectious skin lesions by professional personnel or other contacts, but this latter source of infection is rare. Transplacental syphilis infection of the unborn infant may occur at any time during pregnancy. Because young fetuses are unable to manifest a readily detectable response to early invasion, they formerly were inaccurately considered to be safe by virtue of a special placental barrier until approximately 18 weeks' gestation. The techniques of electromicroscopy and immunofluorescence have proved this concept to be in error. The infective organism cannot live for more than a few hours in an environment deprived of moisture, and is destroyed by drying. It is also killed by many chemicals, including soap.

Stages. The disease has been divided into three

different stages of development, or progression. The first stage—the period of initial body response—usually manifests itself from 10 to 90 days after exposure. The average time is 3 weeks. Classically, the characteristic lesion of the first stage of the disease is a relatively hard, raised, painless area crowned by a craterlike depression found at the site of entry known as a *chancre*. This lesion is not always seen, however. Sometimes it seems to be actually absent; at other times it is present, but hidden from view in the folds of the vaginal or urethral canals. Rarely the chancre may develop on the lips or breast. It is highly infectious. The spirochete may be identified in its secretions in dark-field microscopic studies. However, at this time the serology test is usually negative. The chancre disappears after 3 to 5 weeks. The uninformed victim may think the problem has also disappeared, but such is not the way of syphilis. The organisms have been multiplying and spreading throughout the body. Usually not long after the chancre vanishes, the patient discovers other difficulties, and their advent signals the beginning of the second stage of the infection.

The second stage of syphilis is characterized by a bronze- or rose-colored flat or raised scaly rash that may be quite faint, appearing on different body areas but most significantly on the palms of the hands and soles of the feet. This eruption is often accompanied by enlargement of the lymph nodes. Flattened, moist, wartlike lesions called *mucous patches*, or *condylomata lata*, may also appear on the skin and mucous membranes. These are highly infectious, containing the spirochete. The patient does not feel well and may have a headache, sore throat, and aching joints and muscles. There may be spotty loss of hair. These signs and symptoms may fade away after several weeks, never to return in the same way, or they may reappear at irregular intervals for a period of up to 4 years. During the second stage of syphilis the serology test is routinely positive.

The third stage of the disease may occur anywhere from 2 to 20 years after the initial contact with the spirochete. Although the disease is present, it may produce no visible symptoms. It is then considered to be latent. About 30% of those patients in the tertiary stage do develop widespread serious disorders that interfere greatly with life. Soft tumors called *gummas* develop in the tissues and may ulcerate or form abscesses. Vital centers, such as the brain, spinal cord, large blood vessels, and heart, are often damaged. There may be gastrointestinal symptoms. Patients may become mentally ill; such illness is called *generalized paresis*. They may be unable to walk normally because of central nervous system disease, and have a typical body-jarring gait. Patients are usually not infectious at this stage. Routinely the serology test is positive. Adequate treatment with penicillin in the first or second stages brings an optimistic prognosis. Results of treatment in the third stage are questionable.

Congenital syphilis. Prenatal maternal serology examinations have been successful in identifying most potential cases. Some physicians repeat these blood tests later in pregnancy to combat new, developing infection and fetal damage, since previous maternal infection and treatment does not produce immunity or protection of the fetus.

The syphilitic baby may not be born alive. The untreated syphilitic mother characteristically has a high spontaneous abortion rate. If born alive, the affected child may suffer from various problems. Probably the most common characteristic of the syphilitic infant is the presence of a thick, almost continuous, sometimes blood-tinged nasal discharge associated with a sniffling sound on respiration. For this reason the manifestation is called "snuffles." The skin, especially over the palms of the hands and soles of the feet, may be blistered and peeling. There may be sore fissures around the lips and anus. The joints are sometimes very tender. The liver and spleen are usually enlarged. The causative organism has been found in lesions of the skin and mucous membranes. All syphilitic infants should be isolated until 48 hours after adequate treatment is begun. Other more permanent but later-appearing signs indicating the prior presence of congenital syphilis are notched teeth

(Hutchinson's teeth) and a so-called saddle nose. Penicillin is again the drug of choice in the treatment of congenital syphilis. (See also p. 294.)

GONORRHEA

In many communities gonorrhea has now reached epidemic proportions, particularly among the teen-age and young adult population (see Figs. 30-3 and 30-4). In the United States over 1 million cases were reported in 1980, and many cases were unreported. Many city and county health departments accept minors for free, confidential venereal disease diagnosis and treatment, without parental consent, relying on their right under law to care for persons of all ages suffering from communicable diseases. However, not all states have laws that permit private and hospital physicians to treat minors for venereal disease without parental consent.

Gonorrhea is caused by a coffee bean–shaped diplococcus, *Neisseria gonorrhoeae*. In females it may produce an irritating, purulent, infectious vaginal discharge, and, since it often infects the Skene glands, may initiate burning on urination. The disease may spread up the reproductive tract and cause inflammatory changes. It may produce abnormal narrowing of the fallopian tubes and may be responsible finally for ectopic pregnancy (a pregnancy that develops outside the normal uterine placement) or sterility. In males it generally produces a urethral irritation or discharge. However, asymptomatic carriers of either sex are possible. Gonorrhea may also become a more generalized infection, spreading through the bloodstream and lymphatic system. It is not innocuous, occasionally causing serious complications, spreading abscesses, arthritis, and other inflammations in both sexes.

Previous disease confers no immunity in the event of additional exposures. The incubation period extends from 1 to 14 days. Recommended medications have been aqueous penicillin or ampicillin in conjunction with probenecid to prolong antibiotic activity. A new resistant strain of the gonococcus does not appear to respond characteristically to this routine treatment. Spectinomycin (Trobicin) has been successfully used, but the safety of the drug has not been established for use during pregnancy or with infants and children.

HERPES SIMPLEX VIRUS (HSV) TYPE 2 (GENITAL HERPES)

Herpes simplex virus type 2 is a sexually transmitted disease of the lower genital tract (with possible spread to the urethra and bladder). It can be annoying, painful, and potentially life threatening to a woman and deadly to her unborn or newborn infant. Early maternal infection may cause spontaneous abortion; later disease may be associated with premature birth. Among *infected* newborns a 50% mortality rate is reported, while more than 25% of the remaining half suffer severe neurologic effects. When *active* maternal genital HSV infection is diagnosed, infection of the baby may be prevented by cesarean birth before the membranes are ruptured. The risk of neonatal infection is greater during the initial episode of herpes. Some writers declare that if rupture of the membranes occurs, the significant time interval before a cesarean section is done appears to be 4 hours, after which the intrauterine infection rate rises rapidly. After approximately 6 hours cesarean birth may offer no benefit.

The lesions are similar to those of the related common fever blister, Herpes simplex type 1. They are first seen usually as small blisters, which subsequently rupture to reveal painful ulcerations. The incubation period lasts for 5 to 10 days. The lesions may persist for 3 to 6 weeks, subside, and then reappear at irregular intervals. The virus may be identified by tissue culture or through the detection of special inclusion bodies in a Pap smear. A mother or infant with the disease should be isolated.

Recently the new drug acycloguanosine (Acyclovir, Zovirax) was approved for topical use on herpetic lesions. Tests indicate that application of acycloguanosine shortens initial infections and may render them less painful. It may also reduce the shedding of live virus, especially during recurrent episodes, but it does not cure the disease. Other forms of the drug are being investigated. Currently a vaccine for the *prevention* of herpes is still being sought.

Supportive comfort measures like sitz baths, heat lamps, and povidone-iodine complex (Betadine) irrigations may be helpful. There seems to be an association between genital herpes and later development of carcinoma of the cervix; therefore, follow-up observation is essential.

TUBERCULOSIS

Tuberculosis is still a maternal-child health problem, because the disease may be worsened by pregnancy and postpartum demands, and it may be contracted fairly easily by the newborn infant. Rarely, cases of infection of the fetus have been reported. A pregnant woman with tuberculosis should be under close medical supervision. Drug therapy and newer surgical techniques have made the outlook for tuberculosis patients much more optimistic. As a rule, gas anesthetics at the time of birth are avoided. The care of infants born to women with tuberculosis has to be individualized.

Diseases associated with pregnancy

The following complications are so grouped because they are of major importance and are associated only with pregnancy, labor, and birth. They are not always preventable or predictable.

HEMORRHAGIC COMPLICATIONS

The threat of hemorrhage is a very real consideration during all periods of pregnancy, birth, and even after delivery. In the months of gestation, vaginal bleeding is always considered to be a potential menace to both the fetus and the mother. Hemorrhage, you will remember, is the most common complication of pregnancy.

Abortion. Spotting or bleeding during the early months is often related to *abortion*, defined as loss of the fetus before viability.

Types. Abortions may be *spontaneous*, without any premeditation (called miscarriages by the public), or they may be *induced*. Most communities identify two types of induced abortion: legal abortions, which are done after medical consultation following definite prescribed protocols, and criminal abortions, which have no legal sanction. The problems of sepsis, hemorrhage, and unequal availability to all women are some of the factors that have brought about changes in the laws governing legalized abortion. The problem of induced abortion continues to be a very controversial issue in our society.

Other terminology is also used in describing an abortion. Physicians and nurses often use the adjectives "threatened" and "inevitable." A *threatened abortion* may possibly be halted. It may declare itself by uterine cramping or intermittent backache and spotting, but the loss of blood is relatively small, and the cervical opening remains closed. An *inevitable abortion* is characterized by severe or persistent contractions, moderate to abundant blood loss, and dilatation of the cervix. Loss of the fetus cannot be prevented. An *incomplete abortion* refers to the retention of some of the products of conception, most commonly a portion of the placenta. The uterus usually must be emptied by a mechanical dilatation of the cervix and gentle scraping of its walls by a curet. Such a procedure is called a dilatation and curettage, or "D and C." If it must take place at all, a *complete abortion* is desirable. In a complete abortion, all the products of the pregnancy are eliminated from the uterus. Patients with the diagnosis of inevitable abortion are admitted to the gynecologic service. However, if the viability of the fetus is debatable, the patient may be referred to the obsetric service.

Women who have lost more than three pregnancies at about the same stage of development are said to be victims of *habitual abortion*. Sometimes a very young fetus will die in the uterus and remain there 2 months or longer before it is expelled, either through spontaneous processes or medical or surgical intervention. Such a situation is declared a *missed abortion*. In such cases the placenta usually has remained attached to the uterus for an extended period of time, and the amniotic fluid has been gradually absorbed, producing a type of fetal mummification or even petrification.

Nursing care. The nursing care of a woman who is threatening spontaneous abortion would routinely include bed rest; avoidance of stress; observation for uterine cramping and loss of amniotic fluid; temperature, pulse, and blood pressure records; careful determination of the presence and amount of vaginal bleeding (the physician may wish all pads and soiled linen to be saved to evaluate the extent of blood loss or frequent hematocrit and hemoglobin checks); and watchfulness to secure any passed tissue for diagnosis. Periodic checks for fetal heart tone should be performed if the fetus is over 4½ months' gestation. Vigilance for an elevation of temperature should be maintained. Iron medication or blood transfusions may be indicated. Sedatives and antibiotics may be employed. Inevitable abortion may be speeded by the use of certain drugs (oxytocics) to stimulate the uterus to contract or by surgical intervention, especially in the presence of hemorrhage. A patient who aborts must continue to be closely observed for complications for several hours or days, depending on her general condition and the circumstances of her loss.

About 50% of all threatened abortions terminate as abortions. A large percentage of such fetal loss is associated with some defect in the developing child. Spontaneous abortion seems to be one way that nature tries to rectify a basic error. Attention to certain health measures may at times prevent fetal death from abortion. General improvement of maternal health, previous immunization against infectious diseases, and proper prenatal care are all valuable. If loss is caused by premature dilatation of the cervix (incompetent cervix), the cervix may be closed by various suturing techniques and released only when the fetus is ready for birth (for example, Shirodkar and Würm and Lash procedures). It would appear that spontaneous abortion during the first trimester is not caused by climbing stairs, jogging, exercise, activity, or intercourse.

About 10% to 15% of all pregnancies end in spontaneous abortions with no known causes.

The nursing care of a patient undergoing a voluntary legal abortion in the hospital setting will be determined by her condition, the length of her pregnancy, and the method used by the physician to terminate her pregnancy. Termination may be secured by dilatation and curettage, aspiration techniques, or intra-amniotic saline injections (amniotic fluid replacement); see Chapter 11.

Nurses caring for patients receiving hypertonic intra-amniotic salt injections should observe their patients carefully for signs of saline injection into the bloodstream: localized burning or painful sensations, thirst, nausea and vomiting, and excessive blood sodium levels revealed by mental confusion, changes in the level of consciousness, and shock. Disseminated intravascular coagulation (DIC) is a potentially fatal complication of this procedure. Resuscitation equipment should be readily available.

Because of changes in the interpretation and content of abortion laws, nurses working in gynecologic, delivery, and operating room areas may be requested more frequently to assist in the process of legal abortion. If a nurse's scruples dictate that she not participate, she may decline her services, if by so doing she is not jeopardizing the immediate health or life of a mother (for example, she could secure another nurse to assist for whom abortion did not pose the same ethical problem). However, the nurse who declines to participate may be risking the loss of her employment.

Ectopic pregnancy. The term "ectopic pregnancy" refers to any pregnancy that does not occupy the uterine cavity proper. In the vast majority of normal pregnancies the migrating egg is fertilized by the sperm in the fallopian tube and nests or implants rather high on the walls of the uterine cavity. However, because of the anatomy and physiology involved, this progression does not always occur. Sometimes the tubes are abnormally narrow. This narrowing, or stenosis, may occur because of inflammation or tumor formation, or it may be congenital in origin. The tube may allow the sperm to ascend but be too narrow to allow the passage of the fertilized egg into the uterus. The egg may develop in the tube and cause rupture or eventually drop out the end to perish. Rarely, it may continue growing as an abdominal pregnancy, which in unusual cases produces a full-term child who may survive if delivered through an abdominal incision. Pregnancies have also been found trying to develop in the ovary. The danger of hemorrhage in ectopic pregnancy is extremely serious. The amount of vaginal bleeding observed does not always reveal the true condition of the patient, since much blood loss can be hidden within the abdominal cavity. An ectopic pregnancy is most often tubal. A higher incidence of ectopic pregnancies is associated with failure of intrauterine contraceptive devices.

Symptoms. If tubal rupture or abortion occurs, the patient, who may or may not consider herself to be in early pregnancy, characteristically suffers severe knifelike pain in either lower abdominal quadrant. This may or may not be followed by spotting or bleeding. Shoulder pain from blood irritating the diaphragm or the urge to defecate are classic symptoms. A mass in the cul-de-sac may be palpated or bloody fluid may be aspirated by the physician.

The signs of shock that develop are out of proportion to the amount of blood loss apparent. The patient may exhibit the classic signs of circulatory shock: pallor; cold, clammy skin; rapid, weak pulse, which will slow if shock deepens; falling blood pressure (a systolic reading of 90 mm Hg or under is usually considered "shock," depending on previous readings obtained); apprehension; loss of consciousness; and dilated pupils. Rapid surgical treatment and blood-loss replacement are generally indicated. Estimates vary, but ectopic pregnancy is more common than is usually supposed, occurring approximately once in 200 to 250 pregnancies. It terminates almost invariably with fetal loss, and the maternal mortality in the United States approaches 1 in 800 cases.

Placenta previa (Fig. 9-3, A). Two main types of obstetric hemorrhage are associated with the loca-

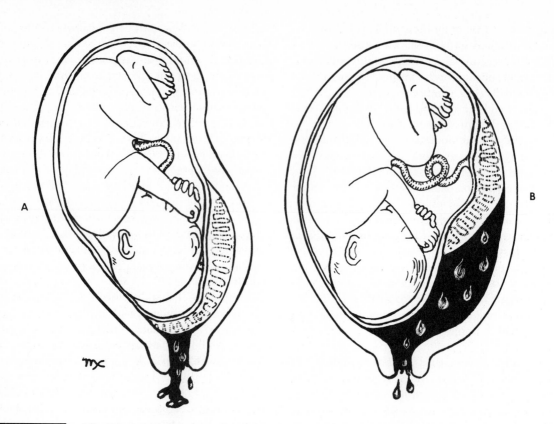

FIG. 9-3   **A,** A type of total placenta previa. **B,** Abruptio placentae, or separation of normally inserted placenta.

tion of the placenta and its attachment. In the condition known as *placenta previa*, the placenta implants low on the interior of the uterine wall. (A *total* placenta previa will cover the cervical opening; a *partial* or *incomplete* placenta previa impinges on but does not cover the cervix; and a *marginal* placenta previa is low lying, close to the dilating cervix.) In the latter part of pregnancy, the uterine contractions, which are always taking place to some degree although they are not always felt by the mother, may loosen the attachment of this abnormally positioned placenta and cause bright red, painless bleeding. The presence of placenta previa in other cases may not be detected until the onset of true labor and the dilatation of the cervical canal. Because of the relative safety of cesarean birth today, it is usually the treatment of choice. However, if the placenta is not implanted too low, bleeding is minimal, and the fetus is well but premature, some obstetricians may adopt a "wait-and-see" attitude and eventually deliver the patient vaginally. The use of electronic fetal monitors has been of real aid in detecting fetal problems in this instance.

Infection and emboli are other possible complications of placenta previa that should be considered. Many hospitals now practice the "double set-up technique" when treating a patient with placenta previa. Because vaginal or rectal examinations may worsen any bleeding present but may be considered necessary for the physician to obtain a proper evaluation, these procedures are delayed until preparations are completed for either a cesarean or a vaginal delivery in the same location as needed. Detection of a low placental insertion by the use of ultrasonic techniques is increasingly available. Placenta previa is more common in women who are multiparous. It occurs once in approximately 200 births.

Abruptio placentae (Fig. 9-3, *B*). The other type of hemorrhage related to placental attachment results from *abruptio placentae*, also called ablatio placentae or premature separation of the placenta. In this condition the placenta is implanted in the correct place, but for some reason—high blood pressure, sometimes as part of the preeclampsia-eclampsia syndrome or glomerulonephritis, vitamin C and folic acid deficiency, local injury, rapid changes in intrauterine pressure, fetal pressure on the maternal vena cava, or other causes—it becomes detached. Although its name implies that the detachment occurs suddenly, this is not always the case. Separation of the placenta from the uterine wall may occur over a period of time. Detachment may occur first at the center of the placenta, resulting in hidden hemorrhage at first, or it may begin at the rim or outer portion, causing vaginal bleeding of varying amounts. Old blood, which has been trapped behind the separating placenta, appears dark when it finally escapes from the vaginal canal. Fresh bleeding usually is bright red (amniotic fluid may become port-wine colored). Bleeding from a premature separation of a normally implanted placenta may be severe enough to cause rapid maternal circulatory shock, death or brain damage to the infant due to lack of oxygen, and even danger of maternal mortality.

Symptoms. The first sign of abruptio placentae during labor may be an alteration in the contraction pattern. The contractions become very strong and almost constant. Little relaxation period, if any, may be detected. The uterus becomes tender and boardlike if enlarged with retained hemorrhage. There may or may not be external bleeding from the vagina. The symptoms of shock may be greater than the amount of visible bleeding would indicate. The fetal heart rate is either greatly accelerated or

slowing. Uteroplacental insufficiency, as noted by late decelerations on the fetal monitor, indicates diminishing placental function. The use of electronic monitoring techniques is encouraged, especially in suspect cases. The fetus, in its struggle to obtain more oxygen, may be very restless and active. If the amniotic sac, or bag of waters, is ruptured, meconium may be seen in the amniotic fluid—another sign of fetal distress. As shock from blood loss develops, the blood pressure falls, and the pulse increases and weakens. Abruptio placentae in its more severe forms is an obstetric emergency. The treatment often, although not inevitably, includes delivery by cesarean birth and blood replacement. A serious complication of abruptio placentae that has been encountered often enough to warrant mention is hypofibrinogenemia, an abnormally low fibrinogen level in the blood that makes normal blood clotting impossible. Treatment may include fibrinogen replacement or use of cryoprecipitate (containing both fibrinogen and clotting factor VIII). A rare but serious associated complication, possible in other obstetric and medical settings as well, is disseminated intravascular coagulation (DIC). This problem begins with the triggering of coagulation mechanisms, probably by incidents such as the introduction of unusual clot-forming substances from the detaching placenta or its associated blood clot into the maternal circulation. Paradoxically, difficulties related to an opposing overprotective anticoagulation response by the body may lead to hemorrhage. Expert medical management and intensive nursing care are needed in these precarious circumstances. (See also p. 177.)

Hydatidiform mole. Another complication that may produce hemorrhage, although it is characterized by a much more unusual series of signs and symptoms, is called *hydatidiform mole* (usually shortened to hydatid mole). It is fairly rare in the United States but relatively frequent in parts of Asia. In this condition, for some unknown reason, the developing embryo and placenta deteriorate and usually lose their identity. Instead, a mass of abnormal, rapidly growing trophoblastic tissue develops. It is theorized that formation of the mole is preceded by the death of the embryo and disappearance of fetal circulation, while maternal circulation continues to sustain residual trophoblastic tissue. However, a mole can coexist with a normal pregnancy. At times this tissue may resemble a cluster of small grapes, or it may be of tapioca consistency. Its presence may be suspected when a pregnancy seems to be growing abnormally rapidly (a 3-month pregnancy may equal the size of a 5-month gestation), when no fetal heart tone or movement is detected, and nausea and vomiting are excessive or persistent. Vaginal bleeding may be intermittent. Quantitative chorionic gonadotropin levels in the urine are greatly elevated. Ultrasonic diagnosis is possible. No fetal skeleton is demonstrated. If part of the abnormal tissue is expelled from the uterus, pathologic examination is indicated. This growth rarely may erode the uterus and cause rupture. It occasionally becomes malignant, spreading to the lungs and other body parts. After the mole's removal, pregnancy tests are continued to see if any tissue is still active in the body and producing hormones. In the event of the diagnosis of hydatid mole, physicians may consider the advisability of removal of the uterus (hysterectomy) because of the possibility of the development of a malignant tumor, choriocarcinoma. Spreading choriocarcinoma, fortunately, is often curable by the use of anticancer chemicals such as methotrexate and actinomycin D.

Other causes. The causes of obstetric hemorrhage previously discussed—abortion, ectopic pregnancy, placenta previa, placentae abruptio, and hydatidiform mole—are those that most often occur during pregnancy or early labor. However, they are not the only causes of significant blood loss associated with childbirth. Obstetric laceration—vaginal, perineal, or cervical—and postnatal uterine inertia (abnormal postpartal relaxation of the uterus) leading to excessive bleeding from the site of former placental attachment can be important intrapartal and postpartal complications.

Care of the bleeding patient. Before leaving the topic of blood loss during pregnancy and labor, let us review the care of these bleeding patients. Presented below are some important do's and don't's that all nurses should know. Although licensed vocational or practical nurses (LVNs or LPNs) should not have the total responsibility for such patients, they should understand the following basic considerations:

1. Never give a bleeding patient an enema as part of the "routine admit." Never examine a bleeding patient rectally or vaginally. The physician performs any needed examination. Unnecessary manipulation of the area may increase the bleeding (especially in patients with placenta previa). Institute a regimen of bed rest and give the patient no food or fluids until ordered otherwise.

2. Observe the patient carefully and frequently:
   a. Take frequent pulse and blood pressure determinations. Compare, if possible, the results obtained with the patient's blood pressure reading on her prenatal record. Check for falling blood pressure and rising pulse.
   b. Check for type and amount of vaginal bleeding or amniotic drainage. If it is possible, save the evidences of bleeding for evaluation by the physician.
   c. Apply the fetal heart monitor routinely in any situation where fetal stress or distress is a potential problem.
   d. Monitor also the character of any contraction and relaxation period by frequent observation. Check for any special uterine tenderness or rigidity and for poor or absent uterine relaxation.

3. Keep the charge nurse and physician informed of changes in the patient.

4. Expect possible orders for intravenous fluids, blood analyses, and cross match for blood transfusion. Record intake and output. Know if any religious scruples would preclude transfusion (for example, if the patient is a Jehovah's Witness).

5. Maintain a calm, supportive manner.

PREGNANCY-INDUCED HYPERTENSION (PREECLAMPSIA-ECLAMPSIA SYNDROME, TOXEMIA OF PREGNANCY)

Definition and importance. Traditionally, toxemia of pregnancy, preeclampsia-eclampsia, or, using its newer name, pregnancy-induced hypertension (PIH), has been described as a serious, statistically important disorder characterized by the development after the twentieth week of gestation of *hypertension*, with *albuminuria* or *edema* or both. These symptoms should be progressive in severity to actually make the diagnosis of PIH. If coma or convulsion—not caused by coincidental neurologic disease—complicates the course of the illness, it is then called *eclampsia*.

Preeclampsia affects approximately 5% of the entire maternity population in the United States, although in some areas, particularly the Southeast and in some other parts of the world, the incidence is considerably higher. About 5% of those demonstrating preeclampsia develop eclampsia. Approximately 8% of those mothers who become eclamptic succumb to the disease or its complications. Preeclampsia-eclampsia, or the older term "toxemia of pregnancy," has long been listed among the first three causes of maternal mortality. Chief causes of maternal death associated with preeclampsia-eclampsia are aspiration (pneumonia), cerebral hemorrhage, cardiac failure with pulmonary edema, or obstetrical hemorrhage associated with premature separation of the placenta. A surviving infant may suffer from intrauterine growth retardation. A perinatal mortality of about 20% has been reported for North America.

Different types of pathologic conditions, especially cardiovascular and renal disorders, may mimic certain aspects of preeclampsia. Considerable effort has been made in recent years to tighten its definition to advance the treatment of the patient and to aid in promoting accurate statistical reporting and analysis. Indeed, when any of the three classic signs of preeclampsia (hypertension, albuminuria, or edema) occur singly during a pregnancy, use of the term preeclampsia is not usually recommended. Instead, current usage advises that the modifier *gestational* precede these signs, denoting a transient condition worthy of interest and consideration but not the label "preeclampsia." Hypertension that predates the twentieth week (except in multiple coexistent or molar pregnancies) is usually not considered to be indicative of true preeclampsia either—although later the trio of signs may be superimposed on a preexisting chronic hypertension causing a particularly dangerous variety of the disorder. Concurrent edema *and* albuminuria with hypertension are not necessary to a diagnosis of preeclampsia. For example, a patient may be quite ill and manifest significant edema but not spill any protein in her urine.

Signs and symptoms. The signs and symptoms of pregnancy-induced hypertension may, of course, extend beyond the classic three manifestations. Table 9-1 includes more possible findings that help determine the relative seriousness (mild or severe) of the disorder, and therefore influence the types of treatment advised. However, some authorities favor abandoning the terms "mild" and "severe," since all preeclampsia is potentially life threatening. It should be pointed out also that a number of clinicians do not consider the usual criteria of hypertension (a BP at or above 140 systolic or 90 diastolic) to be appropriate during pregnancy because blood pressure levels normally are reduced—especially during the second trimester. In midpregnancy, blood pressure readings greater than 120/80 are considered elevated by some investigators.* Blood pressures in mild preeclampsia as described in Table 9-1 are better indications of hypertensive states in pregnancy. The definition of a 30 mm Hg systolic elevation or a 15 mm Hg diastolic rise obtained two different times at least 6 hours apart after a period of rest is not new. The concept represented by a mean arterial pressure of 105 or more, or a rise of 15 mm Hg, has been employed more frequently in research than in clinical practice. Mean arterial pressure (MAP) is obtained by finding the difference between a

---

*O'Shaugnessy, R.D., and Zuspan, F.P.: Managing acute pregnancy hypertension, Contemp. OB/GYN **18:**85, Nov. 1981.

CLASSIC SIGNS OF PREECLAMPSIA-ECLAMPSIA

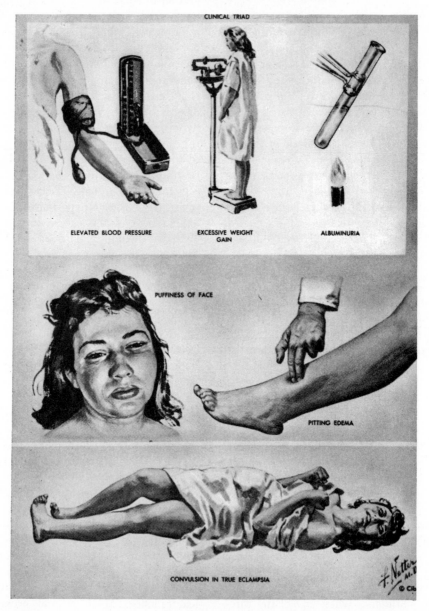

FIG. 9-4   Symptomatology of preeclampsia and eclampsia.

From The CIBA collection of medical illustrations, by Frank H. Netter, M.D. Copyright CIBA.

TABLE 9-1 COMPARISON OF SIGNS AND SYMPTOMS OF MILD AND SEVERE PREECLAMPSIA-ECLAMPSIA*

Characteristics	Mild preeclampsia	Severe preeclampsia
Blood pressure	Greater than 140/90 but less than 160/110 mm Hg 30 mm Hg systolic rise; or 15 mm Hg diastolic rise over baseline readings of early pregnancy Mean arterial pressure (MAP) of 105 mm Hg or more or a rise of 15 or more. (Above readings obtained after rest in a sitting position 2 times at least 6 hours apart.)	Blood pressure greater than 160/110 mm Hg
Proteinuria (albuminuria)	300 mg/L per 24 hours or 2 separate random daytime specimens 6 hours apart (true clean catch) of 1+, 2+	5 g or more per 24 hours, 3+ in true clean catch or catheterized specimen
Edema	More than 3 pounds or 1.4 kg/week gain in the second trimester or 1 pound, or 0.5 kg/week in the third trimester Slight generalized visible edema 1+, 2+	Weight gain advances at accelerated rate Edema more pronounced, especially of hands, face 3+ (as condition worsens, edema of lungs, brain, and other organs)
Urine output	Not below 500 ml/24 hours	Oliguria less than 500 ml/24 hours
Neurological signs and symptoms	Absent or only occasional headaches, blurred vision, or spots before eyes Normal peripheral reflexes	More persistent headaches, blurred vision, and spots before eyes—retinal arteriole spasms on ophthalmic exam Hyperactive knee jerk and other tendon reflexes Irritability, tinnitus
Other organ involvement		Liver involvement causing epigastric or right upper quadrant abdominal pain, nausea, vomiting (often said to precede convulsion/coma or onset of eclampsia) Pulmonary edema manifested by respiratory distress, rales, cyanosis

*These criteria are not uniformly accepted by experts in the field.

patient's systolic and diastolic blood pressure (usually termed the pulse pressure) and adding one third of this value to the diastolic reading (MAP = D + ⅓ [S-D]). For example, if a woman has a blood pressure reading of 138/88, she would have a mean arterial pressure of 88 + 50/3 or 105.

When reviewing only some of the possible signs and symptoms of preeclampsia, one is struck by the total body involvement that this potentially lethal progressive disorder may demonstrate. The kidneys, heart, lungs, liver, and brain may become prominent direct and indirect targets of the disease process, which is characterized by erratic narrowing of the microscopic arteries. This pervasive vasospasm of the arterioles probably accounts for many of the abnormalities found. However, its onset may be very subtle, with no remarkable initial signals that a patient may notice. Pregnant patients should be asked to report any swelling of the hands (tight rings) or puffiness of the face, headache, or visual problems such as blurred vision or "spots before eyes," but these clues of difficulty usually appear late. Regular and frequent prenatal supervision is needed for verification or interpretation of hypertension, albuminuria, and weight gain. Sudden weight gain, often signaling edema, is also associated with a rising hematocrit as more fluid from the blood transfers to the tissue spaces. As fluid leaves the blood stream, less blood is processed by the kidneys, and a fall in urine production occurs. Albuminuria, often the last sign of the three classic clinical findings to be noted, is thought to appear as blood vessel spasm and hypertension affect the kidneys. Some investigators have described unique microscopic renal changes that usually disappear after delivery. Abnormal neurologic signs and symptoms are probably related to lowered blood oxygen levels to the brain, minimal to massive cerebral hemorrhages, and edema. Abdominal pain is said to be associated with swelling and vascular involvement of the liver. This pain and nausea and vomiting are often noted before the onset of convulsion or coma, as is also pulmonary edema. The appearance of fever indicates a general worsening of the patient's status.

Possible etiology. Many theories have been formulated regarding the causes and the mechanisms of preeclampsia-eclampsia. A limited list includes explanations involving uterine overdistention; lack of normal blood supply to uterine and placental tissues, the presence of superabundant chorionic villi or the first exposure to such tissue, malnutrition, hormonal changes, autoimmune mechanisms, and psychologic factors. Most references state that the cause is unknown. Among the most popular current hypotheses is that mechanical factors (that is, the developing fetal-placental unit) impede development or maintenance of a proper blood flow to the uterus and its contents, and that this circulatory

lack (uterine ischemia) favors production of substances that raise the systemic blood pressure and cause the other characteristic symptoms of the disease. Dr. T.H. Brewer* has been most instrumental in promoting the concept that malnutrition is the underlying cause of this syndrome. He believes that malnutrition—particularly protein deprivation—in pregnant women causes impaired liver function which, in turn, interferes with the synthesis of albumin, the metabolism of the increased output of progesterone and estrogen characteristic of pregnancy, and normal hepatic detoxification processes. He cites the low serum protein levels found in many such patients as a cause of the typical edema, lowered blood volume, and reduced placental blood flow that trigger a compensatory hypertension and kidney pathology.

Identification of women at risk. Though much debate still exists regarding the causes of preeclampsia-eclampsia, it is generally agreed that certain groups of mothers are more likely to develop the condition. These include young teenage and older nulliparas; those with multiple pregnancy; those with a history of renal, vascular, or hypertensive disease; diabetics; and those who develop hydatidiform mole. Victims demonstrate an apparent familial tendency toward the disorder. Some researchers think certain tests help predict the onset of preeclampsia later in pregnancy. One is the so-called rollover or supine pressure test (SPT) performed between the twenty-eighth and thirty-second week of gestation. Upper extremity blood pressure is measured while the expectant mother lies flat on her side. The patient is then rolled over to a supine position. Her blood pressure is repeated immediately and again in 5 minutes. A diastolic *rise* of 20 mm Hg or more *after* the woman has turned to the supine position has been said to be a significant prognostic sign. However, inconsistent responses to this maneuver have caused it to lose some support. Tests that have been based on an abnormal rise in blood pressure after an infusion of

---

*Brewer, G.S., and Brewer, T.H.: What every pregnant woman should know, New York, 1977, Random House, Inc.

the substance angiotensin II also continue to be controversial.

Treatment and nursing care. Treatment of pre-eclampsia depends on the severity of the symptoms encountered, the philosophy of the physician, and the understanding and compliance of the patient. She and her family deserve careful teaching regarding her problem, its observation, and its treatment. Regular, adequate prenatal care is the best insurance for control of the complication.

In *mild* forms of preeclampsia, if a patient is conscientious in carrying out her physician's instructions, all treatment may be possible on an outpatient basis, but many physicians prefer to hospitalize these patients until symptoms are controlled. Treatment is directed toward relieving the edema and hypertension and restoring normal kidney function. Bed rest in a left side-lying position to increase placental blood flow is usually helpful in decreasing blood pressure. Bed rest is often very

---

USE OF MAGNESIUM SULFATE (EPSOM SALTS, MgSO₄) IN TREATMENT OF PREECLAMPSIA-ECLAMPSIA

Action and uses	Reduces transmission of nerve impulses from brain to muscles. Used primarily to prevent or treat convulsions. Some vasodilation and smooth muscle relaxation observed but not used chiefly for these effects.
Intent	To administer enough to prevent convulsions but avoid dangerous *nervous system* and *respiratory* depression caused by excessive magnesium serum levels in the body—either respiratory or cardiac arrest could occur.
Administration	May be ordered by IM or IV, intermittent or continuous drip. Introductory (bolus) and maintenance dosages prescribed based on clinical observations and serum levels. *Extreme care* must be used to be sure the concentration and volume of solutions to be given are understood. IM dosage should be given with long (3 inch) needles using Z track technique followed by site massage. With physician approval, lidocaine may be injected with MgSO₄ to relieve pain.
Antidote	10% solution calcium gluconate 10-20 ml, given intravenously, injected slowly (over 3 minutes to prevent ventricular fibrillation).
Monitoring side effects and patient response	Blood pressure, pulse, respiration every 15-30 minutes while on continuous IV infusion; before and after on varying schedules for intermittent IV or IM therapy; an initial decrease in blood pressure may be noted due to vasodilation. Patient may complain of generalized warmth, exhibit diaphoresis. Level of consciousness: anxiety may become disorientation, drowsiness, slurring of speech, coma. Frequency and intensity of uterine contractions may diminish. Repeat doses should not be given and physician notified if any of the below exist: 1. Pateller knee-jerk absent 2. Respirations below 14/minute 3. Urine output for previous 4 hours less than 100 ml. 4. Signs of fetal distress 5. Elevated magnesium serum levels—above 10 mg/dl (therapeutic levels 4-10 mg/dl)

difficult for a mother to maintain at home, especially if she has small children. Attention must be paid to her sources of help and support, or this important ingredient in her care will be lost. Improvement of the diet, emphasizing high-quality protein, vitamin, and mineral intake, and avoidance of empty calories, is to be encouraged. Salt restriction below normal dietary levels (4 to 6 g/24 hours) is usually not recommended. Diuretics, except in select cases, are considered to be of little value and may cause harm to the patient and the fetus.

When these patients are hospitalized, a bed rest regimen in a quiet room is usually advised. Valium may make bed rest more tolerable. Bed rest patients should be observed particularly for sacral edema. Blood pressure and fetal heart rate are taken at least every 4 hours. A daily weight determination and urinalysis are common. Twenty-four-hour urinary protein levels may be ordered, and creatinine clearance tests to measure renal function are favored. Intake and output should be observed. The patients are questioned regarding the appearance of any symptoms, such as headache, blurred vision, abdominal pain, or nausea. Intermittent tests of fetal maturity and well being (see p. 50) will help provide information needed to direct the care of the unborn infant and his mother. Although for many physicians the treatment for this disease currently remains almost as controversial as its proposed causes, all agree that the birth of a viable child as soon as possible is the best therapy. The rationale of treatment is to improve the condition of the mother to allow a vaginal or abdominal delivery at term. However, if her condition continues to deteriorate, induction of labor or a cesarean birth may be carried out.

SEVERE PREECLAMPSIA

Preeclampsia has been defined as "severe" if one or more of the following signs and symptoms are present: blood pressure of 160/110 mm Hg or more, albuminuria 3+ or more, urinary output of less than 500 ml/24 hr, persistent cerebral or visual disturbances, pulmonary edema, or cyanosis.

For a patient with severe preeclampsia, the room should be quiet and dimmed, and the tox-emia tray should be close at hand, containing a padded tongue blade; airway; percussion hammer (to test reflexes); and emergency anticonvulsant, sedative, antihypertensive, diuretic, and heparin-containing drugs, with appropriate equipment for their administration. Probably the most commonly used medication in the tray is magnesium sulfate. Rules regarding its use and that of its antidote, calcium gluconate, are highlighted in the box on p. 175. An oxygen mask or cannula, a suction apparatus, and possibly emergency tracheostomy equipment should be nearby.

Fortunately the occurrence of convulsion is rare today. Increase in blood pressure, severe headache, abdominal pain, apprehension, twitchings, and hyperirritability of the muscles often precede convulsions. As soon as a convulsion manifests itself, a plastic airway, or, if hospital policy allows, a padded tongue blade or soft, rolled washcloth may be placed in the patient's open mouth between the teeth to prevent biting the tongue and help maintain an airway. If possible, the patient's entire body or head should be turned to the side. Suctioning is rarely necessary, but aspiration is a danger. During the periods of rigidity and muscle contraction, the patient should be restrained only enough to keep her from hurting herself or rolling off the bed. The sides of the bed should be padded with pillows. Be aware that labor may progress rapidly and that babies have been suddenly born during a convulsive episode.

To measure urinary output and character more accurately, an indwelling catheter is inserted and attached to a urinometer. The blood pressure cuff is left in place. Frequent blood pressure, pulse, and respiration checks are made. Typically the patient is heavily sedated. An intravenous infusion is instituted for therapy as needed. Electronic fetal monitoring should be ongoing. A severely preeclamptic or eclamptic patient should never be left alone. Certain patients may convulse in response to loud noises, jarring of the bed, or bright lights. Conversation should be minimal. Routine bed baths, unnecessary procedures, or patient stimulation should be avoided.

As soon as the patient's convulsions are controlled, the condition of the fetus (if the seizures occur before birth) is ascertained, and plans for the birth are considered. The patient may deliver spontaneously. If the progress of labor is sufficient and the conditions of the patients (mother and fetus) are satisfactory, vaginal birth may be the procedure of choice. After birth the possibility of convulsion diminishes with the passage of time, and convulsion 72 hours after birth is rare. Intensive nursing must continue during the early postpartal period, but improvement is usually rapid.

RUPTURE OF THE UTERUS

Rupture of the gravid uterus may occur during late pregnancy, but is most often reported during labor and birth. The nurse should know under what circumstances this emergency is most likely to occur, the signs and symptoms most often seen, and the usual treatment pursued.

Uterine rupture is most frequently associated with previous uterine surgery (for example, cesarean births with classic uterine incisions, myomectomies), injudicious use of obstetric forceps or oxytocin, a tempestuous or prolonged labor (for example, fetal-pelvic disproportion), or grandmultiparity.

Typically the patient experiences a period of strong, almost unremitting contractions that, in spite of their force, produce little progress in the descent of the fetus in the birth canal. The uterus becomes extremely tender, and a weakening of its lower segment may cause a distention above the pubic bone, which may simulate the appearance of a full bladder. At the moment of rupture the patient may exclaim that she had a sharp pain and "felt something giving way." If rupture is complete—that is, the wall of the uterus is torn through—contractions will suddenly cease. However, partial ruptures are more common. These may not be detected until postpartal intrauterine palpation.

Classically the patient, after experiencing momentary relief from pain, will develop signs of profound circulatory shock resulting from intra-abdominal hemorrhage. Some of this blood loss may be visible vaginally. Signs and symptoms of rupture depend on the extent and depth of the tear, the location of the fetus, and the stage of labor in which the complication occurs. Occasionally, the onset of symptoms will be delayed. Almost all the unborn babies and one third of their affected mothers die when a classic rupture occurs.

Treatment of severe cases usually consists of immediate laparotomy, possible hysterectomy, antibiotics, and massive blood transfusions.

AMNIOTIC FLUID EMBOLISM

A complication that few women survive involves the spontaneous, accidental infusion of amniotic fluid into the endocervical or uterine veins after the bag of water has ruptured. This may occur any time during the labor-delivery and immediate postpartum period but has been most often reported near the end of the first stage of labor. Amniotic fluid containing particles of meconium, vernix, and lanugo may enter the large blood sinuses in the placenta through defects in the placental attachment. These emboli gain access to the mother's general circulation and lodge in the lungs. Although the entire disastrous mechanism is not clear, it would seem that this foreign matter also produces profound shock and disseminated intravascular coagulation (DIC), leading to lowered fibrinogen levels in the blood and subsequent hemorrhage. It is important to note that this complication is more frequently associated with tumultuous uterine contractions and has been described in an excessively disproportionate number of cases in which oxytocin has been administered to initiate or stimulate labor.

Symptoms manifest themselves suddenly. The patient may complain of chest pain or dyspnea and become extremely restless and cyanotic, occasionally expectorating frothy, blood-tinged mucus. Profound circulatory shock from hemorrhage may occur rapidly. Fetal death may result, and maternal death is almost always the outcome. Fortunately this complication is rare—occurring only once in several thousand births.

Emergency care includes intravenous administration of fibrinogen, blood, and other substances that will help restore normal clotting mechanisms, which paradoxically in DIC may include heparin and epsilon-aminocaproic acid (EACA) and oxygen therapy. If the baby is not yet born, he is delivered as soon as possible.

PROLAPSE OF THE CORD

When the umbilical cord precedes the presenting part of the fetus during labor so that the blood circulating within the vessels of the cord may be clamped off against the pelvis by the continued advance of the fetus down the birth canal, an obstetric emergency exists. This condition, termed "prolapse of the cord," occurs in approximately 0.4% of labors. The nurse should be aware that this complication is more frequent during labors involving multiple pregnancies, an unengaged fetal presenting part, footling breech or shoulder presentations, or small fetuses. It is more common when pelvic distortion or asymmetry is present. To prevent prolapse of the cord, patients in labor whose fetal presentations are not engaged should not ambulate or sit up steeply after cervical dilatation is advanced. Enemas should not be given routinely to these patients. A sudden gush of amniotic fluid may push the cord down into the vagina or to the exterior. This is one of the reasons why the fetal heart tone is always taken after the bag of waters ruptures spontaneously or is ruptured artificially by the physician. Sometimes the cord is clearly visible outside the vaginal canal. In other instances it has prolapsed but is not visible; it may only be felt. As long as pulsations are detected, blood is flowing in the cord. Periodic checks of the fetal heart tone are necessary and continuous monitoring of the FHR preferable, since any compression of the cord would usually cause detectable, abnormal alterations in its rhythm or rate. A constantly monitored patient with cord compression may characteristically reveal variable deceleration patterns. Other signs associated with fetal distress could be the passage of meconium during a cephalic presentation and sudden agitated fetal activity.

Treatment is directed toward removing any real or potential pressure on the prolapsed cord by applying vaginal or abdominal pressure to push the baby away from the cord or by a steep head-down or knee-chest position for the mother. Close observation of the fetal heart tone is maintained. A fetal heart monitor is very helpful. The nurse should never attempt to replace the cord in the birth canal. Oxygen may be administered to the mother; it will not cause harm and may be helpful to her or the infant. Usually the only feasible treatment is cesarean birth, carried out as quickly as possible!

PREMATURE LABOR AND BIRTH

A baby born before the end of the thirty-seventh week of gestation is considered premature. Prematurity involves about 10% of all babies. The incidence of a baby born "before its time" represents a special threat to the life or future health of the infant, special physical, psychological, and economic stress on the family, and a challenge to community resources. Premature babies are more likely to suffer trauma during birth, to be victims of respiratory distress syndrome and other problems, and to require longer supportive hospital care.

For these reasons, in most cases, attempts would be made to halt a premature labor, unless continuing the pregnancy would jeopardize the mother or fetus or the labor is considered to be inevitable. However, if evidence exists of intrauterine infection, hemorrhage, rupture of the bag of waters, or cervical dilatation beyond 3 or 4 cm, these efforts would not be appropriate. Bed rest may inhibit progression. Certain drugs may be used to quiet uterine contractions, among which are intravenous infusions of isoxsuprine hydrochloride (Vasodilan), terbutaline sulfate (Brethine), ritodrine (Yutopar), or ethyl alcohol in a 5% dextrose solution. The alcohol, which causes maternal intoxication, is thought to reduce the release into the circulation of oxytocin, a hormone that stimulates the uterus to contract. Alcohol is now used less frequently since approval of ritodrine, a more effective drug for the same use. Magnesium sulfate ($MgSO_4$) may also be used in the treatment of premature labor. All the drugs mentioned for suppression of labor have important side effects. Patients receiving them should be carefully observed, especially for hypotension and tachycardia. A maternal cardiac monitor may be appropriate.

If labor cannot be terminated, little analgesic medication is given, because the premature infant's body cannot detoxify drugs well, and his respirations at birth must not be depressed. It has been found that the administration of a glucocorticoid, betamethasone (Celestone), will hasten maturity of fetal lungs by promoting earlier formation of lung surfactant. This may enable the infant to avoid respiratory distress syndrome. However, some concern has been expressed over possible subsequent neurologic changes in the baby's brain that may affect his intellectual potential. A type of spinal anesthesia may be given at delivery. A deep episiotomy may be performed to minimize head compression at expulsion. The nursery must be notified of an impending premature birth. Ideally a pediatrician particularly skilled in the immediate care of immature newborns (neonatologist) would be present at the birth. Transport to a special intensive care nursery may be indicated.

Special attention to the psychologic needs of the mother is essential. Her labor is all the more demanding and difficult because her body is not prepared for the event, the outlook is precarious, and analgesic aids are minimal.

Teenage parenthood

Other problems meriting consideration by nurses may be related to special circumstances surrounding the events of pregnancy, birth, and the responsibilities of parenthood. They may not be physiologic or anatomic problems per se, but they represent situations that may be associated with certain obstetric complications and may profoundly affect the entire experience of the patient and her future adjustment to life's challenges. One such situation that is creating increasing concern in American society is teenage parenthood. Teenagers make up approximately 18% of sexually active women capable of becoming pregnant. However, they account for 46% of all out-of-wedlock births

and 31% of all abortions. If no change occurs in the current rates, four out of ten girls now 14 years of age will get pregnant while teenagers; two out of ten will give birth; and three in twenty will have abortions.* Most single teenage mothers are keeping their babies with or without family assistance. Those who receive support from their own families and remain at home fare better educationally and financially than those who live alone.

Numerous teenage marriages take place after pregnancy or birth has occurred. The divorce rate for these unions is very high. This is not meant to imply that no successful marriages begin in the teenage years. It does, however, reveal that the chances for a satisfactory, continuing family relationship are slim. Teenage marriages in modern American society too often are an attempt to solve or escape problems too serious and complex to be corrected by a wedding ring.

Many factors may be related to the incidence of early marriage or out-of-wedlock births. These factors most often involve family conflicts, social and economic deprivation, individual psychological problems, and a lack of education and appreciation regarding the role and responsibilities of sexuality in the family and society. Communities are now becoming more aware of the needs of the young parent, married or not. A number of programs have been instituted that make it possible for the pregnant girl's formal education to continue. These programs also may supervise prenatal care; prepare the girls for their experiences during pregnancy, labor, and birth; possibly provide education in mothering skills; and assist them with needed personal and vocational planning. Attempts are made to avoid repeat pregnancies by unmarried teenagers. Often, although not without exception, such situations involve failure to complete education, dependency on governmental welfare, and family instability. A few agencies make efforts to work with the unwed father, as well as the mother. Much work is still to be done to prevent or treat the

*Teenage pregnancy: the problem that hasn't gone away, New York, 1981, The Alan Guttmacher Institute, pp. 16, 36.

personal and community stress caused by teenage pregnancy.

Physicians and nurses are learning more about the needs of the pregnant teenager, both in and out of the hospital setting. Needless to say, most teenage maternity patients need a great deal of supportive care, careful instruction, and explanation to enable them to gain constructively from their experiences. A punitive attitude toward these patients from the nursing staff does not aid the individual girls or help solve the larger problems involved.

The nurse should realize that the incidence of preeclampsia-eclampsia is higher in this age group, especially for girls in their early teens from lower socioeconomic backgrounds. This increased incidence may be related to the poor nutrition exhibited by many of these young girls. These patients also have an especially large number of low birth weight babies. The delivery room nurse will be interested to know that teenage multiparas are more susceptible to precipitate labor than any other group of obstetric patients. For the unmarried pregnant teenager or teenager who has experienced a forced marriage, the trauma of the situation is mainly psychosocial. Her misdirected search for identity, freedom, love, or recognition places her in a role for which she is ill prepared, faced with decisions the outcome of which will unavoidably influence her the rest of her life.

• • •

This chapter, with its rather dismal recital of the minor and major complications of pregnancy and labor, may seem frightening to the student anticipating marriage and founding a family. However, it is the purpose of a text to point out the unusual as well as the commonplace. It is the business of a nurse to know about the possibility of these problems, although some of them may never be encountered—either personally or professionally.

UNIT 3

SUGGESTED SELECTED READINGS AND REFERENCES

GENERAL

Affonso, D.D., and Harris, T.R.: Postterm pregnancy: implications for mother and infant, challenge for the nurse, JOGN Nurs. 9:139-145, May-June 1980.

Allen, A.: Preoperative teaching for cesarean birth, AORN J. 34:846-854, Nov. 1981.

Aumann, G.M.E., and Blake, G.D.: Ritodrine hydrochloride in the control of premature labor: implications for use, JOGN Nurs. 11:75-79, Mar.-Apr. 1982.

Bettoli, E.J.: Herpes: facts and fallacies, Am. J. Nurs. 8Z:924-929, June 1982.

Bills, B.J.: Nursing considerations: administering labor-suppressing medication, Am. J. Mat. Child Nurs. 5:252-256, July-Aug. 1980.

Bolton, G.C., and Cohen, F.L.: Detecting and treating ectopic pregnancy, Contemp. OB/GYN 18:101-104, July 1981.

Chez, R.A., moderator: Symposium: therapeutic approaches to premature labor, Contemp. OB/GYN 8:58-86, Dec. 1976.

Chez, R.A., editor: The Schirodkar procedure: managing the incompetent cervix, Contemp. OB/GYN 3:137-139, May 1974.

Fort, A.T.: The obstetrics emergency: management of the injured gravida, Contemp. OB/GYN 3:41-46, Feb. 1974.

Howley, C.: The older primipara: implications for nurses, JOGN Nurs. 10:182-185, May-June 1981.

Jones, M.B.: Respiratory distress syndrome and the induction of fetal lung maturity by the use of glucocorticoids, JOGN Nurs. 6:21-27, July-Aug. 1977.

Kantor, G.K.: Addicted mother, addicted baby—a challenge to health care, Am. J. Mat. Child Nurs. 3:281-289, Sept.-Oct. 1978.

Kapstrom, A.: Career woman's dilemma: "How long dare I put off having a baby?" RN 43:60-64, Sept. 1980.

Klein, J.D., editor, Committee on Infectious Diseases, the American Academy of Pediatrics: Control of infectious diseases, pp. 115-118, 277, Evanston, Ill., 1982, The Academy.

Lewis, J.L., et al: How to diagnose, follow, and treat molar pregnancy, Contemp. OB/GYN 17:146-162 Apr. 1981.

McConnell, E.A., et al: Brace yourself: it's an orthopedic delivery, Nurs. '76 6:32-36, Dec. 1976.

McGovern, C.S.: Recognizing a tubal pregnancy, Am. J. Mat. Child Nurs. 3:303-305, Sept.-Oct. 1978.

O'Sullivan, M.J.: Ruptured uterus: still a challenge, Contemp. OB/GYN 18:145-148, July 1981.

Oxorn, H., and Foote, W.: Human labor and birth, New York, 1980, Appleton-Century-Crofts.

Pardve, S.F.: Hydatidiform mole: a pathological pregnancy, Am. J. Nurs. 77:836-838, May 1977.

Umbeck, K., and Diamond, F.: An oxytocin challenge test protocol, JOGN Nurs. 6:29-33, Jan.-Feb. 1977.

LABOR AND BIRTH

Angelini, D.J.: Nonverbal communication in labor, Am. J. Nurs. 78:1220-1221, 1978.

Campbell, A., and Worthington, Jr., E.L.: Teaching expectant fathers how to be better childbirth coaches, Am. J. Mat. Child Nurs. 7:28-32, Jan.-Feb. 1982.

Elsherif, C., McGrath, G., and Symrski, J.T.: Coaching the coach, JOGN Nurs. 8:87-89, Mar.-Apr. 1979.

Friedman, E.A.: Labor: clinical evaluation and management, New York, 1978 Appleton-Century-Crofts.

Kelley, J.V.: Use of the vacuum extractor for delivery, Contemp. OB/GYN 2:69-73, Dec. 1973.

McKay, S.R.: Second stage labor—Has tradition replaced safety? Am. J. Nurs. 81:1016-1019, May 1981.

McKay, S.R.: Maternal position during labor and birth: a reassessment, JOGN Nurs. 9:288-291, Sept.-Oct. 1980.

Meissner, J.E.: Predicting a patient's anxiety level during labor: a two-part assessment tool, Nurs. '80 10:50, July 1980.

Mercer, R.T.: "She's a multip . . . she knows the ropes," Am. J. Mat. Child Nurs. 4:301-304, Sept.-Oct. 1979.

Norr, K.L., et al: The second time around: parity and birth experience, JOGN Nurs. 9:30-36, Jan.-Feb. 1980.

Whitley, N., and Mack, E.: Are enemas justified for women in labor? Am. J. Nurs. 80:1339, July 1980.

Whitley, N.: A comparison of prepared childbirth couples and conventional prenatal class couples, JOGN Nurs. 8:109-111, Mar.-Apr. 1979.

ANESTHESIA AND ANALGESIA

McAllister, R.G.: Obstetric anesthesia—a two-way street, JOGN Nurs. **5**:9-13, Jan.-Feb. 1976.

McLaughlin, M., and Taubenheim, A.M.: Epidural anesthesia for obstetric patients, JOGN Nurs. **10**:9-15, Jan.-Feb. 1981.

Nicolls, E.T., Corke, B.C., Ostheimer, G.W.: Epidural anesthesia for the woman in labor, Am. J. Nurs. **81**:1826-1830, Oct. 1981.

Richart, R.M., et al: Paracervical block-anesthetic hazard to the fetus, Contemp. OB/GYN **17**:97-118, Apr. 1981.

Schultetus, R.R.: Anesthetic emergencies, Contemp. OB/GYN **18**:43-61, July 1981.

Shearer, M.H.: Obstetrical acupuncture, Birth Fam. J. **1**:14-18, Spring 1974.

Vadurro, J.F., and Butts, P.A.: Reducing anxiety and pain of childbirth through hypnosis, Am. J. Nurs. **82**:620-621, Apr. 1982.

BIRTHING ALTERNATIVES

Anderson, S., Bauwens, E., and Warner, E.: The choice of home birth in a metropolitan county in Arizona, JOGN Nurs. **7**:41-45, Mar.-Apr. 1978.

Averitt, S.S.: Adapting the birth center concept to a traditional hospital setting, JOGN Nurs. **9**:103-106, Mar.-Apr. 1980.

Boyd, S.T., and Mahon, P.: The family-centered cesarean delivery, Am. J. Mat. Child Nurs. **5**:176-180, May-June 1980.

Candy, M.M.: Birth of a comprehensive family-centered maternity program, JOGN Nurs. **8**:80-84, Mar.-Apr. 1979.

Faxel, A.M.H.: The birthing room concept at Phoenix Memorial Hospital, Part I: development and eighteen months' statistics, JOGN Nurs. **9**:151-155, May-June 1980.

Gimbel, J., and Nocon, J.J.: The physiological basis for the Leboyer approach to childbirth, JOGN Nurs. **6**:11-15, Jan.-Feb. 1977.

Grad, R.K.: Breaking ground for a birthing room, Am. J. Mat. Child Nurs. **4**:245-249, July-Aug. 1979.

Kieffer, M.J.: The birthing room concept at Phoenix Memorial Hospital, Part II: consumer satisfaction during one year, JOGN Nurs. **9**:155-159, May-June, 1980.

Leboyer, F: Birth without violence, New York, 1976, Alfred A. Knopf, Inc.

Levine, N.H.: Family-centered maternity units—fact or fiction? JOGN Nurs. **9**:116-117, Mar.-Apr. 1980.

Mahan, C.S.: When patients ask about "gentle birth," Contemp. OB/GYN **7**:51-54, Apr. 1976.

Paukert, S.E.: One hospital's experience with implementing family-centered maternity care, JOGN Nurs. **8**:351-358, Nov.-Dec. 1979.

Perez, P.: Nurturing children who attend the birth of a sibling, Am. J. Mat. Child Nurs. **4**:215-217, July-Aug. 1979.

Ritchie-Lee, A.H., and Swanson, A.B.: Childbirth outside the hospital—the resurgence of home and clinic deliveries, Am. J. Mat. Child Nurs. **1**:373-377, Nov.-Dec. 1976.

Sumner, P.E., and Phillips, C.R.: Birthing rooms: concept and reality, St. Louis, 1981, The C.V. Mosby Co.

FETAL MONITORING

Cranston, C.S.: Obstetrical nurses' attitudes toward fetal monitoring, JOGN Nurs. **9**:344-347, Nov.-Dec. 1980.

Cupit, L.: Helping expectant parents understand the fetal monitor, Ped. Nurs. **6**:21-23, May-June 1980.

Hodnett, E: Patient control during labor: effects of two types of fetal monitors, JOGN Nurs. **11**:94-99, Mar.-Apr. 1982.

Langhorne, F.: The fetal monitor: a friend or foe? Am. J. Maternal Child Nurs. **1**:313-314, Sept.-Oct. 1976.

McDonough, M., Sheriff, D., and Zimmel, P.: Parents' responses to fetal monitoring, Am. J. Mat. Child Nurs. **6**:32-34, Jan.-Feb. 1981.

Paper, J.T.: FHR monitoring: answering the critics, Contemp. OB/GYN **17**:163-174, June 1981.

Tucker, S.M.: Fetal monitoring and fetal assessment in high risk pregnancy, St. Louis, 1978, The C.V. Mosby Co.

Wagner, P.G.: Continuous fetal tissue pH monitoring: a preliminary experience, JOGN Nurs. **10**:164-168, May-June 1981.

COMPLICATIONS: DIABETES

Gibbons, J., and Nagle, M.: Assessing fetal health when the mother is diabetic, Contemp. OB/GYN **15**:115-126, June 1980.

Moore, D.S., Bingham, P.R., and Keesline, O.: Nursing care of the pregnant woman with diabetes mellitus, JOGN Nurs. **10**:188-194, May-June 1981.

Schuler, K., et al: When a pregnant woman is diabetic: a case study, Am. J. Nurs. **79**:456-458, Mar. 1979.

Schuler, K.: When a pregnant woman is diabetic: antepartal care, Am. J. Nurs. **79**:448-450, Mar. 1979.

Vogel, M.: When a pregnant woman is diabetic: newborn care, Am. J. Nurs. **79**:458-460, Mar. 1979.

Wimberly, D.: When a pregnant woman is diabetic: intrapartal care, Am. J. Nurs. **79**:451-452, Mar. 1979.

COMPLICATIONS: PREECLAMPSIA-ECLAMPSIA (PREGNANCY-INDUCED HYPERTENSION)

Foster, S.D.: Magnesium sulfate: eclampsia management effects on neonates, Am. J. Mat. Child Nurs. **6**:355, Sept.-Oct. 1981.

Jensen, M.D., Benson, R.C., and Bobak, I.M.: Maternity care: the nurse and the family, ed. 2, St. Louis, 1981, The C.V. Mosby Co., pp. 352-364.

Tichy, A.M., and Chong, D.: Placental function and its role in toxemia, Am. J. Mat. Child Nurs. **4**:84-89, Mar.-Apr. 1979.

Sonstegard, L.: Pregnancy-induced hypertension: prenatal nursing concerns, Am. J. Mat. Child Nurs. **4**:90-95, Mar.-Apr. 1979.

Wheeler, L., and Jones, M.B.: Pregnancy-induced hypertension, JOGN Nurs. **10**:212-235, May-June 1981.

Zuspan, F.P., and Zuspan, K.J.: Strategies for controlling eclampsia, Contemp. OB/GYN **18**:135-142, July 1981.

COMPLICATIONS: TEENAGE PREGNANCY

Abrams, B.: Helping pregnant teenagers eat right, Nurs. '81 **11**:46-47, Mar. 1981.

Admire, G., and Byers, L.: Counseling the pregnant teenager, Nurs. '81 **11**:62-63, Apr. 1981.

Barrett, A.E., and Peoples, M.D.: A model for delivery of health care to pregnant adolescents, Part II: implementation and evaluation, JOGN Nurs. **8**:343-345, Nov.-Dec. 1979.

Bartel, C.H.: Old enough to get pregnant—too young to have babies, Nurs. '81 **11**:44-45, Mar. 1981.

Donlen, J., and Lynch, P.: Teenage mother—high-risk baby, Nurs. '81 **11**:51-56, May 1981.

Foote, J.A.: Special needs of teenage cesarean patients AORN J. **34**:855-858, Nov. 1981.

Kandell, N.: The unwed adolescent pregnancy: an accident? Am. J. Nurs. **79**:2112-2114, Dec. 1979.

McAnarney, E.R., editor: Pregnant adolescent, Ped. Ann. **9**:(entire issue), Mar. 1980.

Mercer, R.T.: Teenage motherhood: the first year, Part I: the teenage mother's views and responses; Part II: how the infants fared, JOGN Nurs. **9**:16-27, Jan.-Feb. 1980.

Moore, K.A., et al: Teenage motherhood: its social and economic costs, Child. Today **8**:12-16, Sept.-Oct. 1979.

Peach, E.H.: Counseling sexually active very young adolescent girls, Am. J. Mat. Child Nurs. **4**:191-195, May-June 1980.

Peoples, M.D.: A model for the delivery of health care to pregnant adolescents, Part I: assessment and planning, JOGN Nurs. **8**:339-343, Nov.-Dec. 1979.

POSTPARTAL AND POPULATION PROBLEMS

CHAPTER 10

The postpartal period

The postpartal period, or puerperium, is usually considered to be the interval extending from the birth of the baby until 6 weeks after. This interval is characterized by the development of lactation and the return of the reproductive organs to their approximate prepregnant positions. Of course, some mothers, not wishing to or unable to nurse their babies, do not experience the full development of lactation. The return of the reproductive organs to the nonpregnant state is called the process of *involution*. The postpartal days are numbered starting with the first day after birth.

ADMISSION

Preparation and transfer

The basic care of the postpartum patient is an extension of the care given in the delivery room after childbirth. Today, many maternity services include a special postpartum recovery room where a new mother is closely observed and cared for during the first 2 to 4 hours after birth or until her condition is considered stabilized. The patient arriving in the postpartum area is put to bed in a unit previously prepared for her. The bed will be turned down, and bed protectors will be in place to catch extra vaginal drainage. Near at hand will be a sphygmomanometer, stethoscope, and individual unit equipment, such as towel and washcloth set, wash and emesis basins, soap, bedpan, back care lotion, breast and perineal pads, perineal irrigation equipment, and newspapers or paper bags for pad discard. If the patient has an intravenous infusion, some sort of support for the bottle will also be needed.

The transfer of the patient from the stretcher to the bed may require two or three persons, depending on her condition and the equipment available. It is important to know the type of delivery (vaginal or abdominal) experienced, the kind of anesthesia employed, if any, and the status of her recovery when planning to move her. Side rails are used. Before the delivery room nurse leaves the area, she checks the patient's fundus and vaginal flow to determine whether the uterus is firm, and she makes sure that any pertinent information concerning the patient is told to the postpartum charge nurse as she transfers the patient's records. Information to be shared is listed below. The patient's personal effects are carefully transferred so that nothing is lost in the move. The description of care that follows relates particularly to the patient who gave birth vaginally.

Observation

The postpartum nurse continues to check the condition of the patient every 15 to 20 minutes for at least 2 hours to determine the following (Fig. 10-1):

1. Blood pressure, pulse, and respiration
2. Type and amount of vaginal discharge (lochia) and the appearance of the perineum
3. Consistency and location of the fundus

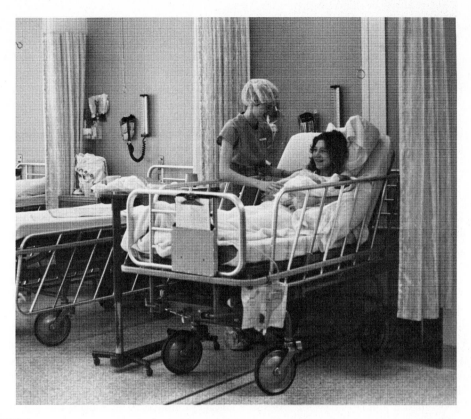

FIG. 10-1 Congratulations to mother and baby—getting acquainted in the postpartum recovery room.

Courtesy Grossmont Hospital, La Mesa, Calif.

4. Signs and symptoms of distention of the urinary bladder
5. General condition of the patient: color, feel of her skin (warm or cold, dry or clammy), level of consciousness (drowsy, apprehensive, unresponsive), and the presence of nausea or vomiting
6. Emotional status: depression, any special complaints or requests (pain, need to see husband and infant, interactions with infant, family, and friends)
7. Rate of flow and condition of any infusion present, and amount and type of medication added

8. Recovery from anesthesia, if any (return of motion, sensation, or consciousness)
9. Nutritional and fluid status

OBSERVATION FOR SIGNS OF HEMORRHAGE

Blood pressure, pulse, and general condition. Occasionally the blood pressure will be elevated at the time of transfer. This condition may be the result of the excitement of the birth and seeing the baby. It may be related to the type of oxytocic the patient received or is still receiving by intravenous infusion. It may be a sign of preeclampsia or be caused by the presence of pain or urinary retention. It is important to know the patient's baseline vital signs and how they have been since the birth. A guideline could be that all blood pressures over 130 mm Hg systolic or 90 mm Hg diastolic should be reported to the charge nurse.

The blood pressure may be low. Any pressure of 100 mm Hg systolic or below should definitely be reported. Other pressures that may not be that low but are not hypertensive compared with the patient's baseline and that continue to fall should be reported for evaluation. Many patients with a systolic reading of 90 mm Hg or below are going into circulatory collapse or shock. Such a falling blood pressure would be accompanied by an initially rising pulse. However, if the patient continues into shock, the pulse will gradually slow, weaken, and have a thready quality. Abnormally dilated pupils, pale, cyanotic, or clammy skin, apprehension, and an unconscious state are also signs of shock.

Some postpartum patients have a relatively slow pulse, but it has a good quality and is not associated with other signs of shock. This pulse rate (usually in the 60s) is not significant.

Lochia. The attending nurse is also interested in the amount of vaginal drainage, or *lochia*. As she checks the patient's drainage, she is sure to check under the patient's hips, since much of the drainage may not be observed on the perineal pad but seeks lower dependent areas. Immediately after birth the lochia should be moderate in quantity and dark or bright red—a quality called *rubra*. (About 2 days later the lochia changes to a pinkish brown, called *serosa*). The patient will usually wear two perineal pads that have to be changed once or at the most twice during her routine 2-hour postpartum check. These should always be removed and applied from front to back to avoid contamination of the perineum. The saturation of a greater number of pads would be considered abnormally excessive. When estimating blood loss and its significance, the nurse must evaluate the general condition and size of the patient. Usually a 450 to 500 ml blood loss is considered hemorrhage.

Fundus. The first consideration related to blood loss is the condition of the uterus. Is the fundus firm and contracted? Is it at or below the umbilicus? If a fundus is large, soft, or boggy (seems to contain excess blood), it should be gently massaged with a circular motion until firm while one hand is held against the top of the pubic bone to prevent the uterus from being inverted or prolapsed. If clots are suspected, once the fundus is *firm* it may be gently grasped and positioned in the middle of the abdomen. Pressure is then exerted in the direction of the pelvic canal to push out to the exterior the clots that were emptied from the uterus into the lower uterine segment and vagina during the massage. The uterus can be overstimulated by excessive manipulation, leading to its relaxation and possible hemorrhage. Students should not attempt to express clots alone until instructed individually. In the event of excessive vaginal bleeding, massage is the first measure employed to control vaginal hemorrhage.

It is surprising how quickly the uterus responds to simple massage in most cases. The nurse can easily feel the uterine muscles tighten. This tightening of the uterine muscle to make a firm fundus is essential. It pinches off the large vessels that brought blood to and from the placental sinuses before the placenta separated and was delivered. Allowing the baby to nurse early will also stimulate uterine muscles to contract.

Postpartum hemorrhage. When the uterus does not contract or remain contracted, the presence of placental fragments in the uterus may be suspected. If bleeding continues to be excessive and the uterus remains firm, a cause other than uterine relaxation must be sought to explain the blood loss. Excessive bleeding may develop because of a previously undetected cervical or vaginal laceration or a defective suture or repair. Frequently an abnormally bleeding patient will be returned to the delivery room to facilitate inspection of the uterus and vaginal canal. In some cases a dilatation and curettage of the uterus or the insertion of vaginal or, more rarely, uterine packing may be undertaken. If no lacerations or abnormal tissue retention are evident, treatment is usually confined to the administration of additional oxytocics such as oxytocin, synthetic injection, ergot, or its modification, methylergonovine (Methergine). Such treatment will combat the lethargy of the uterine muscles known as *uterine inertia*. Blood transfusions may be required. Patients who have had many children, multiple or frequent pregnancies, large babies, long or induced labors, uterine dystocia, or preeclampsia should be especially observed for uterine inertia.

The location and consistency of the fundus are important. A high, soft fundus makes nurses think of possible uterine bleeding; a high, firm fundus more often indicates urinary retention. A distended bladder, located just below the uterus, will cause the fundus to rise (usually to one side and most often to the right). This is an important cause of postpartal hemorrhage. After the completion of the third stage of a normal full-term labor, the fundus should be found below or possibly just at the umbilicus. Any higher position is suspect.

The position of the fundus is usually coded by counting finger widths above or below the umbilicus in the following manner. If the fundus (which usually feels somewhat like a large cantaloupe through the abdominal wall) is two finger widths above the level of the umbilicus, it is recorded as +2. If it is located one finger width below the level of the umbilicus, it is recorded as −1. A recording of 0 may indicate that the fundus is found at the level of the umbilicus, but usually nurses write "@ umbilicus." A typical record of the condition of the fundus would be "Fundus: firm −2 midline." On the first postpartal day the fundus is usually felt at the umbilicus or below at −1 or even −2 position. The location of the fundus may be influenced by the size of the patient's baby, the condition of her uterine muscle, the content of the urinary bladder, and abnormal conditions such as retained placental fragments and the development of uterine infection. Normally the uterus undergoes involution at the rate of about one finger width a day. At the end of 10 days it is usually down behind the pubic bone again and not palpable (Fig. 10-2).

Multiparas often complain of "aftercramps," caused by the contraction of the uterus in the pro-

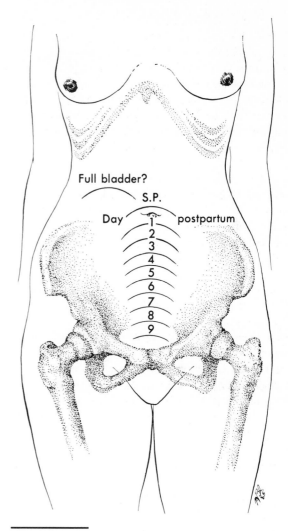

FIG. 10-2

Involution of the uterus, showing the various positions of the fundus. *S.P.,* Level just after the separation of the placenta from the uterine wall before its delivery.

cess of involution. They are more often bothered by cramping than are primiparas, who usually possess better muscle tone. Nursing mothers may experience more aftercramps because of the stimulation of the uterus during the process of nursing. Mild analgesics usually relieve the discomfort.

OBSERVATION FOR SIGNS OF URINARY DISTENTION

The most common cause of a high fundus is a full bladder. Even when a woman is catheterized just before birth, she may have a full bladder fairly soon after admittance to the postpartum area, especially if she is receiving or has had intravenous infusions. Routine catheterization just before birth is now relatively infrequent.

Other signs of urinary distention are a puffy area just above the pubic bone, complaints by the patient that she feels she should void but cannot, or the voiding of small amounts—less than 200 ml. This is called "dribbling" and usually indicates a full bladder that can contract only partially to release limited amounts of urine. A distended bladder is to be avoided because it jeopardizes normal bladder tone and may lead to the development of residual urine, an amount that routinely remains in the bladder and is not voided. Residual urine may become an excellent medium for bacterial multiplication. A distended bladder may also interfere with the normal contraction of the uterus and predispose the patient to hemorrhage. The condition may be painful and add to the aftercramping experienced by some patients.

Encouraging voiding. Voidings of postpartum patients are usually measured until two voidings of over 300 ml are recorded and a fundus check after the voidings indicates that the patient is emptying her bladder well. Thereafter patients are encouraged to void every 3 to 4 hours and to report any associated pain, burning, or difficulty in emptying their bladders. To check the efficiency of a bladder, the physician will sometimes order a catheterization for residual urine. It is important that all the equipment necessary be at the patient's bedside before she voids so that the catheterization may proceed without delay.

If a patient is suspected of having a full bladder, every effort should be made to help her void without resorting to catheterization, which may cause inflammation even in the best of circumstances, especially if repeated. Several techniques to encourage voiding may be useful.

If the patient cannot get up to go to the bathroom because of her general condition, because she has given birth too recently, or because she has had spinal anesthesia and does not as yet have an ambulation order, the problem of initiating natural voiding is more difficult. Many patients find it difficult to use the bedpan. The time that physicians allow their patients to ambulate post partum differs widely. Patients who have received spinal anesthetic may be kept in bed, flat or with a pillow, for 6 to 24 hours after the birth. The restriction in ambulation and posture is chiefly an effort to reduce the possibility of "spinal headache." Whether the restriction actually prevents the headache, however, has been debated. Patients who have had a general anesthetic can usually ambulate at the end of 8 hours. Those who have had local or no anesthetic usually are allowed up with aid as soon as they wish. Sometimes if a physician knows that a choice must be made between catheterization and probable success in voiding, he will choose to order earlier ambulation. Patients who have had spinal or saddle block anesthesia also experience more problems voiding because they have lost normal feeling in the bladder area.

If a metal bedpan must be used, it should be warmed. Patients who have had a spinal anesthesia may be raised just enough so that their hips are not higher than their heads while positioned on the pan. Privacy should be maintained, and, if possible, water should be left running into a washbowl to provide psychological stimulation. If an order is available, giving an analgesic such as oxycodone (Percodan) or acetaminophen (Tylenol) and codeine about 20 minutes before the bedpan is offered often helps solve the problem. Having the patient blow bubbles through a straw into a glass of water or pretend to blow up a balloon while she is on the bedpan sometimes helps relax the sphincter muscle. Some nurses report that placing a few drops of spirits of peppermint or an open ampule of spirits of ammonia in the bedpan may relax the urinary sphincter and safely stimulate a void. Pouring a measured amount of warm water over the perineum, using a sitz bath, or taking a shower, if approved, may help the patient void. If not, it will help clean the area before catheterization. Encouraging the patient to drink amounts of fluid exceeding normal requirements before she has voided normally will add to rather than relieve the problem and is not recommended.

The height of the fundus should always be determined after voiding has been initiated or catheterization performed to evaluate, by change in the position of the fundus, the efficiency of the emptying process and other possible problems with fundal relaxation.

Catheterization technique. If none of the preceding methods brings about the desired result, catheterization must be carried out. The nurse should know whether a specimen should be saved for laboratory analysis. The technique of catheterization and the materials used will differ from hospital to hospital. The following instructions are only general in character to make allowances for the different setups used, but they include principles that should be understood as well as review information for the student.

Individual differences of opinion still exist regarding how much urine should be removed from the bladder during the catheterization of a postpartum patient. The most common current practice appears to be to empty the bladder completely but slowly, even after more than 700 to 1,000 ml of urine are obtained. Although there could be a mild sympathetic response with slightly lowered blood pressure when more than 1,000 ml are removed, this could result from decreased maternal anxiety from the pressure of a full bladder. Lowered blood pressure has not been found to be significant in this type of patient.* If urine remains in the bladder, the problems usually outweigh any mild sympathetic response.

Catheterization: postpartum area

Use hospital procedures, bearing the following principles in mind:

Procedure:

1. Check the physician's order regarding catheterization.

---

*Sands, J.P.: Bladder pressure and its effect on mean arterial blood pressure, Invest. Urol. **10:**14-18, July 1972.

2. Explain in simple terms what is going to be done for the patient and that she will feel better as a result of the procedure.
3. Provide privacy and *lighting*.
4. You *must* get sufficient exposure to identify the urethral meatus, but you must be gentle. Remember, some patients have stitches in the true perineum just below the vagina.
5. Some of the newly delivered "saddle" patients will have little feeling in the area; others will be very sensitive.
6. *Remember,* once your hand has touched the patient, the hand is contaminated.
7. Sometimes holding the labia back with a cotton ball under one supporting finger helps maintain the position.
8. Technically, if you let the labia close after having washed the crucial area with antiseptic, the area must be rewashed, since it has been contaminated by the enfolding tissue; thus it is important to maintain the labia in a drawnback position.
9. The female urethra is about 1½ inches long. No more than 4 inches of the catheter should ever be inserted, to avoid bladder puncture. If obstruction is encountered, the catheter should never be forced. There may be an abnormality of the canal (presence of a tumor, stricture, etc.), or you may not have properly identified the meatus.
10. A slight downward incline of the catheter may aid insertion as the urethral canal slopes downward when the patient is in dorsal recumbent position.
11. Always measure the amount of urine obtained and record it. Note also the color of the urine. Note whether a catheter was left in place and if a specimen was obtained and sent to the laboratory.
12. Assure the patient that the inability to void is usually temporary.

EMOTIONAL STATUS

The patient's emotional status can be an early indication of psychologic or physical problems. Also, this is an important time for the patient to begin the development of *maternicity*, which supplies her with the emotional energy for feeling that her infant occupies an important part of her life. This is a time for developing bonds of affection. But the postpartal woman should have her own needs met so that she may meet those of her baby. She needs to control her own body before she can undertake the mothering tasks ahead.

The labor experience is often one of the most demanding periods for a woman. To use it instructively in her life, she will need to talk about it and relive it. (See also p. 203.)

Assessment for pain. Although most patients will be able to describe discomfort, it is important to make a systematic assessment of the presence, cause, type, and location of pain. Changes in the patient's blood pressure and pulse may also indicate the existence of pain. Perhaps nursing measures, such as emptying the bladder, comfort and cleansing procedures, or positioning, will ease the discomfort. Applications of cold or heat, as ordered, may be indicated. And, of course, analgesics will be used when needed as ordered. Whatever measure is used must be evaluated as to its success in relieving the pain.

CONTINUING CARE

The need for good aseptic technique during all procedures in the postpartum area is readily understood when one realizes that within the uterine cavity, easily accessible to microorganisms from the exterior, is an open "wound," the former place of placental attachment. This diminishing but still easily infected area is well supplied with veins and arteries. It provides an ideal entry into the general body circulation and the possibility of septicemia.

Infection is still a threat if nurses are not enlightened and conscientious in their techniques. In fact, although the maternal death rate is falling, the 1978 statistical reports for the United States list sepsis (infection) of childbirth and the puerperium as the second cause of maternal mortality.

Perineal care

Postpartum perineal cleansing is given in countless ways in maternity services across the nation. Techniques have ranged from the use of separate sterile irrigation setups by a masked nurse each time the procedure is needed by the patient to teaching the mother which way to wipe with a clean washcloth. The acceptance of a technique should be based on whether it is safe, adequate, simple, inexpensive, and aesthetically satisfying to all concerned. The principles involved in perineal care should be the same whether it is done by the nurse or the patient herself.

PERINEAL CLEANSING

Perineal cleansing is performed to prevent infection, eliminate odor, observe the area and lochial flow, and ease the patient. Any equipment used by the patient should be absolutely clean and should not be used by another. Equipment used by more than one patient should be sterilized between patients. Hands should be washed before and after care. Care should be taught in cleansing the perineum and in removing and applying perineal pads so that soil cannot be introduced to the vulva. This means, for both nurse and patient, stroking from front to back once only with each cleansing surface. It means that the nurse will routinely remove and apply perineal pads from front to back, and not touch the surface that adjoins the perineum.

At least once each shift the perineum of the patient who gave birth vaginally should be observed for signs of infection (redness, swelling, or unusual discharge) and for signs of trauma. A hematoma in the area may develop slowly. Sufficient light should be provided to see the area clearly. The perineal pad should be changed each time the toilet is used. Some maternity services issue plastic squeeze bottles for antiseptic solution or warm tap water plus cellulose wipes to each mother for self-care. Water temperature should be tested on the thigh or wrist to promote comfort and prevent burns. Other services issue pitchers and furnish appropriate solutions. Still others provide individually wrapped, moist towelettes impregnated with rapid-drying antiseptic. The use of a clean washcloth when showering would be appropriate, making sure that the mother uses only the front-to-back motion.

In most instances the mother may be taught perineal cleansing and instructed to do it after each

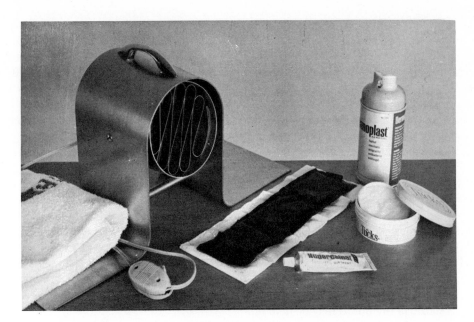

FIG. 10-3 Aids in relieving perineal discomfort through local application: the perineal lamp (the hood is draped with a towel when used), a perineal ice pack (unwrapped for better viewing), Nupercainal anesthetic ointment, Dermoplast antiseptic-anesthetic spray, and Tucks (lightweight witch-hazel-impregnated compresses).

Courtesy Grossmont Hospital, La Mesa, Calif.

trip to the bathroom. This should be continued at least twice a day until the lochial flow has stopped. If a bedrest regimen is necessary, the patient may be placed on a bedpan and warm water poured over her perineum, taking care to avoid entering the birth canal with the water. Then she may be patted dry from front to back with clean tissue.

EPISIOTOMY AND FIRST- AND SECOND-DEGREE LACERATIONS

For patients who have had episiotomies or laceration repairs, perineal care usually involves more than just cleansing. Many hospitals provide an antiseptic, analgesic benzocaine perineal spray such as Dermoplast or Americaine. The physician may also order sitz baths to increase circulation and ease discomfort in the perineum. Most maternity services also routinely offer a perineal lamp ("Peri light") several times a day for 20-minute intervals to improve circulation, promote healing, and ease

discomfort. It is usually not applied until several hours after the birth because it may stimulate additional bleeding if given too early. When perineal lamps are applied, care must be taken that they are no less than 18 inches (41 cm) from the perineum. A 25 to 40-watt lamp is used. The thighs of blondes, redheads, or other fair-skinned women should always be draped before the lamp is used. This is a good time to observe the perineum.

Patients with standard episiotomies and first- and second-degree lacerations usually respond very well to the combination of cleansing, heat lamp, and analgesic spray offered. However, many such women still would prefer to stand rather than sit. Advising the mother to tense her buttocks and tuck in her pelvis before sitting down often helps lessen the pull and discomfort of the perineum.

Other local analgesics may also be ordered, such as dibucaine (Nupercainal) ointment and witch-hazel compresses such as Tucks (Fig. 10-3).

THIRD-DEGREE LACERATIONS

Mothers who have had third-degree perineal laceration (extending into the rectal sphincter) may need more help. Great caution must be exercised in giving patients who have had such problems any type of enema, suppository, or cathartic, since the suture line may not only involve the sphincter but also may extend into the rectum itself. Oral and topical analgesics may be needed.

APPLICATION OF COLD TO THE PERINEUM

Occasionally a patient has a swollen perineum after childbirth, or a physician may consider swelling of the perineal tissues likely in a certain patient. An order for the application of cold compresses or ice packs may be written. An ice pack should be wrapped with clean, waterproof material and a fairly thin, absorbent outer layer and intermittently applied directly to the perineum. It may be held in place by its own attachments or by an encircling sanitary pad. Various commercial clean and sterile perineal ice packs are now available. They need to be fairly comfortable, durable, and able to provide cold for reasonable periods. If no such pads are available to the nurse, she may fill a rubber glove with cracked ice and water, close it tightly and wrap it in a light, disinfected plastic covering and a clean towel. Ice packs must be changed frequently. The perineal area should be frequently observed for developing hematoma or increased swelling. Application of ice is usually limited to the first 24 hours, when it is most effective in preventing edema.

Ambulation

As previously stated, the ambulation of the postpartum patient is determined by the orders of the attending physician and depends on the type of anesthetic given during delivery and the general condition of the patient. Early judicious ambulation of postpartum patients lessens the incidence of respiratory, circulatory, and urinary problems, helps prevent constipation, and promotes the rapid return of strength. But whenever the patient is first allowed out of bed, *the nurse should not leave her alone!* These patients often become dizzy and faint. If the patient does become faint, ease her onto a chair, her bed, or even gently to the floor, but do not leave her to seek help. If she is on a chair, support her with her head lowered to her knees. No matter how many days post partum, the nurse should always evaluate her ambulating patient.

The first time the postpartum patient gets up she may experience a sudden temporary gush of vaginal discharge. If it is dark red, it is probably not significant. It reflects the patient's change in posture after being recumbent for several hours when the uterine drainage was not as efficient. However, the patient should be evaluated for shock.

Bath and breast-care procedures

The postpartum bed bath given in the recovery room or patient's unit after delivery is a procedure designed to permit observation and instruction as well as provide comfort and protection against infection. The postpartum patient is likely to perspire profusely. It is one way the body has to rid itself of excess fluids. In most cases mothers have only one such bed bath during their hospital stay. After that they usually are allowed to take showers.

The postpartum bed bath differs from the routine bed-bath procedure followed in other hospital areas. It recognizes that the new mother's body includes two areas that are easily infected, the breasts and the perineum, which leads to the internal reproductive tract. If the patient had a cesarean delivery, the incision line would constitute a third area susceptible to infection.

Postpartum bath procedure

A modified hospital procedure for bed bath would be used. During the bath the following changes would be incorporated:

1. Start washing the breast area first, whether the mother is nursing or not. Often only clear water is used to help prevent the formation of cracked nipples.
   a. Wash in a circular manner from the nipple outward.

b. Instruct the mother to follow this same order of bathing during her shower the next day.

c. If the mother is nursing, especially observe the nipples for inversion, fissures, and cleanliness.

d. Dry the area and cover with a clean towel. If the mother is nursing, exposure of the nipple to the air for short periods (15 minutes) will help maintain healthy tissue. The application of lanolin or breast cream, if ordered, following air exposure and nursing is advocated by many.

2. Apply bra and breast pads, if needed.

a. If patients may wear their own bras, be sure they are large enough and clean.

b. All patients should have some type of adequate breast support and breast pads if appropriate.

c. In applying the bra, be sure the breasts are not pushed down against the chest wall. They should be elevated and lifted toward the opposite shoulder.

3. When washing the feet and legs, do not rub vigorously or massage because of the danger of emboli.

4. Perineal care is usually done after the bath as a separate procedure. At this time the principles of perineal self-care may be taught.

ANATOMY OF THE BREASTS

A greater understanding of the basics of breast care, the technique of nursing an infant, and the principles involved in pumping the breasts may be gained at this time by a brief description of the anatomy involved.

The breasts, or mammary glands, are divided into segments, or lobes, which in turn are divided into lobules (smaller lobes). These contain the actual milk-producing glands known as *acini*, or alveoli (Fig. 10-4). The breasts are richly supplied with blood vessels, lymphatics, and nerves.

Each segment of the breast radiates from the central colored portion, known as the *areola*, which in turn rings the sensitive erectile tissue known as the *nipple*. Milk ducts from the acini travel toward the areola and open out onto the surface of the nipples. Usually each nipple has 15 to 20 such openings.

As each major milk duct approaches the areola, it widens temporarily, forming a small reservoir, or sinus. When the baby begins sucking, oxytocin from the posterior pituitary is released. Its action stimulates the contraction of muscles around the milk ducts, allowing the milk to flow into the sinus to be readily available to the baby. This physiologic response is called the *let-down reflex*. It may be accompanied by a tingling or shivering sensation. It occurs in both breasts, even though the baby is only nursing at one. The oxytocin also stimulates the uterine muscles to contract, thus lessening the possibility of hemorrhage and increasing the rapidity of involution. When a mother pumps her breasts manually, she obtains the best flow if she first presses the breast tissue back with her thumb and fingers and then squeezes the breast. Properly holding the breast with one hand during nursing not only allows the baby to breathe more comfortably but also encourages the secretion of milk. For more information on breast-feeding see p. 239.

BREAST ENGORGEMENT

Breast engorgement may occur about the third day post partum and is often regarded by mothers as the result of the milk "coming in." However, not all the tenderness and swelling result from the presence of more milk. It results, for the most part, from the increased venous and lymphatic congestion in the breast tissue.

Engorgement may be avoided or lessened by breast massage techniques and manual expression of colostrum during the prenatal period. It also will be greatly reduced or eliminated by frequent early (on-demand) feedings of the newborn. With engorgement the breasts may feel hard and nodular. Lay people have called this "caked breasts." This uncomfortable and painful condition can sometimes be eased for nursing mothers by the manual expression of a small amount of milk. Good breast support worn continuously, warm, moist compresses, a warm shower, or the use of an oxytocin nasal spray prescribed to enhance the let-down reflex and the flow of milk may be helpful. Analgesic drugs may also be prescribed to relieve the pain. Many medications can pass through the milk to the nursing infant with varying effects.

Nonnursing mothers may be made more comfortable by supportive bras, the application of ice

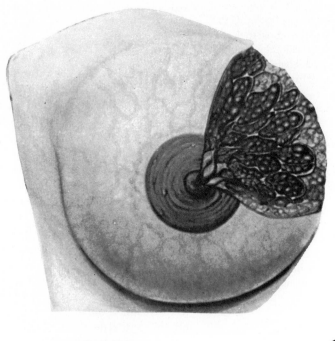

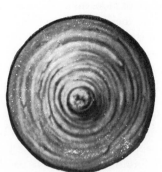

In the lactating breast the nipples
become characteristically erect

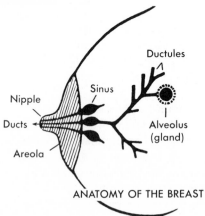

ANATOMY OF THE BREAST

FIG. 10-4   Lactating breast.

Courtesy Carnation Co., Los Angeles, Calif.

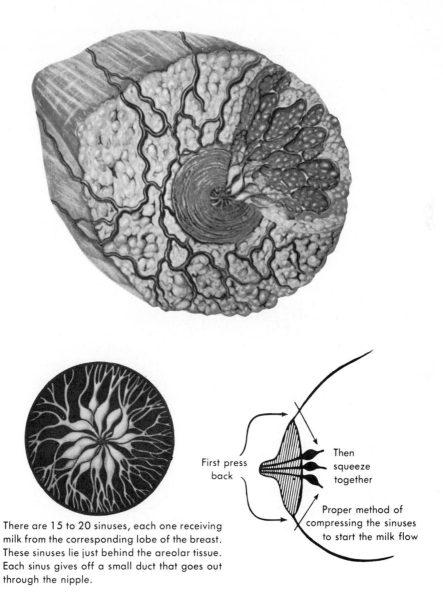

There are 15 to 20 sinuses, each one receiving
milk from the corresponding lobe of the breast.
These sinuses lie just behind the areolar tissue.
Each sinus gives off a small duct that goes out
through the nipple.

First press
back

Then
squeeze
together

Proper method of
compressing the sinuses
to start the milk flow

**FIG. 10-4,
cont'd**

Lactating breast.

"caps," analgesics, and perhaps the prescription of oral estrogenic or androgenic compounds, such as stilbestrol and chlorotrianisene (Tace). A single intramuscular injection of testosterone enanthate (Deladumone OB), best given from late first stage to the third stage of labor, may have been prescribed.

Recent research has indicated that a causal relationship may exist between the later development of endometrial cancer and the use of lactation suppressants, as well as an increased occurrence of thromboemboli following the use of estrogens, especially after cesarean birth; therefore, informed patient consent is required by the Federal Drug Administration before estrogens are administered.

PUMPING THE BREASTS

When the order is given that a mother's breasts be pumped, it is usually done to maintain or encourage her milk supply. This procedure is not advised routinely to relieve engorgement in non-nursing mothers, since emptying the breasts stimulates more milk production.

A mother may pump her breasts manually as described or use a hand or electric pump as shown in Fig. 10-5. Whatever method is used, she should be supported comfortably in a sitting or side position with her hands and breasts freshly washed. Any equipment that would touch her breasts should have been sterilized before use. If the milk is to be saved for the baby, it should be collected in a sterile container, using aseptic technique. The mother should be instructed how to empty her breasts using the method that is ordered or preferred. If the electric breast pump is used, the nurse must make sure that the suction is not too great. It should be increased gradually—4 to 6 inches of pressure is plenty! A record of the amount of milk obtained should be kept in the patient's chart. Mothers sometimes are distressed at the color of their milk. They should be assured that although human breast milk looks more bluish than cow's milk, it is perfectly suited for the baby. Colostrum, the first secretion from the breast, is more creamy or orange in appearance.

BREAST INFECTIONS

Infections of the breast are not as common today as formerly, but occasionally they still occur. Most infections are introduced at the nipple area, which may be fissured or cracked because of poor nursing techniques or exceptionally fragile breast tissue. Such a complication is usually not found while the patient is in the postpartum area because of early discharge practices. It becomes the subject of an office call and, rarely, an admission to another part of the hospital for excision and drainage of an abscess. Fortunately, most cases of mastitis do not progress as far as abscess formation. The nurse should always observe the patient's breasts or inquire about their condition. Signs of inflammation or cracked and bleeding nipples should always be reported. Exposure to air and application of an antiseptic analgesic breast cream may be advised. Breast infections are most often caused by the organism *Staphylococcus aureus*. Any patient with such an infection should be isolated and moved from the maternity service. The application of cold or heat to the breasts may be ordered. The treatment prescribed will depend on the stage of the infection. Systemic antibiotics are commonly given. Nursing the infant is usually continued, and an antibiotic is chosen that is not harmful to the infant.

Elimination

Constipation may be a problem to the postpartum patient; it may be caused by diminished intestinal and abdominal muscle tone. Physicians often order a mild laxative the evening of the first or second postpartum day. If this medication does not produce results, a suppository or a gentle enema is often scheduled. Since many of these patients suffer from hemorrhoids or have adjacent episiotomy or laceration repairs, one must be very careful in the insertion of the suppository or well-lubricated enema tip. Early ambulation, increased fluids, and a diet containing roughage and cereal food fiber may prevent constipation. If stools are difficult to pass, a stool softener may be prescribed. During

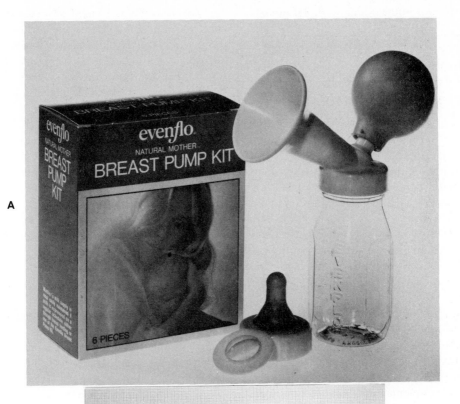

FIG. 10-5 **A,** Manual breast pump-bottle combination. **B,** Electric breast pump.

A courtesy Evenflo Products Co., Ravenna, Ohio. **B** courtesy Grossmont Hospital, La Mesa, Calif.

the second day the patient may experience diuresis with a urinary output as high as 3,000 ml.

Supportive care and educational opportunities

AIMS OF POSTPARTAL HOSPITALIZATION

The postpartal hospital stay should ideally provide safety, rest, constructive encouragement to the recent parturient, and opportunities to initiate parent-infant bonding. However, in some areas the actual hospitalization period is so brief that it is difficult to realize the ideal. Discharge on or before the third postpartum day is almost routine in many parts of the United States, and short stays of 24 hours or less are increasing. The pendulum has swung a long way since the time of mother or grandmother, when 5 and 10 days passed before the new mother stirred from her bed!

The fact that the pendulum of postpartum management needed to swing is not debated. Certainly early ambulation and self-care techniques have reduced the incidence of many complications associated with prolonged bed rest, such as thrombophlebitis, pneumonia, and subinvolution of the uterus. However, the shortened postpartal stay necessitates a prenatal reevaluation of the needs of the new mother and her provisions for help in the home setting. The average primipara has had less opportunity than her counterpart of past generations to learn the art of child care in her own family circle while growing up. Often her first responsible contact with a newborn infant arrives the day she takes her own baby home from the hospital, unless she has had the benefit of rooming-in with her baby. Many times she has adequate and loving help at home. Too many times she does not.

EDUCATIONAL RESOURCES

There do not seem to be enough hours in the hospital day to teach a new mother what she needs to know about herself and her baby and still give her sufficient time to regain her strength and composure. Of course, for a multipara perhaps educational needs are not as great, but the primipara cannot gain the assurance desired in a 3-day period even if hospital classes and practice sessions could be held all day long, and she could attend them all.

At present one answer seems to lie in the introduction of parentcraft courses into the regular school curriculum. Also, greater use of the prenatal and postnatal courses offered by such community agencies as adult school programs, childbirth education associations, YWCA, Red Cross, or public health departments and wider involvement of the visiting nurse should be encouraged. Further, more rooming-in facilities in hospitals, an increased awareness by all postpartum-staff members of their teaching roles, and the possibility of family telephone contacts with postpartum and nursery personnel following discharge are needed.

The vocational nurse may not find herself involved in any formalized classroom teaching, but the quality of nursing care given, the importance she places on personal hygiene (her own and her patient's), and the skill she develops in observing, listening to, and responding to her patient's needs will make her an important teacher nonetheless. With the advent of primary nursing and care of the mother and infant together, opportunities for teaching a mother to care for her own infant are increased.

Of course, in places where postpartum stays are longer and facilities and staff are available, actual classes in baby care, bathing, formula preparation, and nursing techniques may be offered to mothers. Some maternity departments have started closed-circuit television classes. If the prerequisites are present, the maternity department should not neglect its opportunity. (See Fig. 10-6.)

At her arrival on the postpartum unit, assessment of the mother's teaching needs should begin. It is important to focus on the individual mother's needs, since the time available is often short. The box on p. 199 offers possible areas of teaching needs. After teaching it is important to gain feedback from the mother to evaluate what learning has taken place. Listening to the mother describe in

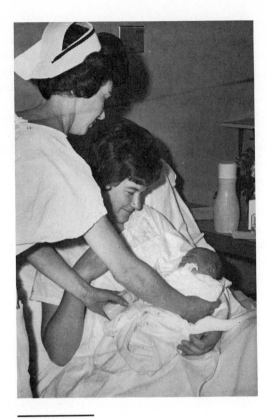

FIG. 10-6

Nurses can do a great deal to reassure new mothers.

Courtesy Grossmont Hospital, La Mesa, Calif.

PARENT EDUCATION NEEDS OR TEACHING TOPICS

1. Recognition of postpartum complications and what is normal
2. Perineal and breast care
3. Fluid needs, nutrition, and weight loss
4. Rest and exercise
5. Birth control concerns (if wished)
6. Anticipating and dealing with postpartal "blues"
7. Physician's appointments
8. Prevention of infection
9. Infant care and feeding (Chapter 13)
10. Prevention of accidents

---

her own words what she learned or observing her as she performs the skill are two ways to evaluate her learning.

ROOMING-IN

The so-called rooming-in plan is especially well adapted for providing learning opportunities for the new mother who desires to have this closer contact with her infant. The baby is kept at the mother's bedside or in an adjoining cubicle close at hand most of the day. If the mother so desires, her baby may be returned to a special part of the newborn nursery for the night or specified periods. A nursery nurse may be assigned to go to the patient's unit, bathe the baby, and help with any questions that the mother may have. She may return at feeding times and when called to assist in any way necessary. As the mother feels stronger and more confident, she is invited to participate in her child's care. The postpartum nurse washes her hands and wears an overgown when caring for the mother, her unit, or the baby. Visitors are usually restricted to the father or chosen companion. He must wear an overgown during the visit and wash his hands when entering. In this way he, too, is able to know his child better before discharge. Rooming-in is not desired by all parents. Some mothers, especially multiparas, welcome the brief period when they will have little direct responsibility for child care. Others may feel too tired to have the baby at the bedside for extended visits. However, this method of care when available, offers excellent training and learning possibilities.

• • •

The new mother is usually an exceptionally good source of questions. Some the nurse will be able to answer immediately. Others she must refer to the physician.

One of the first things the mother wishes to investigate after she has seen her baby and recovered some of her strength is her own weight loss. She is usually dissatisfied with her initial loss the first time she steps on the scale and needs to be reassured that under normal conditions she will approximate her prepregnant weight in about 1 month. However, to help regain a good figure, she must regulate her caloric intake to her metabolic needs. The weight gained during pregnancy in normal conditions is caused by the size of the infant, the weight of the placenta (about 1 pound), the amniotic fluid (about 2 pounds), the increased size of the uterus (about 2 pounds), breast enlargement (about 3 pounds), and increased circulating and tissue fluids and reserves.

Sometimes students are taken aback when they see postpartum patients ambulating for the first time. They confide to one another that Mrs. Smith does not look as though she has delivered yet! Multiparas, because of the repeated stretching of the abdominal muscles, particularly need time and effort to regain a nonpregnant appearing shape. Occasionally a hernia develops because of the separation of the rectus abdominis muscles, which are supposed to support the abdominal contents. This condition adds to the "pregnant look." A number of years ago the use of straight or many-tailed scultetus abdominal binders for support was common. Now they are seldom ordered unless the abdomen is particularly pendulous. If a scultetus binder is ordered in the postpartum period, it should be applied upside down with the wrapping starting at the top to avoid forcing the uterus up and out of place.

Nowadays it is thought better to rely on the abdominal muscles for support and to build up their strength instead of advocating indiscriminate use of abdominal binders. Various postpartum exercises are recommended to restore muscle tone as well as improve circulation, promote involution, and regain general strength. These exercises are graded according to difficulty, ranging from deep breathing and gentle range of motion to pelvic tilts,

leg lifts, and the knee-chest position. The progression of exercises should be directed by the attending physician because some may be too strenuous or even dangerous if done too early. (The knee-chest position done in early puerperium has been associated with a few cases of air embolism.)

Mothers often ask what they may do when they return home. They should be advised to increase their activities gradually and to avoid fatigue, lifting heavy objects and older children, and climbing stairs. They should be encouraged to have midmorning and midafternoon rest periods and arrange to have extra help at home. Newly delivered mothers have a tendency to try to do too much and then regret it. Even while in the hospital the provision for rest is sometimes limited. Nurses should make every effort to provide their patients with a restful environment and periods of relaxation. Showers and shampoos at home are allowed as soon as desired. Many physicians allow tub bathing equally as early. Douching should be deferred until after the routine postpartum examination by the physician in 3 to 6 weeks, *if resumed at all*. (See p. 159.) The physician's advice should be asked regarding resumption of sexual intercourse. Couples are usually asked to wait until lochial discharge has stopped and discomfort has minimized.

In the interim women should be made to feel welcome to contact their physicians if any problems arise. Accessible and knowledgeable nursing staff members, a good physician-patient chat, and the distribution before discharge of printed instructions and hints for a smooth adjustment to life with the baby helps solve some of the predictable difficulties. Problems that should be reported when noted include pain or localized tenderness in the legs, increased vaginal flow, painful breasts or cracked nipples, painful urination, backache, and fever.

In nonnursing mothers, menses usually return in 5 to 8 weeks. The nursing mother may not experience menstruation until several weeks after the weaning of her infant. This does not mean, however, that she cannot become pregnant during this period. Success in nursing the infant may be enhanced by support groups such as La Leche

League and the federally sponsored food supplementation program for Women, Infants and Children (WIC).

DISCHARGE

The discharge of the mother and child from the maternity service is an exciting time for the family. A calm and, literally, collected patient the morning of discharge is rather the exception despite all efforts to smooth the departure. Before the patient leaves, any instructions that are to be carried out after discharge concerning the mother or baby must be clarified.

The baby is brought to the room after all other arrangements have been completed and the mother is ready to go. Her bags are packed, and she is dressed as she wishes. Great care should be taken that all her belongings leave with her.

The baby is identified again and dressed for the short trip outdoors to the car. The mother is usually discharged in a wheelchair. The nursing staff sincerely wish to both a "bon voyage."

SPECIAL CONSIDERATIONS

Postpartum hemorrhage, the most common serious problem in the postpartum period, has been previously discussed on p. 186. Preeclampsia has been discussed on pp. 171 to 177.

Cesarean birth patient

If a cesarean birth is anticipated, the mother may be admitted initially to the postpartum unit and prepared for surgery by its staff. For a review of what this preparation entails and other related information, see p. 143.

NURSING CARE POSTSURGERY

The physical care of the postcesarean-birth patient is similar to that of any patient who has had abdominal surgery. However, in addition, this patient has become a mother. She needs special attention to her postpartal needs.

Immediate observation. Blood pressure, pulse, and respiration rate should be taken at least every 15 minutes for a minimum of 2 hours and until stable. A falling blood pressure and a rising pulse are among the first signs of difficulty. Other signs of shock include pallor, cold, clammy skin, apprehension, disorientation or unresponsive behavior, and dilated pupils. But do not wait to observe all the classic signs of shock before seeking help. The dressing should be observed for drainage and any staining reported. The lochia must be observed and evaluated. As a rule cesarean birth patients have less lochial flow. After the placenta is extracted during surgery, the uterus is inspected and gently sponged, emptying the cavity of some of the drainage that would otherwise be expelled vaginally. The fundus may be gently palpated after surgery to determine its position, but it should not be massaged.

The patient usually receives intravenous fluids during the first 24 to 48 hours. The first ordered fluids may contain an oxytocic to cause the uterus to contract. The intravenous infusion should be frequently observed for rate of flow and signs of infiltration. An indwelling Foley catheter is usually maintained for 12 to 24 hours or until the IV fluids are discontinued. The catheter should be checked for rate of flow and the type of urine being expelled, and approved catheter care given. The tubing must be stabilized, without dependent loops.

Psychologic and postpartal support. Although the initial physical care of the new cesarean birth mother is perhaps one's primary priority, the emotional and maternal needs of the patient must not be forgotten. According to her strength and desires, she should be given opportunity to see, handle, and nurse her infant. Communication with the nursery should be frequent. If the infant can be brought to the bedside for care by the nursery nurse, perhaps this should be recommended. Often the "section patient" feels very isolated and fearful regarding her offspring.

Dietary considerations. Although orders may vary considerably, at first, the patient is usually given nothing by mouth, and then she is gradually given a progressive surgical diet based on her toleration of oral feedings. This would mean progressing from sips of water to a clear liquid, to a soft diet, and then to a regular diet, over a period of approximately 3 or 4 days. Because of their reputations as gas-formers, milk, ice water, and citrus juices are often omitted from the diet along with other notorious foodstuffs such as green peppers, cauliflower, and brussels sprouts. Some observers believe that drinking through straws may also increase flatus. A new surgical patient or one with an IV infusion or an indwelling catheter should have intake and output determinations taken.

Ambulation. Although orders to ambulate the patient may not be written until the day after surgery, planned movement in bed should be carried out. The patient is periodically encouraged to breathe deeply and cough as soon as she is put to bed from surgery. She is turned at least every 2 hours. How long she remains flat depends on the anesthetic used, her general condition, and her physician's orders. When she is first allowed out of bed, she should briefly dangle her feet and then stand and march in place; during the second attempt, she walks with the nurse's support. Walking the patient to a chair two steps away for a 15-minute period of sitting is not considered the best interpretation of "ambulate the patient"! The sitting position does not aid the circulation in the lower extremities. It is important to follow orders for progressive ambulation. Just because a patient is hesitant does not mean that ambulation should not be carried out. The nurse does not need to reiterate all the complications the physician seeks to avoid by early ambulation. Usually if the nurse simply states that it will help the patient feel stronger faster and prevent or relieve flatus, the needed motivation will be provided.

Some physicians are allowing cesarean section patients to shower relatively soon after delivery, with a plastic protector over their abdominal dressings.

Abdominal distention. Abdominal distention caused by trapped flatus can be distressing to any patient who has undergone abdominal surgery. Frequently it is the chief complaint of the cesarean

birth patient. Although medications such as morphine or meperidine hydrochloride (Demerol) may be used for postoperative pain, it is still much better to try to prevent or eliminate the distention. As part of her care, the nurse should evaluate the condition of the abdomen. Is the area just above the dressing hard, bloated, and tender, or is it soft and relatively flat? Ambulating the patient may help relieve distention—so may intermittent, small enemas, the Harris flush technique, or insertion of a rectal tube. Also helpful are suppositories, laxatives, or the use of neostigmine. Occasionally, strange to say, the use of carbonated drinks helps the patient to "bring up air" more easily and gain relief. In severe cases a nasal gastric tube connected to suction may be inserted.

Sutures. The cesarean patient will receive perineal irrigations for cleanliness and comfort, but no sprays or heat lamps are used, since no suturing or trauma occurred in the perineal area. But abdominal sutures, clips, or adhesive "butterflies" are usually removed about the fifth or sixth postoperative day.

COMPLICATIONS

Cesarean births result in a relatively low maternal mortality. Neonatal mortality, however, is higher. The results depend on the condition of the mother and the fetus, the equipment available, and the skill of the operator and nursing staff. Related maternal problems reported include sepsis, hemorrhage, thrombosis formation, embolism, and complications of anesthesia. Occasionally afibrinogenemia complicates the recovery.

The sorrowing mother

Not all mothers admitted to the postpartum area leave with healthy babies. Some leave without a child because the infant did not survive birth or died in the early hours of life. Some leave alone because their infant is premature or has some abnormality. Still others leave alone because they are not going to keep their babies, who will be placed for adoption. It is especially sad when a new mother who has waited for her child with anticipation finds that for all her waiting and care she has either no child or a child with gross deformities. Parents also need each other at this time. For the nurse to give parents the support they will need in this crisis, she must acknowledge her own feelings. Only then can she really begin to understand the parents' reactions. Nurses are in a position to give a great deal of help and support to parents during infant sickness or death. Most parents have an over-whelming need to talk about the experience and should be allowed to do so with whomever they choose to share. Some of the things a nurse can do to facilitate the parents' acceptance of the deformity or death are showing concern, allowing the parents to cry, relaxing visiting hour regulations, supporting the parents in their need to see and touch the infant, providing adequate and appropriate information, and allowing expressions of anger (recognizing these to be part of the grief process). Listening is probably the most important part of emotional support; platitudes are not helpful. Groups of bereaved parents are being organized in some settings to allow parents to share feelings and benefit from group counsel. Supportive nurses who are available, who listen, who recognize the stages of mourning, and respond to the patient's cues, by touch or voice, will be much appreciated by these parents.

Nurses on the postpartum unit should be alerted by the nursery when a baby is not "doing well." Team members need sharing of information by everyone working with the family. Early parental contact with the infant usually should be encouraged. (See p. 284.) Referral to helping agencies may be needed.

The unwed mother

At times, conditions surrounding pregnancy and birth call for "confidential" or "no information" treatment of a patient. For numerous reasons, knowledge of the presence of the patient in the hospital may not be wished to be shared. The patient may be unmarried. Her child may have been conceived before marriage took place. Her husband may not have fathered the child. A patient may simply want a quiet hospital period without undue publicity attached to pregnancy. Some of these women will choose to have their babies adopted; others will keep them.

Various church-related and public organizations are engaged in helping the unwed mother and her child, although with changing attitudes and mores, special homes for these maternity patients are less frequently used. Public welfare departments assist with adoption arrangements when desired. It is not the function of the nurse to judge the circumstances under which a woman has become pregnant. The nurse's function is to meet these patients' postpartum needs as well as possible. The circumstances in which most of these women find themselves are symptoms and not the cause of basic difficulties in their lives. These patients need kindness, probably as never before. Constructive help from professional social work personnel to aid the woman in facing the situation and evaluating its causes may be indicated.

If the mother is planning to give up her baby for adoption, individual assessment of each mother should be made when determining if she should be separated from the baby. An emotionally healthy mother with the support of friends and family may work through this crisis better when given an opportunity to do caretaking activities for her baby.

Maternal postpartal challenges and tasks

It has been said that all postpartum patients, regardless of their different individual backgrounds and specific strengths and problems, must respond successfully to certain challenges related to changes in body image, roles, and responsibilities before they can develop a satisfactory sense of progress, wellness, and fulfillment. Ramona Mercer, in her excellent article "The Nurse and Maternal Tasks of Early Postpartum"* speaks of the mother's need to review her childbirth experience and integrate it into her total self-concept and to put aside the fantasies that she may have entertained regarding her unseen baby by identifying, claiming, and learning to care for her real infant. She indicates that as the mother undertakes the tasks of adapting to the reality of her changing body and her new role as both mother and mate, the mother is performing a type of necessary "grief work." The nurse can be an important force in helping the mother cope with these changing perceptions and developing "duties" in a realistic and progressively successful manner. Ideally the nurse listens, teaches, reassures, and reinforces the mother's efforts as she moves from a role of dependency to one of greater independence and autonomy.

Postpartum "blues"

As body hormonal levels change and the responsibilities of an enlarging family and infant care rather suddenly make themselves felt, many new mothers experience at least some degree of depression, commonly called postpartum "blues." The nurse may enter a patient's room for a routine check and find the previously exuberant mother trying to wipe away some tears. While providing some tissues and gently asking what she may do to help, the nurse is often told that the patient does not really know why she is crying. "The tears just come." The knowledge that mothers sometimes are a bit depressed from 1 to 7 days after childbirth is usually reassuring to the patient. "Blues" commonly are not prolonged.

Postpartum psychosis

Labor and birth often comprise a physically and emotionally exhausting period even for the normal, healthy woman. For a small minority the entire

---

*Mercer, R.T.: The nurse and maternal tasks of early postpartum, Am. J. Mat. Child Nurs. **6:**341-345, Sept.-Oct. 1981.

period of pregnancy is a great strain because of other basic unresolved psychologic problems. During the postpartum period these patients may show the development of definite signs of mental illness. They may become withdrawn and disinterested or belligerent and suspicious. They are often victims of unreasonable fears. In severe cases they may become dangerous to themselves and others. Any signs of such behavior or inability to cope with reality should be reported and evaluated by the patient's physician. Psychiatric help may be indicated. Often these patients have had histories of previous emotional instability or mental illness. It is important to recognize and report early signs of possible difficulty—for example, rejection of infant or spouse, excessive depression, anxiety state, amnesia, or distorted perceptions.

Puerperal infection

The term "puerperal infection" may be used to describe any infection of the reproductive tract during the puerperium. More technically speaking, a patient has been considered to have a puerperal infection if she has a temperature of 100.4° F (38° C) or more on 2 successive days during the first 10 days' post partum, excluding the first 24 hours—unless another source of the temperature is determined. However, this definition has been found to be inadequate by critics, since many infections may be masked by the use of antibiotics.

The appearance of a puerperal infection is always a serious development. It may involve the perineum proper, the uterine lining (endometritis), or the pelvic area outside the uterus (parametritis). It may extend by means of blood vessels and lymphatics to areas relatively far removed, as in the case of septic thrombophlebitis of the leg. It is most often localized, but it can become a generalized peritonitis or septicemia. It can be caused by several different organisms, but the usual microorganism implicated is the streptococcus or staphylococcus. If such an unfortunate complication should occur, all efforts should be made to determine the orginal source of the infection. This involves a knowledge of the history of the patient, the personal health of attending personnel and visitors, and the nursing and medical techniques used.

Use of aseptic technique (careful hand washing, perineal care, etc.) by patients and other caregivers can decrease the number of infections.

ACCOMPANYING SIGNS AND SYMPTOMS

Along with the appearance of fever, pelvic infection is often accompanied by abdominal tenderness or pain, foul-smelling lochial drainage, an abnormally large uterus, and the presence of chills. The patient may complain of general malaise and lack of appetite and display a rise in pulse rate. Such signs and symptoms should be reported immediately. Detection of a puerperal infection should initiate the use of isolation procedure and again, if possible, the removal of the patient from the maternity service proper. Such a diagnosis may also affect the nursing procedures in the care of the infant, and the infant would usually not be allowed to visit its mother while she is deemed contagious.

Treatment of a case of puerperal infection will depend on the extent of involvement. Antibiotics to which the causative organisms are sensitive will be ordered. In cases of pelvic infection the patient will most often be placed in Fowler's position to encourage drainage of the affected area.

EXTENSION OF INFECTION

Observation for signs of the extension of the infection or generalized peritonitis should be constant. Such indications would be increased abdominal tenderness and distention, and nausea and vomiting, as well as those previously listed.

Thrombophlebitis. Not all cases of thrombophlebitis involve the presence of infection, but many do. Clots may form anywhere in the body where a slowdown in circulation, a repair of damaged tissue, or a plugging of bleeding vessels occurs. During the postpartum period, clots or thrombi may form in the pelvis or the lower extremities. They may stay localized and interfere with local circulation, set up areas of inflammation, or actually become foci of infection. Rarely, they may break away from the original site of formation and travel

about in the circulation. Then they are called emboli (singular, embolus). These clots are particularly dangerous, because they may enter some small but vital vessel and cause grave damage or sudden death. This most often occurs in the case of an embolus or emboli to the lung field or brain.

A common site of thrombophlebitis is the thigh or calf. Sometimes circulation is so impeded that the leg swells considerably, is extremely painful, and may demonstrate red streaks or locally inflamed areas. The skin may be so tense that it appears lighter in color.

Treatment of femoral thrombophlebitis varies considerably, depending on the philosophy and experiences of the physician in charge. Some will order elevation and the application of heat with a heat cradle or pad. Others will order ice packs. Antibiotics may be indicated. Some may prescribe anticoagulants to cut down on the formation of further thrombi. The nurse must recognize that use of anticoagulants for a postpartum patient increases the possibility of postpartum hemorrhage significantly. Her observations of any abnormal bleeding would need to be quickly reported. Blood pressure should be taken periodically. Prothrombin determinations by the laboratory would be expected.

An order for support stockings is common. Applied correctly, they help speed the venous circulation back to the heart and discourage the formation of clots. No massage of the legs is permitted for fear of dislodging previously formed clots. Ambulation is only ordered after assessment of the day-by-day progress of the patient revealed by the presence or absence of fever and her general condition. Thrombophlebitis may occur in all degrees of severity. Some physicians automatically order elastic stockings applied to the legs of their patients who have had difficulties with varicosities, as a preventive measure.

• • •

The postpartum hospital stay is brief in many parts of the United States. However, the nurse can do much, even in this short interval, to help the patient face her increased responsibilities with added knowledge, skill, energy, and assurance.

CHAPTER 11   Population, ecology, and reproduction

Any modern maternal and child health text would be neglecting a crucial area of concern and controversy if it did not include at least a brief consideration of population growth, natural resources, and environmental protection. These subjects are vitally linked with maternal and pediatric interests such as genetic counseling, birth planning, abortion, sterilization, fertility, and adoption. Because discussion of birth planning has often been part of postpartal counseling, these topics are included in this unit. However, the student can readily understand that these represent a much broader area of concern, involving more than this particular interval in a woman's life.

For many centuries some of these subjects were deemed irrelevant, irreverent, or simply outside the possibility of human control. The idea that the entire earth could become seriously impoverished or poisoned by mankind was foreign to most human thought. A rather simple optimism existed that as one resource became scarce, another would be prepared to take its place. Problems of ecology, such as the balance of nature, were considered to be largely theoretic or curiosities of only local importance.

Today, human beings are showing an increasing awareness of the changing ecologic balance and their role in it. Complex ecologic issues have become concerns at both local and international levels. In many areas legislation has been affected. The impact of this focus on impending ecologic cri-

sis is beginning to have a wide range of effects on individual and collective life-styles in the Western world.

If people of this generation are to be deemed responsible ancestors by future generations, they must realize that although the earth's resources are finite, or limited, the demands for its bounty are steadily increasing.

The world's population currently stands at approximately 4.5 billion, with a projection of 6.5 billion at the end of the century. Although population projections are extremely difficult to construct, the following observation is indeed sobering. It took the earth's human inhabitants until approximately 1850 to form a living group of 1 billion persons; only 80 years passed before a second billion was present. Forty-five years later, the population had doubled to 4 billion.

The predictable impact of population growth of this magnitude on food supply, natural resources, and political stability is ominous. A nation whose population is rapidly increasing and whose vital resources are curtailed has frequently become a militant nation. As populations double and triple, goods and services and natural resources are stretched to the point where they can no longer meet basic human needs, and more mental and physical illness is to be anticipated. Is mankind expecting famine, war, and disease to automatically solve the population problem? There must be other more acceptable alternatives!

The options would all seem to involve a conscious, orderly limitation of the number of persons who are to inherit the earth. Such a limitation may be achieved in various ways, and much debate focuses on the efficiency and ethics of the techniques employed. The basic methods, all of which have been used at some time, are (1) abstinence, (2) contraception, (3) planned abortion, (4) sterilization, (5) infanticide, and (6) adult murder.

Of these methods infanticide and adult murder are, of course, unacceptable to all modern societies. Abstinence, although highly efficient when practiced, appears difficult to maintain. Its use within the context of marriage, except for special circumstances for agreed periods, may be questioned. Justified alarm that the world is rapidly becoming overpopulated and recognition of the right of individuals to control their fertility have resulted in considerable modification of attitudes, both public and private, concerning the desirability and methods of birth planning. Three methods seem to have gained some acceptance by segments of today's society. They are contraception, abortion, and sterilization. Indeed, governmental agencies—local, state, national, and international—are now obligated to try to provide birth control services for those individuals who desire them and cannot otherwise obtain them. This is a far cry from former years, when many public institutions, by inaction if not by proclamation, effectively impeded application of birth control practices.

Not all human beings accept the same explanation of the origin and meaning of life, nor do they agree concerning the order of life's priorities. Philosophic differences in viewpoint cause various groups or individuals to endorse, tolerate, or condemn certain techniques of population control or family planning. These philosophic considerations include convictions regarding (1) the ultimate purpose and potential of the individual and mankind as a whole, (2) how the developmental state of the unborn child affects his status as a person or soul, (3) the rights of the unborn vis-à-vis those who have already begun extrauterine existence, (4) the purposes of the marriage relationship and sexual intercourse, (5) the responsibility and ability of the individual to make and implement decisions involving personal conduct, and (6) the role of Deity in the affairs of human beings.

In the area of birth control the function of the health professional is to counsel, reassure, and give information allowing an individual to decide his or her own course of action. Each potential set of parents should consciously make the decision whether or not to have children and the method of birth control they will employ. This decision should be appropriate for them and in accordance with their own personal, societal, and religious values and beliefs.

CONTRACEPTION

Contraceptive techniques or methods used to prevent birth temporarily are usually considered to fall into three main categories: (1) those that prevent conception, (2) those that prevent ovulation, and (3) those that prevent implantation. Strictly speaking, the last is not a method of contraception, since the egg may be fertilized but unable to embed itself into the uterine lining to maintain life. A brief description of these methods follows.

Methods used to prevent conception

NATURAL METHODS

Coitus interruptus. This is probably the oldest type of birth control practiced. The method employed is that of premature withdrawal of the penis before ejaculation during intercourse. Although the method is used by many couples, its reliability is low because sperm are emitted in varying quantities in the normal lubricating fluid secreted throughout intercouse.

Rhythmic abstinence. The human ovum is susceptible to fertilization for approximately 18 to 24 hours after ovulation. Sperm deposited in the vagina are ordinarily capable of fertilizing the ovum for no more than 72 hours. These are the principles

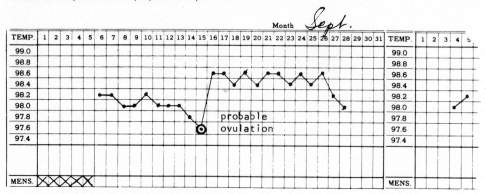

FIG. 11-1   Basal body temperature graph. Normally, ovulation is signaled by a drop in basal body temperature of about 0.5° F followed by a rise of 1° F or more. This relative elevation continues until about 2 days before the menstrual flow reappears. If pregnancy occurs, the temperature remains within a relatively high range. Basal body temperatures must be taken consistently, either rectally or vaginally before *any* activity directly on awakening each morning.

underlying the various "rhythm methods" for preventing pregnancy.

Calendar rhythm. Use of mathematical calculations to predict the probable time of ovulation is the basis of this method. If the menstrual cycle were consistently 28 days in length, ovulation would predictably occur at midpoint. It is known that ovulation most often takes place about 14 days before the onset of the next menstrual period. But, unfortunately, there is little consistency in the number of days between the onset of the last menstrual period and ovulation. Thus, since menstrual cycles differ so much from woman to woman and, indeed, at various times in the experience of any one woman, use of a calendar alone to estimate the time of ovulation to avoid the period of greatest fertility is unreliable and reduces protection considerably.

Temperature rhythm. This method relies on "slight" changes in basal body temperature that may occur just before ovulation (Fig. 11-1). An extended, careful calendar history of menses and daily basal body temperature patterns do not predict ovulation but identify the "safe" luteal phase of the menstrual cycle. This method involves temporary abstinence from the end of menstruation until

the slight increase (usually 1° F) in basal temperature is observed for 3 consecutive days. The temperature rhythm method is much more likely to be successful if during each cycle intercourse is restricted to well after the identified temperature rise. The Catholic Marriage Advisory Council recommends abstinence during days 10 through 19 of the menstrual cycle.

Potential problems with this technique stem from the fact that basal body temperature may vary with sleeplessness, illness, digestive disturbances, immunizations, alcohol ingestion, fever, emotional upset, and medications to induce sleep.

Cervical mucus rhythm. (Also called "Billings" or "ferning" method.) This method depends on identifying fertile periods by awareness of "dryness" and "wetness" in the vagina as the consequence of changes in amount and kind of cervical mucus formed at different times in the menstrual cycle. This approach is gaining in popularity and is explained in detail in the book *Natural Family Planning: The Ovulation Method.**

Natural family planning (NFP) is characterized

---

*Billings, J.J.: Natural family planning: the ovulation method. Collegeville, Minn., 1975, The Liturgical Press.

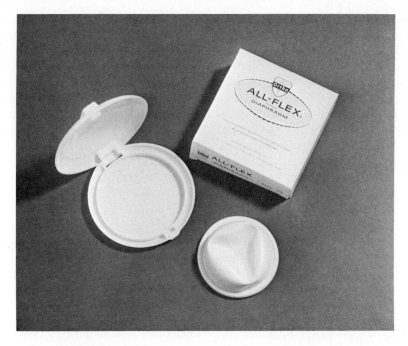

FIG. 11-2   Rubber spring diaphragm with case.

by avoidance of intercourse during fertile periods, and the "fertility awareness method" (FAM) employs a barrier method of birth control during fertile intervals.

Symptothermal method. This is the newest of the rhythm methods and is currently being actively promoted by an organization called Couple to Couple League (CCL). Its effectiveness depends on periodic abstinence during fertile periods identified by a combination of factors. Records are kept of menstrual cycle, basal temperature, changes in vaginal mucus, disturbances in normal routine, and many other special notations (spotting, pains, moods, cervical softening, and other so-called secondary signs).

LOCAL BARRIER METHODS

*Condom.*The most widely used birth control device in the world, the condom, was probably first employed to prevent the spread of venereal disease. Made of rubber or animal tissue and shaped

like a large finger cot, it is worn over the penis during intercourse to prevent semen from entering the vaginal canal. It must be carefully applied to the penis after erection. To prevent the condom from breaking during ejaculation, a half-inch "pocket" should be maintained at its end. Petroleum jelly should never be applied to a condom, as this product weakens rubber. It can be used in conjunction with chemical contraceptives, which may also serve as lubricants. Condoms should be stored away from heat and never reused.

Cervical caps and diaphragms. Use of these devices was first reported in the 1800s. Cervical caps may be made of rubber, metal, or plastic. They fit closely over the cervix. Diaphragms are latex domes with spring rims (Fig. 11-2). They are positioned over the cervix between the pubic bone and posterior vaginal wall. Both devices must be used in conjunction with spermicidal cream or jelly. They hold these chemicals in place over the mouth of the uterus. Caps and diaphragms must be fitted by a physician or technician. The woman's ability to insert them properly must be checked, and detailed education regarding their use is necessary. Because of anatomic differences, not all women can be fitted satisfactorily. Some women find it distasteful to insert the device. These barriers are most effective when inserted no longer than 1 hour before intercourse, since the spermicidal application becomes less powerful with the passing of time, and should remain in place at least 8 hours after intercourse.

Intravaginal contraceptives used alone. These substances are available in the form of creams, jellies, suppositories, foams, aerosols, and foam tablets. Such preparations work by providing a physical barrier to sperm penetration as well as chemical spermicidal action. They must be applied immediately before intercourse, since the maximum duration of their spermicidal action is 15 to 60 minutes, and they must be allowed to remain in the vagina for 8 hours after intercourse. The most recent substance in this category of contraceptives is the foam tablet (Encare Oval), a potent spermicidal ovoid tablet with an effervescent barrier that blocks penetration of sperm into the cervical canal. The advantage of this tablet is a prolonged duration of spermicidal action (minimum of 2 hours). It becomes effective *after* it melts from body heat. Therefore a minimum delay of 10 minutes between insertion and coitus should be observed.

Higher pregnancy rates are attributable chiefly to inconsistent use rather than to failure of this category of contraceptive method.

Douches. Vaginal irrigations are not recommended as a means of contraception. Sperm may enter the cervix 10 to 90 seconds after ejaculation. Douching may help to force sperm into the uterus.

Methods used to prevent ovulation

In recent years various combinations of estrogens and progesterone-like compounds have been introduced in tablet form that, when taken orally as directed, are designed to prevent the escape of the ovum from the ovary. They simulate pregnancy in this regard. Another associated action of these substances that helps to prevent pregnancy in the rare instances when ovulation is not inhibited involves (1) the decrease in and the thickening of cervical mucus, making the uterus less hospitable to spermatozoa and (2) the altered maturation of the uterine endometrium, rendering it inappropriate for successful implantation. "The pill" was first accepted for general use by prescription in the United States in 1960. It is now one of the most popular methods of contraception in this country. If the standard technique of administration is followed, a woman is given a special dispenser to help her keep a record of her medication.

There are two main types of pills and programs that may be prescribed. One prescription uses one type of tablet (the combination), which includes both estrogens and progesterones, to be taken daily for 3 weeks and omitted for 1 week, during which time withdrawal uterine bleeding normally occurs. Correctly followed, this method of contraception is 99% to 100% effective. The second type is the all-progestin Mini Pill (norethindrone), which is taken *every* day. Perhaps technically it should not be placed in this category, since it does not necessarily inhibit ovulation but seems to prevent sperm transport by causing cervical mucus to thicken. One of three patterns of menstrual response may occur: (1) no change in menstruation may be experienced—and ovulation will still take place; (2) irregular menstrual-type bleeding may occur associated with lack of or reduced ovulation; or (3) the woman may become completely amenorrheic. If menstrual flow seems excessive or prolonged or if pregnancy is suspected, a physician should be consulted. The method is claimed to be 96% effective. The so-called morning-after pill, designed to be taken after unprotected intercourse, often contains diethylstilbestrol in large doses. Its effectiveness has been established, but because of its suspected role in causing cancer, its use is seriously questioned at this time. Combined birth control pills have also been used for postcoital contraception. Ethinyl estradiol 50 μg and norgestrel 0.5 mg is taken within 72 hours of intercourse, and the same dosage is repeated exactly 12 hours later.

Frequently reported problems associated with oral contraception include nausea, occasional vomiting, breast tenderness, acne, headache, increased weight gain, and irregular vaginal bleeding. Certain vascular phenomena that are induced or enhanced by oral contraceptives, although rare, can be serious. In various studies the risk of increased incidences of blood clot formation and embolism has been estimated to be three to eleven times greater in women who used oral contraceptives than in similar women who did not. The risk is dramatically increased in women who smoke—especially in those over 30 years of age. Also, a small percent (less than 5%) of women using oral contraceptives have developed hypertensive problems. For most this side effect is mild and reversible; the blood pressure returns to normal in 1 to 3 months after discontinuing the pill. The much-publicized concerns that oral contraceptives might induce cancer appear at this time to have been unfounded.

Disadvantages involved in the use of oral contraceptives also include (1) the need for ability and motivation to proceed with their administration faithfully, (2) their expense, and (3) possible interference in lactation, causing insufficient milk supply and unknown absorption of the drug by the baby. However, some physicians are prescribing low-dose contraceptives to lactating mothers. Probably the best hormonal contraceptive during lactation is progestin alone, which appears to have no effect on the milk supply. Advantages of the pill include its high reliability, the fact that its use is removed from the actual sex act, and the woman's ability to stop therapy when she chooses to conceive.

Because of their convenience and high level of effectiveness, oral contraceptives will probably continue to be one of the most popular forms of reversible contraception. Careful screening to determine women who are at risk, use of the lowest acceptable dosage pill for each woman, and careful follow-up to detect any developing problems will help ensure that they will be as safe as they are convenient and effective.

Methods that may prevent implantation

Authorities are not agreed as to how the intrauterine devices (IUD) may control pregnancy. It would seem, however, that the mechanism involved interferes in some way with the fertilization process, the readiness of a fertilized ovum to implant, or the ability of the uterine wall to receive the egg. IUDs are not new, but only within the last 15 years have they been used with much success. Those inserted in the early 1900s often caused tissue damage and infection because of their placement or design. Their use was largely abandoned by physicians. However, since the advent of polyethylene and improved designs, including the tiny 7-shaped copper-containing "Cu 7" IUD, they have been a particularly popular method for controlling birth in populations who lack the finances, skill, or opportunity to use other techniques. (See Fig. 11-3.) IUDs must be positioned by a proficient physician or technician. They may still be associated with uterine cramping and bleeding and, in rare instances, infection and perforation. However, considering the many IUDs that have been inserted, the incidence of complications appears to be low—less than that reported for "the pill." IUDs may be spontaneously expelled. However, once inserted they require little care and, unless expelled, they may remain in place for months or years without untoward symptoms. Ectopic pregnancies occur more frequently among wearers of IUDs than among pregnant women in general, not because the device causes these abnormally placed pregnancies but because it prevents uterine pregnancy much more efficiently than it does extrauterine gestation. If intrauterine pregnancy does occur, it is recommended that the IUD be removed as soon as possible to prevent the risk of septic abortion.

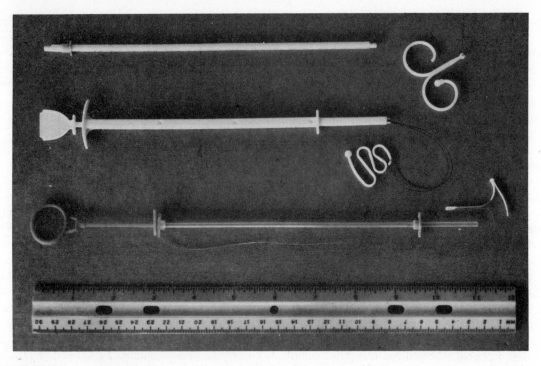

FIG. 11-3   Types of intrauterine devices (IUDs) with their inserters. From top down: Saf-T-Coil, Lippes Loop, and "Cu 7."

Reliability of contraceptive methods

An evaluation of the efficiency or reliability of the various methods of contraception is difficult to present in statistical terms because in some instances data collection and analysis have posed particular problems. Contraceptive techniques perhaps can be ranked for effectiveness as follows,* with the recognition that more research is needed:

Most reliable   "The pill"
Condom used with spermicidal agent

Highly reliable	Intrauterine devices
	Condom
	Diaphragm used with spermicidal agent
	Cervical cap used with spermicide
Moderately reliable	Aerosol vaginal foam
	Rhythm, using basal body temperature, cervical mucus indicators, or combination techniques
	Intravaginal agents alone
	Gels or creams
	Suppositories
	Tablets (foaming and nonfoaming)
Less reliable	Coitus interruptus
	Calendar rhythm
Least reliable	Douche

Several exciting prospects are being explored for future contraceptives. They include synthetic substances that correspond to a luteinizing hormone-releasing hormone (LHRH) that are being consid-

*Chart adapted from data from the following sources: Ryder, N.B.: Contraceptive failure in the United States, Fam. Plan. Perspectives **5**:133-142, 1973; Tanis, J.: Recognizing the reasons for contraceptive nonuse and abuse, J. Mat. Child Nurs. **2**:364-369, Nov.-Dec. 1977.

ered for both male and female contraceptive control; a contraceptive one-size-fits-all sponge, time-release contraceptive implants or microcapsules, and improved tailless IUDs.

Clearly no perfect method exists that is applicable to all persons and circumstances, and research continues. Equally clear is the trite observation that a method must be used consistently to be effective. It is important to note that the maternal death rate associated with pregnancy and childbirth is greater than that associated with the use of any of the types of contraceptives previously discussed and more than that of legal first-trimester abortion.

ABORTION

If a pregnancy occurs that for medical, psychologic, economic, or social reasons is unwanted by those who would have the responsibility of bearing and caring for the child, the possibility of terminating the intrauterine life before it is supposedly capable of extrauterine survival is sometimes considered. From the mid-1800s when abortion was outlawed until 1967 the only way that a woman could procure a legal abortion in most states was through a statement of medical agreement that continuation of the pregnancy would be a threat to her life. (A few states also considered the *health* of the mother in the wording of relevant legislation.) Laws condemning abortion were written more than a hundred years ago when the operation was dangerous, even under the best auspices, and in unskilled hands was often catastrophic. Community concepts concerning population growth, the roles of women and children, and meanings and rules surrounding sex, pregnancy, and childbirth also influenced this legislation. In the time between 1967 and 1973, several states modified their statutes to include other reasons for abortion: the mother's physical and mental health, probable serious deformity of the baby, and cases of incest or rape. A few made abortion, with certain reservations, a private decision between a woman and her physician.

In January 1973 the U.S. Supreme Court ruled that the decision to have an abortion in the first trimester of pregnancy rests only with the woman in consultation with her physician. In the second trimester the state recognizes a vested interest in the health of the woman and can regulate the conditions under which an abortion is performed but cannot prohibit the procedure. In the third trimester, because the fetus may be viable, the state may prohibit abortion based on its interest in the life and health of the fetus. Most states do prohibit third trimester abortions except to save the life of the pregnant woman.

The judicial decision has not been unchallenged, and practical compliance with the law appears uneven, although 25 attorneys general simply declared their former state legislation "null and void." Organizations such as the Right to Life Committee and the National Youth Pro-Life Coalition, which favor abortion only when the mother's life is in danger, are supporting efforts to overturn the Supreme Court decision by a constitutional "Human Life" amendment. They also support other antiabortion legislation such as states' rights laws that would allow each state's legislature to determine its own abortion regulations. Meanwhile, the National Abortion Rights Action League (NARAL) is working to maintain the impact of the 1973 court action.

First-trimester abortions may be performed in physicians' offices, separate clinics, or hospitals. Medical personnel should be familiar with the regulating laws of the area where they practice. The question of professional participation in abortion when not done for obvious health needs of the mother is, for many individuals, emotionally charged, morally disturbing, and legally complex. As the legal abortion rate has risen, maternal and infant mortality rates have dipped, but reported embryonic and fetal deaths have, of course, climbed.

Nurses should be familiar with the laws of the area in which they practice and how these laws have been interpreted. Legal sanctions and funding regulations regarding this problem are currently undergoing rapid change.

The following methods of abortion are employed in hospital settings if the pregnancy is of less than 3 months' duration.

1. *Aspiration*. The uterine contents are dislodged by the use of a specially designed suction catheter or vacuum apparatus. The procedure is rapid (approximately 5 minutes), and blood loss is minimal. It is now the most common method used and has the least complications.

2. *Dilatation and curettage*. The cervical canal is progressively dilated, and the products of conception are gently scraped from their uterine attachments.

Methods used if the pregnancy is of greater duration are as follows:

1. *Dilatation and evacuation*. This procedure, performed under local anesthetic between the thirteenth and twentieth weeks of pregnancy, involves a gradual dilatation of the cervix and removal of the fetus by alternating suction and curettage.

2. *Amniotic fluid replacement*. Techniques vary. Amniotic fluid is withdrawn from the amniotic sac. This fluid is usually replaced by an equal amount of approximately 200 ml concentrated (20%) saline solution. The hypertonic salt solution kills the fetus, and large doses of oxytocin (Pitocin) administered by IV infusion usually initiate uterine contractions within a day. Complications have included inflammation of the uterine lining, retained products of conception, hemorrhage, and cardiovascular collapse. The risks of mortality are not negligible. Amniotic fluid can also be replaced with a solution of urea and prostaglandin. The urea causes fetal death, and the prostaglandin initiates uterine contractions. Uterine contractions begin within 2 to 10 hours. The most common side effects are nausea and fever.

3. *Hysterotomy*. This is a type of cesarean birth, but it is performed when a nonviable fetus is judged present. It usually involves a hospitalization and recovery period similar to that of a cesarean birth patient.

Obviously, termination of a pregnancy after 3 months is a more difficult and hazardous procedure. The incidence of second-trimester abortions

has dropped dramatically with increased public awareness of abortion availability. Of women seeking abortions, 90% do so in the first trimester. In 1979, 1.5 million women in the United States, representing 30% of those who were pregnant, obtained abortions; about 3% of women aged 15 to 44 had abortions—a large percentage of whom were teenagers.

The psychologic impact of abortion, although perhaps not immediately apparent, is an important consideration. Clearly, contraception is a better solution than abortion. Nursing care of a patient having an abortion is discussed briefly in Chapter 9, p. 167.

STERILIZATION

In some instances an individual or couple, for health, genetic, social, or personal considerations, may wish to permanently discontinue the capacity to have children. Any process that produces this result may be termed *sterilization*. Many couples in the United States now complete their desired families at an early age. Rather than practice long-term use of contraception, many more couples are now requesting sterilization after they have had their desired number of children. Procedure for permanently discontinuing the capacity to have children may be performed on either the man or woman. Such procedures do not interfere with the ability to participate in sexual relations nor do they diminish any masculine or feminine characteristics previously present.

In the past 5 years many advances have been made in techniques and social acceptance of female sterilization. Following is a brief description of the three broad types of procedures.

1. *Laparotomy* or "mini-laparotomy" involves abdominal incisions to visualize and ligate or otherwise occlude the fallopian tubes.

2. *Laparoscopy* ("Band-Aid") surgery has been widely publicized and accepted as an inexpensive, safe, and effective method of sterilization. Under general or local anesthesia the physician observes

the operative site through a laparoscope introduced into the abdominal cavity through a small incision at the base of the umbilicus. The fallopian tubes may be occluded by electrocoagulation or the placement of several types of clips or rings. This procedure may be performed in the hospital on an inpatient or outpatient basis.

3. *Vaginal tubal sterilization* may be performed by entering the peritoneal cavity through the posterior vaginal fornix (colpotomy) with or without a scope similar to the laparoscope. The basic sterilization procedure is as described for the laparoscopy technique. This technique is associated with an increased risk of infection.

Sterilization of the man by *vas ligation* or vasectomy is accomplished without entry into the abdominal cavity. It may be an office procedure. Twin surgical incisions are often made in the area where the scrotum joins the body, just over the vas. The ducts are tied and separated. Portions may be excised. After the operation the man does not become sterile immediately, and follow-up sperm counts should be made to determine when contraceptive techniques are unnecessary.

Although sterilization procedures are performed to be permanent, occasionally a man or woman may regret his or her decision. In some cases the tubes may be rejoined and reproductive ability regained, but sterilization should be viewed initially as a lasting intervention. Occasional spontaneous failures of sterilization techniques have been reported, but attempts to provide temporary sterility using various devices have been disappointing.

GENETIC COUNSELING

Advances in understanding genetic disorders have been rapid in the last few years, and with them the need and desire for genetic counseling have grown. Genetic screening offers the possibility of reducing suffering resulting from genetic defects. Large screening programs have been initiated to detect people who may be carriers of harmful genes, such as those of Tay-Sachs disease and sickle cell anemia. There is no coercive action associated with the information given. What persons do with the knowledge they gain is a personal choice. Through the use of the services of a genetic counselor, the genealogy of the client or couple may be investigated. Such a study is particularly helpful when a hereditary problem has been identified in a person's family, but the potential incidence of the defect is unknown. The investigation may include pedigree analysis and tissue studies to determine chromosomal patterns and biologic constituents. Genetic screening may also be of value in cases of possible alteration or damage of an individual's genetic components.

Whether the subjects of screening tests are found to be carriers of genetic problems or not, psychologic problems may confront them, and the nurse must be aware of this. Regional genetic counseling is available in most areas to aid the client who has difficulty in understanding the concept of probability, psychologic defense reactions, and differences in individual values. A wide range of psychologic, ethical, and financial considerations are involved in genetic counseling. (See also p. 308.)

SUBFERTILITY OR INFERTILITY

In a world where population increase is a major problem, it may seem inconsistent to be concerned about the inability of a man and woman to conceive. Yet the capacity to have children of one's own lineage is particularly desired by and meaningful to most persons, even if they are not ruling monarchs! Some authorities have stated that a marriage may be regarded as infertile when pregnancy has not occurred after a year of periodic intercourse without the use of contraception.

Couples who come to a fertility clinic have two outstanding needs. The first is for education about reproduction and about procedures used to evaluate fertility. The second is for counseling to help them maximize their potential for conceiving. Knowledge about reproduction provides the client with a basis for understanding the circumstances necessary for conception and reasons for evaluating fertility.

The first step in evaluating the infertile couple is a complete physical examination to rule out related endocrine problems, emotional conditions, or disease entities that may be interfering with conception.

The next step in the evaluation is usually an evaluation of the reproductive capacity of the man. Recent semen samples are examined microscopically to detect abnormalities in the number, form and motility of his sperm. If few or no sperm are found, hormone analysis, a testicular biopsy, and x-ray studies may determine whether the spermatozoa are being manufactured but lack transport because of a blockage in his reproductive system. If this is the case, surgery to relieve the obstacle is sometimes possible. If sperm are not being produced or are limited in quantity, hormonal therapy may be helpful.

Evaluation of the capacity of the female to conceive is more complex because of the difference in anatomy. A complete physical examination is usually followed by a determination of the ability of the woman to ovulate. Several methods may be used; these include detection of a characteristic pattern of basal body temperature readings (Fig. 11-1), microscopic examination of a biopsy of the endometrium, or lining of the uterus, and investigation of the viscosity of the cervical mucus. If ovulation is established, examination of the patency of the fallopian tubes through dye and gas studies may be performed. The uterine cavity, the vaginal canal, and the type and action of cervical and vaginal secretions may also be investigated.

If ovulation does not occur, hormonal therapy as well as general measures to improve health may be helpful. One example of a hormonal product that stimulates ovarian function is a follicle-stimulating hormone called menotropins (Pergonal). Another medication that has been used to promote pregnancy is clomiphene citrate (Clomid). Perganol particularly has been known to promote the maturation of more than one ovum during the menstrual cycle, causing the development of multiple births (for example, quadruplets and quintuplets). Since these infants are usually of low birth weight and very fragile, multiple births are a mixed blessing to even the most eager parents.

Surgical intervention to open blocked passageways that must be traversed by the ascending sperm or the descending egg may also be performed with varying success, depending on the area to be treated. sometimes the diagnostic procedures used to detect fallopian tube obstruction also serve as therapy, causing the removal of minor blocks in the oviducts. The 1978 birth of the first "test tube" baby has added yet another alternative for selected clients previously unable to conceive because of oviduct defect. Medical treatment of pelvic inflammatory disease may enable conception to occur.

How intensively solutions for infertility will be sought depends on the ages of the couple, their continued interest, cooperation, and financial resources. At times, persistent failure to conceive because of certain male defects can be circumvented through artificial insemination techniques using the husband's sperm. More rarely, semen from an anonymous, healthy, normal man may be employed. Adoption or foster parenthood, although sometimes not available to couples and often involving long waiting periods, may be a satisfying solution. There are certainly many children already on earth who need loving care.

• • •

Never before in the history of this world have the questions of population, ecology, and reproduction appeared more critical than in this last half of the twentieth century. All persons should be informed concerning the problems to be faced and their possible solutions. All those engaged in the provision of maternal and child health, whether within or outside the hospital setting, need to be especially involved in striving to increase the possibility that a newborn boy or girl will not only be well and well formed, but also welcome.

THE POSTPARTAL PERIOD

Affonso, D.D., and Stichler, J.F.: Cesarean birth: women's reactions, Am. J. Nurs. **80**:468-470, Mar. 1980.

Breuer, J.: Sharing a tragedy, Am. J. Nurs. **77**:758-759, May 1977.

Brown, B.: Maternity patient teaching: a nursing priority, JOGN Nurs. **11**:11-14, Jan.-Feb. 1982.

Brown, M.S., and Hurlock, J.T.: Mothering the mother, Am. J. Nurs. **77**:438-441, Mar. 1977.

Burd, B.: Encouragement counts in breast feeding, Am. J. Nurs. **81**:1491, Aug. 1981.

Carr, K.C., and Walton, V.E.: Early postpartum discharge, JOGN Nurs. **11**:29-30, Jan.-Feb. 1982.

Dibble, J.C.: ABC for teens: parent education after the baby comes, Pediatr. Nurs. **7**:21-23, July-Aug. 1981.

Foster, S.D.: Bromocriptine: suppressing lactation, Am. J. Mat. Child Nurs. **7**:99, Mar.-Apr. 1981.

Hames, C.T.: Sexual needs and interest of postpartum couples, JOGN Nurs. **9**:313-315, Sept.-Oct. 1980.

Hart, G.: Maternal attitudes in prepared and unprepared cesarean deliveries, JOGN Nurs. **9**:243-245, July-Aug. 1980.

Hedahl, K.J.: Cesarean birth: a real family affair, Am. J. Nurs. **80**:471-472, Mar. 1980.

Inglis, T.: Postpartum sexuality, JOGN Nurs, **9**:298-300, Sept.-Oct. 1980.

Jarrett, G.E.: Childbearing patterns of young mothers: expectations, knowledge and practices, Am. J. Mat. Child Nurs. **7**:119-124, Mar.-Apr. 1982.

Lockhart, B.: When couples adopt, they too need parenting classes, Am. J. Mat. Child Nurs. **7**:116-118, Mar.-Apr. 1982.

Lucas, W.E.: Bleeding after giving birth, Emergency Medicine **15**:172-179, Mar. 1981.

Ludington-Hoe, S.M.: Postpartum: development of maternicity, Am. J. Nurs. **77**:1170-1174, July 1977.

Marecki, M.P.: Postpartum follow-up goals and assessment, JOGN Nurs. **8**:214-218, July-Aug. 1979.

McCarty, E.: Early postpartum nursing care of mother and infant in the home care setting, Nurs. Clin. North Am. **15**:361-372, June 1980.

Mercer, R.T.: Crisis: a baby is born with a defect, Nurs. '77 **7**:45-47, Nov. 1977.

Mercer, R.T.: The nurse and maternal tasks of early postpartum, Am. J. Mat. Child Nurs. **6**:341-345, Sept.-Oct. 1981.

Minkoff, H.: Steps to reduce postcesarean infection, Contemp. OB/GYN **18**:165-174, Nov. 1981.

Mynick, A.: Instituting a postpartum self-medication program, Am. J. Mat. Child Nurs. **6**:422-424, Nov.-Dec. 1981.

Ojofeitimi, E.O.: Effect of breast-feeding on postpartum amenorrhea, Pediatrics **69**:164-168, Feb. 1982.

Pellegrom, P., and Swartz, L.M.: Primigravidas' perceptions of early postpartum, Pediatr. Nurs. **6**:25-27, Nov.-Dec. 1980.

Poole, C.J., and Hoffman, M.: Mothers of adolescent mothers: how do they cope? Pediatr. Nurs. **7**:28-31, Jan.-Feb. 1981.

Roux, J.F., and Brauerman, J.: Forecasting the afterbirth blues, Emergency Medicine **12**:118-119, May 1980.

Tentoni, S.C., and High, K.A.: Culturally induced postpartum depression: a theoretical position, JOGN Nurs. **9**:246-249, July-Aug. 1980.

Wong, D.L.: Bereavement: the empty-mother syndrome, Am. J. Mat. Child Nurs. **5**:384-389, Nov.-Dec. 1980.

POPULATION, ECOLOGY AND REPRODUCTION

Aby-Nielsen, K.: Physical sensations during stressful hospital procedures: a preliminary study of saline abortion, JOGN Nurs **8**:105-106, Mar.-Apr. 1979.

Ausubel, F., Beckwith, J., and Janssen, K.: Stimulus/response: the politics of genetic engineering: who decides who's defective, Psychol. Today **8**:30-43, June 1974.

Berger, J.M.: The relationship of age to nurses' attitudes toward abortion, JOGN Nurs. **8**:231-233, July-Aug. 1979.

Bibb, B.N.: The effectiveness of nonphysicians as providers of family planning services, JOGN Nurs. **8**:137-143, May-June 1979.

Billings, J.J.: Natural family planning: the ovulation method, ed. 3, Collegeville, Minn., 1975, The Liturgical Press.

Bradbury, B.A.: Preventing the "diaphragm baby syndrome": a matter of technique, teaching and time, JOGN Nurs. **4**:24-32, Mar.-Apr. 1975.

Britt, S.S.: Fertility awareness: four methods of natural family planning, JOGN Nurs. **6**:9-17, Mar.-Apr. 1977.

Burbach, C.A.: Contraception and adolescent pregnancy, JOGN Nurs. **9**:319-325, Sept.-Oct. 1980.

Calderone, M.S.: Sex and social responsibility, J. Home Economics **57**:499-502, Sept. 1965.

Draegenmueller, W., Weinstein, L., and Milzer, G.: Low-dose prostaglandins for second trimester abortion, Contemp. OB/GYN **15**:19-23, June 1980.

Ehrlich, P.R.: The population bomb, New York, 1968, Ballantine Books, Inc.

Gara, E.: Nursing protocol to improve the effectiveness of the contraceptive diaphragm, Am. J. Mat. Child Nurs. **6**:41-45, Jan.-Feb. 1981.

Gilbert, S.: Artificial insemination, Am. J. Nurs. **76**:259-260, Feb. 1976.

Gorline, L.L.: Teaching successful use of the diaphragm, Am. J. Nurs. **79**:1732-1735, Oct. 1979.

Greydanus, D.G.: Contraception in adolescence: an overview for the pediatrician, Pediatr. Ann. **9**:52-63, Mar. 1980.

Grimes, D., and Cates, W.: The brief for hypertonic saline, Contemp. OB/GYN **15**:29-38, June 1980.

Gromko, L.: Intrauterine devices, Nurse Practitioner **5**:17-26, July-Aug. 1980.

Henshaw, S., et al: Abortion in the United States, 1978-1979, Fam. Plann. Perspect. **13**:6-18, Jan.-Feb. 1981

Huxall, L.K.: Update on IUDs, Am. J. Mat. Child Nurs. **5**:186-190, May-June 1980.

Kilker, R., and Wilkerson, B.: Eight-point postpartum assessment, Nurs. '73 **3**:56, May 1973.

Kreutner, A.K.: Adolescent contraception, Pediatr. Clin. North Am. **28**:455-474, May 1981.

Machol, L.: Oral contraceptives: what's new? Contemp. OB/GYN **18**:31-40, Nov. 1981.

McRae, M.J.: Condemned to loneliness: a necessary maternity care decree? Am. J. Mat. Child Nurs. **2**:374-377, Nov.-Dec. 1977.

Menning, B.E.: Resolve: a support group for infertile couples, Am. J. Nurs. **76**:258-259, Feb. 1976.

Olson, M.: Helping staff nurses care for women seeking saline abortions, JOGN Nurs. **9**:170-173, May-June 1980.

Pomerance, J.: Steroid contraception and its effects on lactation are a public health dilemma, Health Serv. Rep. **87**:611-616, Aug.-Sept. 1972.

Rosenthal, T.: Voluntary childlessness and the nurse's role, Am. J. Mat. Child Nurs. **5**:398-402, Nov.-Dec. 1980.

Stewart, F.H., et al: My body, my health: the concerned woman's guide to gynecology, New York, 1979, John Wiley & Sons, Inc.

Swenson, I.: Psychologic considerations in vasectomy: a review of the literature, JOGN Nurs. **4**:29-32, Nov.-Dec. 1975.

Tyrer, L.B., and Granzig, W.A.: The new morality, ethics and nursing, JOGN Nurs. **2**:54-55, Sept.-Oct. 1973.

THE NEWBORN INFANT

CHAPTER **12**   The normal newborn infant

The newborn infant is a marvelous creation, the result of approximately 40 weeks of intensive growth and development never to be equaled at any subsequent period of his life. A passive participant in the drama of birth, the infant, for the present and near future, is almost totally dependent on the physical care, emotional support, and mental stimulus given his inborn potential by his immediate environment. The human newborn does little for himself. In his egocentric way he waits impatiently for his needs to be met by others as if no other needs exist, and indeed, as far as he knows, they do not.

Although newborn infants have occupied similar environments during their approximately 9 months of prenatal life, even this basic experience is not identical. True, all lived in the warm, watery environment of the amniotic sac, but not all infants receive identical portions of nourishment or oxygen. Their genetic backgrounds, greatly influencing basic body strengths and weaknesses, are very unlike. The stresses and strains of each birth are not always duplicated. Babies are individuals; each is different, and a wide range of shapes, sizes, and behavior patterns, despite their variations, must still be labeled "normal." So although one often speaks of the typical newborn infant, it must be realized that in reality such a child exists only within the pages of textbooks.

QUALIFICATIONS OF NURSERY PERSONNEL

The nurse caring for the newborn infant has a tremendous responsibility. Because of the newborn's inability to verbalize his needs, the nurse must be a keen observer. Technique, skills, and a gentle approach must be based on sound scientific principles and high ethical standards. The nurse's health must be evaluated frequently to verify the absence of infection.

THE TYPICAL NEWBORN INFANT

Having explained that a baby is really an individual, we will now describe the general appearance, anatomy, and physiology of the "representative" newborn infant. For unknown reasons approximately 106 male infants are born to every 100 female infants. It can be said, however, that the male newborn infant appears to be more fragile than the female, having a higher mortality. The average male newborn infant weighs about 7½ pounds (3.400 kg), whereas the average female weighs about ½ pound less, or 3.180 kg. The average male length is 20 inches (50.8 cm), ½ inch longer than his female counterpart. Of course, these figures are just averages, and much depends on the hereditary background of the child. Blacks and Orientals usually have smaller babies, whereas whites tend to have larger children.

219

When uninitiated persons first see a newborn infant, certain reactions are fairly standard: "He seems to be all head." "Where is her chin?" "Nurse, my baby has flat feet!" "Boy! She sure is red." "Will his skull always be that shape?"

The head

The head of a newborn infant represents one fourth of its total length (Fig. 12-1), but in adulthood the head equals only one eighth of the individual's total height. The newborn infant's head circumference equals or exceeds that of its chest or abdomen, and the normal limits of its head size are from 33 to 37 cm (13.2 to 14.8 inches). No wonder the relative size causes comment!

The shape of the baby's head can also cause a mother or father needless concern. Cesarean-born babies and even breech babies usually have rounded, "normal-appearing" heads. But infants who are born vaginally in cephalic presentations, particularly those who are firstborn, usually undergo considerable head sculpture, or _molding_. This molding is caused by the compression of the head in the birth canal during labor. The infant skull, because of the soft membranous seams separating the skull bones, can become shaped in its journey through the canal. In response to the pressure of the cervix and bony pelvis, the head usually elongates, and the skull bones may even overlap in places. This phenomenon is called _overriding_; the molding lasts for only about a week or less.

The fontanels, or soft spots, where sutures cross or meet, are particularly noteworthy. Two are easily felt and identified: the anterior diamond-shaped fontanel, through which a pulse is sometimes visible (hence the name fontanel, or "little fountain"), and the smaller posterior fontanel just in front of the occiput. The larger fontanel closes at 9 to 18 months of age. Occasionally it is the site of "cradle cap," or "milk crust," also called seborrhea. This occurs when the mother or nurse is fearful of cleaning this soft area, and secretions from the oil glands

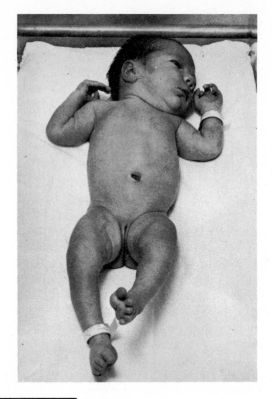

FIG. 12-1

Representative newborn infant, 3 days old. Note the size of the head relative to total length.

Courtesy Grossmont Hospital, La Mesa, Calif.

and cellular debris build up. Actually the cartilage covering the fontanels is tough; the mother should be assured that no harm will come from shampooing the area well. The posterior fontanel is so small, averaging 1 cm by 1 cm, that it is closed at 1½ to 3 months of age.

Two other temporary conditions involving the head may manifest themselves and cause parental anxiety. These are usually caused by the continued pressure of the undelivered head against the partially dilated cervix. The first and less important is called _caput succedaneum_, or caput. Caput is an abnormal collection of fluid under the scalp on top of the skull that may or may not cross suture lines,

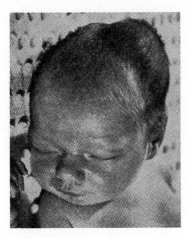

FIG. 12-2

Cephalhematoma over the parietal bone.

From Davis, M.E. and Rubin, R.: DeLee's obstetrics for nurses, ed. 17, Philadelphia, 1962, W.B. Saunders Co.

depending on its size. The accumulation is usually absorbed over a period of days and requires no treatment. The second condition is *cephalhematoma* (Fig. 12-2), caused by a collection of bloody fluid under the first covering layer (the periosteum) of a flat cranial bone. It is normally restricted to one bone. If it crosses a suture line, a skull fracture may be indicated. It usually develops when labor is particularly prolonged and the passageway is tight in relation to the needs of the passenger, causing bruising against the pelvis. As a result of the trauma, small blood vessels under the periosteum break. A cephalhematoma may not be apparent at the time of birth because of the presence of a more inclusive caput. Like caput, cephalhematoma, although temporarily disfiguring, is not harmful and requires no treatment. However, it is important to note the infant's blood values, since excess bleeding into the cephalohematoma may cause some lowering of hemoglobin and hematocrit levels.

General body proportions

Parents are often amazed to see the small size of the child's face compared with the total head size. The facial bones are underdeveloped, and the chin is almost nonexistent. The baby's neck is usually short and creased and difficult to clean unless the head is tipped backward and unsupported while the child is held at the shoulders. The torso of the normal newborn infant displays a relatively small thorax and a soft, rather protuberant abdomen. The genitalia are small but may be swollen. The extremities are short in relation to body length. The feet are always flat because of the presence of a fatty pad that normally disappears as the child begins to exercise and purposefully use his feet.

Ears and eyes

The ears may be folded and creased and may seem out of shape because they contain little hardened cartilage. The infant usually responds to sound at birth.

The eyes may not track properly and may cross (strabismus) or twitch (nystagmus). These symptoms are usually not considered significant unless they persist beyond the age of 6 months. The irises of white infants are slate blue, and true eye color is seldom determined until 3 to 6 months of age. It is difficult to tell what a baby is able to see. The pupils do react to light, and the infant can focus on objects (for example, on another person's eyes) at about 8 inches (20 cm) away. Blinking is an inborn protective reflex. The lacrimal glands evidently function only minimally at birth, and the newborn infant's cries are characteristically tearless. Occasionally, an eye discharge is apparent, caused by eye irritation initiated by the prophylactic against *ophthalmia neonartorum* (a condition that results from a gonorrheal infection in the mother). The prophylactic, which is required by most states, is usually silver nitrate, 1%. Because of sensitivity problems, penicillin is seldom used for this purpose. The reason for the eye irritation or conjunctivitis should be explained to the parents. It is important to note the time of onset of any neonatal conjunctivitis to help determine its cause.

Skin   ✗

The skin of the newborn infant is subject to numerous conditions and manifestations that always elicit questions.

Vernix caseosa. The skin of the fetus is protected from its watery environment by a soft, yellowish cream named *vernix caseosa,* or "cheesy varnish." This is an accumulation of old cutaneous cells mixed with an early secretion from the oil glands. Sometimes the baby is thickly covered with vernix at birth. Sometimes it is found in abundance only in the body creases. Some nursery units believe that vernix is a good culture medium for bacterial growth and now meticulously remove all of it from their newborn patients.

The skin of the newborn infant is thin. The more immature the baby is the less developed will be the layer of subcutaneous fat. For this reason babies not many hours after birth, when oxygenation is optimal, tend to be red. The smaller the baby the more tomato-colored he will tend to be—especially when the newborn is upset and crying. Nurses should be aware that black babies are light colored at birth and darken gradually.

Lanugo. A relatively long, soft growth of fine hair called *lanugo* is often observed on the shoulders, back, and forehead of the newborn infant. In fact, the infant at times may seem to have sideburns. The more premature the infant, the more conspicuous this extra growth of hair tends to be. This hair falls away and disappears early in postnatal life.

Toxic erythema. Another skin manifestation that can be puzzling but is probably harmless is a condition known to the nursery staff as "newborn rash." *toxic erythema.* The adjective "toxic" perhaps should not be used, since no poison has ever been proved to be the cause. In fact, the cause is unknown. Some authors list it as a possible allergic response and call it instead *erythema allergicum.* The lesions consist of red blotches that quickly develop hivelike elevations, which may later become blisters containing clear fluid which, when cultured, reveal eosinophil concentrations. These may appear on the day of birth and persist for hours or days. They are most often seen on the trunk but may appear elsewhere. They are not contagious and are most frequently seen on vigorous, healthy babies. No treatment is needed.

Mongolian spots. Babies of black, Indian, Mongolian, or "Mediterranean" ancestry often exhibit blue-black colorations on their lower backs, buttocks, anterior trunks, and, rarely, fingers or feet; they occur less frequently on white babies. These are not bruise marks or signals of ill treatment, nor are they associated with mental retardation. These so-called *Mongolian,* or *Asiatic, spots* disappear in early childhood.

Jaundice. The skin of the infant on about the third day may begin to take on a yellow cast. This icterus, or jaundice, is not usually considered to be of pathologic origin but is thought to be associated with the destruction of red blood cells that are no longer needed in as great a number as when external respiration by means of the lungs was impossible in utero. However, if jaundice is present before 36 hours of age, the possibility of Rh factor or main blood group incompatibility (AB-O) most certainly should be recognized and determined. Indeed, no matter what the age of the baby, the fact that the baby is jaundiced should be reported and evaluated because the number 36 is not magical, and although it is not common, difficulty could occur later. The jaundice caused by the expected erythrocyte destruction, seen to some extent in almost all newborn infants, has been termed *physiologic jaundice,* and is characterized by a rise in the serum bilirubin to 7.5 to 8 mg/100 ml blood by the fourth day of life.

Petechiae. Another possible signal of skin trouble that usually turns out to be a false alarm is the presence of petechiae, or small blue-red dots on the body, caused by the breakage of minute capillaries. If present, these dots are usually seen on the face as a result of the pressure exerted on the head during birth. Nevertheless, if petechiae are accompanied by jaundice or begin to increase measurably after birth, one may consider a diagnosis of blood disease. True petechiae do not blanch on pressure.

Milia. Small pinpoint white or yellow dots are common on the nose, forehead, and cheeks of the newborn infant. They are clogged sweat and oil glands that have not yet begun to function normally and are called *milia*. They will disappear with time and under no circumstances should they be expressed.

Birthmarks. Small reddened areas are sometimes present on the eyelids, midforehead, and nape of the neck. They are probably the result of a local dilatation of skin capillaries and abnormal thinness of the skin. Because of the frequent involvement of the nape of the neck, they are sometimes called "stork bites," but another name often heard is *telangiectasia*. Some writers term such an area *nevus flammeus,* an unfortunate choice, since this term is also used for the so-called port-wine stain, which is disfiguring and difficult to treat. Whatever the choice of terms, however, the parents should be told that these small areas usually fade and disappear altogether. Some are noticeable only when the person blushes, is extremely warm, or becomes excited.

Other birthmarks are sometimes seen. The so-called strawberry mark may not be present at birth but may develop days or weeks later. It is characterized by a dark or bright red raised, rough surface. Since it is formed by a collection of capillaries at the skin's surface, it may be classed as a blood vessel tumor, or *hemangioma*. The first signs of a strawberry mark may be a grouping of red dots that eventually coalesce, forming the clear-cut raised lesion. Many times this mark will disappear spontaneously in early childhood without treatment. However, some such hemangiomas tend to increase in size rather than subside, and some seem so disfiguring to the parents that efforts to remove the lesion are made at an early age. Although rarely used, the application of dry ice at

brief intervals or actual surgical excision, depending on the location of the strawberry mark, are methods of removal. A "wait-and-see" attitude is advocated, since many such lesions regress spontaneously.

Additional birthmarks that may sometimes cause concern are various flat or raised, frequently pigmented irregularities of the skin that are generally termed moles, or *nevi* (singular, nevus). For the most part, these lesions are benign, causing only occasional cosmetic difficulties. Nevertheless, one type of blue-black mole is considered precancerous, and any such lesion must be evaluated by the physician to ascertain its true character.

Vital signs in the newborn infant

Temperature. The newborn infant's body temperature drops immediately after birth from a reading about 1° F higher than that of the mother to a subnormal range. The internal organs of the neonate are poorly insulated, and the skin is relatively thin. The newborn infant's heat-regulating center and circulatory system have not yet matured, and his body temperature rapidly reflects that of his environment.

The newborn does not raise or maintain body temperature by shivering but is aided in his efforts to increase body temperature by a special tissue found only in neonates called *brown fat*. It is located principally between the scapulae, in the neck region, behind the sternum, and near the adrenals. This tissue produces a chemical, noradrenaline, which helps burn fats in the presence of oxygen to increase heat. When the neonate is placed in a warm incubator or wrapped in warm blankets, his temperature usually reaches "normal range" within 8 to 12 hours. Maintaining body warmth as much as possible in the immediate postnatal period may be critical to the well-being of an infant; therefore, special efforts have been initiated to provide warmth to newborns in many delivery rooms. (See also p. 231). A newborn infant's feet and hands are bluish (acrocyanotic) for about 6 to 12 hours after birth, and circulation is particularly poor in the extremities. For this reason one should not attempt to judge an infant's temperature by feeling the feet or hands. Evaluating the warmth of the trunk is more accurate. Newborn infants are sometimes overheated by overzealous nurses or mothers who put too much clothing or bedding on or around them. Since the newborn infant is not yet able to perspire effectively (the sweat glands are not functioning adequately), the baby breaks out in a pinpoint reddish rash. This is sometimes called *prickly heat*, or *miliaria*.

Pulse. It is very difficult to take a radial pulse on an infant. For this reason all "pulse" readings are routinely taken with a stethoscope over the heart (precordial) region through the chest, or possibly the back. The reading is called an *apical pulse*. Newborn infants' pulse rates usually range between 120 and 160 beats per minute (the same as the fetal heart tone range).

Respirations. A newborn infant's respirations are irregular and usually abdominal or diaphragmatic in character, typically ranging from 30 to 80 breaths per minute, depending on the baby's activity. If respirations at rest are persistently 45 or more per minute, the rate is usually considered abnormal, and further respiratory evaluation is required. At no time are costal or sternal retractions considered normal in the newborn infant. Retraction, or a sucking in of the chest wall in the rib or sternal area on inspiration, is an indication of respiratory distress. (See p. 527).

In many hospitals the blood pressure of the newborn is recorded routinely once following birth. Measured with a cuff 1 inch wide, the average blood pressure at birth is 80/46 mm Hg. If blood pressure is abnormal, the physician is notified and serial determinations are made. If available, a Doppler blood pressure device greatly improves accuracy. Otherwise, a systolic reading may be obtained by noting the pressure when palpating the return of the brachial pulse if the blood pressure is inaudible using standard techniques. Students should know that as a person grows older, pulse and respiratory rates decrease, whereas blood pressure readings rise.

Survey of the newborn infant's body systems

GASTROINTESTINAL SYSTEM

Mouth. The newborn infant's mouth is of great interest to parent and physician and should be carefully examined for gross abnormalities such as cleft lip and palate. However, certain small structural differences in the normal newborn infant may need to be explained to the first-time parent to alleviate anxiety. Near the center of the hard palate little, white, glistening spots may be occasionally observed. These are called *Epstein's pearls*. They mark the fusion of the halves of the palate and will disappear in time.

Sometimes the mother has heard of an oral infection called *thrush* and thinks that Epstein's pearls are an indication of this infection. Thrush, or oral moniliasis, caused by a fungus called *Candida (Monilia) albicans*, is a coating on the tongue and cheeks that looks something like milk curds (Fig. 12-3). But it does not disappear when water is given to the infant as do true milk curds. The white patches adhere to the mucous membrane, but when they are forcibly lifted by an applicator, a raw, red, sore surface is revealed.

The gums of the newborn infant may at times appear somewhat jagged, and the rear gums may be whitish. Although the primary teeth are semiformed, they are not erupted. If a tooth is present at birth, it usually is an "extra," which has little root. These so-called rice teeth are sometimes pulled to prevent aspiration when they loosen.

The cheeks of the newborn infant have a chubby appearance because of the development of fatty sucking pads that persist until food is obtained in ways other than sucking.

Mothers may be worried about the possibility of tongue-tie, or a restrictively short frenulum at the base of the tongue. Actually problems in food manipulation or speech because of this condition are rare.

Stomach and intestines. The fetus has no need for a digestive system of its own. All its food is provided predigested by the placental circulation. A

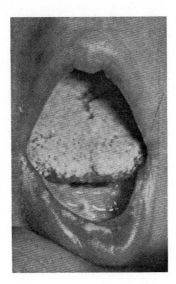

FIG. 12-3

Thrush.

From Potter, E.L.: Pathology of the fetus and the newborn, Chicago, 1952, Year Book Medical Publishers, Inc.

good share of the waste products created are eliminated through the same circulation. After birth, however, digestion is a different story.

The capacity of the newborn infant's stomach at birth probably varies from 1 to 2 ounces (30 to 60 ml) and increases rapidly. The feeding usually begins to leave the stomach before the total taken is completed. It is common for infants to swallow air as they feed, especially when bottle fed. Swallowed air in the stomach may cause difficulty in continuing the feeding, or it may cause vomiting later. Air passing into the intestines may cause colic (abdominal cramping). Bottle-fed babies need to be bubbled frequently. Newborn infants are usually bubbled after every ounce of formula. The older infant is bubbled once halfway through the feeding and again at the end of the feeding. Nursing babies are usually bubbled once or twice during a feeding. Immediately after the feeding, a small amount of milk (less than an ounce) may come up with a bubble. This is termed a "wet burp," "spitting up," or a small regurgitation. Within limits this is a natural

occurrence. It usually subsides by 8 to 9 months of age as the gastrointestinal tract matures.

The first stool of the newborn infant is meconium, a greenish black, tarry, odorless, but very tenacious material. It consists of old lining cells of the gastrointestinal tract, swallowed amniotic fluid debris, and early tract secretions. The first stool should appear in a maximum of 24 hours. If it does not, malformation of the gastrointestinal tract is strongly suspected. Meconium continues to be the normal stool for about 2 days, then the products of digestion of the offered milk begin to change the color of the stool. It becomes first brown and then yellow-green and more loose in consistency. These are the *transitional* stools. Later the stool will become yellow as more milk-product digestion takes place. The stools of formula-fed babies are characteristically lemon yellow and curdy. The stools of breast-fed babies have a more yellow-orange color, are usually softer, and during the first few weeks are more frequent. The wide range of normal stool patterns should be explained to the mother.

CIRCULATORY SYSTEM

In fetal life the circulatory system serves also as a modified respiratory system, since oxygen is not obtained through the breathing of air into the lungs of the baby but through the successive pulsations of the vein in the umbilical cord leading from the placenta attached to the uterine wall. Carbon dioxide is also eliminated through this attachment by way of the two umbilical arteries.

At birth, of course, this type of respiratory function is not continued, since the cord is cut or the placenta soon becomes detached. The fetal circulation, which is designed to channel blood flow to functioning organs and largely avoid the lung fields, is rerouted after birth. (See discussion of fetal circulation, p. 48.) The two fetal shunts that direct blood flow away from the pulmonary circulation normally close, apparently because of changes in internal pressures and vascular reflexes resulting from loss of the maternal oxygen source and subsequent lung expansion. The opening between the two atria of the heart, the *foramen ovale*, shuts, closing off the blood flow to the left atrium from the right heart and forcing more blood into the right ventricle. The *ductus arteriosus*, the fetal vessel between the pulmonary artery and aorta, collapses, obliging the pulmonary artery to send its total contents on to the lungs.

The circulation of blood in the baby at birth is not at the same stage of development throughout the body. The hands and feet are typically blue. At times the entire body of a baby at birth may be blue because the fetal blood has a relatively low oxygen content, and a momentary disturbance of the placental circulation may occur before expansion of the lungs is possible. However, as soon as the airway is cleared and a healthy cry is elicited, the skin "pinks up" dramatically. Although significant, color is the least important of the characteristics or vital signs to be considered when using the Apgar scoring method in evaluating a newborn infant's need for resuscitation aid. (See Table 7-4, p. 134.) If a newborn infant is chilled or inactive for a period of time, a mottled pattern may be seen on the skin—particularly on the extremities. This purplish mottling called *cutis marmorata* is transitory in nature and soon disappears.

For a discussion of newborn infants' blood pressure readings and pulse rates, see p. 224.

Vitamin K is routinely given to newborn infants in many nurseries to prevent hemorrhage because of the natural low prothrombin level in this period of life. It is especially recommended for those suffering from hemorrhagic disease of the newborn, infants born of complicated deliveries, or premature infants. However, it has been found that too high a dosage (usually over 5 mg) may be accompanied by an increase in jaundice and in some cases kernicterus (the yellow staining of the basal ganglia of the brain, causing possible cerebral damage).

Three blood vessels are found in the umbilical cord—one vein and two arteries. These are fairly easily seen in the cut umbilical stump. Considerable interest has developed in counting these vessels at the time of the nursery admission, since if only two vessels are found, there seems to be a significant incidence of internal congenital defects (malformed kidneys, heart, etc.).

The vessels of the umbilical cord are fairly soon occluded by clot formation and shrinkage. However, if the cord is manipulated often, the clot may become dislodged, and bleeding through the cord stump may occur if the ligature or cord clamp is loose. Large cords that contain a great amount of gelatinous connective tissue, called *Wharton's jelly*, must be especially watched for bleeding, since the cord will shrink in diameter and the clamp or ligature may become ineffective. The cord has no sensory nerves; the baby does not feel it when the cord is clamped or cut. The umbilical cord drops off, and the place of attachment heals in about 7 to 10 days.

RESPIRATORY SYSTEM

Although the fetus may make some occasional shallow lung movements in utero, the lungs serve no respiratory function, since the oxygen supply is secured through the placental circulatory system from the mother. Until the first breath of air is taken, the air sacs (alveoli) in the lungs are in an almost total state of collapse, or *atelectasis*. This is as it should be, however, because the lungs must not fill with amniotic fluid or other liquids. In fact, one of the physician's main concerns at birth is the possible aspiration by the baby of thick secretions before the airway can be cleared, thereby plugging or irritating the respiratory tree. Newborn respiratory rates and patterns have been previously discussed on p. 224.

Babies normally are nose breathers and do not breathe through open mouths. Cyanosis of other than the hands and feet, costal or substernal retractions, flaring nostrils, and expiratory grunts heard with or without a stethoscope are all possible signs of respiratory distress.

The most frequent cause of respiratory difficulty in the first few minutes or hours of birth in the United States has been the too liberal use of sedatives, tranquilizers, analgesics, and anesthetics, which not only affect the mother but also pass over the placenta to the baby, making the newborn sleepy and disinclined to take a first breath. Because of this, a real effort has been made in the last few years to reduce the use of these agents.

It is not known exactly why a baby takes that first breath, but the following factors are believed to be significant:

1. The buildup of carbon dioxide in the fetal bloodstream caused by the beginning separation of the placenta from the uterine wall and the pressure of the uterine contractions
2. The decrease of oxygen in the fetal bloodstream.
3. The rapid change in the baby's environment at the moment of birth
4. The direct handling of the baby for the first time in his life

URINARY SYSTEM

The newborn infant's renal system does not have the ability to concentrate urine to the degree of the older child or adult. Water is not reabsorbed as freely by the nephrons, and a newborn infant may become dehydrated rather easily. A newborn infant with profuse diarrhea or vomiting is in imminent danger of dehydration.

Uric acid is found in relatively large amounts in the urine of the newborn infant. Occasionally this substance may "crystallize out" as it cools in the diaper, leaving a pink stain like "brick dust."

All infant voidings in the newborn period should be recorded. Although newborn infants may not void a large amount or often at first, it is very important to note the fact that they are able to void normally.

ENDOCRINE SYSTEM AND GENITAL AREA

The endocrine system of the newborn infant is supplemented by maternal hormones that have crossed the placental barrier. These maternal contributions—presumably the estrogenic hormone, luteal hormone, and lactogenic hormone—when withdrawn from the baby through the act of birth, bring about certain phenomena that may cause parents concern and should be explained. The maternal hormones crossing to the fetus may affect the breasts of both male and female infants, causing swelling, which is particularly noticeable about the third day of life. The breast secretion sometimes seen has been given the interesting name of *witch's*

milk. The breasts may continue to be edematous for 2 or 3 weeks, but gradually the congestion subsides without treatment. The breasts should not be squeezed; this only increases the possibility of infection and injures the tender tissue.

Maternal hormones acting on the miniature uterus of the female newborn infant may set the stage for *infantile menstruation*. The hormones help thicken the infant's tiny endometrial lining. Withdrawn at the time of birth, these hormones no longer maintain this thickened uterine lining, and a tiny menstrual flow may be observed. Usually only a few blood spots are seen on the diapers. The entire process may terminate in 1 or 2 days. This bleeding should not be profuse, and any considerable blood loss may be an indication of hemorrhagic disease. White mucoid vaginal discharge in the newborn infant is also thought to be stimulated by maternal endocrine secretions. The genitalia of both the boy and girl may be swollen. Hymenal tags that regress spontaneously may be seen on girls. Breech infants may have particularly swollen genitalia because of the prolonged pressure on the area. In male infants the scrotum most often contains the testes, although sometimes the descent of one or both is delayed. The foreskin of the uncircumcised infant is normally tight. Few are retractable at birth, and only about 50% are retractable at 1 year. They should not be forced. If adherence of the prepuce (phimosis) persists, circumcision may be advised to facilitate gentle cleansing.

At birth the thymus gland, located under the sternum and above the heart, is larger than a baby's fist. The thymus, long a mysterious lymphoid tissue difficult to classify, has recently been reevaluated as an endocrine gland. It seems that a hormone, thymosin, has been identified, which in cases of thymus lack can be administered to help prevent or control infection. It is now thought to initiate the body's complex immune reactions by producing special defensive cells that are distributed to the spleen, bone marrow, and lymph nodes. After puberty, however, the thymus atrophies, and the change in the gland's size is thought either to stimulate or reflect the development of sexual maturity. Pressure on the respiratory tract from a large thy-

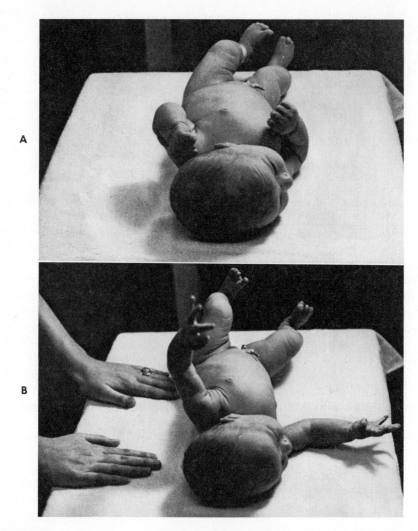

FIG. 12-4   **A,** Infant at rest. **B,** Typical Moro reflex, stimulated by jarring the table.

Courtesy Mead Johnson Laboratories, Evansville, Ind.

mus has, in the past, been cited as the cause of occasional infant suffocation. This has not been adequately substantiated. Although many theories have been advanced, the primary cause of so-called crib death, or sudden infant death syndrome (SIDS), is still unknown.

NEUROMUSCULAR SYSTEM

The nervous system of the normal newborn infant is immature. Essential activities for maintenance of life and protection are largely reflex in character—inborn reactions making life possible until the nervous system and associated muscles can "grow up" to the demands of more complex living. Inborn reflexes that normal newborn infants possess include the rooting, sucking, and swallowing reflexes employed in eating and the protective reflexes, such as coughing, sneezing, gagging, blinking, and perhaps crying. Other muscular reactions in newborn infants are also reflex.

The most commonly tested muscular reflex is a total body response known as the Moro reflex, normally present during the first 3 months of life. This response is elicited when the baby is startled, usually by a sudden jarring of his support such as occurs when someone abruptly pounds on the examining table with a fist. The infant responds symmetrically, throwing out his arms sideways and drawing up his legs with the soles of the feet in opposition. The absence of the Moro reflex in the newborn infant may indicate brain damage (Fig. 12-4).

Another often-seen reflex position is called the tonic neck reflex. The child assumes a modified fencer's position while on his back. The arm and leg on one side of the body are extended while the opposing arm and leg are flexed. The fists are shut and the toes curled. The head is turned toward the extended arm, which incidentally is usually the dominant side. This reflex position may be seen commonly until about 4 months of age. Grasping is also an inborn reflex. (See Figs. 17-1, A, and 17-2 A, on pp. 329 and 330.)

The immaturity of the nervous system is demonstrated by the unstable temperature regulation of the newborn infant and his limited ability to pursue purposeful activity. The baby sees and may discriminate patterns and shapes but probably is unable to interpret much of what he sees. A newborn may turn his head, blink, or grimace in response to sound but be unable to sort out the sound and make it meaningful. The sense of taste is well developed. The sense of smell is rather hard to evaluate, but evidently some newborn infants can detect the smell of breast milk. Cutaneous sensation is highly developed. Pressure, temperature, and pain are increasingly felt by the infant. The newborn reacts to cuddling, caresses, and skillful, gentle handling with greater relaxation and acceptance of care. The neonate responds especially to stimulation by parents and caregivers during the "alert state," or hour following birth.

The newborn infant at first sleeps about 20 hours a day, waking to be fed, bathed, changed, repositioned, and briefly entertained.

A baby's level of consciousness ranges between deep sleep and crying. Recent literature often mentions the so-called quiet-alert state, which affords an especially rewarding opportunity for infant-parent interaction. Usually a newborn infant stays in the position in which he is placed, since he seldom has the ability to turn himself. However, no baby should be left alone on an unguarded table or bed. Accidents can happen!

The order of peripheral nervous system development and muscular coordination proceeds from the head region to the arms and then the legs. Later, the finer activities of the hands and feet are perfected.

Intellectual development is difficult to assess in the newborn infant, but we are reassured when all the normally present reflexes are active. We are concerned when a baby fails to suck well, lacks good muscle tone, or is lethargic and unresponsive to care.

• • •

All in all, the newborn infant is quite an invention, and the succeeding months of his life will include some of the most perplexing, exasperating, and wonderful hours ever experienced by any family lucky enough to welcome him or her into their home.

CHAPTER 13

Care of the normal

newborn infant

UNIVERSAL NEEDS

Today in the United States the trend in the care of the newborn is toward specialization, particularly in centers that serve a large high-risk maternity or infant population. One encounters recovery or transition nurseries devoted to the care of the infant less than 24 hours old or the newborn surgical patient, special care nurseries designed for care of small premature or sick infants (Chapter 15), and intermediate or progressive care units for those infants whose nursing needs are not as intensive. Such care opportunities now enable the survival of many babies who formerly would have died or suffered severe damage. But no matter what the circumstances or locale of birth or the type of care facilities available, all newborn infants have certain needs that must be met for them to thrive and take their place in society. Some of these needs take priority, some can be met simultaneously, and still others are important but need not be rushed. Following are listed nine universal needs of the newborn infant; the first two must be met in order, but the others do not demand such high priority:

1. A clear airway
2. Established respiration
3. Warmth
4. Protection from hemorrhage
5. Protection from infection
6. Identification and observation
7. Nourishment and fluids
8. Love—parent-infant attachment (bonding)
9. Rest

A clear airway

The first two needs must be met immediately or the baby will not survive, and no amount of oxygen, mouth-to-mouth resuscitation, or intermittent positive pressure will stimulate a newborn infant to breathe if its airway is not open. Conversely, if the airway is not clear but filled with amniotic fluid, meconium particles, or blood, and the infant does try to take a breath and inhale, the respiratory tree may become plugged, irritated, or contaminated. The airway may be cleared by using these methods:

1. Wiping off the child's face at the time of the birth of the head
2. Gently suctioning first the mouth and then the nose with a small, soft, short bulb aspirator or a soft catheter attached to a trap before birth is complete
3. Holding the child's head down to drain immediately after birth while gently compressing the throat toward the mouth to milk out secretions

4. Visualizing the larynx with a laryngoscope and suctioning the trachea by trained personnel for unresponsive infants

Established respiration

With the introduction of closed-chest cardiac massage techniques and appliances to stimulate the heartbeat electrically, perhaps "established respiration" should read "established respiration *and* heartbeat." However, for this discussion it will be assumed that heart action is present and adequate. (For cardiopulmonary resuscitation of the newborn infant see p. 522.) If respiration does not occur spontaneously after the airway is clear, the child should be stimulated to cry. This may be done by slapping the heels, lightly spanking the buttocks, rubbing the back gently, or gently suctioning the nose with a soft catheter. Any rough treatment or procedures such as alternating hot and cold baths is now considered to add to the child's problems rather than offer a solution. If breathing is not initiated soon, methods of breathing for the infant must be employed. Sometimes this means the use of intermittent positive pressure by means of orotracheal tube or mask and bag. Sometimes the operator will blow directly through a patent endotracheal tube. Mouth-to-mouth resuscitation also may be attempted. No matter what method is used, it should be emphasized that an airway must be maintained through proper head positioning or the use of a small oropharyngeal airway to keep the infant's tongue from falling back and obstructing the pharynx.

When a child is being resuscitated, is breathing poorly on his own, has generalized cyanosis, or a heart rate under 100 beats per minute, supplementary oxygen should be administered.

Warmth

Newborns may suffer from depressed body temperature not because they produce heat poorly but because they are so vulnerable to heat loss. They lose heat easily because the body surface area is so great in relation to weight, and they have relatively little subcutaneous fat to provide insulation. Heat is provided for the infant in most delivery room settings through the use of unenclosed infant warmers that provide easy accessibility for care by utilizing overhead radiant heat panels. The baby should be dried immediately after birth with a warm towel or blanket to decrease heat loss. An interesting study by Phillips, comparing heat loss in heated cribs with heat loss in the mothers' arms, confirmed that the mother is a reliable source of heat for the normal, dry, wrapped infant placed on the mother's chest.* This has implications for early maternal-infant bonding techniques.

The importance of maintaining an infant's body heat immediately after birth and in the extended neonatal period has been emphasized because the temperature of the infant affects the amount of calories the baby must burn to keep warm, as well as his oxygen consumption, the incidence of apnea, and the acid-base balance of his blood. In circumstances when the infant is sick, the provision of appropriate heat might be critical. (See also p. 554.)

The way in which the baby is dressed will depend on the temperature of the nursery or rooming-in area. Current recommendations are that nursery air temperature be 22 to 25° C (72 to 76° F) with a relative humidity in the range of 35% to 60% for personnel comfort. Some babies are perfectly warm in only a cotton shirt and diaper, covered by a light cotton blanket. Except for an initial reading when a check is made for imperforate anus, 3-minute axillary rather than rectal temperature determinations are now advocated more often in the nursery.† An electronic thermometer may be employed. Axillary temperatures for the normal newborn should range from 36 to 37° C (96.5 to 98.6° F).

---

*Phillips, C.R.N.: Neonatal heat loss in heated cribs vs. mother's arms, JOGN Nurs. 3:11-15, Nov.-Dec. 1974.

†Committee on the fetus and newborn: Standards and recommendations for hospital care of newborn infants, ed. 6, Evanston, Ill., 1977, American Academy of Pediatrics.

Protection from hemorrhage

Today most babies born in hospitals have their cords clamped with some type of compressive band rather than tied with the woven cotton umbilical tape used for so many years. These commercial clamps have proved to be satisfactory, and although the cord must still be frequently observed for bleeding, incidences of difficulty are extremely rare. When a ligature of any kind is being used, it is usually tied twice approximately 1 inch from the abdominal wall in a depression in the cord made by a previously placed hemostat, if one is available. The tie is secured by a square knot for stability and checked frequently during the first few hours to detect any loosening or bleeding.

Protection from hemorrhage in the newborn infant also becomes important when caring for the male infant after circumcision, to be discussed later in this chapter.

In an effort to decrease the possibility of abnormal cerebral pressure and subsequent intracranial bleeding, newborns following delivery are not placed in a prolonged steep head-down position.

Vitamin K to decrease coagulation time is routinely administered in many hospitals (p. 226).

Protection from infection

Protecting the newborn infant from infection is a constant challenge to delivery room and nursery nurses. It involves the entire environment of babies and the techniques used in handling and nourishing them. It even can be said to reach back to the prenatal period when efforts are made to prevent any contamination of the fetus by organisms that are able to pass over the placental barrier (viruses, spirochetes). The baby, while in the hands of the delivering physician, is considered and maintained sterile. The physician clamps and cuts the cord aseptically. Then the baby is usually handed to a circulating nurse who, having carefully washed her hands and put on a clean overgown, receives him for further care without contaminating the physician's sterile gloves.

In most states of the United States, protection of the infant from infection involves the use of some prophylactic against ophthalmia neonatorum caused by the gonorrheal organism. Usually 1 to 2 drops of silver nitrate 1% is instilled in each eye in the delivery room. Care must be taken in administering the drops or ointment; no pressure should be put on the eyeball itself. Occasionally, if the eye area has not been previously touched, shading the baby's eyes from the light will cause them to open spontaneously, making instillation comparatively easy. If this helpful reaction does not occur, the nurse pulls down on the lower lid to instill the agent into the conjunctival sac (Fig. 13-1). All the while the nurse guards the child from cold and continues to observe skin color and respiration patterns. Parents should be told that the eye drops may cause some swelling and drainage within the next 24 hours. (See also p. 132.)

In the nursery the infant has his own individual bassinet and should also have his own bath equipment, supply of linen, and layette (Fig. 13-2). Infants should be bathed in their own beds and not on a common bathing table. The scale used for determining weight should be protected and balanced and handled in such a way that no cross-infection could take place. Technique papers may be used if necessary. Any instruments or appliances that must be used for more than one infant because it is not feasible to supply individual equipment must be carefully disinfected or sterilized after use. This would apply to stethoscopes, circumcision boards and instruments, resuscitators, and other equipment.

Staff members should wear simple, hospital-supplied and laundered scrub gowns on duty, keep their fingernails short, restrict jewelry, and evaluate their own health. No personnel should assume responsibility in a nursery if suffering from a contagious respiratory condition, a skin infection, or diarrhea.

Personnel entering the nursery should wash their hands and arms above the elbow with an anti-

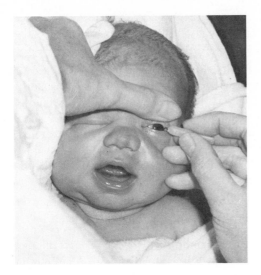

FIG. 13-1

The nurse stabilizes the head with one hand and pulls down on the conjunctival sac with one finger of the other hand while dropping in the silver nitrate.

Courtesy Grossmont Hospital, La Mesa, Calif.

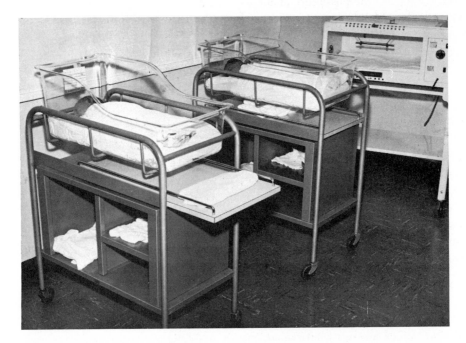

FIG. 13-2   Individual nursery units reduce the possibility of cross infection.

Courtesy Grossmont Hospital, La Mesa, Calif.

bacterial product such as Betadine before starting patient care. Hand washing is mandatory after the care of each baby or individual unit and in the care of the same baby after changing a soiled diaper and proceeding with further needs. The hands should always be washed before treating the cord, since it can become the site of serious infection. It should be observed for signs of inflammation and drainage. A nurse who leaves the maternity area should wear a cover gown to protect her clean nursery gown. If her gown should become soiled in the nursery with urine, regurgitation, or stool at any time, it should be changed. Unless wrapped in a protective blanket or on a protective cover, the infant should be held away from the nurse's gown during care and feedings to protect the nurse's dress from becoming a source of cross-contamination to other infants. Precautions not necessary at home are essential when many infants from many backgrounds and families are being cared for in a small area, such as the hospital nursery.

Parents and ancillary staff (x-ray personnel, and so on) should also be taught the importance and technique of hand washing when visiting the nursery or caring for infants in the mother's hospital room or in the home.

Professional organizations such as the American Academy of Pediatrics, hospital accreditation boards, and local public health and safety officials take an active part in making recommendations and requirements governing the construction, maintenance, and operation of the nursery as well as other parts of the hospital. They are concerned about the floor space available, distance between bassinets, type of ventilation, control of temperature and humidity, provision for adequate lighting, safety of electrical appliances, elimination of possible fire hazards, appropriate dressing and handwashing facilities, and safe formula preparation as well as optimum techniques.

The maternity unit should be separated from other hospital services, and personnel should not be borrowed from other services where infectious sources may exist.

Identification and observation

Identification of the infant may be accomplished in various ways, but it should always be done beyond doubt before the baby leaves the delivery room. In multiple births, the infants should be identified immediately after birth so that no confusion will result. Identification that can be easily counterchecked, such as the use of double or triple bands, is recommended.

ADMISSION BATH

Although some newborn infants receive their first bath in the delivery room or its annex, most infants have their "admission bath" in the nursery after being checked in, identified, weighed, and measured. Many infants are not bathed completely until several hours after birth when the body temperature is higher. Newborn infants are covered with varying amounts of vernix and blood. They may also be soiled with meconium. During the admission bath the nurse usually seeks to remove this soil, reaffirm identification, inspect the infant more carefully than was possible in the delivery room, take his temperature, dress him appropriately, and tuck him into bed. An admission bath usually employs a mild soap solution or an antibacterial product. The following description outlines procedures for the admission bath, although details may differ from hospital to hospital. The nurse's hands are freshly washed before she starts.

Admission bath

Materials:
1. Basin of warm water
2. Mild soap or antibacterial product
3. Paper mesh squares
4. Sterile cotton balls
5. Alcohol, 70%, or other antiseptic for cord care
6. Applicators for cord care
7. Two towels or soft diapers for covering and drying
8. Individual thermometer
9. Small plastic comb

10. Laundry hamper
11. Appropriate clothing, diaper, shirt, and receiving blanket

Procedure:

1. The newborn infant is usually wrapped partially with a towel or coverlet to prevent chilling.
2. The eyes may be wiped with cotton balls moistened with water if necessary.
   a. Irrigation or wiping starts at the nose and proceeds outward to try to prevent unwanted drainage from the inner canthus of the eye from entering the lacrimal duct leading to the nose. (One cotton ball is used for each wipe.)
3. The face is cleaned with a paper mesh square or cotton balls dipped in clear water. No soap is used, since it may be drying to the skin.
   a. If necessary, the opening of the nose is cleared with water-moistened, firmly twisted wisps of cotton (remember, babies are nose breathers).
   b. The external ears may be gently wiped with water-moistened cotton balls, but the canal is never probed.
4. The head is gently but efficiently sudsed and rinsed over the washbasin.
   a. A football hold on the baby is best.
   b. A small comb, gently used, helps to lift out particles of vernix that are difficult to dislodge.
5. The bath is continued, washing, rinsing, and drying the neck, chest, arms, hands, abdomen, and back.
   a. The recently clamped cord and its base are usually avoided until later when an antiseptic is applied. Many nurseries today put no gauze dressing whatsoever on the cord and have found that it dries much faster and has no greater incidence of infection for having been left exposed.
   b. Most nurseries now remove all vernix found in skinfolds as well as all blood and meconium at the time of the initial bath. Special attention should be paid to the neck creases.
   c. After turning the baby on his side to wash, rinse, and dry, a clean, dry, partially folded towel may be placed under the washed portion of the infant to be completely unfolded when the "bottom half" is clean.

d. A small undershirt may be put on at this time, rolled up away from the cord to conserve warmth until the bath is completed.

6. The temperature is taken.
   a. If a rectal temperature is to be taken, it should be completed before bathing the buttocks and genitalia, since the stubby rectal thermometer used often initiates a stool.
   b. Usual time is 3 minutes or until the mercury stops rising.
7. The bath is continued, washing the legs, feet, and then the buttocks and perianal region.
8. The nurse's hands are again washed, and any ordered antiseptic is applied with an applicator to the cord end and the inner rim of the skin cuff surrounding the base of the cord. The vessels in the cord may be counted at this time.
9. The genitalia are inspected and cleansed with cotton balls previously moistened with clear water.
   a. For a baby girl the cotton balls may be wiped gently from front to back between the labia, never using a ball more than once.
   b. For a baby boy pediatric urologists are not recommending retraction of the foreskin of the newborn until about 5 months of age—since most are adherant. The glans that is visible should be gently cleansed with a moistened cotton ball.
10. The diaper is put on and the infant is tucked into bed. The crib identification card is checked against the infant's personal identification.
    a. Newborn infants are frequently propped on their right sides with a rolled blanket. In the older infant a right-side position is supposed to be better because of the aid that gravity gives to the flow of food from the stomach and because any air or bubble remaining will rest near the entrance of the stomach and be more easily expelled.
    b. No newborn infant should be left unattended on his back because of the danger of aspiration.
    c. In some hospitals the newborn infant is not dressed until shown to the parents and waiting relatives through a nursery window.
11. Notations regarding voidings, stool, or any pertinent observations should be appropriately recorded.

All during the bath procedure the nurse is inspecting and evaluating the infant. As she cleans the eyes, she watches for discharge, conjunctival hemorrhage, or areas of opacity. As she feels the head, she checks the contour, the relative size of the fontanels, and the presence of areas of swelling. Pushing down on the chin, she peers into the mouth. Continuing the bath procedure, the nurse evaluates respirations, counts and separates fingers, and judges skin turgor and muscle tone. As she washes each part, she inspects the infant. She is not trying to diagnose, but she wants to be able to report significant findings so that the pediatrician or general practitioner may be called if necessary. Every new baby should be completely examined by a physician within 24 hours of birth, and the condition of some may necessitate a much earlier examination.

INSPECTION BATH

On the following days the bath of the newborn infant serves two main purposes—inspection and stimulation. An example of this procedure follows. Details of possible eye care and genital cleansing are similar to those observed during the admission, both described previously.

Daily inspection bath

Materials:
1. Each infant should have its own individual unit including:
   a. Thermometer
   b. Diapers, shirts
   c. Linen supply
   d. Blankets
2. Paper mesh squares or two washcloths
3. Mild soap
4. Alcohol, 70%, or other cord antiseptic
5. Applicators for cord care
6. Scales and scale paper, technique paper
7. Scratch paper and pencil
8. Laundry hamper
9. Disinfectant for equipment cleanup
Procedure:
1. Wash your hands; check crib for materials needed.

2. Identify the baby.
3. Undress the baby as necessary to take temperature and drop clothing into hamper.
4. Take the temperature (axillary or rectal) following appropriate technique.
5. Place the baby on a clean paper mesh square on scale; weigh, using technique papers to handle scale weights and pencil.
6. Apply alcohol or other ordered antiseptic to the cord at the base by the skin margin and at the tip.
7. Replace the baby in the crib on the scale paper and wash the face with a paper mesh square and clear water. Wash the rest of the baby with mild soap and water solution in the following order: external ears, head, neck, arms, front of body (avoiding the cord), back, legs and feet, lower back, and anus. Pat dry. (Genitalia are cleansed as necessary with newly washed hands and a separate paper mesh square or cotton ball.)
8. Dress the baby and change the bed as necessary.
9. Place the baby on his abdomen, head to one side. Tuck one or more blankets over the infant.
10. Record weight, temperature, general condition, stool, and urine on work paper as appropriate. Loose, watery stools should be reported.
11. Hands should be washed before and after each baby's care and after caring for the anal-genital area before proceeding with additional tasks with the same child. Hands should also be washed before removing a cord clamp.
12. Avoid chilling the baby during the procedure.
13. All equipment that becomes contaminated while weighing should be washed with disinfectant before it is reused. Scales, cart, and all equipment are washed with disinfectant at the end of daily care.
14. As you bathe the infant, inspect for the following:
    a. Color—jaundice
    b. Rash
    c. Petechiae
    d. Bruise marks
    e. Swellings on the head
    f. Condition of the mouth—excess salivation
    g. Condition of the eyes (cleaned only if a discharge is present)
    h. Condition of genitalia

i. Condition of the cord (signs of inflammation, discharge, bleeding)
j. Signs of possible paralysis or spasticity
k. General level of alertness and activity
l. Indications of respiratory distress
m. Possible congenital malformations

"Cuddle bathing," a technique developed at the University of Arizona, is based on the concept that exposure of the infant's skin before, during, and after the bath causes much of the crying at bath time. It also has helped conserve newborn body heat. The procedure is described by Iles and McCrary.*

LIFTING AND HOLDING

The positioning, handling, and transporting of young babies can sometimes be alarming to new mothers or beginning student nurses. It is almost as if they expect to see sawdust leaking out of a tiny joint after touching the child. Both need to be reassured of their ability to learn to care for their charges and to learn comfortable and safe methods of handling a baby. A baby does not break, and knowledge of certain principles will help to give the infant greater support and confidence.

The newborn infant usually tries to maintain a fetal position. With a little coaxing—a pat here, a little pressure there—the child usually readily assumes his unborn posture. This is sometimes useful to the pediatrician or general practitioner who is trying to evaluate the placement of a foot or the line of a mandible.

The newborn infant has one continuous anteroposterior spinal curve and no real control of head movements, although in prone position the baby may raise its head slightly and briefly. Whenever the baby is lifted or transported, the head, being so large and heavy in relation to the rest of the body, must be supported for comfort and to prevent muscle strain. For safety all lifts must have at least two contact points so that if one fails, another is still

*Iles, J.P., and McCrary, M.: Cuddle bathing can be fun: the rewards of research, Am. J. Mat. Child Nurs. 1:350-354, Nov.-Dec. 1976.

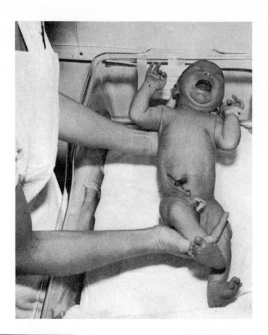

FIG. 13-3

One method of lifting a baby, starting from a side position. The head and upper back are supported by one hand, the legs by the other. Note that the baby is gently grasped.

Courtesy Grossmont Hospital, La Mesa, Calif.

available. Babies, even small ones, can be wriggly and sometimes slippery. Following is one of the most common methods of lifting an infant on his back from a bed.

1. Facing the soles of the feet, lift the legs and buttocks slightly with one hand by grasping the feet, ankles separated by a finger.
2. Slide the opposite hand, palm up, under the full length of the baby until finally the entire back and head are supported.

A second method follows (Fig. 13-3):

1. Facing the baby's side, slide one hand from the side under the head and neck to grasp the farther arm. The head is supported by the forearm, or the head and neck may be supported by the grasping hand.

2. With the other hand reach under the legs to grasp the farther thigh, or grasp the feet holding one finger between the ankles. This is a good lift for weighing the baby or putting him into a tub.

A baby should not be lifted by the arms. When head stability is attained at about 3 months of age, the child may be lifted by grasping the trunk with both hands below the arms. A newborn infant should not be left alone flat on his back. The baby may be propped with a rolled blanket along his back to maintain a side position or may be placed on its abdomen with the head turned to one side. Some newborn infants, when placed in this position for protracted periods, seem to object and rub their knees up and down on the linen, causing reddened shins. Baby beds should have firm mattresses regardless of the style. No pillow should be used. A child should not always be placed in the same position, since this can distort the shape of his head or chest or cause localized baldness.

Babies have been carried in many ways; some are more comfortable for the one who carries and give the baby a greater sense of safety and support. Three ways are common in the United States and are recommended:

1. The traditional cradle hold (Fig. 13-4): The child's head is cradled in the bend of the elbow; the forearm reaches around the outside of the body to grasp the outer leg with the fingers. The nurse's opposite hand and forearm helps support the back and buttocks. This additional support may be momentarily withdrawn if the hand is needed for a task.
2. The football hold (Fig. 13-5): About half the length of the baby's body is supported by the nurse's forearm with the head and neck resting in her palm. The rest of the body, legs, and buttocks are firmly wedged between the nurse's elbow and hip. This is a fine secure hold, and it was definitely designed to provide the mother or nurse with a free hand. However, one should not carry the baby in this position, since the head is somewhat unprotected.

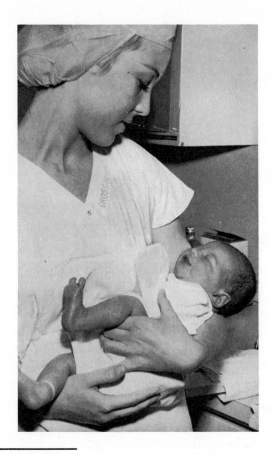

FIG. 13-4

Traditional cradle hold. This baby was a wriggler!
Courtesy Grossmont Hospital, La Mesa, Calif.

3. The shoulder hold (Fig. 13-6): The baby is held up against the chest and shoulder. The palm of one hand supports the baby's buttocks. The other hand keeps the head and back from sagging. Two hands are needed to support the baby's back correctly. This is the old hold used often for bubbling the baby.

Most newborn infants love to be cuddled, and the way they are handled, touched, and fed are ways nurses and caregivers can show love and respect for them as individuals and as very important members of humanity.

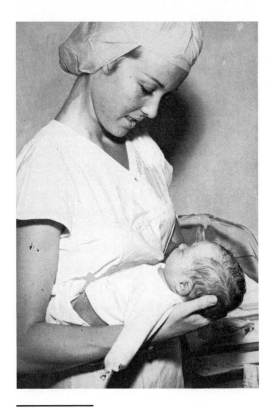

FIG. 13-5

Football hold.

Courtesy Grossmont Hospital, La Mesa, Calif.

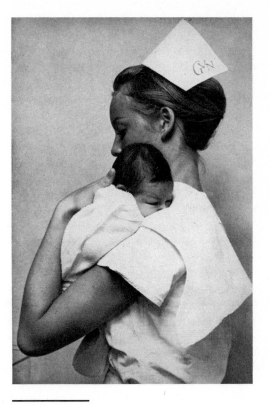

FIG. 13-6

Shoulder hold.

Courtesy Grossmont Hospital, La Mesa, Calif.

Nourishment

Nourishment is the least pressing of a newborn infant's needs, but eventually it becomes paramount. In modern society there are two ways of meeting this need—breast-feeding and formula feeding.

BREAST-FEEDING

Breast-feeding, of course, has an ancient biologic basis and is still the most universally recommended way of providing infant nourishment. A mother should carefully consider its advantages when deciding how she will feed her infant.

Advantages. Putting the baby to breast contributes to the mother's well-being in that the stimulation of the infant's nursing causes the recently emptied uterus to contract and helps in the return of this organ to its proper size and position, a process called involution. Many investigators believe that the baby receives certain immune factors through the breast milk that help protect the baby against diseases to which the mother may have been previously exposed. It is agreed that as a general rule breast-fed babies have fewer respiratory tract infections and alimentary tract disturbances. Certainly, when environmental hygiene is poor, breast feeding is to be preferred over the great possibility of the contamination of artificially prepared feedings because breast milk is normally sterile.

The observation that cow's milk was first designed for calves, whereas' mother's milk is specifically designed for babies, is indisputable. The curd of human milk is softer than that of cow's milk and is easier for a baby to digest. Breast-fed babies have fewer allergy problems. At first, breast-fed babies have more frequent stools than formula-fed youngsters. The stools are yellow-orange and aromatic but not necessarily offensive. Later on they may have fewer stools than their formula-fed counterparts. No prolonged preparation time is necessary except that of washing the breasts, and in the long run, successful nursing is less expensive. Obesity is seen less often in children who have been breast-fed. If the mother nurses her baby, the return of menstruation will probably be delayed until several weeks after weaning, but nursing is no guarantee that pregnancy will not occur. However, the nursing mother may experience such a sense of fulfillment and motherliness that this becomes the primary reason she continues to nurse.

Other considerations. The nursing mother must have a good diet to maintain her resources and provide sufficient nourishment for her infant. She produces approximately 30 ounces of milk a day when lactation is fully established. She needs more calories—approximately 500 to 1,000 more calories per day than when she is not pregnant. (Caloric needs increase as stores of maternal fat built up during pregnancy are depleted in about 3 to 4 months after delivery.) She also needs increased fluid intake to maintain her milk production. Her diet should also include at least 1½ quarts of skimmed or whole milk in liquid form or cooking mixtures a day to protect her personal calcium supply and to avoid possible *osteoporosis*, or weakening of the bony skeleton. Calcium in the form of

medication can be supplied if necessary, but a balanced diet containing calcium-rich foods would give her other healthful nutrients, benefit the whole family, and eliminate the need for pills. She should maintain a daily protein intake of about 64 g (which is 20 g higher than indicated for the *nonpregnant* woman). Recommended intakes of vitamins A, some B complex, C, and E and minerals zinc and iodine are expanded above those advised during pregnancy. (See RDA allowances for lactation, p. 64.) Some foods eaten by the mother have been said to cause the nursing baby abdominal distress, such as cramping or diarrhea, but no one food seems to affect every baby. Probabilities are chocolate and "strong" vegetables such as cabbage, brussels sprouts, and asparagus. Other notorious "gas formers" should be approached with an attitude of caution, but some babies do not seem aware of any deviation in diet.

Most, if not all, drugs taken by the mother may pass through the milk to the baby. The drug thiouracil used in treating hyperthyroidism actually becomes more concentrated in the maternal milk and may affect the infant severely. Certain laxatives are equally as effective on baby as on the mother and should be avoided or used only very judiciously. Common medications to be avoided include cascara, milk of magnesia, Epsom salts, and Ex-lax, but not inert mineral oil. It is wise to counsel mothers to remind their physicians that they are nursing when receiving new prescriptions. Concern has been expressed regarding the amount of DDT and other environmental contaminants found in some human milk samples. However, discontinuance of breast-feeding is not recommended by authorities unless the level of DDT is judged to be high.

Some cultures teach that an intake of low-percentage beer or, for those more affluent, the addition of champagne to the diet increases milk production. Their benefit is probably caused by increased fluid intake and a feeling of relaxation. It is true that a tense, worried mother may have difficulty in maintaining an adequate milk supply.

Mothers who must or who prefer to work outside the home may find it difficult to maintain breast-feeding, depending on the demands of their employment. To maintain a milk supply, the breasts must be stimulated and emptied at fairly frequent intervals. A nursing mother may manually empty her breasts when unable to feed her infant because of separation, but this procedure may not always be convenient. The nursing mother needs good breast support. The typical nursing bra, with the lift-down cup, is efficient and easily used. Many mothers use freshly laundered or paper handkerchiefs or soft-cellulose pads strategically placed to absorb leakage.

To be completely successful most nursing mothers must really want to nurse, have supportive family members, be convinced of its advantages, and receive instruction in the prenatal period regarding the care and normal function of their breasts as well as encouragement and assistance in the postpartum period. If a woman has flattened or inverted nipples, they should be treated during this period of preparation by massage and possibly suction as directed by her physician. In some localities groups of mothers particularly interested in promoting breast-feeding have formed organizations to help the new mother or mother-to-be. La Leche League International, founded in Illinois in 1956, is an organization that is dedicated and active in this field. The League's address is 9616 Minneapolis Avenue, Franklin Park, Illinois, 60131.

Contraindications. Even though some mothers may want to nurse, occasionally the condition of the mother or baby makes it inadvisable. Maternal illness that is particularly protracted, severe, or contagious in nature may preclude breast-feeding. Chiefly because of the high susceptibility of the infant, a diagnosis of maternal tuberculosis used to preclude breast feeding. Currently a new mother found to have tuberculosis who is desirous of nursing her baby is individually evaluated. Her own health, the communicability of her disease, and the needs of her infant are all considered. A woman with cardiac disease or established renal disease may be discouraged from nursing because of the demands on her own body resources that nursing may make. Mentally disturbed mothers would

probably not be allowed the close contact needed for feeding their infants either artificially or by breast unless closely supervised. A mother with severely cracked nipples or breast abscess may find it best to terminate nursing. However, many authorities recommend continuation of breast-feeding while antibiotics and other remedies are used. With proper initial management such conditions are avoidable.

The condition of the baby may influence the decision of whether or not to nurse. Small premature infants usually do not have the strength to suckle at breast, but they may benefit from the expressed maternal milk. For this reason, mothers of premature infants may wish to maintain their milk supply for the immediate use of the baby in the hospital (to be given by means of gavage) and for later use when the baby goes home. Other babies, unable to suckle, may benefit from maternal milk; a child with a cleft lip or palate may be able to breast-feed, depending on the extent of the defect.

In a few communities maternal milk banks have been established for the benefit of babies with special feeding problems. Milk that is expressed for feeding a baby must be carefully handled to safeguard its purity, and a mother expressing milk to be used by her baby needs to be instructed meticulously to prevent contamination. If household freezing techniques are used, maternal milk may be stored for 1 to 2 weeks. Longer storage necessitates quick-freezing and deep-freezer storage.

Techniques. The breast-feeding mother and her baby should be comfortably positioned. The mother may lie on her side with her lower arm raised to shoulder level, helping support the baby. If sitting up in bed, she usually finds it more comfortable to place the baby on a pillow in her lap. This brings the infant closer to the breast with less strain. Because soaps, detergents, and antiseptics used routinely are drying to the nipples and may cause fissures or cracking, many hospitals have changed their breast-care procedures. Often the nipples are wiped with cotton balls saturated only with water and then gently dried prior to nursing. The moth-

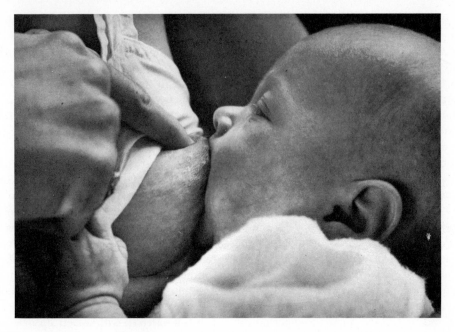

FIG. 13-7   Feeding time for a breast-fed baby. Note that the nipple and almost all the areola are within the baby's mouth.

er's hands should be previously washed. In her own home she will probably find that a clear water wash to the nipple and breast area once a day is sufficient unless a protective cream or ointment used on the nipples requires removal before nursing.

With breast-feeding the nurse and mother have some powerful allies—inborn reflexes and hunger. If it is the first time at breast or a relatively new procedure for the baby, gently expressing a drop of milk on the tip of the nipple will serve as an appetizer and help give the baby the basic idea. If the breasts are engorged, expressing some milk before beginning to nurse will relieve the tension of the breast and make it easier for baby to grasp the nipple. Most babies resent having their mouth shoved at the breast to begin nursing and protest such attempts. It is infinitely better to rely on the rooting reflex. When the baby's cheek is touched by the nipple, the baby almost invariably turns his open lips to seek the nipple. The mother should compress the breast with her thumb and forefingers while the baby nurses to regulate flow and draw the breast away from the nose, making it easier for the baby to breathe. The baby must nurse with the nipple plus almost the entire areola in its mouth to suck successfully and preserve the good condition of the nipple. (See Fig. 13-7.) Cracked or fissured nipples may originate by allowing the baby to chew on the end of the nipple or to nurse too long in one position at one time, by routinely using drying soaps and antiseptics, or by allowing the nipples to stay covered and damp for extended periods.

Different maternity services have different nursing schedules, but most do not advocate allowing the baby to nurse more than 3 to 5 minutes at a time the first day. Each succeeding day the nursing time is gradually increased to 5 or 10 minutes or longer, depending on the state of the nipples and

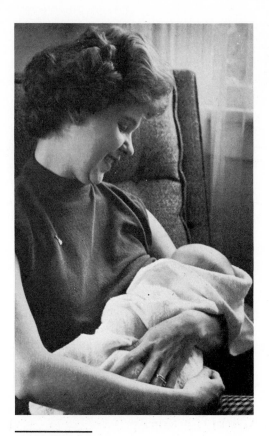

FIG. 13-8

It is possible to nurse an infant unobtrusively.

the baby's desire. In many hospitals the baby is put to breast for the first time on the delivery table. Fair-skinned, blonde, and redheaded mothers should be especially careful about nursing placement and duration, because their delicate skin may need greater protection. Once nursing has been established, the infant gets most of his nourishment in the first 10 minutes. The rest of the time the baby spends satisfying his sucking reflex and enjoying the whole procedure. Twenty minutes is usually the maximum time recommended. The first few days the baby obtains an "introductory milk," called colostrum, which has a laxative effect and contains protective antibodies. Maternal milk becomes "complete"—that is, possessing its char-

acteristic content—several weeks later. (See Fig. 13-8.)

When removing the baby from the breast, remember that babies are capable of considerable tenacity. To convince an infant that it is best to let go, gently pull down on the chin, the corner of the mouth or cheek, or press the breast away from the baby's mouth, but please do not just pull!

It must be emphasized that the greatest aid to milk production is frequent stimulation and emptying of the breasts. If the breasts are not emptied, milk production may dwindle. probably the ideal maternity accommodations for a nursing mother, particularly if the child involved is her first, is the rooming-in plan or a modification of rooming-in. In this setting the baby may be put to the breast as desired and is not limited to the 4-hour feeding schedules followed by most hospitals without family-centered postpartum care programs. Nursing infants are often fed every 2 to 3 hours when breast-feeding is being initiated. Recommended breast-feeding methods also differ in various hospitals. Some suggest alternating the breasts, emptying one side for one feeding and the other for the next. Other maternity services advocate putting a child to the breast on one side, allowing the baby to empty the breast, and changing to the other breast for a few minutes to stimulate milk production. Perhaps the most important consideration is that the breast be emptied. If it is not emptied by the baby, the mother should empty it manually or with the aid of a pump to maintain milk production. For a brief presentation of breast anatomy and more details of breast care, see the section on postpartal care (pp. 193 to 196).

Breast-fed babies, like formula-fed babies, must be bubbled to get rid of swallowed air. Sitting the infant up or holding him over a protected shoulder while gently rubbing his back, plus patience, produces results for both breast and bottle babies.

ARTIFICIAL FEEDING

Today, with present knowledge of nutrition and increased understanding of food processing and preservation, the bottle-fed baby need not be threatened with malnutrition or disease in developed countries. Although mothers should be told the advantages of breast-feeding, they should not be considered or made to feel like maternal failures if they cannot or choose not to nurse. To assume such a position is unrealistic and unkind. To force a mother to nurse against her will may cause an unhappy cycle of rebellion, failure, and regret and make those few mothers who cannot or should not nurse feel lacking in maternal virtue. Some have schedules that are difficult to combine with nursing; some are concerned that their youngsters are not getting enough to eat; and some have felt like failures in past nursing experiences. For others the process of nursing is physically unattractive and may lack approval from their mates. Many healthy children have been formula fed in this society. A loving mother cuddling her baby while tilting a milk-filled bottle need not consider herself to be a "poor mother."

Comparison of cow's milk and human milk. A comparison of the components of cow's milk and human milk gives a clue to formula preparation in the event that breast feeding is not undertaken.

	Cow's milk	Human milk
Protein	3.3%	1.25%
Fat	3.5 to 4%	3.8%
Carbohydrate	4 to 5%	7.0%
Salts (calcium, phosphorus, and potassium principally)	0.75%	0.20%

Most formulas seek to modify cow's milk to make it as much as possible like human milk. To do this, cow's milk is usually diluted to decrease the protein, and more carbohydrate is added. Formula composition and amount is determined by the infant's body weight, growth, activity, and specific dietary needs. (See Fig. 18-3 for relative calorie requirements of children.)

Human milk, when "complete," has approximately the same caloric count as whole cow's milk, 20 calories per ounce. However, some young babies do not tolerate the proportions of ingredients found in whole cow's milk and must have a modification. In the past, 20-calorie-per-ounce formula using evaporated milk (which is twice the strength of whole cow's milk) was frequently used. (Infants drinking this formula needed additional sources of iron and vitamin C.) Its contents per quart is as follows:

> 13 ounces evaporated milk
> 19 ounces water
> 4 tablespoons Dextri-Maltose No. 1, or 2 tablespoons Karo syrup

The physician should guide the selection of formula. The American Academy of Pediatrics recommends that non-breast-fed infants receive iron-fortified formula during the first year of life. Numerous commercially prepared proprietary formulas are available that contain the necessary iron and vitamins (see Table 13-1). These may come in liquid or powder form. Directions must be carefully followed since some are ready to use and others must be diluted or mixed. Their use saves preparation time and bother. The cost involved differs with the type, form, and vendor. The less modification needed before use, the more expensive the product. A number of companies are manufacturing disposable prefilled nursing units. Most hospitals use commercial baby formula.

Preparation of formula. If the more costly ready-to-feed bottle formula is not purchased, the most frequently recommended method of formula preparation today is the so-called tap water method, using prepared formula in the form of liquid concentrate, or powder, or evaporated milk.

Tap water method—formula preparation

This method of formula preparation has become popular because of its simplicity. Used conscientiously, it is safe. Abused by lack of cleanliness or improper technique, it may be associated with infant illness.

Materials:

Capped formula bottle	Sauce pan
Nipple	Can opener
Bottle brush	Spoon
Soap or detergent	Formula as prescribed: ready-to-use, liquid concentrate, powder, or evaporated milk and carbohydrate mixture.

TABLE 13-1 COMPOSITION OF MILK AND OF VARIOUS INFANT FORMULAS*

Product	Common usage	Calories/ (100 ml)	Protein (g/100 ml)	Carbohydrate (g/100 ml)	Fat (g/100 ml)	Minerals (g/100 ml)	Sodium (mEq/L)	Potassium (mEq/L)	Calcium (mEq/L)	Phosphorus (mEq/L)	Iron (mg/L)
Whole cow's milk	After first 12 months	67	3.3	4.8 (lactose)	3.7	0.72	25	35	60	62	1.0
Human milk	First 12 months or longer	67	1.2	7.0 (lactose)	3.8	0.21	7	14	17	9	1.5
Similac with iron	When breast milk unavailable	67	1.8	7.1 (lactose)	3.4	0.4	12	20	30	26	12.0
Enfamil with iron	When breast milk unavailable	67	1.5	7.0 (lactose)	3.7	0.3	11	19	32	32	12.7
SMA with iron	When breast milk unavailable Lower in sodium	67	1.5	7.2 (lactose)	3.6	0.25	7	14	21	21	12.7
Similac PM 60/40	For renal and cardiac disease	67	1.5	7.2 (lactose)	3.4	0.2	7	14	17	10	2.6
ProSobee	Soy formula; for allergy to cow's milk	67	2.5	6.9 (corn syrup solids)	3.4	0.5	24	23	47	42	12.7
Isomil	Soy formula; for allergy to cow's milk	67	2.0	6.8 (corn sugar, sucrose)	3.6	0.38	13	18	35	29	12.0
Cho-Free	CHO-free, soy formula	67	1.8	13% solution added	3.5	0.5	17	25	47	47	8.4
Premature	For infants less than 2,500 g	67-100	2.8	9.0 (sucrose, lactose)	3.7	0.6	-	-	49	49	Trace
Pregestimil	For fat or CHO malabsorption	67	2.2 (hydrolysate)	8.8 (glucose)	2.8 (MCT)†	0.6	18	48	48	47	12.7
Nutramigen	For protein hypersensitivity	67	2.2 (hydrolysate)	8.5 (sucrose)	2.6	0.6	14	27	48	43	12.7
Portagen	For pancreatic or liver disease (poor fat absorption)	67	2.7	7.7 (sucrose, maltodextrins)	3.2 (MCT)†	0.7	17	27	35	36	12.7
Advance	For interim between breast milk or formula and whole milk; lower in calories	56	3.6	6.6 (sucrose)	1.6	0.7	17	32	50	47	18.0

Modified from Fitzgerald, J.F., Infant feeding, Postgrad. Med. **56:**49, July 1974.
*Commercially prepared formulas are vitamin fortified. Consult individual labels for detailed vitamin content.
†MCT: Medium-chain triglycerides

Procedure:

1. Use a clean formula bottle that has been *meticulously washed* in warm, sudsy water, rinsed in *hot* water, and air dried.
2. Use a nipple that has been carefully washed and rinsed. Make sure that the nipple holes are open. (Some references also recommend boiling the clean nipple 3 to 5 minutes).
3. Measure the ingredients needed for one feeding into the bottle. Be sure that you understand what dilution (if any) is to be made because formula is sold in many different forms and concentrations. Read the directions! Babies have become ill and even died because caretakers have not realized this. Add warm water from the tap to the bottle in the amount the formula directions indicate. (Boil tap water which is unapproved.) Mix with clean spoon.
4. Feed *immediately;* do not save formula from one feeding to the next or for more than an hour.

Special handling of infant formula is necessary because milk is such an ideal medium for the nourishment and growth of other living things in addition to human babies. Microorganisms not at all compatible with the baby's digestive system may multiply rapidly in milk if it is improperly bottled or is left open to air and warmed for an extended period. Typhoid organisms were fairly common contaminants of milk and milk products before pasteurization became widespread. Because of the baby's susceptibility, certain methods of disinfection or "sterilization" of the formula (aseptic or terminal) were considered necessary until fairly recently. Now it is believed that in most instances conscientious clean technique is sufficient unless formula must be prepared in advance and stored. However, hospitals usually use sterile precautions until an infant has reached 3 months of age. Plastic bottles employed for older infants who "hold their own," if reused, should be sterilized between patients.

Techniques of feeding. Feeding an infant his formula can be a very enjoyable experience. The hands should be clean; the milk usually should be tepid (no sensation of hot or cold) falling on the inside of the parent's or nurse's wrist.

Experiments using cold formula for feeding the newborn have demonstrated no undesirable effects, even on premature babies. However, personally we find it psychologically difficult to give a young infant a *cold* meal. Many nurseries have discarded formula warmers because of problems with elevated bacterial count on the equipment. Feedings are offered at room temperature. The rate of nipple flow should be almost one drop per second when the bottle is inverted. Nipple holes may be enlarged by a hot needle mounted on a cork. Vigorously sucking babies should be given a resistant nipple. Babies who tire easily and premature babies do better on a soft, pliable nipple (Fig. 13-9).

Be sure the nipple is on top of the tongue, and do not push it too far back—it may stimulate the gag reflex. Babies seem to drink best when held closely on a definite incline. Studies indicate that such positioning minimizes the possibility of retrograde infection through the eustachian tubes to the middle ear and helps prevent aspiration. (See Fig. 13-10.) The neck of the bottle should always be tipped so that it is full of milk. Air in the baby's stomach may cause pain, decrease appetite, or promote regurgitation. Bubbles may be expelled by rubbing the baby's back in an upright position. This may be done after each ounce with newborn babies or halfway through and at the end of the feeding for older babies. It may be best to bubble some babies, particularly finger suckers, before feedings as well. (See Fig. 13-11.) Newborns should be carefully observed before and during feedings for indications of any abnormality in the digestive or respiratory tracts. Prefeeding coughing, cyanosis, and excessive mucus may be associated with anatomic abnormalities. Regurgitation of a feeding through the nose and mouth should be reported at once. Many babies are offered water before they are put to the breast or fed formula to evaluate their ability to drink without difficulty.

After feeding the infant should have his diaper changed if needed and be placed on his right side or abdomen to sleep. The amount taken should be recorded in nursery records. The newborn infant may take only 1 ounce the first day and 2 or 3 ounces per feeding on the second and third days.

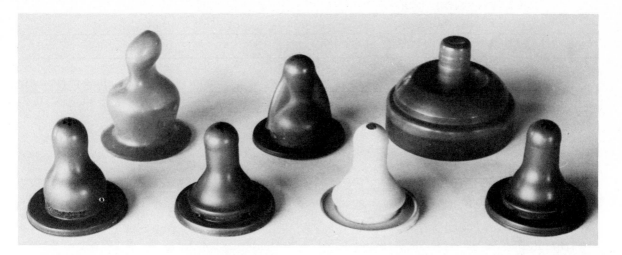

FIG. 13-9   Various types of nipples. Back row, left to right: Nuk, winged, Playtex. Front row: regular three-hole, cross-cut, cereal (large-hole), and soft rubber for premature infants.

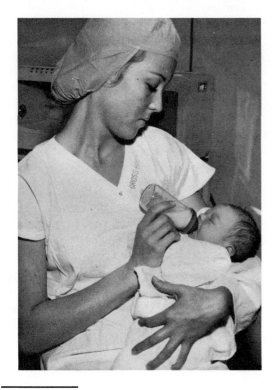

FIG. 13-10

The "en face" position. The nipple should always be full of formula and the infant preferably upright.

Courtesy Grossmont Hospital, La Mesa, Calif.

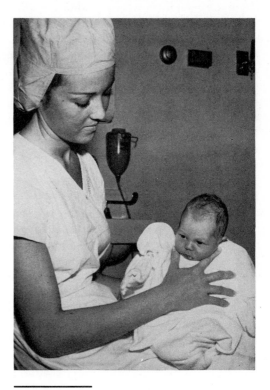

FIG. 13-11

Let's hear a "thank you!"

Courtesy Grossmont Hospital, La Mesa, Calif.

TABLE 13-2   SUGGESTED SCHEDULE ON AN APPROXIMATE 4-HOUR BASIS FOR AVERAGE-WEIGHT INFANT

Age	Milliliters per feeding	Ounces per feeding	Number of feedings	Time of feedings
First week	60-90	2 to 3	6	6, 10, 2, 6, 20, 2
Two to four weeks	90-150	3 to 5	6	6, 10, 2, 6, 10, 2
Second to third months	120-180	4 to 6	5	6, 10, 2, 6, 10
Fourth and fifth months	150-210	5 to 7	5	6, 10, 2, 6, 10
Sixth and seventh months	210-240	7 to 8	4	6, 10, 2, 6
Eighth to twelfth months	240	8*	3	7, 12, 6

Modified from Williams, S.R.: Nutrition and diet therapy, ed. 4, St. Louis, 1981, The C.V. Mosby Co., p. 409.
*120 ml (4 ounces) milk may be given midafternoon.

See Table 13-2 for usual formula amounts and number of feedings.

EVALUATION OF NUTRITIONAL STATUS

There are numerous ways of judging if a newborn infant, whether formula- or breast-fed, is receiving enough to eat.

1. Observing his behavior; does he seem content, or is he a short sleeper and irritable? (Note that babies cry for reasons other than hunger pangs; for example, if they are wet, too tightly bundled, too warm, have gas pains, or want to be held.)
2. Watching for signs of dehydration from poor fluid intake.
   a. Dark, concentrated urine; dry, hard stools.
   b. Dry skin with little "bounce."
   c. Low-grade fever. (Note that the most common cause of low-grade fever is dehydration, although the nurse does not want to overlook the possibility of infection.)
   d. Elevated specific gravity (above 1.020).
   e. In severe cases, sunken fontanels.
3. Measuring intake.
   a. This is routine with bottle-fed babies.
   b. If measuring is ordered, breast-fed babies are weighed dressed and wrapped directly before the feeding and directly after the feeding, before any diapers are changed with the same clothes and blankets. (1 g = 1 ml).
   c. Intake should be evaluated in terms of a 24-hour period and not individual feedings.

4. Measuring weight gain.
   a. This method is of little use in the nursery because of the short hospital stays of most newborn infants in the United States (approximately 3 days).
   b. All babies lose weight directly after birth, which should cause no concern unless the weight loss approaches 10% of the birth weight. Bottle-fed babies regain their birth weight more rapidly than most breast-fed babies.
   c. After weight gain is reestablished, a gain of about an ounce a day is average, equaling about 6 ounces a week; at the end of 5 months most babies have doubled their birth weight.

Love—parent-infant attachment (bonding)

The birthday of a child is a special occasion, and although the child needs to be protected against infection and overhandling, the way that the child is introduced to the parents and siblings is of great importance. Both the father and the mother should have an opportunity to see and handle the infant without hurry directly after birth.

The importance of this early postpartum period to the formation of positive mother-child and mother-father-child relationships is being explored attentively. The newborn has been reported to be often more alert during the first hour after birth than in the immediately subsequent hours. Many researchers agree that birth and the immediately postpartum period when the baby is first seen, touched, and cared for are sensitive periods in the development of attachment (bonding). If the mother is also alert and willing and the circumstances of the labor and birth are conducive, an early parent-child interaction followed by frequent visits would appear to help young parents develop gratifying maternal-paternal identities.

Long-term studies of maternal attachment to normal and high-risk infants in the early postpartum period, its manifestations, and long-term influence on the child are now underway.* The nurse is in an excellent position to assess and facilitate attachment. Numerous investigators have described the typical initial exploratory behavior of human mothers and fathers. Gentle fingertip touching of the hands and feet progresses to massagelike motions of the palm on the baby's trunk. Eye-to-eye contact is remarkable, and a characteristic "en face" position is often demonstrated (the mother's face poised directly in front of and in line with that of her infant). This eye-to-eye observation helps establish the newborn's identity as a person and provides rewarding feedback to the mother. These activities appear to be particularly significant because some evidence already suggests that increased maternal attention seems to facilitate later exploratory behavior in infants. Could the early postpartum interval be a possible critical period in the growth and development of the human offspring as it is in some other species?

Nurses must recognize that many expectant fathers want to be involved not only in the preparation for parenthood but in the actual birth and care of the infant. Mothers must be helped in understanding that just as they have many adjustments to make, so do new fathers. A father often has a need to handle and touch his newborn. Typically he has experienced various concerns including the health of his wife, the outcome of the pregnancy, changes in sexual practices, and increased financial responsibility.

If the newborn's siblings, grandparents, and other family members visit, they should be able to see the baby and visit with the new mother according to her wishes. Newborn infants may receive all other things, but if they do not receive true love, they will not thrive.

Rest

Although it is important that newborns receive stimulation, they also need times of relative little input to "organize" their world and to grow. Overstimulated babies are likely to be more nervous, with shorter attention spans.

SPECIAL NEEDS

Parent education

The new mother will have a lower level of anxiety if she is equipped with a comprehensive knowledge of her child. Although she is in the hospital for a brief time in the postpartum period, it is the nurse's responsibility to initiate or build on teaching in the following areas:

Importance of stimulation
Possible sibling rivalry
Infant care
    Bathing
    Skin care
    Cord care
    Circumcision care
Nutrition
    Breast feeding
    Formula preparation
    Introduction of solids
Sleep patterns
Elimination patterns
Safety
    Car seats
    Never leaving child unattended

---

*Klaus, M.H., and Kennell, J.H.: Parent-infant bonding, ed. 2, St. Louis, 1981, the C.V. Mosby Co.; Lamb, M.: Second thoughts on first touch, Psychol. Today **16**:9-11 Apr. 1982.

Cool vs. hot mist vaporizer
Pacifiers
Cribs
Available community resources

Additional teaching can be begun or continued in high school family education classes, prenatal and postnatal parent education programs, clinic and office waiting rooms, and well-child visits.

Baptism

Sometimes other occasions of special meaning and deep significance occur in the nursery. Catholic parents and occasionally Protestant families may request the baptism of their child while the baby is in the nursery. Efforts should be made to comply with the religious practices of parents of any faith. When the child is in no immediate danger, a member of the clergy involved should always be called. Most hospitals have appropriate utensils available. If doubt exists concerning what should be in readiness, the clergy may always be consulted. Some will bring their own articles. Most require only a pitcher of pure water. If the child is a member of a Catholic family and appears to be in immediate danger of death, a nurse may baptize the baby. It is preferable that a nurse of the Catholic faith should do this task, but any adult may do so. In performing the baptism, she should pour water on the head or face of the child while saying, "I baptize thee in the name of the Father, and of the Son, and of the Holy Spirit." A record of the baptism should be made in the nurse's notes and the parents notified. This simple but deeply meaningful act can be of great comfort to the family.

Circumcision

Circumcision involves the slitting or surgical removal of all or part of the foreskin, or prepuce, of the penis. Advocates of the procedure believe that it makes hygiene easier and decreases irritation of the area from an accumulation of cellular debris (smegma) under the foreskin and may help to avoid cancer. Other practitioners declare that circumcision is unnecessary and a possible source of infection, hemorrhage, and meatal stenosis. The outcome of this ancient surgery appears to be frequently dependent on the skill and technique of the operator. The American Academy of Pediatrics has stated that there are no valid medical indications for circumcision in the newborn period. Routine circumcision of all male infants appears to be decreasing.

The circumcision of a Jewish infant has religious import. Among Orthodox Jews it is undertaken by an ordained circumciser called a "mohel." This ceremony is usually performed after the child leaves the hospital on the eighth day of life. The child is then officially named.

Physicians usually have individual preferences regarding the technique used, but the following setup list and procedure may be helpful.

Circumcision procedure

Materials:
1. Sterile setup including:
   a. One circumcision drape
   b. Two 4 × 4 squares (flats or gauze compresses)
   c. Two cotton balls
   d. Three small hemostats (mosquito clamps)
   e. One Yellen (Gomco) clamp, 1.3 to 1.1 cm in diameter or plastic bell circumcision device
   f. One scalpel handle and added blade
   g. Possibly needle holder, needle, and suture materials (chromic 3-0)
   h. One grooved director and probe
   i. One thumb forceps
2. Sterile gloves, appropriately sized
3. Ordered antiseptic for skin preparation
   a. Povidone-iodine (Betadine)
   b. Tincture of thimerosal (Merthiolate)
4. Dressing materials
   a. Petrolatum-impregnated gauze
   b. Tincture of benzoin application
5. A circumcision board, diapers, pins, or special restraining halter that ties over the board

Procedure
1. Preliminary
   a. Obtain a signed informed consent from parent before procedure.

b. Properly identify the baby. Check for possible reasons for not proceeding with the operation (presence of inflammation, tendency to bleed). Clean diaper area.

c. Restrain the baby gently but firmly on a padded or plastic circumcision board.

d. Assure good light. A stool or chair may be appreciated by the operator.

e. Use of a pacifier may comfort the baby during the procedure.

2. Technique

a. The technique of circumcision differs considerably from physician to physician. Rarely local anesthetic will be given, but most physicians seem to feel it may cause more problems than it solves (distortion of tissues) and consider the operation of such short duration, performed in an area that, at this age, has a low level of sensitivity, that is is not truly necessary.

b. The Yellen (Gomco) clamp may be used to cut off circulation, and the foreskin excised. Sutures may or may not be used.

c. The foreskin may be freed from the glans with probe, cut away, bleeders controlled and sutured.

d. A nonconstrictive dressing is applied. Petrolatum-impregnated gauze is often used.

3. Aftercare

a. Notice of the recent circumcision should be attached to the crib.

b. Frequent checks should be made to determine possible swelling and bleeding.

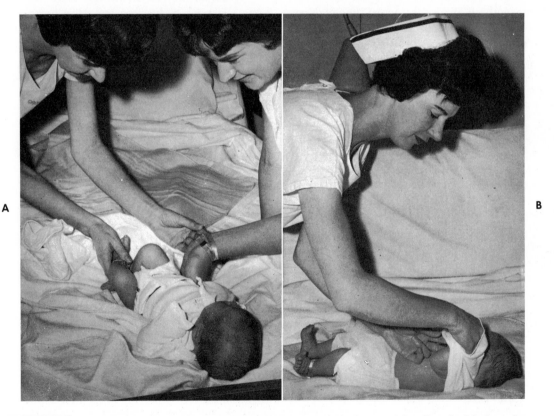

FIG. 13-12   **A,** Identification of the baby before hospital discharge using the double-banding technique. **B,** Dressing the baby in his own clothes for discharge. (Note the method of placing the sleeve over the infant's hand and arm.)

Courtesy Grossmont Hospital, La Mesa, Calif.

c. Voidings, especially the first after the procedure, should be carefully charted. There is a danger of urinary retention.

d. The area should be kept clean; soiled or displaced dressings should be replaced with clean materials.

e. The infant is positioned on his side.

Sometimes circumcisions are performed not long before the baby's discharge home. In this event the mother should be carefully instructed regarding observation and care of the area.

DISCHARGE PROCEDURE

Discharge is an exciting, somewhat trying time for most mothers. Before the actual time of departure, the physician's order for discharge is checked and home orders are reviewed. The mother's belongings are packed, and clothes are put out for the infant. Mothers should have ready at least two diapers, pins, a baby shirt, kimono, and receiving blanket or comparable wardrobe. Identification should be established, the baby viewed, and dressed in his own clothes (Fig. 13-12). The discharge record should be signed and witnessed. If the mother wishes it, a supply of formula may be available to take home. Before saying goodbye to the family, the nurse should make sure discharge instructions are understood and preferably written out and any questions answered. Ideally, the baby's first car ride home from the hospital should be in an approved automobile safety restraint. Many hospitals are making this item available to new parents, some at cost.

Before leaving the infant, the nurse should take one last peek at his face to assure herself of his condition. Then, no matter what she may desire, she must let the baby go.

CHAPTER 14   Infants with special needs:
prematurity and abnormality

This chapter is included to help students appreciate some of the more common abnormalities or conditions encountered during their practical experience and to help them assist more intelligently in the care of infants who have these conditions. Some of the conditions discussed are found and treated in the nursery and pose few or no problems later. Other anomalies by their very nature call for prolonged therapy and correction long after the neonatal period, infancy, or, indeed, childhood has passed.

THE PREMATURE (PRETERM) INFANT (Figs. 14-1 and 14-2)

Among those babies with special needs, the first to be discussed are the premature infants. In the past the most common definition of prematurity was based on weight. For a long time, babies having a birth weight under 5½ pounds (2,500 g) were all considered to be premature. However, in reality some of these babies had completed a term gestation and were underweight because of genetic or intrauterine factors. In fact, the term *premature*, referring to the infant born before the end of the thirty-seventh week of gestation, is now often being replaced by the more accurately descriptive adjective *preterm*. In this chapter the two words, preterm and premature, are used synonymously. Infants who are small at birth for other reasons are

called small for gestational age (SGA). Babies may be of *low birth weight* because of an abbreviated gestation, unfavorable prebirth conditions, or both. Following is a more complete, newer classification of newborns based on gestational age and birth weight:

preterm or premature Any infant born before the end of 37 weeks' gestation regardless of weight.
term Any infant born between the beginning of the thirty-eighth week and the end of the forty-second week of gestation *regardless of weight.*
post-term or postmature Any infant born after the end of 42 weeks' gestation *regardless of weight.*
small for gestational age (SGA) Any infant weighing less than 90% of the babies of the same gestational age.
appropriate for gestational age (AGA) Any infant weighing less than the heaviest 10% and more than the lightest 10% of the babies of the same gestational age.
large for gestational age (LGA) Any infant weighing more than 90% of the babies of the same gestational age.
low birth weight infants Any preterm and small for gestational age infant weighing less than 2,500 g, or 5½ pounds.

Actually, in determining the status of the small infant, birth weight, heredity, possible length of gestation, clinical appearance, and behavior all must be considered. Although some babies cannot be classified premature by the scale or calendar, they are judged underdeveloped and treated as "premies."

The mortality percentages related to birth weight and gestational age have improved signifi-

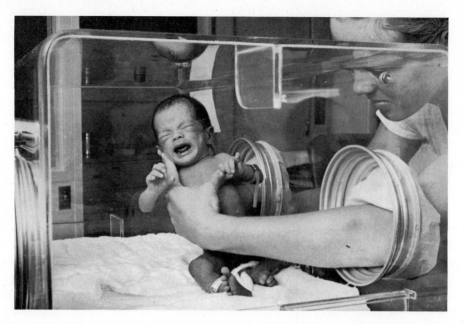

FIG. 14-1   This baby would have been technically premature if only his birth weight were considered. However, his Oriental ancestry influenced his size; he was probably a "finished product," although he weighed less than 5½ pounds (2,500 g).

Courtesy Grossmont Hospital, La Mesa, Calif.

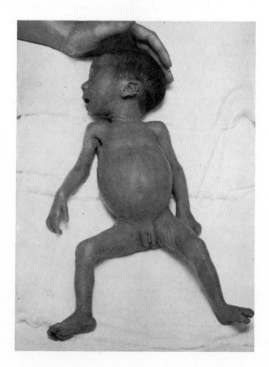

FIG. 14-2

Typical premature infant.

Courtesy Grossmont Hospital, La Mesa, Calif.

cantly in modern perinatal centers as a result of advanced knowledge, sophisticated equipment, and increasingly skilled personnel. However, survivals of 26-week gestations or infants weighing less than 750 g are very rare.

Role of the nurse

The student nurse who wishes to work with premature babies should seek more supervised advanced training than is possible in her basic course. The nursery care of these infants must be extremely gentle, deft, and precise, and the ability to evaluate their behavior and reactions properly takes an extended period of time to acquire. However, although as a student she may not have the opportunity to be involved in the direct nursing of many premature infants, she should understand the nature of the problems encountered in such nursing. Some of these babies will be cared for in an intensive care setting, others in the pediatric area. A leading cause of neonatal mortality, remember, is prematurity.

Causes

The causes of low birth weight infants are not always known. However, it is recognized that low birth weight infants are more frequently born to mothers of lower socioeconomic status. This may be related to the nature of prenatal care, the obstetric complications encountered, nutrition, and general health practices. Young teenage mothers also have a higher rate of low birth weight babies. Multiple births are almost always associated with prematurity. Heavy smoking seems to be an etiologic factor.

Appearance and activity

The typical premature infant has a "wrinkled old man" appearance resulting from a lack of subcuta-neous fat. The baby has a good supply of long, soft body hair called "lanugo", the head and abdomen are relatively large, and the thorax is small. There is little molding of the skull. (See Fig. 14-3.) Respirations are usually irregular, and the premature infant may be surprisingly active. (See Table 14-1.)

Nutrition

Sucking and swallowing reflexes may be weak or absent in very small infants, necessitating feedings by gavage (the insertion of a stomach tube) or by intravenous feedings. Intravenous feedings are now commonly given, especially to infants weighing less than 1,200 g or classified as "sick" prematures. These feedings may be given by umbilical catheter or peripheral veins. Stronger "premies" may do well when fed with a soft rubber nipple.

Premature feeding schedules and techniques are controversial at the present time. However, after a period of evaluation of feeding tolerances for glucose water, oral feedings generally progress to formulas richer in calories than those normally fed to full-term infants because of the premature infant's lack of nutritional reserves and the great need for rapid growth. Often breast milk is used. Later the diet is supplemented by iron administration. Often the premature infant is also given vitamin E, which is believed to help protect lung structures, help prevent eye problems such as retrolental fibroplasia, and preserve red blood cell integrity.

Most premature infants are put on a 2- or 3-hour feeding schedule. Nourishment is offered in extremely small amounts of 3 to 5 ml at a time, since the danger of overfeeding the premature baby is very real. Overfeeding may increase abdominal distention, cause respiratory embarrassment, and trigger vomiting, which may involve aspiration. The infant must be bubbled frequently. After a feeding the baby's head and chest are elevated by tilting the incubator mattress tray, and the infant is positioned on his side to discourage emesis and aspiration.

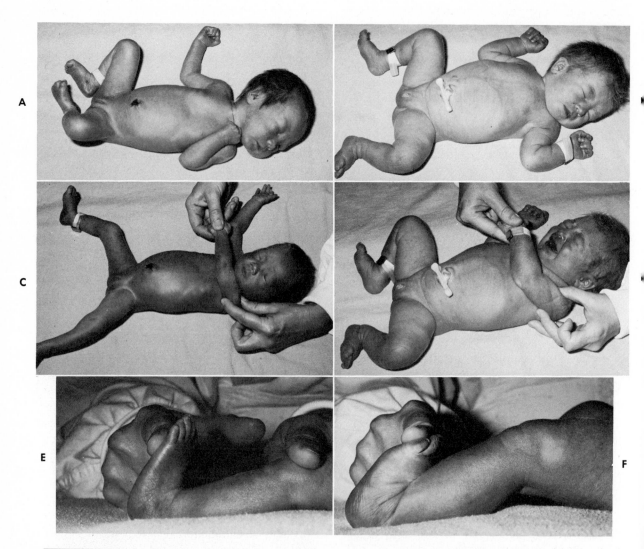

FIG. 14-3   Illustrations on the left show a premature infant; those on the right show a mature infant. **A** and **B**, Typical body contours and postures. **C** and **D**, Scarf sign: immaturity seen when the elbow passes the midline. **E** and **F**, Prematurity is seen when the heel cord is short and sole crease is scanty.

Courtesy U.S. Naval Regional Medical Center, San Diego, Calif.

TABLE 14-1 POSTNATAL ESTIMATION OF FETAL AGE BASED ON SIGNS OF MATURITY ASSUMING NORMAL GROWTH

	28 weeks	32 weeks	36 weeks	40 weeks
Skin	Thin, red, gelatinous	Smooth, dark pink; many vessels visible	Pink, tender; few vessels visible	Pale pink; no vessels
Breasts	Flat, areolae barely visible	Well-defined areolae	Areolae raised; 1 to 2 mm breast tissue	7 to 10 mm breast tissue
Sole creases	None	One anterior transverse crease	Creases on anterior two thirds of sole	Creases on heels
Ears	Pinna soft, flat; stays folded	Slight incurving at top; returns slowly from folding	Incurving upper two thirds; springs back from folding	Incurving to lobe; firm, stands out from head
Genitalia Male	Testes undescended; scrotum smooth	Testes high in canal; few scrotal rugae	Testes high in scrotum; more rugae	Testes low in pendulous scrotum; rugae complete
Female	Labia majora widely separated; clitoris, labia minora prominent	Labia majora becoming closer, nearly cover labia minora		Labia majora completely cover labia minora
Neurologic posture	Hypotonic, arms and legs extended	Partial leg flexion	Froglike; flexion all limbs	Hypertonic
Recoil	None	Partial leg recoil	Partial arm and leg recoil	Prompt recoil

Special needs

The maintenance of body temperature is a real challenge in the care of premature infants. Because of the immaturity of the temperature-regulating center in the brain, little stability is seen. The baby must be specially assisted in his efforts to keep warm. This aid may be provided by the open-type infant warmer or an enclosed plastic incubator.

Oxygen levels above that of room air (21%) may be required to meet the infant's metabolic needs. The most accurate way to evaluate a baby's oxygen status is through the use of intermittent arterial blood gas determinations. Although some babies may approach oxygen toxicity levels when the environmental oxygen reaches 40%, others with diminished respiratory function will need higher levels of environmental oxygen to achieve correct blood concentrations. Environmental oxygen concentrations together with blood gas analysis are very important. They are monitored to evaluate the infant's general condition in response to therapy and to prevent the blindness or visual loss called *retrolental fibroplasia*, which can be produced by extended high oxygen concentrations in the blood. The immature blood vessels in the retinas of the eyes hemorrhage. The retinas partially or completely detach from the inner surfaces of the posterior chambers of the eyes. They become fibrous masses behind the lenses, unable to receive visual stimuli.

Premature infants are especially susceptible to injury and must be handled with extreme gentleness and discretion. (They need their rest to grow!) They are particularly susceptible to injury at the time of birth and may suffer from intracranial hemorrhage and brain damage. A large percentage of cerebral palsied children, who exhibit some form of spasticity, or lack of muscle control, were premature. Lack of muscular coordination and mental retardation may stem from brain injury, prolonged lack of oxygen caused by delayed or interrupted breathing at the time of or subsequent to birth, or bilirubin deposits in the brain tissue resulting from the inability of the immature liver to handle red blood cell breakdown satisfactorily. Jaundice is a significant finding.

"Premies," because of their abrupt debut, are said to be deprived of antibody protection given by mothers to full-term infants. They are also less prepared to manufacture their own antibodies. They are easy victims of infection and must be scrupulously guarded.

Significant immaturity of the respiratory system is an often encountered finding. Failure of lung tissue to expand, or atelectasis, is frequently reported. *Hyaline membrane disease, or respiratory distress syndrome,* is found in a high percentage of premature babies, particularly those delivered by cesarean section, and in children of diabetic mothers. (These babies, although large, appear to be physiologically immature and should be treated similarly to premature infants.) This disease is the commonest cause of death in premature infants and is discussed on pp. 289 to 292.

• • •

The care of the premature infant is a heavy responsibility; life is enclosed in a fragile package.

Yet some of the celebrated figures of history, who have made vast contributions to mankind, entered the world in just such an unfinished state—such men as Sir Isaac Newton and Sir Winston Churchill. Do not underestimate the "premie"!

ABNORMALITIES OF THE NEWBORN INFANT

One would wish that each baby born were perfect in every detail—physically, intellectually, and emotionally ready to meet the challenge of life without an initial obstacle or defect. Sadly, such is not the case. Approximately one in fourteen of all children born has some kind of abnormality, causing disfigurement or resulting in physical or mental handicaps or a shortened life, although not all these problems may be noted at birth.

The birth of a handicapped or ill child is always a distressing time for the family. Feeling of failure, anxiety, guilt, frustration, anger, and exhaustion are common. Parents at first may be unable to believe that their child is abnormal, and when the realization comes, grief may be intense. Problems in organizing the family to meet the unexpected demands created by the necessary trips to the hospital, physician, and therapist and the extra financial burden it all entails can seem almost without end to the often perplexed and unprepared parents.

Although the vocational nurse is not in a position to give professional guidance to people to mobilize the total resources of the family and community to meet the needs involved, she should recognize the pressures under which they are operating. She should know how much has been told the parents regarding their child and be extremely discreet in her conversations. She should be supportive in allowing the parents to express themselves and in relaying any problems that seem to be causing worry to the charge nurse or physician. It is *very important* that the parents not feel alone in their attempt to adjust to the reality of their child's imperfection. In an attempt to prevent such feelings the nurse can be a vital liaison between the family and medical staff, clergy, and community resource personnel. Guided participation in the care of their child usually helps reduce feelings of isolation.

Birth injuries

Cerebral hemorrhage. The most common type of birth injury is *intracranial hemorrhage*. As noted previously, it is most often seen in premature infants but can be diagnosed in full-term babies as well, particularly those who had a traumatic passage to this external world. Symptoms or signs of hemorrhage within the skull may manifest themselves suddenly or gradually. They may include irritability, listlessness or cyanosis, marked irregular respiration, varying degrees of paralysis, lack of appetite or poor sucking reflex, tremors, convulsions, projectile vomiting, unequally dilated pupils, tense or bulging fontanels, and a high, shrill cry. These kinds of symptoms could arise from other causes, such as intracranial abscess, cerebral edema, tumor, or developing hydrocephalus—in fact, from anything that would increase the pressure within the skull. Diagnosis is usually made through the history and observation of the infant or by computerized transaxial tomography (CTT) (p. 650). Sometimes the bleeding is mild and stops spontaneously, and the child recovers with little or no effects. Sometimes pressure is so intense that it must be relieved by aspiration of the subdural space or by surgery. Sometimes brain damage is permanent, or death results from the condition.

The infant is usually placed in an incubator with his head slightly elevated in an attempt to relieve pressure. Rarely, a spinal tap may be done for the same reason or as a diagnostic aid. Vitamin K to relieve bleeding tendencies may be prescribed. Sedatives such as phenobarbital may be ordered for tremor. It is very important for the nurse observing the infant to be able to describe accurately the type of tremor, convulsion, or abnormal behavior pattern seen; her description of the part of the body affected—one or both sides—how long it lasted,

and what event, if anything, occurred just beforehand may help the physician localize the area of bleeding. The child is kept as quiet as possible.

Fractures. Fractures may occur at birth. The most frequently broken bone is the clavicle, or collarbone. It usually heals without treatment. Fractures of long bones are uncommon; they may be splinted. All broken bones normally heal rapidly during infancy.

Facial paralysis. Temporary or even permanent paralysis occasionally results from nerve injury during childbirth. Facial paralysis may be caused by forceps pressure. The affected side of the face does not move, and the eye may remain open. This condition usually disappears gradually.

Erb's palsy. Injury to the brachial plexus, the network of nerves that branches to supply the nervous control of the upper extremities, may cause the arm on the affected side to hang limply from the shoulder and rotate internally. With this condition, the Moro reflex is asymmetric. The infant cannot raise his arm. This injury, called Erb's palsy, is usually not permanent. Treatment consists of immobilizing the arm in an abducted, externally rotated position with flexion at the elbow.

Hydrocephalus

Hydrocephalus is a defect that results from the accumulation of abnormally large amounts of cerebrospinal fluid within the cranium, causing abnormal enlargement of the immature skull (Fig. 14-4).

Types. There are a variety of causes of hydrocephalus. A congenital structural defect may exist in the cerebrospinal fluid drainage system, preventing the flow of the fluid from the ventricles, of the brain where it is produced, into the subarachnoid space and the venous system where it is reabsorbed. Such blockage may also occur as the result of a brain tumor or abscess. This type of blockage produces noncommunicating hydrocephalus. Occasionally the flow of cerebrospinal fluid from the ventricles to the subarachnoid space is normal, but

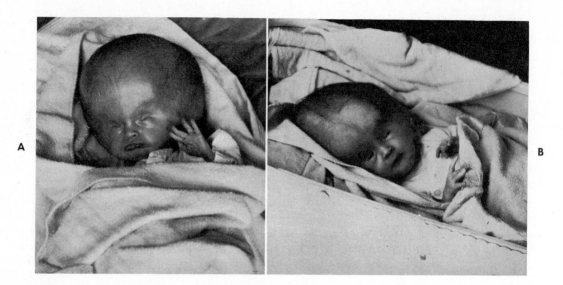

FIG. 14-4   **A,** This baby with advanced hydrocephalus was 4½ weeks old. He was delivered 7 weeks early by cesarean section. **B,** The same child at 3 months of age. The cranium has collapsed. He died at 5½ months of age. (Shunting procedures available today would have prevented such enlargement.)

the absorption of the fluid into the venous system is inadequate, usually as the result of damaged absorbent surfaces, causing excessive fluid collection. This situation, as described, is called communicating hydrocephalus and may occur as a sequela to meningitis or intracranial hemorrhage. It often coexists with a congenital defect called *myelomeningocele*, a herniation of a part of the spinal cord elements and its coverings through an abnormal opening in the back of the bony spine. The hydrocephalus usually becomes more evident after the myelomeningocele is surgically repaired. Circulation pathways outside the brain for the cerebrospinal fluid that had previously been available may be disturbed or unavailable.

Early recognition and treatment. The infant responds to mounting cerebrospinal fluid pressure by an abnormal symmetric increase in head size. Other manifestations noted shortly after birth include bulging of the fontanels, separation of sutures, distended scalp veins, irritability, and vomiting. A downward displacement of the eyes

and skin tension, giving the pupils a "setting-sun" appearance, is a late symptom.

Early reduction in ventricular size is essential if the child is to have the best chance of becoming a useful individual. The treatment of hydrocephalus is influenced by the degree of intracranial pressure, the level of obstruction, and any associated major congenital defects found. Spontaneous arrest occurs in 30% to 40% of children affected but usually does not occur until the hydrocephalus is well advanced. By this time a useful existence may be impossible.

Hydrocephalus is usually treated by insertion of a tube or shunt that drains the ventricular fluid into a body space outside the skull. The well-being of the child depends on the continuous functioning of the shunt. Ventriculoperitoneal and ventriculoatrial shunt systems are the most effective.

Ventriculoperitoneal (VP) shunt. The ventricular catheter is inserted into the lateral ventricle through a small burr hole. The distal catheter is passed beneath the skin down the neck and may

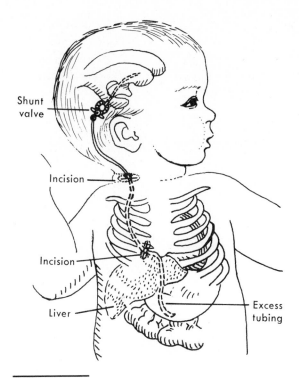

FIG. 14-5

Ventriculoperitoneal shunt with the multipurpose valve designed by the Heyer-Schulte Corp. Provides a sophisticated system for the control of hydrocephalus. Can be used with any of the various Heyer-Schulte ventricular and distal catheters.

tunnel across the front of the chest to enter the abdomen over the liver. Several inches of coiled catheter are left in the peritoneal cavity in an effort to provide the necessary increased length automatically as growth proceeds. The ventriculoperitoneal shunt is commonly inserted in infants because of the ease with which it can be surgically revised, if necessary, to compensate for the growth of the child (Fig. 14-5).

Ventriculoatrial (VA) shunt. The insertion of tubes and valves that allow one-way flow of fluid has led to the successful shunting of cerebrospinal fluid into the right atrium as well as the peritoneal cavity. A burr hole is made in the skull, and a small tube is directed into the lateral ventricle of the brain. Through a small neck incision the cardiac tube is inserted into the right atrium by way of the internal jugular vein (Fig. 14-6). Both VP and VA shunts are connected to the flushing device situated beneath the skin and behind the ear. The flushing device is shaped to fit into the burr hole with its flange overlying the surrounding skull. The entire device is covered with skin. Under normal operating conditions cerebrospinal fluid flow is unobstructed. The flushing devices differ on the various tubes used. In the Pudenz-Mishler double-lumen device, both the ventricular and distal tubes are flushed when the reservoir is compressed. Pumping the functioning shunt permits highly effective flushing in both directions. Obstruction of the ventricular tube, the commonest cause of shunt malfunctions, may be cleared by occluding the easily felt distal catheter with finger pressure and compressing the reservoir. Thus the flushing device serves a dual purpose: It flushes and checks the operation of the entire system. In postoperative care a daily check by manually depressing the skin (pumping) over the reservoir of the flushing device and watching for refill will determine if the shunt is functioning properly.

Postoperative care. When the infant is wide awake, dextrose in water is offered by mouth. If it is tolerated, breast milk or formula may be given. It is important that the nurse observe the baby before the shunting procedure to compare and evaluate his postoperative condition. To avoid respiratory complications, the child must have his position changed at least every 2 hours. His head should be placed carefully to avoid pressure on the cranial wound, which might predispose the skin to break down. The fontanel should be less tense and slightly depressed. If the fontanels are sunken, the child is kept flat. If the fontanels are full or bulging, his head is elevated. Pulse and respiration determinations and pupil equality checks are done frequently. The nurse must be constantly alert for any signs of increased intracranial pressure such as slowed pulse and respirations, lethargy, irritability, vomit-

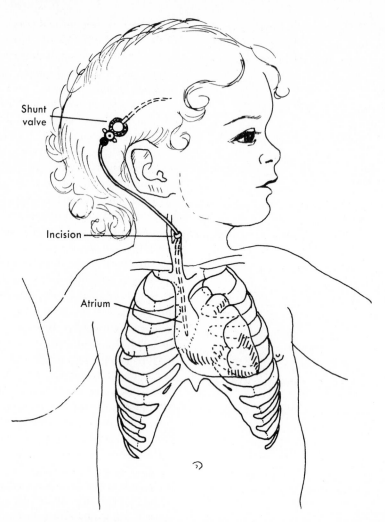

Shunt
valve

Incision

Atrium

FIG. 14-6   Ventriculoatrial shunt drains cerebrospinal fluid from the ventricles of the brain to the right atrium.

ing, and tense fontanels. Head circumference should be measured daily at the widest diameter. Any abnormalities detected by those observations, signs of faulty functioning of the flushing device, or an elevated temperature indicating a postoperative infection should be recorded carefully and immediately called to the attention of the attending physician.

Complications. Infections continue to be the major problem in both types of shunts. Despite all methods of parenteral antibiotic therapy, including injections into the spinal canal, bacteremia, which is a complication especially associated with ventriculoatrial shunts, can be cleared only by the replacement of a new shunt mechanism in a different site. Debilitated infants seem to be susceptible to infection. Other problems include obstruction of the shunt system caused by plugged tubing by debris at the ventricular end, thrombus formation at the cardiac end, and adhesion formation at the peritoneal end. Improved methods of controlling this problem continue to be sought.

Continued care. When surgical intervention cannot be considered, nursing care of the child with advanced hydrocephalus takes considerable gentleness and patience. The head may be extremely large with widely separated cranial bones, broad sutures, and bulging fontanels. Despite the plasticity of the infant skull, injury to the brain usually causes some degree of mental retardation. There may be wide swings in body temperature, tremors or convulsions, lack of appetite, or vomiting. The tension of fontanels and other signs of increasing intracranial pressure should be checked daily.

Attention must be given to preventing pressure sores on the scalp by frequent turning and soft pillow supports. When not being supervised directly, the child should be positioned on his side or abdomen with his head turned to the side to prevent aspiration. Support for the head must always be given during feedings, and the nurse may find it more comfortable for the baby and less tiring for herself to place a pillow on her arm for head support and to rest her elbow on the chair arm. After feeding and bubbling, the infant should be left as quiet as possible to prevent vomiting. Malnutrition and infection are frequent complications for these unfortunate babies.

Cranial stenosis

Other congenital deformities of the skull may be found, but happily they are rare. The sutures of the skull may prematurely close (cranial stenosis), causing abnormal pressure on the brain and possible mental retardation, as well as an asymmetric distorted appearance of the head, if unrelieved. Very rarely a child may be born without a developed brain and lack the usual cranial covering of the brain. This condition is called *anencephaly;* the infant soon dies.

Mental retardation

Mental retardation is an extremely common problem. If affects approximately 3% of the general population. Good prenatal and delivery care helps prevent some of the possible causes (birth injury, anoxia). Some types of mental retardation can be prevented or aided by dietary supervision, hormonal therapy, or genetic counseling.

Intelligence classifications. Because of the many problems that have been identified in trying to determine a person's intellectual capacity by testing devices, the concept of IQ, or intelligence quotient, has lost much of its former significance. The mental age score attained by an individual in testing may be influenced by motivation and environment, as well as the test presentation itself. Nevertheless, IQ scores are still often obtained. They represent a special testing score (mental age) divided by the individual's chronologic age multiplied by 100. Table 14-2 shows certain ranges of IQ, representing various degrees of intelligence.

Down syndrome. A common (1 in 650 live births) type of mental retardation associated with certain physical characteristics that has undergone considerable investigation is that of Down syndrome, or mongolism. The most common of the three types known, called "standard trisomy 21," is associated with an abnormal chromosome count in all the baby's body cells. (See p. 307.) These children range from profoundly to mildly retarded.

Infants with Down syndrome are usually identified in the nursery, but some are diagnosed later. Characteristically, these infants are short; they have relatively small skulls, flattened from front to back; their birth weights are usually low; and their behavior is lethargic. The most reliable signs of mongolism are exaggerated epicanthic folds, which make the eyes slant up and out; short hands and fingers with the little finger bent in (clinodactyly); a deep, horizontal crease across the palm (simian crease); and a large space between the great and small toes. Physicians will examine the eyes in an effort to detect small white dots on the iris, which,

TABLE 14-2   INTELLIGENCE CLASSIFICATIONS*

Classification	Intelligence quotient (IQ)	Performance level
Profound retardation	0 to 24	Unable to attend to personal needs; always requires supervision; 0- to 2-year-old intellectual ability
Severe retardation	25 to 50	May be trained to meet personal needs but not self-sustaining; 3- to 7-year-old intellectual ability (trainable mentally retarded)
Moderately severe retardation	50 to 79	Self-sustaining in simple jobs with supervision; 8- to 11-year-old intellectual ability (educable mentally retarded)
Dull normal	79 to 89	
Average	90 to 110	What most of us are
Above average	110 to 130	What most of us would like to be
Gifted	130 to 150	These people may have problems in adjustment, emphasizing that social competence and intellectual ability each contribute to individual success in society
Genius	150 and above	

*One of many classifications of intelligence used.

when present, are helpful in making a diagnosis. Decreased muscle tone and excessive joint mobility are also significant findings (Figs. 14-7 and 14-8).

After the newborn period, other signs manifest themselves, such as delayed eruption of teeth, fissured tongue, and retarded intellectual and physical development. These youngsters often have congenital heart malformations, umbilical hernias, and duodenal atresia. If they survive long enough, they usually possess rather affectionate, placid personalities. Frequently, depending on home circumstances and the individual needs of the child, he can remain with the family, and care outside the home community is not necessary. No one knows for sure the true cause of this condition, but standard trisomy 21 is found most often in cases in which the mother is near the end of her reproductive life. The translocation type of Down syndrome may be hereditary.

Phenylketonuria. Another type of mental retardation that is much less common and has been publicized a great deal is that produced by an inherited error in metabolism of a certain essential amino

acid, or protein, called *phenylalanine*. The disease is called PKU, a short way of saying phenylketonuria. It results when an enzyme normally produced by the liver is missing or inadequate. Unless appropriate measures are taken, poisons build up in the bloodstream that, after a few months, begin to produce noticeable damage to the brain. A high level of the potentially poisonous substance can be detected in the blood serum of the newborn infant, but a few weeks are usually needed before the offending chemical is found in the urine. Blood tests to detect the disease may be done on the third or fourth day of life. Early discharge practices necessitate conscientious follow-up. Treatment consists of eliminating as much of the offending protein as possible from the diet for an indeterminate time. Since phenylalanine is found in many protein foods, the diet is extremely curtailed, and synthetic protein foods are necessary. Results of early treatment have been gratifying.

Galactosemia. Galactosemia, which is another rare metabolic error that may produce mental retardation, involves the metabolism of the sugar galactose.

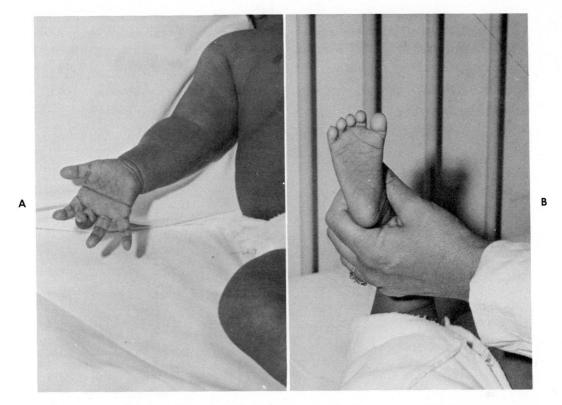

Cretinism. Cretinism, or infantile hypothyroidism, may also be a cause of mental retardation. The thyroid hormone is absent from the time of birth. Prenatally the infant is supplied with thyroid by the mother. The signs of hypothyroidism develop gradually.

The typically affected baby has a large tongue that, because of its size, may protrude from the mouth, causing problems in feeding. The child's cry is hoarse; its hair is course, and the skin is dry (no perspiration is observed); constipation is a continuous problem; and growth is retarded if the condition is untreated.

If cretinism is diagnosed early and hormone replacement therapy is undertaken, the child usually progresses fairly normally, although slight intellectual retardation may persist. Routine newborn screening often includes T_4 and TSH blood analyses to diagnose and treat hypothyroidism, thereby reducing the incidence of mental retardation and thyroid problems (p. 477).

About 15% of retardation results from brain injury associated with birth or from infection in utero. Another 5% is caused by chromosomal abnormality such as Down syndrome, or specific single gene defects like PKU. The remainder, or about 80%, results from unfavorable polygenetic combinations from the general gene pool. This group accounts for

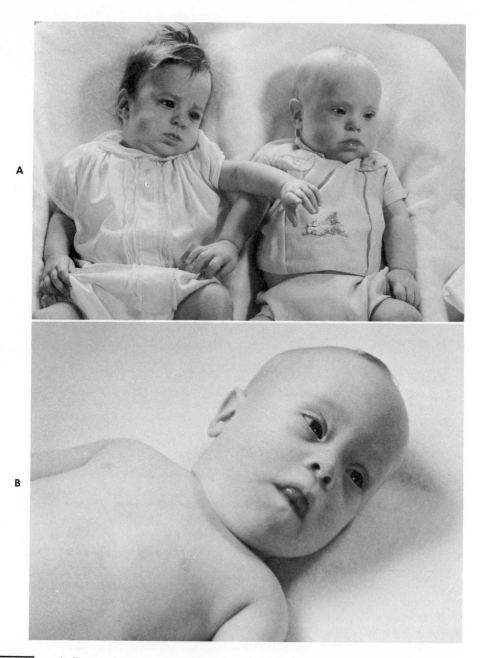

FIG. 14-8   **A,** These children are brother and sister (fraternal twins). The little boy manifests Down syndrome; his sister is unaffected. **B,** Close-up of the male twin. Note the large tongue and typical eyes.

most of the milder forms of retardation, while the more severe forms are usually caused by brain injury, chromosomal abnormalities, or single gene factors producing metabolic disorders.

Spina bifida

Spina bifida, a condition briefly noted in the discussion of hydrocephalus, may exist in several degrees of severity. The term "spina bifida" simply means "divided spine," or that a portion of the posterior wall of the spine is missing.

Types. The defect may be so small that it offers no difficulty and is discovered only when an x-ray examination of the spine is done for other reasons. This type of defect is called "spina bifida occulta," or "hidden divided spine." Another type is termed "spina bifida cystica," because it exhibits a cystlike structure. There are two kinds of spina bifida cystica. A *meningocele* involves a protrusion of only the covering meninges of the spinal cord and cerebrospinal fluid. The child usually develops normal

urinary and intestinal control and has no paralysis, but the sac, until removed, is a cosmetic problem, and its possible injury always poses the problem of infection of the nervous system. The second and more serious kind of spina bifida cystica is called *myelomeningocele* or *meningomyelocele*. In this condition the meninges protrude through the spinal opening, and nerve tissues are also found in the herniated sac. Children with this problem are often troubled with persistent urinary and fecal incontinence, partial or complete lower extremity paralysis, and sensory disturbance. Hydrocephalus frequently accompanies this defect (Figs. 14-9 to 14-11).

Nursing care. The nursing care of the child with either meningocele or myelomeningocele is challenging. Before surgery the sac, or mass, as it is sometimes called, must be protected from injury and infection. The child must be adequately nourished and should be assured of loving care. To protect the sac, the child is usually positioned on his abdomen or carefully propped on his side. Because of the usual position of the sac, no diapers are

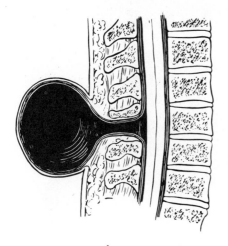
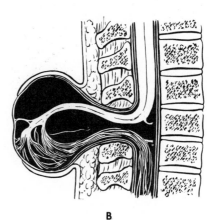

A   B

FIG. 14-9 **A,** Section of the spinal cord and vertebral column showing a meningocele. Note that no nervous tissue protrudes through the defect into the sac. **B,** Section of the spinal cord and vertebral column showing a myelomeningocele. Nervous tissue is found in the herniated meningeal sac.

From Benz, G.S.: Pediatric nursing, ed. 5, St. Louis, 1964, The C.V. Mosby Co.

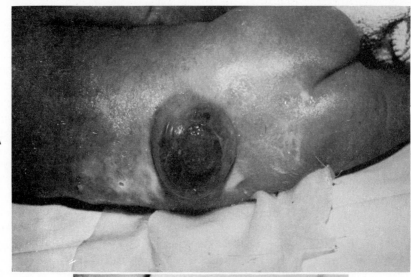

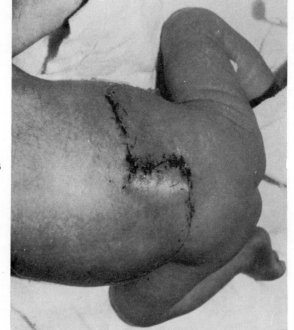

FIG. 14-10   **A,** Myelomeningocele before surgery. (An antibacterial dressing was used.) **B,** Repair of the same patient.

Courtesy M.C. Gleason, M.D., San Diego, Calif.

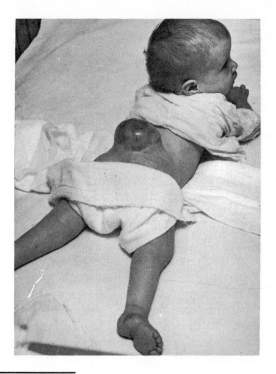

FIG. 14-11

This youngster's myelomeningocele was repaired shortly after this photograph was taken.

Courtesy Children's Hospital and Health Center, San Diego, Calif.

pinned in place. To avoid putting strain or pressure on the sac, the nurse must be extremely careful in lifting the infant. Slipping her hands and forearms palms up under the leg and chest area to grasp the farther thigh, arm, and shoulder seems to be a safe, effective way of lifting and moving the smaller infants. Caution must be taken when putting these children in a sitting position, even if no direct pressure is exerted on the sac. Sometimes the sac is so low on the spine that the sitting position puts too much tension on the area. A positioning device called a Bradford frame may be used, consisting of a metal framework that rests on the bed and ele-

vates the baby on a divided, padded canvas support. The perineal area and sac are placed directly over splits in the canvas, and a bedpan is positioned directly underneath. Plastic strips hanging from the opening of the frame help direct urine and feces into the pan. This device helps protect the area from soil and pressure.

When being fed, the infant may be propped on his side with his head elevated; held by one nurse with his head over her shoulder while fed by another nurse holding the bottle or, the child's condition permitting, held in a sitting position with no pressure on the sac.

Meticulous skin care must be observed and pressure areas prevented. Occasionally, to avoid infection, the sac may be covered by sterile petrolatum or medicated strips and gauze compresses. A foam rubber ring with a hole large enough to admit the sac may be placed over the sterile compresses and wrapped in place with an elastic bandage. Treatment depends on the size, location, and condition of the sac, but surgical closure is usually planned early to avoid the problem of infection. The sac should be observed for variance in size and tenseness as well as ulceration. Any leaking of fluid should be reported immediately. The head of a child with any type of meningocele usually is regularly measured to try to detect developing hydrocephalus. The sensation and movement of the lower extremities are evaluated as care is given.

After surgery (usually a flap-type procedure is done), the prone position is maintained, at least until the sutures are removed. There may be no dressing over the incision, and a dry incision and body warmth may be maintained by a carefully positioned gooseneck lamp or the use of an incubator. Although surgery rarely improves function, it certainly improves the child's appearance and facilitates care. The care of a patient with spina bifida, complicated by a herniation of nerve tissue elements, continues for life. Many orthopedic procedures may have to be completed before the child achieves even the ability to walk with braces. Many spina bifida babies have clubfeet, and some have flexion contractures of the hips. Urinary complications are the rule rather than the exception. To avoid the problems created by continued long-term use of indwelling catheters, a urinary diversion may be made from an excised part of the ileum into which the ureters have been placed. It drains continually through an opening on the abdominal wall. However, intermittent self-catheterization is preferred over the surgical creation of a urinary diversion (see p. 416). The prevention or treatment of decubiti is a real concern. The child needs constant psychologic and emotional support, as well as physical assistance, to become a healthy personality capable of giving to as well as receiving from his environment. To meet the many specialized needs of these patients, many communities have multidisciplinary clinics available.

Cleft lip and cleft palate

Cleft lip and cleft palate are common congenital malformations, appearing approximately once in every 750 births. They constitute a failure in the embryonic development of the child, and a hereditary factor is often found to be significant. Cleft lip is found more often in males, whereas females more often have cleft palates. Cleft lip, sometimes called harelip, may vary from a single notching of the border of the lip to a deep split extending through the lip to or into the nose. It may exist on only one side of center or be found on both sides. It does not create a problem in feeding. The major problem involves the infant's appearance. For this reason a cleft lip is usually repaired as soon as the child's condition is sufficiently stable, at approximately 2 months of age or before. A second repair may be necessary when the child is 4 or 5 years of age to correct scar irregularities and nasal asymmetry. A cleft palate may involve lack of fusion of only part of the hard or soft palate or may extend along the entire roof of the mouth. Cleft palate is repaired at about 18 months of age or according to the child's individual needs.

Before taking their baby home to await surgery for cleft palate, the parents must receive detailed instructions regarding the infant's care and have several opportunities to feed the infant with supervision. The baby with a cleft palate usually has difficulty sucking normally, since he cannot create the necessary vacuum in his mouth. The baby may be fed slowly with a rubber-tipped medicine dropper, or syringe, no faster than the baby's capacity to swallow. Rarely, a specially molded cleft-palate nipple with an extra built-in hump that fits the cleft in the palate and makes sucking possible is employed. Occasionally soft, long lamb's nipples are tried, or the child may be fed from the end of a small spoon. Sometimes the defect is so placed or is so small that a regularly shaped soft nipple may be used. The baby is fed in an upright position to help prevent aspiration and regurgitation through the nose. The method of feeding that is most successful and closest to that used by a normal baby is the method of choice. Since these babies swallow more air than usual, they should be bubbled frequently. This will lessen the possibility of emesis or unattended "wet burps" and subsequent aspiration. Some children with cleft palate are fitted early with a prosthesis to help guard against nasal regurgitation, aid in the formation of speech patterns, and maintain anatomic relationships important to the final repair.

The success of plastic surgery depends on the extent of the defect, the developmental stage of the individual, the repair techniques available, the skill of the surgeon, the standard of nursing care, and the cooperation of the parents. A cleft palate is much more difficult to repair, and the child may have to undergo several procedures at different ages (Fig. 14-12).

Postoperative care of the child with cleft lip. After surgery for a cleft lip the infant should have his arms restrained to prevent damage to the suture line. Elbow restraints may be used. The nurse can adequately restrain the arms of very young infants by pulling their long shirt sleeves past their hands and pinning the sleeves to their diaper. Periodically these restraints should be removed one at a time to provide needed exercise and inspection of the arms.

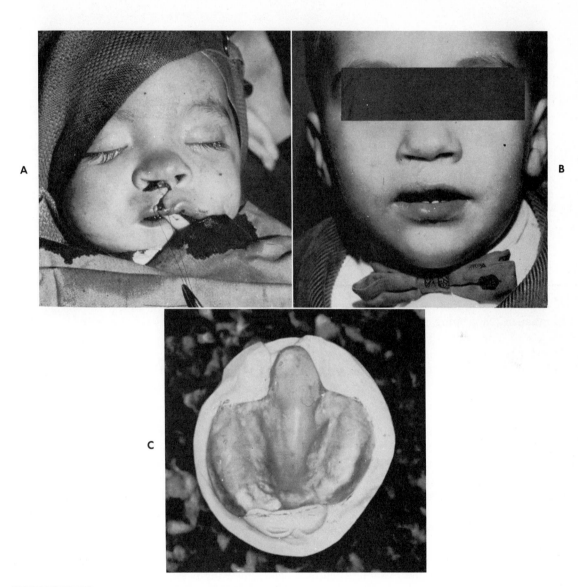

FIG. 14-12 **A,** Closure of a unilateral complete cleft lip. **B,** Same child 13 months later. **C,** Palate prosthesis resting in a plaster-of-Paris mold. The prosthesis is used until a child is old enough for optimal palate repair.

Courtesy M.C. Gleason, M.D., San Diego, Calif.

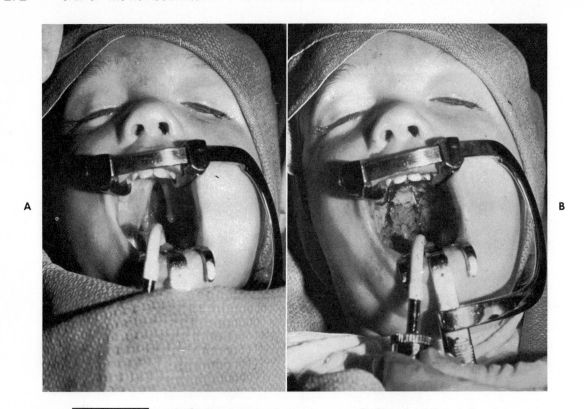

FIG. 14-13   **A,** Cleft palate just before surgery. **B,** Closure of the cleft palate.

Courtesy M.C. Gleason, M.D., San Diego, Calif.

The suture line should be kept clean, and no crust should be allowed to form because crusting enlarges the scar. Various solutions are used for cleaning, depending on the physician's preference. Tightly wrapped, sterile cotton applicators saturated with hydrogen peroxide, warm sterile water, or physiologic saline solution may be used to remove the blood or crust. Such maneuvers must be done gently but persistently. Soaking the area for a brief period with a saturated applicator or sponge before any motion over the area is attempted aids considerably. Afterward the lip should be gently dried. Sometimes an antibiotic ointment may be left on the suture line.

Every effort should be made to keep the child happy because a happy child cries less and puts less strain on the repair. The parents should be encour-

aged to cuddle the infant and, as soon as feasible, participate in feedings under supervision. The child may be fed by a small medicine cup or a rubber-tipped medicine dropper and graduated to a soft nipple when sucking is allowed.

Postoperative care of the child with cleft palate (*Fig. 14-13*). A cleft palate is a much more serious defect than a cleft lip, considering the impairment of function it produces. Not only is feeding difficult, involving possible problems of aspiration and dental placement, but speech is often nasalized, and infections of the respiratory tract and middle ear are common. The child who has undergone palate surgery is usually fed from a cup or side of a spoon. Nothing is introduced into the mouth that may endanger the suture line, and unless the child is old enough to understand and cooperate, arm restraints must be used. The diet progresses from clear liquid to full liquid to soft food over a period of approximately 2 weeks. The mouth should be rinsed with water at the end of a meal.

The problems of the child with cleft lip, cleft palate, or both are occasionally so complex that the combined therapy of a plastic surgeon, pediatrician, orthodontist, speech therapist, child psychiatrist, and medical social worker may be needed. For this reason, clinics for those with cleft lip and palate are found in most large cities.

Other digestive tract abnormalities

Other abnormalities of the digestive tract are found with enough frequency to merit mention, especially since they are so serious in nature.

ESOPHAGEAL ATRESIA AND
TRACHEOESOPHAGEAL FISTULA (FIG. 14-14)

Esophageal atresia refers to the congenital absence or closure of the esophagus at some point. The upper portion usually ends in a blind pouch. Tracheoesophageal fistula represents an open connection between the trachea and the esophagus. A frequent association exists between esophageal atresia and tracheoesophageal fistula as a result of the nature of embryonic development.

Several varieties of these malformations are known, but the following three major types are (1) tacheoesophageal fistula with esophageal atresia (80% to 95% of cases), in which the upper esophagus ends in a blind pouch and the lower esophageal segment connects with the trachea; (2) esophageal atresia alone; and (3) tracheoesophageal fistula alone. These anomalies are relatively common. About 25% of the infants with digestive tract abnormalities are premature. Another 25% usually have associated defects (primarily other gastrointestinal malformations, such as imperforate anus). Maternal polyhydramnios is frequently noted in these infants as a result of the inability of the fetus to dispose of swallowed amniotic fluid. The malformations are slightly more common in male infants.

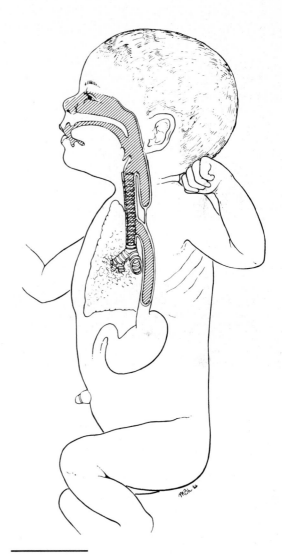

FIG. 14-14

The most common type of esophageal atresia involves an upper esophageal segment ending in a blind pouch and a lower tracheoesophageal fistula. There is great danger of aspiration.

Symptoms. The infant usually cries at birth, breathes well, and becomes a normal, healthy color. Soon, however, saliva accumulates in the pharynx and mouth, and the infant is noted to be frothing or drooling. The mucus is thick and seems excessive, but it is actually a normal amount of mucus that simply cannot pass through to the stomach and therefore pools in the esophageal pouch. Respirations become noisy, gurgling, and rapid. The cry is hoarse. Respiratory difficulty increases, and cyanosis occurs. If the infant is fed, he will repeatedly cough, gag, and regurgitate. Feeding is usually followed by aspiration of breast milk or formula into the lungs, which leads to pneumonia and often to atelectasis. All of the pulmonary symptoms are caused by the drainage of secretions into the lungs from the stomach or mouth by way of an esophageal fistula or overflow from an esophageal pouch.

Diagnosis. Diagnosis can be easily made in the delivery room or nursery by the inability to pass a catheter into the stomach. X-ray films positively confirm the diagnosis.

Treatment. Surgical repair is the only method of treatment and should be instituted within 12 to 24 hours after birth. The chest is opened, and the tracheoesophageal fistula is tied off (ligated). Connection of the esophageal segments is also performed, if possible; otherwise, this is accomplished at 1 to 2 years of age. A gastrostomy is performed, and a chest tube is inserted.

Nursing care. Preoperative care is directed toward rapid stabilization of the infant. The baby is kept in a head-up position and given oxygen with humidification to thin the secretions; constant gentle suction is applied to the esophageal pouch by means of a specialized (sump) tube. The baby is handled minimally and receives nothing orally. Fluids are administered intravenously by way of a peripheral vein or by umbilical catheter. Postoperative care is much the same but includes proper care of the surgical incision, chest tube, gastrostomy, and frequent turning. Initially the gastrostomy is allowed to drain freely into a collection bag. When feedings are begun through the gastrostomy

in 2 to 3 days, the tube is elevated and left open. An esophageal sump tube is not used postoperatively—suctioning is performed very gently only as needed.

Prognosis depends largely on the initial condition of the infant at the time of diagnosis, degree of prematurity, presence of other malformations, and whether or not feedings had been given. Once the surgical repair is complete and recovery has taken place, these infants generally develop normally. They do, however, have a higher incidence of pulmonary infections during their first year and usually a harsh cough for some time. Continued medical supervision is essential.

IMPERFORATE ANUS

Occasionally the infant's rectum ends as a closed or blind pouch or connects to an adjacent canal (urethra, vagina) by means of a fistula (Fig. 14-15). The possibility of this defect is one reason that observation of the stools of the newborn is so important. Often a temporary colostomy, an abdominal exit for the contents of the colon, must be made. Later the creation of a normally placed functional rectal opening will be attempted surgically.

ABDOMINAL HERNIAS

An absence of the normal abdominal wall in the region of the umbilicus that allows a portion of the intestinal contents to be clearly observed, virtually unprotected, and subject to herniation and strangulation is called an *omphalocele* (Fig. 14-16). The defect may be small or exaggerated. Its repair is usually considered a surgical emergency. Another type of hernia, involving the abdominal contents and causing respiratory distress as well as digestive problems, is the *diaphragmatic hernia*. In this condition an abnormally large opening is present in the diaphragm that allows part of the contents of the abdominal cavity to displace upward into the chest. Sometimes the entire stomach, as well as portions of the intestine, is found in the thorax, crowding the heart and lungs. This situation, too, is a surgical emergency.

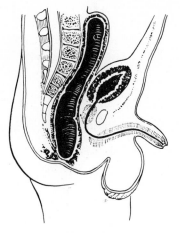 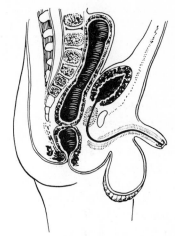

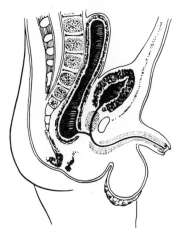 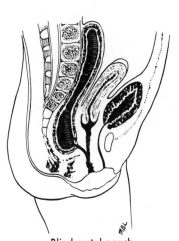

FIG. 14-15

Types of imperforate anus in the newborn infant.

Thin membrane over anus
Both sexes

Blind rectal pouch with
normal anus
Both sexes

Blind rectal pouch
Rectourethral fistula
In males

Blind rectal pouch
Rectovaginal fistula
In females

Hypospadias

A fairly common malformation of the urinary system that is found in male infants is hypospadias (Fig. 14-17). The urethra, instead of traveling the entire length of the penis, opens out on the underside of the penis, either at its base or at varying distances from the tip. Sometimes the presence of

hypospadias, coupled with other irregularities of the external genital organs, leads to confusion in determining the sex of the infant, and cell studies and exploratory operative procedures may be necessary. The repair of well-defined hypospadias by the extension of the urethral canal is usually accomplished by a series of operative procedures before the child is of school age. Minor positional devia-

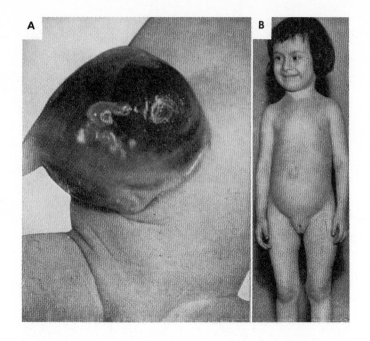

FIG. 14-16

A, Omphalocele before repair.
B, After corrective surgery.

From Potter E.L.: Pathology of the fetus and
the newborn, Chicago, 1952, Year Book
Medical Publishers, Inc.

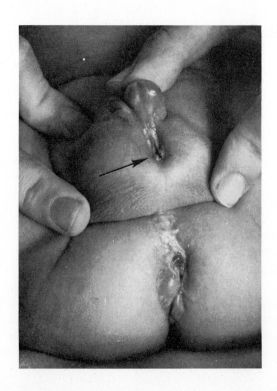

FIG. 14-17

This infant suffers from multiple congenital
anomalies. The arrow indicates the opening of the
urethra at the base of the penis (hypospadias). An
imperforate anus was previously repaired.

tions of the urethral meatus may not require treatment.

Congenital heart deformities

Congenital cardiac conditions frequently stem from the persistence of some part of the fetal circulation pattern, so it would be of benefit to review the basic circulation that is present before birth (Fig. 4-4). The foramen ovale may fail to close, resulting in an _atrial septal_ defect. The _ductus arteriosus_ may persist. However, real structural deviations may also exist in many different combinations (See pp. 686 to 691 for more detail.) Open-heart surgery, with the use of the heart-lung machine, now gives more hope of survival and the possibility of a more normal life for victims of congenital heart defects.

Hemolytic disease of the newborn infant

A number of conditions can cause blood destruction in the fetus or newborn infant. Probably the most well-known cause is Rh factor incompatibility, which may initiate the condition _erythroblastosis fetalis_. The Rh factor was first identified in the blood of Rhesus monkeys. Actually the Rh "factor" has been found to be a group of related protein antigens that under certain conditions may be capable of causing the formation of potentially dangerous antibodies. The two antigens that seem to cause difficulty clinically are D and its genetic variant D^u. Approximately 85% of the white population and higher percentages of the nonwhite population have these substances in their blood (Fig. 14-18).

Rh INCOMPATIBILITY

If a woman who lacks the Rh protein in her blood marries a man who also lacks it, no problem will exist because of the Rh factor for their offspring. However, if her husband is Rh positive and their child inherits Rh-positive blood from his father, trouble may occur.

Probable mechanism. Some of the baby's blood cells carrying the Rh protein may pass through a microscopic tear in the placental barrier and reach the mother's bloodstream. The mother's body automatically manufacturers antibodies (protective substances) designed to destroy the foreign protein in her body. These antibodies may then find themselves in the fetal circulation. There, they do just what they were designed to do: They destroy the Rh protein, or factor, and, in so doing, also destroy the red blood cell to which it is attached. The fetus suffers from the effects of anemia. Making a valiant effort to supply more red cells, it forces out into its bloodstream immature, inadequate forms of red blood cells called erythroblasts. This is the reason that the resulting disease is termed _erythroblastosis fetalis_. In severe cases congestive heart failure associated with enlargement of the spleen and liver occurs. If the pregnancy is not successfully terminated before advanced damage results, the unborn child will die.

Shortly after birth, toxicity caused by the large amount of red blood cell breakdown products (chiefly bilirubin) circulating in the baby's body may lead to brain damage known as _kernicterus_. This condition causes neurologic impairment, such as spasticity, deafness, or mental retardation, or may even lead to death.

One of the first clinical manifestations of Rh factor sensitivity in the infant is the appearance of jaundice within 24 to 36 hours. The baby with a more severe case may be lethargic, suck poorly, and manifest spasticity.

However, not all mothers with Rh-negative blood have such sick babies. Sometimes the baby is also Rh negative and no such problem arises. Sometimes the number of antibodies the mother has produced in response to the baby's cells in her bloodstream is so small that no damage to the baby is detected. Usually trouble is not encountered until the second or third infant. After several pregnancies the titer of antibodies in the blood usually increases greatly. This titer may be measured during pregnancy; also, the progress of the disease may be estimated by analyzing amniotic fluid aspirated from the sac surrounding the baby. These

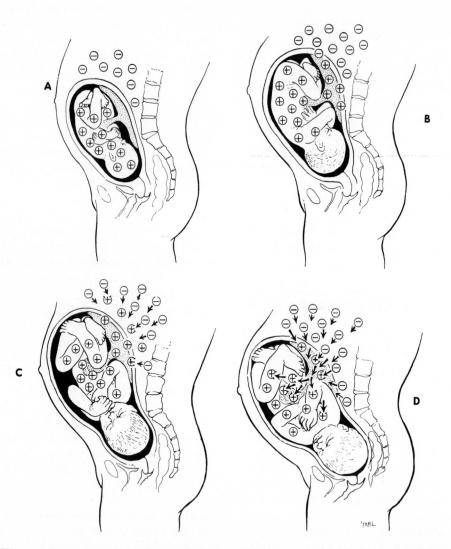

FIG. 14-18   Mechanism of erythroblastosis fetalis, which is caused by Rh incompatibility. **A,** Rh-positive child is carried by Rh-negative mother. **B,** Rh protein crosses the placental barrier and invades the mother's bloodstream. **C,** Mother's system manufactures antibodies to destroy the foreign Rh protein. **D,** Antibodies cross back over the placenta and destroy the baby's blood cells, which are intimately associated with Rh protein.

tests allow the physician to evaluate the health of the fetus and plan for the baby's birth and care.

Often the question is asked, "Why doesn't an Rh-positive mother become ill when her unborn child is Rh negative?" The answer seems to be in the relative inability of the fetus to produce enough antibodies to attack the mother's blood cells in sufficient number.

Treatment. When the presence of erythroblastosis fetalis is determined in a newborn infant, exchange transfusion is carried out. The umbilical vein is used to achieve access to the baby's bloodstream by means of a polyethylene catheter. A carefully measured amount of blood is slowly withdrawn and discarded by a syringe equipped with a complex of stopcocks. Then crossmatched, Rh-negative donor blood with a low Rh antibody titer, warmed to room temperature, is pushed slowly by syringe back into the baby's body as a replacement. This process is repeated many times until complete replacement is estimated to have occurred. During the procedure, close observation of the baby's vital signs and the blood volume exchange is essential. The baby must be kept warm, and oxygen may be administered. This treatment must occasionally be repeated, but the results are usually highly successful, and the child born in good condition and receiving prompt transfusion when needed has an excellent prognosis.

Intrauterine transfusion of those unborn infants, who show signs of not being able to survive until viable is now available at a few research centers. It is not without risk but may be considered when no other hope for the fetus exists.

The exposure of infants with elevated blood bilirubin levels to blue or fluorescent light to reduce the amount of circulating bilirubin is now frequently used. The naked infant is positioned under the lamps with protective eye shields in place, is turned periodically to increase body surface exposure, and is given increased fluids.

Prevention. For the Rh-negative patient who has never been sensitized (that is, formed detectable levels of Rh antibodies) because of a previous contact with the Rh protein, protection is now available that, when properly used, is essentially 100% effective in preventing the detrimental effects of Rh incompatibility. It has been found that passive immunization or ready-made antibody protection, given within 72 hours after birth of an Rh-positive infant or abortus, will destroy the invading Rh protein and inhibit the natural formation of antibodies by the individual. This special passive immunization, Rh immune globulin, first marketed as RhoGam, unfortunately does not aid Rh-negative women who have already actively developed their own immunization against the Rh factor.

It must be administered to the woman at risk *after each exposure* to Rh-positive blood. In certain instances fetal-to-maternal hemorrhages take place that are too large for the normal dose of 300 μg of Rh-immune globulin to provide adequate protection. The number of fetal cells in the maternal circulation can be estimated by the use of the Kleihauer-Betke test or the more recent commercially available Fetaldex technique and the dosage increased as necessary. Some physicians, in an effort to protect a small but important group of Rh-negative women who have unknown antepartal bleeds that may cause early sensitization, administer the immune globulin to all Rh-negative women at 28 weeks' gestation as well as after birth.

A mechanism similar to the Rh problem, but usually of a less serious nature, can operate when the mother has type O blood and the baby has type A, B, or AB. Such a situation is called "ABO incompatibility."

Orthopedic abnormalities

Orthopedic abnormalities are common in the newborn nursery. As a general rule, the earlier they are treated the better the prognosis.

CONGENITAL DISLOCATION OF THE HIP (CDH)

There are two main types of congenital dislocations of the hip: (1) *teratologic*, which develops during life in utero and is commonly associated with other orthopedic problems; and (2) *typical*, which occurs just before, during, or shortly after birth, probably caused by the softening effects of the maternal hormone relaxin on the baby's ligaments and the stress of labor and birth. The hip joints of every newborn should be examined within 24 hours of birth for congenital dislocation. They can usually be successfully treated by simple manipulation. There are 1.5 cases of CDH per 1,000 live births. It affects girls eight times more frequently than boys. Dislocation, or luxation, is present when the femoral head is completely displaced from the socket, or acetabulum. Subluxation, or partial displacement, is more common, occurring in approximately 1 in 60 births. A subluxated hip may become completely dislocated during a baby's care unless certain types of maneuvers are avoided. These infants should never be lifted by their feet for diapering. Their legs should never be pulled, nor should their hips be completely extended when wrapped in a blanket. Since one does not always know which child may have incipient hip problems, these cautions should apply to the care of all babies. Barring complications, the subluxated hip of 88% of the affected newborns become normal by 2 months of age.

Physical findings that the licensed practical or vocational nurse can detect include asymmetry of the thigh folds, limited abduction of the affected hip, and shortening of the femur when the knees and hips are flexed at right angles and when abduction is attempted with the child lying supine on a firm table. The diagnosis is usually confirmed by x-ray examination. Since the socket becomes progressively more distorted if reduction is delayed, the goal of treatment is the immediate return of the femoral head to the acetabulum. A normal hip joint can be obtained when treatment is begun in the first few weeks of life. Reduction of the hip is not difficult and involves maintenance of the hip in a stable position of flexion and abduction. The Frejka pillow-splint allows some hip motion in a relatively normal position while at the same time maintaining flexion and abduction. Semirigid abduction devices are more practical and preferred by some orthopedists. The child's orthopedic condition is frequent-

ly evaluated on an outpatient basis. Early treatment may reduce therapy to about 3 months' duration. If the child's x-ray film indicates normal location of the hip at 2 years of age, the condition may be considered cured. Treatment after 6 months of age varies. It may involve traction for a few weeks followed by casting or operative reduction. However, when CDH is diagnosed at 2 years of age, the outcome is seldom optimal. In children over 8 years, even the most extensive operative procedures cannot produce a functionally satisfactory hip. About one third of the degenerative hip joint disease found in adults is caused by the residual effects of CDH. In adults such conditions may be helped by a total hip arthroplasty. For information regarding the nursing care of the child with congenital dislocation of the hips see Chapter 27, Progressive abduction traction (Figs. 27-1).

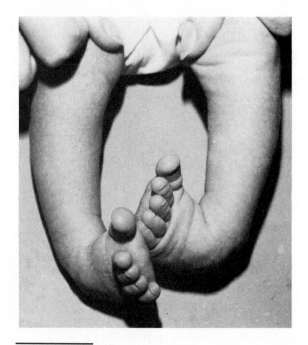

FIG. 14-19

Talipes equinovarus.

Courtesy William C. McDade, M.D., San Diego, Calif.

CLUBFOOT (TALIPES)

Clubfoot is the most common congenital anomaly of the lower extremity. In the most common form of this condition (talipes equinovarus), the anterior one half of the foot is adducted and inverted. The medial border of the foot is concave, the lateral border is convex, and the heel is drawn up (Fig. 14-19). Its cause is unknown, but it has been postulated that clubfoot results from arrested or abnormal development of a particular part of the germ plasm during embryonic life. One or both feet may be involved. It is twice as common in males as in females.

The feet of the newborn infant must be carefully evaluated. Not all apparent deformities are true clubfoot. Some distortions are simply caused by intrauterine positions and not real structural differences. These feet can be corrected to neutral position in all elements of the deformity by manipulation during examination. A true clubfoot cannot.

The treatment of clubfoot should be started as soon as the baby's condition is stable. Treatment

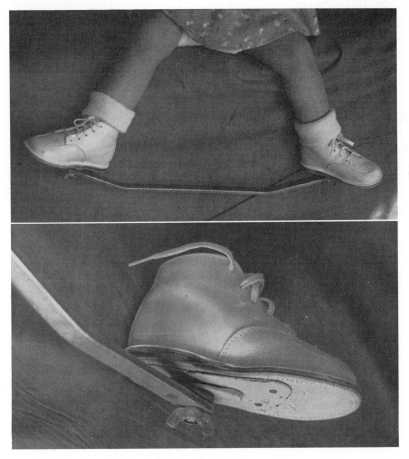

FIG. 14-20 Modified Denis Browne splint is often used to help maintain corrected positions of the feet.

From Larson, C.B., and Gould, M.: Orthopedic nursing, ed. 9, St. Louis, 1978, The C.V. Mosby Co.

may be divided into three stages: (1) correction, (2) maintenance of correction, and (3) long-term follow-up. Correction usually consists of stretching and strapping or casting. Strapping or casting is changed as often as every 3 to 7 days over a period of about 10 weeks. Maintenance of correction may be accomplished by wearing a Denis Browne splint as directed day and night for several months (Fig. 14-20). Follow-up must continue for several years after completion of active treatment to guard against recurrence of the deformity and a less than satisfactory outcome.

SYNDACTYLY AND POLYDACTYLISM

Syndactyly, or webbing of the fingers or toes, is a very interesting anomaly, usually responding well to surgical separation. Syndactyly may accompany another digital abnormality called *polydactylism*, or the presence of extra fingers or toes. At times,

these extra digits have no bony connection with the hand or foot and, when a ligature is tied around the fleshy stalk, cutting off circulation, the digit soon drops off. When a bony connection exists, surgery is necessary.

Effect of contagious diseases

The effect of contagious diseases on the fetus and newborn infant is discussed in Chapters 9 and 15. Those considered are syphilis, gonorrhea, tuberculosis, rubella (German measles), toxoplasmosis, cytomegaly, and herpes simplex virus infections.

• • •

Many abnormalities are possible in the newborn infant, but considering the intricacies of life, the miracle is that more of them do not occur.

CHAPTER 15

Intensive care

of the newborn

THE SPECIAL CARE NURSERY

Neonatology, the study and treatment of the sick newborn, has rapidly become a highly specialized area of pediatrics. Continuing advances in detection, prevention, and treatment of disorders of the newborn have led to the development of specialized neonatal units with highly trained personnel. Basic nursing courses do not attempt to equip the vocational nurse to work in these units. However, with further training and education, selected licensed vocational and practical nurses may be part of these specialized units. Students may have a period of observation and closely guided participation during their obstetric or pediatric experiences. This chapter is designed to help these students better understand the types of patients, conditions, and procedures they may encounter, and to help nurses better comprehend the histories of small patients who are transferred from special care areas to other sections of the hospital.

Objectives and characteristics

The main objective of the neonatal intensive care unit, or special care nursery (SCN), is to provide the earliest and maximum degree of medical and nursing care for the infant at risk so that each infant attains the best possible outcome. As neonatal mortality is reduced, continuing efforts must also be made to decrease the incidence of long-term problems such as chronic lung disease, intestinal disorders, and neurologic sequelae, such as mental deficiency, blindness, and deafness. Awareness of the causes and prevention of residual damage is therefore necessary for the SCN nurse.

Prematurity and its various complications are the most frequently encountered problems in the SCN. Other patients have birth defects, infection, jaundice, hypoglycemia, perinatal asphyxia, or one of many less common disorders. Furthermore, since most hospital recovery rooms are poorly equipped and staffed to care for small infants, the SCN must provide postoperative care for neonates recovering from general anesthesia and various surgical procedures.

SCN patients require many types of specialized care to meet their various needs. Mechanical ventilation, intravenous fluid therapy, continuous monitoring of vital signs, body temperature regulation, and even such mundane tasks as feedings require specially trained SCN physicians and nursing personnel and sophisticated biomedical equipment. The SCN nurse must become comfortable in handling tiny, fragile infants, and she must be proficient with the many mechanical aids used in their care.

The regional perinatal center

Because intensive care facilities are very expensive and are seldom necessary in smaller general hospitals, the concept of the regional perinatal center has evolved. In addition to the SCN, such a center provides an obstetrical-perinatal service for both outpatient and inpatient care of high-risk mothers and their unborn babies. The center usually serves a defined geographic region, accepting referrals of patients with complicated conditions from other hospitals. It often operates a newborn transport system to bring critically ill neonates born elsewhere to the SCN.

Other responsibilities of the comprehensive perinatal center include the supervision of continuing education for health professionals of the region, long-term follow-up of infants treated in the SCN, and ongoing research in perinatal-neonatal medicine. Many perinatal centers are associated with schools of medicine, nursing, and other health professions.

Neonatal transport

When neonatal problems are anticipated, the mother should be transferred to the perinatal center for delivery if possible. Such an "in utero transport" is not only safer for the infant but also avoids the undesirable separation of mother and baby. However, since many infants with serious problems are born at hospitals without neonatal intensive care facilities, the regional center must be able to provide safe, immediate transfer to the SCN when necessary. The neonatal transport team usually consists of a pediatrician or a neonatal nurse clinician or practitioner, a respiratory therapist, and one or more SCN staff nurses. Reliable ambulance and, in some areas, helicopter or airplane service are necessary. Special equipment is needed, including a transport incubator (Fig. 15-1) capable of maintaining the infant's body temperature, a portable monitor, intravenous infusion device, and

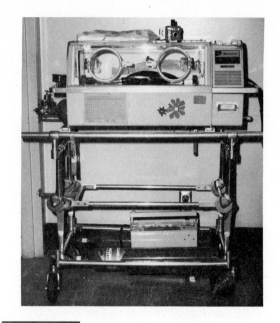

FIG. 15-1

Infant transport equipped with oxygen, resuscitation, and temperature control apparatus.

Courtesy Louis Gluck, M.D., University Hospital, San Diego, Calif.

ventilation equipment to provide care in transit.

The infant must be evaluated quickly. Laboratory tests, x-ray examinations, or procedures may be necessary. Intubation, umbilical catheterization, chest tube placement, administration of antibiotics, glucose, or fluids, and warming or other maneuvers may be required. No infant should be transported until its condition is stable.

Before the transport team leaves the referring hospital, they should talk with the infant's parents, telling them about the child's condition and what will be done in the SCN. Visiting hours should be discussed and telephone numbers given, as well as directions to the SCN. If at all possible, both parents should be allowed to see and handle the infant before it is transported, and a photograph of the baby should be given to them. They should be encouraged to visit their infant as soon and as frequently as possible.

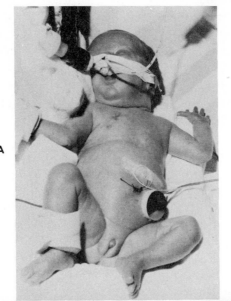

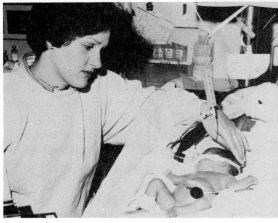

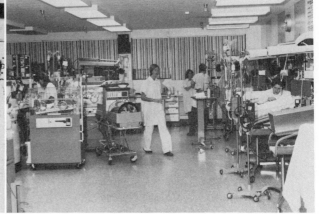

FIG. 15-2   Neonatal intensive care or special care nursery from three perspectives. **A,** This tiny infant was 1 month old when the photograph was taken. Born weighing 2¼ pounds (1,022 g), she was first ventilated mechanically because of respiratory distress syndrome. A heat sensor and umbilical catheter are present. She had a patent ductus arteriosus repair when 6 days old. **B,** Mother came in almost every afternoon. She progessively participated in the care of her daughter as she improved. **C,** One corner of a busy neonatal ICU showing mother at the side of her baby who was receiving maximum care.

Photograph by Bob Burgin; courtesy Children's Hospital and Health Center, San Diego, Calif.

Intensive care of the parents

Separation of an infant from its parents in the immediate postpartum period, although necessary to provide adequate treatment for critically ill babies, can be extremely disruptive to the establishment of normal parent-infant interaction. For this reason the SCN personnel must be extremely supportive of the parents and make every effort to help them adapt to this stressful situation. Visiting should be restricted only when absolutely necessary while procedures are performed, the medical staff is making rounds, or during emergencies. Parents should be encouraged to touch and hold their infant as much as possible, and they should help with bathing, feeding, giving vitamins, and other daily routines as soon as the infant's condition permits.

Ominous terms such as "brain damage," "cerebral palsy," and "blindness" should not be used. Parents whose children have suffered setbacks should be informed and counseled appropriately, but the practice of telling them to "expect the worst" can severely interfere with the bonding process and must not be allowed. Open lines of communication between parents and staff should keep them aware of their child's progress and alleviate unfounded apprehensions. Although the parents' presence in the SCN and frequent questions can sometimes be a nuisance, their feelings must be respected. In this way the psychologic trauma of having their baby in the SCN may be minimized.

Staffing in the SCN

Because of the critical nature of the SCN patient's condition, constant vigilance is necessary to anticipate crises—preventing them, if possible—and being prepared when they inevitably occur. Early detection of deterioration of the infant's vital signs improves the chances for successful intervention. The nurses work closely with the physicians, some of whom must be immediately available at all times.

Since potentially life-threatening conditions may be heralded by subtle changes in the patient's behavior or appearance, the SCN nurse must develop astute powers of observation. A clear understanding of each infant's disease process is imperative, and preparation must be made for any emergency situation that might result from the disease itself or from the treatment (for example, a pneumothorax that develops in an infant's receiving mechanical ventilation). The nurse must also be familiar with the technical equipment (such as monitors and ventilators and be able to interpret alarms and spot malfunctions quickly.

The ideal nurse-patient ratio is 1:1 for infants who are critically ill or in an immediate postoperative phase. (See Fig. 15-2.) The average ratio is 1:2 for most sick infants and up to 1:4 during the convalescent phase. Some hospital settings provide a separate progressive care unit where staffing ratio can be increased.

Nursery personnel use a separate cover-gown technique for each infant. Handwashing is of major importance; personnel wash meticulously before and after handling any infant or piece of equipment. Caps and masks are not used. Cover gowns are worn over street clothing by physicians, parents, and other personnel. In some hospitals persons may freely enter the SCN without gowning or washing as long as no infant or equipment is touched.

THE CRITICALLY ILL NEONATE

Anticipation of the need for care

Prompt recognition and treatment of the sick infant is of utmost importance in obtaining the best possible outcome for each patient. The majority of SCN patients are the products of a relatively small number of high-risk pregnancies; therefore, a knowledge of certain predisposing factors often allows anticipation and early treatment when appropriate, including transfer of the mother to the perinatal center for delivery when possible. An increased incidence of neonatal disease is seen in infants whose mothers have any of the following risk factors: (1) lack of prenatal care, poor nutrition, or other socioeconomic problems; (2) previous history of obstetric complications, such as abortion, stillbirth or neonatal death, premature delivery, prolonged infertility, toxemia, placenta previa, placental abruption, or blood group incompatibilities; and (3) medical illnesses, such as diabetes mellitus, hypertension, infection, alcoholism or drug addiction, and cardiac or renal disease. Complications of labor and birth may also adversely affect the infant. These include premature rupture of membranes, abnormal presentation or fetal size, multiple births, meconium staining of amniotic fluid, and inappropriate maternal analgesia or anesthesia.

These infants deserve special attention, usually including the presence of the pediatrician at the birth and frequently requiring a period of observation in the SCN.

Maintenance of body temperature

Close and continuous monitoring of the infant is a most important duty of the nurse. Axillary temperatures are usually taken with an electronic thermometer. Many neonates, especially low birth weight premature infants, have difficulty with body temperature regulation. They have thin skin that is not insulated by the subcutaneous fat of full-term infants, increased proportion of body surface area to body mass, and immature central nervous system temperature regulation centers. For these reasons they have increased heat losses caused by conduction, convection, radiation, and evaporation. The infant's environmental temperature should be kept in the neutral thermal range so that normal body temperature can be maintained with the least expenditure of energy. This decreases the baby's requirements of oxygen, calories, and fluid and also reduces the production of carbon dioxide. It is an extremely important measure, particularly in the small premature infant with little reserve capacity.

Open radiant heaters provide easy access to the infant who requires frequent intervention and close observation. Treatments, x-ray examinations, procedures, and nursing care can be performed without moving the infant. The bed can be tilted up or down. Special enclosed infant care units (incubators) are used for the infant at risk who needs to be isolated or does not require such frequent direct contact.

Monitoring other body processes

Pulse and respirations are monitored continuously by an electronic cardiorespiratory monitor with audible alarms for apnea, bradycardia, or tachycardia. Blood pressure is measured by the Doppler method, by a standard infant blood pressure cuff, or by means of a pressure transducer connected to an indwelling arterial catheter (usually umbilical).

With each voiding the infant's urine is measured and tested for blood, glucose, protein, pH, and specific gravity. Since fluid volume administered is usually small and must be measured precisely, some type of automatic infusion pump must be used for regulating the intravenous flow. Accurate intake and output charts must be maintained and must include blood withdrawn for diagnostic tests. Daily weights should also be recorded. (Small infants with fluid balance problems are sometimes weighed every 12 hours.)

Infants with respiratory problems require particularly careful observation. The oxygen content of the inspired gas ideally should be monitored continuously or at least checked hourly. For patients receiving either continuous positive airway pressure (CPAP) or mechanical ventilation, the nurse must also check the ventilator pressure settings, endotracheal tube position, and infant's respirations and breath sounds. The chest should be transilluminated periodically if premothorax is likely. Equipment failure or malfunction occasionally occurs and must be detected and corrected quickly. Although all the modern, highly developed equipment being used today in the SCN is a great asset, *the nurse is the most important and accurate monitor* of the infant's condition, and the tendency to rely on mechanical devices must be avoided.

Fluid therapy and feeding

The fluid requirements of the newborn are highly variable and depend on many factors. In the healthy full-term infant an intake of 75 to 90 ml/kg/24 hr is usually adequate during the first 24 to 48 hours of life, increasing to about 150 ml/kg/24 hr over the next few days. The premature infant, however, has increased insensible water losses and may normally require 140 to 160 ml/kg/24 hr. Water losses are also increased by tachypnea, abnormal gastrointestinal losses, administration of a concentrated solution (either orally or intravenously), and fever. The frequently used overhead radiant heater further increases evaporative loss of water, as does the use of phototherapy for hyperbilirubinemia. Thus a small infant in whom several of these factors are operative may need 200 ml/kg/24 hr or even more. On the other hand, fluids should be restricted in some cases, depending on the infant's particular problems. The most important aspect of fluid therapy management is constant monitoring of the infant's state of hydration and appropriate readjustment of fluid intake. This is done by following daily weights, intake and output charts, and urine specific gravities (normal range 1.002 to 1.010).

Caloric requirements are also somewhat variable and are higher in the low birth weight infant (120 to 150 cal/kg/24 hr) than in the full-term infant (110 to 130 cal/kg/24 hr). Increased metabolic rate, for any reason, increases caloric requirements. The presence of disease, environmental temperature above or below the neutral thermal environment, and increased physical activity all increase the baby's needs.

Fluids are administered to the patient either orally, by nipple or gavage, or intravenously. Intravenous fluids may be given through a peripheral vein, an umbilical artery catheter (if one is needed for blood gas sampling), or a central venous line. The use of an umbilical venous catheter for routine fluid maintenance should be avoided. In gavage feeding the stomach must be aspirated before each feeding to check for residual contents from the previous feeding. The amount per feeding is gradually advanced as tolerated; care must be taken not to exceed the capacity of the stomach, because an excess may cause regurgitation and possible aspiration. Nipple feedings may be attempted in the vigorous infant with intact gag and suck reflexes. The breast-feeding mother is encouraged to begin nursing as soon as the baby's condition permits. Until then, she is asked to express milk manually or with a breast pump and bring it to the nursery, where it is usually frozen for storage, to be given to the baby by gavage at a later time.

New techniques for administering fluid and calories include continuous infusion of breast milk or formula into the stomach or, more recently, into the jejunum by way of a transpyloric tube. Parenteral hyperalimentation can provide carbohydrate, protein, and fat by the intravenous route. This is usually given via peripheral veins but may be infused through a central venous catheter. Hyperalimentation is used for infants who are unable to tolerate oral feedings for extended periods of time, such as after bowel surgery. Complications, primarily infection and metabolic imbalance, are frequent, and a team effort involving the pharmacist, nurse, pediatrician, and occasionally a surgeon is necessary for success.

Chest physiotherapy and suctioning

Chest physiotherapy (CPT) and suctioning assist the infant in clearing secretions from his lungs and airway when his own mechanisms are compromised. CPT is indicated in infants with respiratory disorders or those requiring mechanical ventilation for any reason. It is usually done every 2 to 6 hours, depending on the amount of secretions and on the infant's condition. (Some infants' toleration for handling is very poor.) CPT includes 1 or 2 minutes of percussion or vibration. This can be done manually or mechanically using either an electric toothbrush covered with foam rubber or a small portable vibrator. Suctioning (oropharyngeal, nasopharyngeal, and endotracheal) must be gentle; no more than 5 to 10 seconds of intermittent suction is applied as the catheter is withdrawn. Sterile technique must be observed during suctioning through an endotracheal tube but is unnecessary for the mouth, nose, and pharynx. Sterile physiologic saline solution (0.5 ml) may be instilled into the endotracheal tube before suctioning to thin the secretions if necessary. The infant should be hand ventilated with an Ambu or anesthesia bag for a few breaths before and after suctioning to minimize resultant hypoxia or atelectasis.

The infant with pulmonary disease should have his position changed approximately hourly from side to side and from back to abdomen. This helps prevent the pooling of secretions in any one area of the lungs. Even with an umbilical catheter in place, the infant may be placed on the abdomen.

Care of the umbilical catheter

Umbilical arterial catheters are frequently used in the SCN, usually for monitoring of arterial blood gases and aortic blood pressure in critically ill patients who have not yet been stabilized. Umbilical venous catheters are used only on rare occasions in most SCNs, primarily for exchange transfusions, emergency administration of fluids or blood, or for monitoring of central venous pressure. Either type of catheter may lead to serious complications if proper precautions are not observed. Hypovolemic shock or death may result from sudden blood loss if the catheter is accidentally removed or if loose connections at the stopcock or extension tubing allow leakage. Infection or emboli (air or blood clots) may be introduced with careless withdrawal of blood samples, administration of medications, or changing of tubing. Finally, clot formation in the aorta or

other major arteries may lead to infarction of the kidneys, intestines, or lower extremities. The nurse should watch for discoloration of the legs and should never allow the catheter to be opened directly to room air. The physician must be informed of any difficulty in the withdrawal of blood or in the infusion of fluid.

COMMON PROBLEMS ENCOUNTERED IN THE SCN

Respiratory distress syndrome

Respiratory distress syndrome (RDS), or hyaline membrane disease, is the most common problem in the SCN, and, before recent advances in ventilator management, was the leading cause of neonatal mortality (Fig. 15-3). It is most frequently seen in premature infants (less than 36 weeks' gestation), although an occasional full-term baby is affected.

The onset of symptoms often occurs in the delivery room where the baby has low Apgar scores and requires assistance in establishing respirations. In other cases the infant may appear normal initially but begin to have expiratory grunting and nasal flaring in the first few hours of life (usually less than 6 hours). Respiratory distress becomes increasingly obvious with the onset of tachypnea, retractions, and cyanosis in room air. A chest x-ray film is diagnostic, revealing characteristic granular density, air bronchograms, and diminished lung volume. Arterial blood gases show hypoxia and usually a combined metabolic and respiratory acidosis.

Etiologic factors. The cause of RDS is somewhat controversial, but it is definitely a developmental disease (that is, related to natural maturational changes) with many contributing factors. Lung and airway structure, cardiac and pulmonary circulation, and development of surface-active phospholipid compounds in alveoli are all important in the pathophysiology of RDS.

The surface-active compounds, collectively referred to as surfactants, begin to appear in the fetal lung early in development but are not usually fully

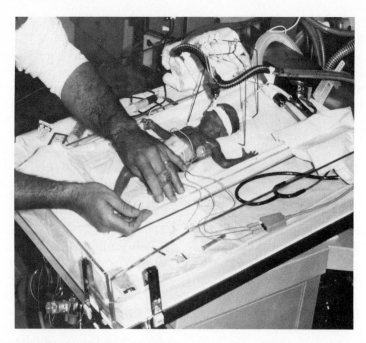

FIG. 15-3   Another blood gas determination for a small representative of humanity who has respiratory distress syndrome.

Courtesy Louis Gluck, M.D., University Hospital, San Diego, Calif.

functional until about 36 to 37 weeks' gestation. Surfactant opposes the natural tendency of alveoli to collapse completely at the end of each expiration and thereby keeps the lung partially expanded at all times.

Infants in whom these substances are deficient or absent must completely reexpand their lungs with each breath, greatly increasing the work of breathing. Extreme stiffness of the lungs (decreased compliance) and progressive atelectasis (collapse of alveoli) result, leading to hypoxia, fatigue, and decreased ventilation, all of which cause acidosis. The acidosis further decreases the lung's ability to synthesize surfactant and also decreases pulmonary blood flow, thus worsening the RDS and creating a vicious cycle.

The presence of surfactant in the lungs depends on enzyme systems that normally increase activity at approximately 33 to 34 weeks' gestation. Certain factors, such as chronic placental abruption, prolonged rupture of membranes, maternal hypertension, and possibly maternal narcotic drug usage, induce earlier activation of these enzymes and therefore protect the infant from RDS. On the other hand, maternal diabetes and erythroblastosis fetalis appear to delay lung maturation.

Treatment. The treatment of RDS is aimed at supporting the infant by assisting oxygenation and ventilation until the baby's lungs begin to produce surfactant (usually within 2 or 3 days). The measures used depend on the severity of the disease. Mild to moderate cases are treated with increased concentration of environmental oxygen, usually given by hood. More severely affected infants require continuous positive airway pressure (CPAP) to prevent the atelectasis that occurs at the end of expiration. This in turn improves oxygenation and decreases the work of breathing. This

BLOOD GAS ANALYSIS

Indications
To monitor oxygenation, ventilation, and acid-base balance

Methods of obtaining
1. Umbilical arterial or other indwelling arterial catheter
2. Arterial puncture (radial, temporal, or other)
3. Arterialized capillary blood sample drawn from heel, ulnar aspect of hand, or digit (extremity is first warmed for 5 to 10 minutes)

Blood gas analysis can be performed on as little as 0.1 ml of blood drawn into a heparinized capillary tube, depending on the particular blood gas analyzer used. Care must be taken not to allow air bubbles or blood clots to enter the sample; sample should be placed on ice unless it is analyzed immediately.

Normal values for arterial blood of newborns in room air
(Normal values in the first hours after birth are different)

pH	7.35 to 7.45
P_{O_2}	70 to 100 mm Hg
	(40 to 50 mm Hg for capillary sample)
P_{CO_2}	35 to 45 mm Hg

pressure is usually applied by means of nasal prongs or an endotracheal tube. Alternatively, the same effect may be accomplished by applying negative pressure to the infant's body, leaving the head open to atmospheric pressure. This is done with the negative pressure respirator and is referred to as continuous negative airway pressure (CNAP).

If the infant develops hypoxia, respiratory failure, or recurrent apnea despite continuous positive airway pressure, mechanical ventilation is instituted with any of several infant respirators. The machine then takes over essentially all ventilatory functions for the baby. Appropriate adjustments must be made for respiratory rate, expiratory pressure and time, inspiratory pressure and time, and concentration of oxygen.

It must be remembered that all of these forms of treatment carry certain risks to the baby. High concentrations of inspired oxygen are known to be toxic to the lungs, whereas high arterial P_{O_2} (exact critical levels are unknown) in the retinal arteries can cause blindness in premature infants as the result of retrolental fibroplasia. Infants receiving increased pressure therapy (CPAP or mechanical ventilation) are at risk for pneumothorax and cardiovascular disturbances. Endotracheal intubation predisposes the infant to infection, or the tube itself may become occluded with secretions. Because of these potential complications, the infant with RDS must be carefully evaluated, and the risks of therapy balanced against the benefits.

General supportive measures, such as proper regulation of fluids, acid-base status, and thermal environment, are of great importance in the infant with RDS. An umbilical artery catheter is often used for frequent arterial blood gas sampling as well as administration of parenteral fluids, medications, and transfusions (blood drawn for samples must be replaced periodically). Antibiotics are not effective against the disease itself but are often used as a prophylactic measure.

Complications. Aside from the risks of therapy just mentioned, the complications of RDS include hypoglycemia, hypocalcemia, hyperbilirubinemia, intracranial hemorrhage, and patent ductus arteriosus (PDA). Intracranial hemorrhage is more common in infants of less than 32 weeks' gestation and is replacing RDS as a major cause of death as newer therapeutic measures improve the prognosis of RDS. The onset of symptoms resulting from patent ductus arteriosus usually coincides with the recovery phase of RDS. Typical congestive heart failure may occur with enlarged heart and liver and tachycardia. More often, however, an infant who has been improving clinically simply stops making progress and becomes dependent on oxygen, continuous positive airway pressure, or a respirator. A trial of medical therapy with digitalis may be attempted, although success is rare. The PDA may close spontaneously, but some require surgical ligation or pharmacologic closure with indomethacin.

Prevention. Prenatal assessment of lung surfactant maturity can be done by performing an amniocentesis and analyzing surfactant compounds in the amniotic fluid. The now-familiar L/S ratio compares the content of lecithin, an important surfactant, to sphingomyelin, an inactive phospholipid. An L/S ratio of 2.0 usually indicates lung maturity, as does the presense of another important compound, phosphatidyl glycerol (PG). Elective delivery (cesarean section or induction) should be delayed until these studies are obtained to minimize the risk of RDS.

Aspiration of meconium

Staining of the amniotic fluid with meconium, the stool of the fetus, occurs in approximately 10% of all births. It may indicate intrauterine distress, and in some instances the infant may make gasping respiratory efforts before the head is delivered and thus aspirate the meconium into the lungs. Although normal amniotic fluid is virtually harmless to the lungs, the particles of meconium produce obstruction of the airways and cause respiratory difficulty. The infant may be vigorous and breathing easily, but if significant intrauterine asphyxia has occurred, he will be depressed and require assistance in establishing respirations. In the latter case, intubation and direct tracheal suction must be performed before the use of positive pressure ventilation. Ideally this will avoid forcing meconium into more distal airways and reduce the severity of the disease. Suctioning of the baby's oropharynx after delivery of the head but before delivery of the shoulders and chest may also minimize the inhalation process. Symptoms of respiratory distress occur in about 15% of meconium-stained infants and vary from mild to very severe. In most cases symptoms resolve by 48 hours of life, but occasionally respiratory assistance must be continued for much longer periods. Treatment consists of oxygen, CPT and suction, and general support-

ive measures. Antibiotics may be used, and mechanical ventilation is sometimes necessary for severe cases. Pneumothorax is a common complication.

Pneumothorax

Many newborns (possibly 1% of all babies) develop pneumothorax (free air in the pleural space), but the great majority of them remain asymptomatic, and the condition is resolved without treatment. Pneumothorax usually occurs spontaneously as a result of the high intrathoracic pressures that infants generate when expanding their lungs with the first few breaths. Other cases may be caused by positive pressure ventilation or aspiration of meconium or blood. Premature infants are more susceptible to pneumothorax than full-term infants. Clinical signs include respiratory difficulty, tachypnea, cyanosis, shifting of the cardiac impulse, decreased blood pressure, and irritability. Transillumination of the chest is significantly increased by a tension pneumothorax. The diagnosis is confirmed by chest x-ray examination.

Treatment of the infant with pneumothorax depends on the severity of the symptoms. The infant with mild or no symptoms needs only careful observation or may be placed in 100% oxygen to speed absorption of the free air. If severe distress is present, the pneumothorax should be aspirated and a chest tube inserted into the pleural space. The chest tube is usually connected to suction by means of a water seal. Follow-up x-ray examinations are indicated to determine the position of the chest tube and reexpansion of the lung. Patency of the tube must be maintained by preventing kinking, clotting, and looping. The chest tube can usually be removed within a few days as the respiratory status improves.

Hyperbilirubinemia

Hyperbilirubinemia occurs to some degree in normal newborns and is often exaggerated in the premature or sick neonate. Bilirubin, most of which is formed from the breakdown of hemoglobin, is taken up by liver cells, where it is modified and excreted through the bile ducts into the intestine. The so-called physiologic hyperbilirubinemia that occurs in normal newborns results from several factors: (1) increased destruction of red blood cells, (2) decreased blood flow to the liver, (3) decreased uptake of bilirubin into the liver cells, (4) decreased activity of liver enzymes in metabolizing bilirubin, and (5) increased absorption of bilirubin from the intestine (enterohepatic circulation).

Hyperbilirubinemia is considered to be pathologic if the serum bilirubin level exceeds 12 mg/100 ml or if obvious jaundice appears in the first 24 hours. The most common cause is hemolytic disease (for example, Rh or ABO blood group incompatibility of the fetus and mother). Other causes sometimes encountered are polycythemia, excessive bruising, hemolytic anemias, sepsis, intrauterine viral infection, or metabolic disorders.

The treatment of hyperbilirubinemia, in addition to treatment of the underlying cause, is the use of phototherapy and exchange transfusions. The effect of phototherapy (cool white or blue lamps) is the breakdown of bilirubin pigments in the skin. In an exchange transfusion, the infant's blood is simply replaced, ideally removing much bilirubin from the baby. The objective of treatment is the prevention of kernicterus, a neurologic condition caused by deposition of bilirubin in the basal ganglia of the brain. Hearing loss may result from bilirubin toxicity to the auditory nerve. The exact serum bilirubin level at which damage occurs varies widely, depending on the maturity and clinical condition of the infant.

Neonatal sepsis

The newborn infant has incompletely developed immunologic responses and therefore has increased susceptibility to infection—bacterial, viral, and other types. Once an infection is acquired, it may quickly invade the bloodstream (neonatal sepsis or septicemia) and lead to meningitis, pneumonia, urinary tract infection, osteomyelitis, or other infections. Certain factors predispose infants to infection, including prematurity, prolonged rupture of membranes, maternal infection (chorioamnionitis, urinary tract infection), difficult labor with fetal distress, and special procedures, such as resuscitation, intubation, and umbilical catheterization. Presenting signs include respiratory distress with grunting and tachypnea, poor feeding, vomiting, lethargy, temperature instability, unexplained jaundice, and apnea.

Group B streptococcal infections have been most often identified in the past few years, but many other bacteria may cause sepsis, including other streptococci, Staphylococcus aureus, Listeria, and gram-negative organisms. In long-term SCN patients less common pathogens such as Citrobacter, Serratia, Pseudomonas, or viruses may be encountered.

Early treatment is of extreme importance in obtaining a favorable outcome. Once infection is suspected, cultures should be taken promptly of blood, urine, spinal fluid, stool, tracheal aspirate, and additional sites as indicated. Antibiotic therapy with two drugs, one for gram-negative and one for gram-positive organisms, should be instituted immediately. Subsequent choice of antibiotics is determined by identification of the offending organism and its sensitivity patterns.

Intrauterine infection

Although the fetus is protected by the mother from most infectious diseases, some microorganisms have the ability to cross the placenta and may cause significant damage. If a pregnant woman becomes infected at a time when her fetus is susceptible, intrauterine infection may result. These infections are commonly referred to as the "TORCHES" (TOxoplasmosis, Rubella, Cytomegalovirus, HErpes, and Syphilis), although other agents are now known to affect the fetus.

Rubella (German measles) is probably the best known and most feared intrauterine infection. Rubella infection occurs in up to 50% of fetuses of mothers who acquire the disease during the first 8 weeks of pregnancy. The fetal infection rate then declines and is very low after the first trimester. Affected infants have demonstrated a variety of manifestations from the most severe congenital rubella syndrome (intrauterine growth retardation, cardiac defects, cataracts, deafness, anemia, jaundice, and mental retardation) to the apparently normal newborn with mild hearing loss. Diagnosis can be confirmed by viral cultures of the infant's pharynx, urine, or stool and by antibody titers on the mother and infant. Immunization programs to prevent infection of pregnant women are of utmost importance, since no proven treatment exists for the disease.

Cytomegalovirus (CMV) is the most common intrauterine infection and, like rubella, may cause a variety of effects in the infant. Most infants are asymptomatic, but others may have microcephaly, growth retardation, hepatitis, low platelet count, seizures, and pneumonia. Diagnosis is confirmed by cultures and by antibody studies.

Toxoplasmosis is a protozoan disease that may be contracted by the ingestion of raw meat or food contaminated with cat feces. The disease is relatively uncommon in the United States and may be entirely asymptomatic in the infected mother. The infection primarily affects the fetal central nervous system and may cause mental retardation, blindness, deafness, convulsions, and hydrocephalus. These infants should be treated with sulfadiazine and pyrimethamine, although much of the damage is probably irreversible.

The incidence of *syphilis* is increasing in the United States as well as other countries, and consequently more babies with the congenital infection are being seen. The infant's risk is greater if maternal infection occurs in the latter part of pregnancy, or infection may be acquired during the birth process. Infected infants usually appear normal in the immediate postpartum period, although prematurity and stillbirths sometimes result. Most cases of congenital syphilis exhibit a typical rash, profuse nasal discharge, radiologic defects of the long bones, and hepatitis in early infancy. Congenital syphilis is most often detected by screening for maternal disease with routine VDRLs on all pregnant women. Treatment with penicillin eradicates the disease, although mental retardation and other sequelae may not be totally prevented. (See also pp. 162 and 164.)

In recent years viruses other than rubella and CMV have been discovered to infect fetuses, including hepatitis B virus and Coxsackie viruses. Herpes simplex virus may be transmitted from maternal genital infections to the infant during birth and cause a rapidly fatal illness (p. 71).

Chlamydia trachomatis, recently identified as an important sexually transmitted pathogen, is also acquired by the infant during birth. Conjunctivitis or pneumonitis may result during the first few weeks of life. As screening techniques and virology studies become more sensitive and widespread, knowledge of these fetal infections will increase as will their relative importance in SCN patients.

Neonatal drug addiction

Infants whose mothers are addicted to heroin, barbiturates, amphetamines, or other drugs inherit the drug dependency. These babies usually appear normal at birth but begin to show symptoms of withdrawal after 8 to 12 hours. Extreme irritability with constant crying and jitteriness, poor feeding, emesis, diarrhea, respiratory distress, and seizures may occur. Symptoms are alleviated by administration of paregoric, phenobarbital, or tranquilizers (chlorpromazine, diazepam) and by keeping the infant well wrapped in a quiet, dimly lit environment. Intravenous fluids may be necessary to prevent dehydration or hypoglycemia. Medication is gradually decreased over several days and eventually discontinued.

Fetal alcohol syndrome

The fetal alcohol syndrome has been well documented in infants born to mothers with excessive alcohol intake during pregnancy. These infants may exhibit intrauterine growth retardation, microcephaly, mental deficiency, cardiac defects, and characteristic anomalies of the face and extremities. Lesser effects may occur in babies born to moderate drinkers and may be difficult to recognize, although intellectual impairment may result. (See also p. 71.) These infants may experience withdrawal symptoms similar to those of infants of drug-addicted mothers.

Infants born to diabetic mothers

Infants born to diabetic mothers (IDMs) are predisposed to a number of neonatal disorders and are frequently encountered in the SCN. Late intrauterine fetal deaths occur more commonly in diabetic mothers so that their pregnancies must be monitored carefully by the physician. Amniocentesis is usually performed at weekly intervals after about 36 weeks' gestation, and the baby is delivered as soon as the L/S ratio indicates lung maturity. Lung maturity is often delayed in these infants, and if the L/S ratio is not performed, an infant may be born who will have severe RDS. If delivered at term, the infants may be very large (10 or more pounds) and therefore susceptible to birth injury unless a cesarean section is done.

Once born, these babies exhibit a high incidence of hypoglycemia, usually during the first 12 hours. Dextrostix determinations or blood glucose levels should be done at intervals and the infants fed early to prevent its occurrence. Infants unable to tolerate feedings or who become hypoglycemic despite feedings require intravenous glucose water at a 10% or greater concentration. Glucagon may temporarily raise blood glucose while intravenous therapy is being started. IDMs are also susceptible to hypocalcemia, hyperbilirubinemia, polycythemia, congenital anomalies, and renal vein thrombosis.

Infants born to mothers with severe or long-standing diabetes suffer intrauterine growth retardation and are usually very small rather than large for their gestational age. Their lungs appear to mature early, and they may be protected from having RDS. The severity and duration of the mother's diabetes and her control during pregnancy are the most important factors influencing the infant's neonatal problems. (See also p. 160.)

Necrotizing enterocolitis

Necrotizing enterocolitis is an acute, often lethal, intestinal disorder in the newborn and is most commonly seen in the premature infant. Clinical signs include abdominal distention, vomiting, diarrhea with blood in the stool, apnea, lethargy, hypothermia, and shock. Positive diagnosis is established by abdominal x-ray examination, which may show pneumatosis intestinalis (air in the intestinal wall) or free air in the peritoneal cavity.

Initial treatment consists of nasogastric suction, intravenous fluids, antibiotics, and transfusions. Serial abdominal x-ray examinations are done at frequent intervals to detect progression of the disease or perforation of the bowel, either of which is an indication for surgery. At surgery the areas of necrotic bowel are resected and a colostomy is usually performed. Anastomosis of the intestine is then done as an elective procedure after the infant has recovered.

The cause of necrotizing enterocolitis is unknown, but lack of oxygen supply to the intestinal mucosa and bacterial infection are two possible factors. Breast milk may be protective against the disease and is therefore used for feeding of premature infants in some centers in the hope of decreasing the incidence of the disease.

Postmaturity

Postmature infants are those who are born after 42 or more weeks' gestation. They have dry, parchmentlike skin, long fingernails, and a wide-eyed, alert expression. Meconium staining of the skin is not uncommon, and meconium aspiration occurs more frequently than with normal term infants. Mortality of the postmature infant is nearly twice as high as that of the term infant. Postmature infants have diminished glycogen stores and are therefore susceptible to hypoglycemia. They should be fed early (at 3 to 4 hours) and have periodic Dextrostix or blood glucose determinations.

• • •

It is important to remember that the material presented here represents only some of the highlights of neonatal intensive care nursing. The student interested in this area should refer to one of the many books now available on the subject.

SUGGESTED SELECTED READINGS AND REFERENCES

GENERAL

Andrews, B.F., editor: Symposium on the newborn, Pediatr. Clin. North Am. **24:**entire issue, Aug. 1977.

Bacon, K.K.: Care of the neonate after cesarean section, AORN J. **34:**860-882, Nov. 1981.

Bliss, V.J.: Nursing care for infants with neonatal necrotizing enterocolitis, Am. J. Mat. Child Nurs. **1:**37-40, Jan.-Feb. 1976.

Committee on Fetus and Newborn, American Academy of Pediatrics: Standards and recommendations for hospital care of newborn infants, ed. 6, Evanston, Ill., 1977. The Academy.

Erickson, M.P.: Trends in assessing the newborn and his parents, Am. J. Mat. Child Nurs. **3:**99-103, Mar.-Apr. 1978.

Finnegan, L.P., and Macnew, B.A.: Care of the addicted infant, Am. J. Nurs. **74:**685-693, Apr. 1974.

Foley, K.L.: Caring for the parents of newborn twins, Am. J. Mat. Child Nurs. **4:**221-226, July-Aug. 1979.

Frankenburg, W.K.: To screen or not to screen: congenital dislocation of the hip, Am. J. Public Health **71:**1311-1313, Dec. 1981.

Holaday, B.: Changing views of infant care 1914-1980, Ped. Nurs. **7:**21-25, Jan.-Feb. 1981.

Iles, J.P., and McCrary, M.: Cuddle bathing can be fun: the rewards of research, Am. J. Mat. Child Nurs. **1:**350-354, Nov.-Dec. 1976.

Irwin, E.C., and McWilliams, B.J.: Play therapy for children with cleft palates, Child. Today **3:**18-22, May-June 1974.

Jenkins, R.L., and Westhus, N.K.: The nurse's role in parent-infant bonding: overview, assessment, intervention, JOGN Nurs. **10:**114-118, Mar.-Apr. 1981.

Klaus, M.H., and Kennell, J.H.: Parent-infant bonding, ed. 2, St. Louis, 1982, The C.V. Mosby Co.

Klaus, M.H., and Robertson, M.O., editors: Pediatric round table No. 6: birth, interaction and attachment, Skillman, N.J., 1982, Johnson & Johnson Baby Products Co.

LaFranchi, S.: Newborn screening for hypothyroidism, Pediatr. Ann. **9:**54-65, Oct. 1980.

Lum, B., Lortz, R., and Barnett, E.: Reappraising newborn eye care, Am. J. Nurs. **80:**1602-1603, Sept. 1980.

Moore, M.L.: Newborn, family and nurse, ed. 2. Philadelphia, 1981, W.B. Saunders Co.

Nugent, J.K.: The Brazelton neonatal behavioral assessment scale: implications for intervention, Pediatr. Nurs. **7:**18-21,67, May-June 1981.

O'Brien, J.S.: The high-risk pregnancy: Tay-Sachs disease, prenatal diagnosis, Contemp. OB/GYN **3:**73-76, Feb. 1974.

Patton, B., editor: Symposium on neonatal care, Nurs. Clin. North Am. **13:**1-84, Mar. 1978.

Schwartz, J.L., and Schwartz, L.H.: Vulnerable infants—a psychosocial dilemma, New York, 1977, McGraw-Hill Book Co.

Sholder, D.A.: Portrait of a newborn, JOGN Nurs. **10:**98-101, Mar.-Apr. 1981.

Smith, D.W., and Wilson, A.A.: The child with Down's syndrome, Philadelphia, 1973, W.B. Saunders Co.

Specht, E.E.: Congenital dislocation of the hip, Am. Fam. Physician **9:**88-96, Feb. 1974.

Stranik, M.K., and Hogberg, B.L.: Transition into parenthood, Am. J. Nurs. **79:**90-93, Jan. 1979.

Zurawski, G., and Shnider, S.: How anesthetic drugs affect neonatal neurobehavior, Contemp. OB/GYN **17:**179-189, June 1981.

CIRCUMCISION

Gibbons, M.B.: Why circumcise? Pediatr. Nurs. **5:**9-12, July-Aug. 1979.

Grimes, D.A.: Routine circumcision reconsidered, Am. J. Nurs. **80:**110-112, Jan. 1980.

Perley, J.M.: Avoiding the complications of circumcision, Contemp. OB/GYN **10:**77-79, Sept. 1977.

Poole, C.J.: Neonatal circumcision, JOGN Nurs. **8:**207-211, July-Aug. 1979.

FEEDING

Arafat, I., Allen, D.E., and Fox, J.E.: Maternal practice and attitudes toward breast-feeding, JOGN Nurs. **10:**91-95, Mar.-Apr. 1981.

Bishop, W.S., and Bishop, P.A.: Father assisted breast-feeding, Pediatr. Nurs. **4:**39-41, Jan.-Feb. 1978.

Broome, M.E.: Breast-feeding and the working mother, JOGN Nurs. **10:**201-202, May-June 1981.

Dutton, M.A.: A breast-feeding protocol, JOGN Nurs. **8:**151-155, May-June 1979.

Gunn, S.: The bottle-feeding mother needs your help too, RN **42**:53, Feb. 1979.

Olson, J.: Breast-feeding: common problems and practical answers, Pediatr. Nurs. **4**:32-35, Jan.-Feb. 1978.

Riordan, J., and Countryman, B.A.: Basics of breast-feeding, Part I: infant feeding patterns past and present; Part II: the anatomy and psychophysiology of lactation, JOGN Nurs. **9**:207-213, July-Aug. 1980.

Riordan, J., and Countryman, B.A.: Basics of breast-feeding, Part III: the biological specificity of breast milk; Part IV: preparation for breast-feeding and early optimal functioning, JOGN Nurs. **9**:277-283, Sept.-Oct. 1980.

Riordan, J., and Countryman, B.A.: Basics of breast-feeding, Part V: self-care for continued breast-feeding; Part VI: some breast-feeding problems and solutions, JOGN Nurs. **9**:357-366, Nov.-Dec. 1980.

Riordan, J., and Rapp, E.T.: Pleasure and purpose: the sensuousness of breast-feeding, JOGN Nurs. **9**:109-112, Mar.-Apr. 1980.

Tibbetts, E., and Cadwell, K.: Selecting the right breast pump, Am. J. Mat. Child Nurs. **5**:262-264, July-Aug. 1980.

Zimmerman, A.W., et al: Milk and lactation among 1,000 infants, Pediatrics **69**:193-196, Feb. 1982.

Zimmerman, M.A.: Breast-feeding the adopted newborn, Pediatr. Nurs. **7**:9-12, Jan.-Feb. 1981.

TEMPERATURE CONTROL

Britton, G.R.: Early mother-infant contact and infant temperature stabilization, JOGN Nurs. **7**:84-86, Mar.-Apr. 1980.

Capobianco, J.A.: How to safeguard the infant against life-threatening heat loss, Nurs. '80, **10**:64-67, May 1980.

Davis, V.: The structure and function of brown adipose tissue in the neonate, JOGN Nurs. **9**:368-372, Nov.-Dec. 1980.

Gardner, S.: The mother as incubator—after delivery, JOGN Nurs. **8**:174-176, May-June 1979.

Phillips, C.: Neonatal heat loss in heated cribs vs. mother's arms, JOGN Nurs. **3**:11-15, Nov.-Dec. 1974.

PARENTS AND THE ILL INFANT

Cagan, J., and Meier, P.: A discharge planning tool for use with families of high-risk infants, JOGN Nurs. **8**:146-148, May-June 1979.

Elsas, T.L.: Family mental health care in the neonatal intensive care unit, JOGN Nurs. **10**:204-206, May-June 1981.

Goldson, E.: Parents' reactions to the birth of a sick infant, Child. Today **8**:13-17, July-Aug. 1979.

Hawkins-Walsh, E.: Diminishing anxiety in parents of sick newborns, Am. J. Mat. Child Nurs. **5**:30, Jan.-Feb. 1980.

Opirhory, G.J.: Counseling the parents of a critically ill newborn, JOGN Nurs. **8**:179-182, May-June 1979.

Schraeder, B.D.: Attachment and parenting despite lengthy intensive care, Am. J. Mat. Child Nurs. **5**:37-41, Jan.-Feb. 1980.

Spenner, D.: When the baby is sick and the mother's concerns are ignored, Am. J. Nurs. **80**:2222-2224, Dec. 1980.

Wooten, B.: Death of an infant, Am. J. Mat. Child Nurs. **6**:257-260, July-Aug. 1981.

ABNORMALITIES (MISCELLANEOUS)

Brueggemeyer, A.: Omphalocele: coping with a surgical emergency, Pediatr. Nurs. **5**:54-56, July-Aug. 1979.

Burnett, J.: Congenital adrenocortical hyperplasia, Am. J. Nurs. **80**:1304-1311, July 1980.

Gennaro, S.: Necrotizing enterocolitis: detecting it and treating it, Nurs. '80 **10**:52-55, Jan. 1980.

Hazle, N.: An infant who survived gastrochisis, Am. J. Mat. Child Nurs. **6**:35-40, Jan.-Feb. 1981.

Sherk, H.H., Pasquariello, P.S., and Wattero, W.C.: Congenital dislocation of the hip, Clin. Pediatr. **20**:513-520, Aug. 1981.

CENTRAL NERVOUS SYSTEM ANOMALIES

Bejar, R. et al: Diagnosis and follow-up of intraventricular and intracerebral hemorrhage by ultrasound studies of the infant's brain through the fontanelles and the sutures, Pediatrics **66**:661-673, 1980.

Bernardo, M.L.: Craniosynostosis: the child's care from detection through correction (pictorial), Am. J. Mat. Child Nurs. **4**:234-237, July-Aug. 1979.

Bernardo, M.L.: When your caseload includes a hydrocephalic child, Pediatr. Nurs. **5**:27-29, May-June 1979.

Braney, M.L.: The child with hydrocephalus, Am. J. Nurs. **73**:828-831, May 1973.

Floyd, C.C.: A defective child is born: a study of newborns with spina bifida and hydrocephalus, JOGN Nurs. **6**:56-62, July-Aug. 1977.

Humphrey, P.A., Britt, P.H., and Peter, C.R.: Craniofacial malformations, Am. J. Nurs. **79**:1230-1234, July 1979.

Jackson, P.L.: Ventriculo-peritoneal shunts, Am. J. Nurs. **80**:1104-1109, June 1980.

MacLaughlin, J.F., and Shurtliff, D.B.: Management of the newborn with myelodysplasia, Clin. Pediatr. **18**:463, Aug. 1979.

McElroy, D.B.: Hydrocephalus in children, Pediatr. Clin. North Am. **15**:23-34, Mar. 1980.

FETAL ALCOHOL SYNDROME

Bartlett, D., and Davis, A.: Recognizing fetal alcohol syndrome in the nursery, JOGN Nurs. **9**:223-225, July-Aug. 1980.

Lindor, E., McCarthy, A., and McRae, M.G.: Fetal alcohol syndrome: a review and case presentation, JOGN Nurs. **9**:222-228, July-Aug. 1980.

Powell, J.: The tragedy of fetal alcohol syndrome, RN **44**:32-35, 92-96, Dec. 1981.

Stephens, C.J.: The fetal alcohol syndrome: cause for concern, Am. J. Mat. Child Nurs. **6**:251-256, July-Aug. 1981.

INFECTIONS

Bond, G.B.: Serratia: an endemic hospital resident, Am. J. Nurs. **81**:2183-2186, Dec. 1981.

Lumicao, G.G., and Heggie, A.D.: Chlamydia infections, Pediatr. Clin. North Am. **26**:269-282, May 1979.

Ridenour, N.: Chlamydia, Nurs. Pract. **5**:45,48, Sept.-Oct. 1980.

Sever, J.L.: Reducing the risk of congenital herpes, Contemp. OB/GYN **17**:191-195, June 1981.

Stagno, S.: Toxoplasmosis, Am. J. Nurs. **80**:720-722, Apr. 1980.

Starr, S.E.: Cytomegalovirus, Pediatr. Clin. North Am. **26**:283-293, May 1979.

Veda, K. et al: Low birth weight and congenital rubella syndrome: effect and gestational age of time of maternal rubella infection, Clin. Pediatr. **20**:730-733, Nov. 1981.

SUDDEN INFANT DEATH SYNDROME

Deal, A.W., and Bordeaux, B.R.: The phenomenon of SIDS, Pediatr. Nurs. **5**:48-50, Jan.-Feb. 1980.

Favorito, J., Pernice, J.M., and Ruggiero, P.: Apnea monitoring to prevent SIDS, Am. J. Nurs. **79**:101-104, Jan. 1979.

Sharer, P.S.: Helping survivors cope with the shock of sudden death, Nurs. '79 **9**:20-23, Jan. 1979.

Sperhac, A.M.: Sudden infant death syndrome, Nurs. Practitioner, **7**:38-44, Sept. 1982.

NEONATAL ICU

Butterfield, L.J.: Can society afford to save babies? Contemp. OB/GYN **10**:110-111, Oct. 1977.

Carey, B., Larson, B., and Goold, G.: A neonatal teaching tool: working with umbilical catheters, Am. J. Mat. Child Nurs. **5**:393-397, Nov.-Dec. 1980.

Curran, C.L., and Kachoyeanos, M.K.: The effects on neonates of two methods of chest physical therapy, Am. J. Mat. Child Nurs. **4**:309-313, Sept.-Oct. 1979.

Dingle, R.E., et al: Continuous transcutaneous O_2 monitoring in the neonate, Am. J. Nurs. **80**:890-893, May 1980.

Ellenberger, D., Kennedy, A.H., and Chase, C.: An education program for nurses from referring hospitals in a perinatal regionalization system, JOGN Nurs. **8**:158-161, May-June 1979.

Endo, A.S.: Using computers in newborn intensive care settings, Am. J. Nurs. **81**:1336-1337, July 1981.

Glassanos, M.R.: Infants who are oxygen dependent—sending them home, Am. J. Mat. Child Nurs. **5**:42-45, Jan.-Feb. 1980.

Greene, H.L.: Nutritional support of the sick infant, Pediatr. Ann. **10**:63-79, Nov. 1981.

Hansen, F.H.: Nursing care in the neonatal intensive care unit, JOGN Nurs. **11**:17-20, Jan.-Feb. 1982.

Hawkins, M.M.: Nursing and regionalization of perinatal services, JOGN Nurs. **9**:215-217, July-Aug. 1980.

Kanto, Jr., W., Maples, J.C., Goldberg, G.H., and Miller, M.D.: Evaluation and need of education programs for community hospital nurses providing neonatal care, JOGN Nurs. **8**:98-103, Mar.-Apr. 1979.

Korones, S.B.: High-risk newborn infants: the basis for intensive nursing care, ed. 3. St. Louis, 1981, The C.V. Mosby Co.

GROWTH, DEVELOPMENT, AND HEALTH SUPERVISION

CONCEPTS OF GROWTH AND DEVELOPMENT

As children grow up they are constantly changing physically and functionally. This is the main factor that distinguishes the child from the adult. Growth is exhibited by all healthy children, although it may be impaired by malnutrition and disease. Growth is the one feature that sets apart pediatrics as a specialty.

Every nurse interested in the care of children needs to have a basic understanding of human growth and development. Such an understanding will be of great help in evaluating the physical, intellectual, emotional, and social behavior of the dynamic child patient.

Terminology

The terms "growth" and "development" are closely bound together and sometimes used interchangeably. Increases in structure (growth) are accompanied by increases in function (development). As children grow in size they grow up or mature mentally, emotionally, and socially. Differences in the way a child thinks, feels, or acts are just as real as changes in size.

As growth and development proceed, various levels of maturity are observable. *Maturation* is the process whereby inherited tendencies begin to unfold, independent of any special practice or training. All children have their own built-in growth pattern. Some children have patterns that allow them to mature rapidly; other children are very slow physically, mentally, and emotionally and are called late maturers. A wide range can exist in the growth and development rates of normal children. Mary enjoyed walking at 12 months of age; her sister was 15 months old when she took her first steps. Each child will advance physiologically toward maturity at his own rate.

Because of similarities in children, cultures, learning methods, and child-rearing practices, generalizations can be made concerning growth and development. Although these generalizations are not applicable in every case, they do provide valuable points of departure in understanding and dealing with groups. This discussion of growth and development follows the child through an orderly sequence beginning with the prenatal phase and continuing through babyhood, childhood, and adolescence.

Principles

The normal growth and development of a child through the successive periods of babyhood, childhood, and adolescence are guided by certain basic principles, five of which follow (Table 16-1).

TABLE 16-1 PROGRESSIVE STAGES OF DEVELOPMENT

Stages of life	Divisions of life stages	Chronologic age
PRENATAL		
Conception to birth	Germinal	Conception to 10 days' gestation
	Embryonic	10 days to 2 months' gestation
	Fetal	2 months' gestation to birth
BABYHOOD		
Birth to 1 year	Newborn (neonate)	Birth to 1 month
	Infancy	1 month to 1 year
CHILDHOOD		
1 to 12 years	Toddler	1 to 3 years
	Preschool	3 to 6 years
	School	6 to 10 years
	Preadolescence (puberty)	10 to 12 years
ADOLESCENCE		
12 to 19 years	Early adolescence	12 to 16 years
	Late adolescence	16 to 19 years

Growth and development (1) occur in an orderly sequence; (2) although continuous, are characterized by spurts of growth and periods of relative rest; (3) progress at highly individualized rates from child to child; (4) vary at different ages for specific structures; and (5) represent a total process involving the whole child.

Orderly sequence. Growth and development occur in an orderly sequence and are continuous. The sequence of development is the same for all children, even though some children do things earlier than others. Children generally creep before they stand and stand alone before they walk. *Average* children talk before they read and usually read before they can write. One child will read at 4 years

of age, and another will read at 6 years of age. What happens at one stage influences what happens in the next stage; each stage in the development of the individual is an outgrowth of an earlier stage. During the first year babies babble; as they grow, they begin to say simple words. The toddler uses words in phrases, and the preschooler uses words in short sentences. No child speaks clearly before babbling, and each stage in the sequence can surely be anticipated.

Continuity. Growth and development continue from the moment of conception until the individual reaches maturity, but at no time is growth even and regular. Spurts and rest periods occur within the same child even though no real interruptions occur until growth is completed. Growth is greatest during the prenatal period and is still rapid during babyhood (infancy) and early childhood. The rate is slow but constant in middle childhood. It shows a spurt during early puberty and then tapers off in the latter part of puberty.

Differences in growth rates. All children have their own unique growth timetables. A child who develops rapidly at first will continue to do so. Jimmy sat unaided at 6 months of age and walked alone at 9 months of age. His brother John sat unaided at 8 months and walked alone at 15 months. Even in the same family no two children grow at the same rate.

Variation of growth rates for different body structures. Not all parts of the body mature at the same time. The brain attains its adult size when the child is about 6 or 7 years of age, but it certainly does not attain organization until many years later. Different phases of physical and mental growth occur at their own individual rates and reach maturity at different times.

Growth and development as a total process. The child does not grow physically one day and mentally the next day, but grows physically, mentally, socially, and emotionally at the same time. The child develops as a whole being. Changes in interest and mental growth are closely related to growth in walking and talking. Growth is a total process involving the whole child, not just the body, mind, or emotions. Each child passes slowly and almost imperceptibly from stage to stage, preserving a patterned integration of behavior throughout life.

GENETIC AND ENVIRONMENTAL INFLUENCES AND LIMITATIONS

Every child's growth and development (pattern, rate, rhythm, and extent) are governed by genetic and environmental forces. Within the broad categories of genetic and environmental influences may be found overlapping and diverse factors such as sex differences, endocrine gland function, racial ancestry, cellular mutations, and other inherited strengths and weaknesses; psychologic and cultural milieu, nutritional and physical advantages or disadvantages; and intercurrent malformation or disease. For many years controversy raged regarding the respective importance of genetics and environment, or "nature versus nurture." Today this interest has been somewhat tempered, and most writers in the field contend that both are important and try to determine ways that both can be improved to enhance the individual and society. The first main category to be discussed is that of genetics.

Genetic influences

A child's cellular inheritance and early embryonic growth may be a lifetime asset or a continuing liability. About one fourth of all hospitalized children have diseases or defects with genetic components. The science of genetics is based on principles of inheritance first described in the mid-1880s by the Augustinian monk scientist, Gregor Mendel. Mendel's law explains certain aspects of gene activity in humans during the formation of gametes (eggs and sperm) and during fertilization (the union of an egg and spermatozoon).

Genes, the ultimate and, as yet, invisible particles of inheritance, are strands of deoxyribonucleic acid (DNA) in structures called chromosomes, which are found in every cell's nucleus. Twenty-three chromosomes from each parent, combining to make a total of 46, endow the offspring at fertilization. Each of 22 chromosomes donated by one parent has a microscopically similar counterpart that is donated by the other parent. These chromosomic counterparts can be paired whether the developing individual is a boy or a girl. They are called *autosomes*. Each pair of autosomal chromosomes is different in its genetic content and appearance. Two other, different chromosomes, labeled X and Y, determine sex. They are called *sex chromosomes*. Each parent donates only one. The mother is able to contribute only an X chromosome, while the father may give to his child either an X or a Y chromosome. Babies having an XX inheritance are girls; those with XY are boys.

Genetic problems are of three major types: (1) mendelian patterns of inheritance involving only one or two defective genes; (2) multifactorial disorders related to multiple gene defects and environmental factors; and (3) gross genetic imbalances caused by chromosomal abnormalities. Defects in chromosomal structure or numbers can be considered *packaging* defects. The chromosomes are the "packages" that carry the genes from generation to generation. Defects in individual genes—the *contents* of these packages—are not evident on inspection of the chromosomes themselves but are evidenced by disease and abnormalities in the affected person.

A brief discussion of the various modes of inheritance will provide the student with an understanding of the basic characteristics associated with each inheritance pattern.

The Mendelian disorders may be subdivided into four distinct patterns of inheritance listed further below. Each involves one or two defective genes. In order to observe the distribution pattern of a specific trait in a family, it is essential to have detailed background information of the child's relatives. The construction of a chart that utilizes standard symbols to designate family members, their relationships, and other pertinent information is called a pedigree or "family tree." Pedigrees are valuable in helping to demonstrate the various

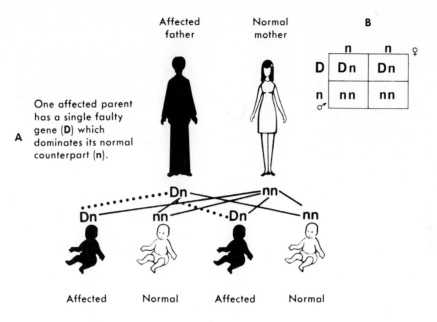

Affected father   Normal mother

One affected parent has a single faulty gene (**D**) which dominates its normal counterpart (**n**).

A

Affected   Normal   Affected   Normal

Each child's chances of inheriting either the **D** or the **n** from the affected parent are 50%.

FIG. 16-1   **A**, Dominant inheritance. **B**, Different method of expressing probability of dominant inheritance exemplified in **A**.

A courtesy The National Foundation–March of Dimes.

modes of inheritance for a given disorder in a particular family. By reviewing various genetic pedigrees, it has been established that certain disorders thought to be transmitted in a specific manner may not be. For example, a disorder called osteogenesis imperfecta may be transmitted in either a recessive or a dominant pattern. A pedigree will then be most helpful in determining the type of inheritance patterns present.

Two terms are often used to describe an individual's gene inheritance from each of his parents. They are *heterozygous* and *homozygous*. When a specific gene controlling certain characteristics is contributed by one parent, while the other parent donates a nonmatching gene for the characteristic, the inheritance for that trait is said to be heterozygous. If both parents donate matching genes, it is said to be homozygous.

AUTOSOMAL DOMINANT INHERITANCE

An autosomal dominant genetic disorder will express itself even though the defect is limited to a single gene on one of two paired autosomal chromosomes. It is usually found that one parent will have a single gene defect that dominates its normal gene partner (an example of heterozygous dominant inheritance). As the parent will either give the normal or abnormal gene to the offspring, each of that parent's children has a 50% chance of being affected. Males and females are affected equally, and if the offspring does not inherit the dominant gene, then that person will not transmit the trait or disorder. Usually the first affected individual in a family is a new mutation. This genetic change, depending on the individual's reproductivity, will either be transmitted to the next generation or will end with the original person affected (Fig. 16-1).

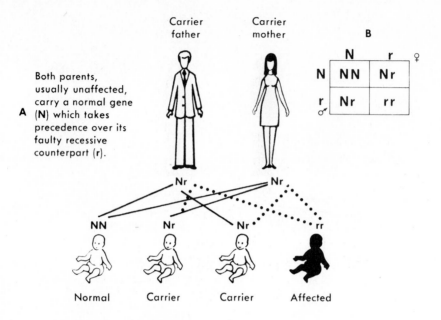

A, Recessive inheritance. **B,** Different method of expressing probability of recessive inheritance exemplified in **A.**

FIG. 16-2

A courtesy The National Foundation—March of Dimes.

AUTOSOMAL RECESSIVE INHERITANCE

Autosomal recessive disorders are expressed only when the individual has two affected paired genes for the particular disorder (homozygous inheritance). Since both parents contribute one gene for each trait, these disorders are inherited from both parents. Most often, the parents are carriers of one abnormal gene that is dominated by its normal paired gene. The parents have an essentially normal appearance and, as a result, are unaware of the gene's presence until an offspring inherits both genes and is affected. It should be emphasized that the probability of having a child with an autosomal recessive disorder increases when the parents share a common ancestor and thus share a

common gene pool. This is referred to as *consanguinity*. Males and females are affected with an equal frequency. Each child has a 25% chance of being affected, a 50% chance of being a carrier, and a 25% chance of not inheriting the gene from either parent. Affected children whose mates do not carry this gene will have unaffected children who will all be carriers of the gene. (See Fig. 16-2.)

X-LINKED INHERITANCE

Each individual has two sex chromosomes that differ from the autosomal chromosomes in that they are not alike in both sexes (males = XY, females = XX). A female may be homozygous for genes located on the two X chromosomes, but a male can only

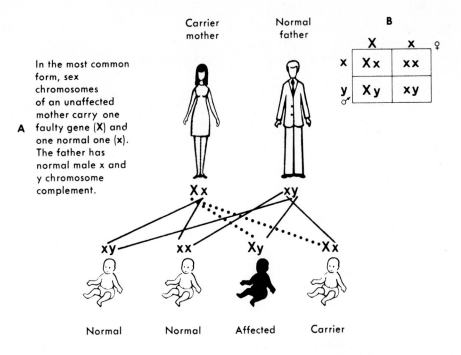

In the most common form, sex chromosomes of an unaffected mother carry one **A** faulty gene (**X**) and one normal one (**x**). The father has normal male x and y chromosome complement.

Carrier mother   Normal father

X x   x y

B

	X	x	♀
x	Xx	xx
y	Xy	xy

xy   xx   Xy   Xx

Normal   Normal   Affected   Carrier

The odds for each *male* child are 50/50:
1. A 50% risk of inheriting the faulty X and the disorder
2. A 50% chance of inheriting normal x and y chromosomes
For each *female* child, the odds are:
1. A 50% risk of inheriting one faulty X, to be a carrier like mother
2. A 50% chance of inheriting no faulty gene

FIG. 16-3   **A,** X-linked inheritance. **B,** Different method of expressing most common form of X-linked inheritance exemplified in **A.**

A courtesy The National Foundation–March of Dimes.

be heterozygous, because he carries only one X chromosome.

X-LINKED RECESSIVE INHERITANCE

X-linked recessive inheritance involves genes located on the X chromosome. The defective X-linked gene of an affected male must come from his mother, who is a carrier, because fathers give male offspring only a Y chromosome. A recessive X-linked gene in a female would usually be matched by a normal dominant gene on the paired X chro-

mosomes, and the disorder is not expressed. However, a male who inherits a recessive X-linked gene on his one X chromosome will always be affected, since there is never a matching gene on the Y. Females affected with an X-linked recessive disorder are rare, because they must carry affected genes on both their X chromosomes. Each male child of a female carrier has a 50% chance of being affected; each female offspring has a 50% chance of being a carrier. No male-to-male transmission occurs, but the female offspring of an affected male will all be carriers, since they inherit the father's only X chromosome with the defective recessive gene. Transmission occurs from one generation to the next with only males affected in the majority of families; a generation may be skipped if only females inherit the recessive gene and the males are unaffected. (See Fig. 16-3.)

X-LINKED DOMINANT INHERITANCE

In X-linked dominant disorders, females will be affected if they carry a single abnormal gene on one of the X chromosomes. The inheritance pattern of an X-linked dominant trait resembles autosomal dominant inheritance with one exception—the trait is transmitted from an affected male to all his daughters, but to none of his sons. An affected female's offspring will each have a 50% chance of being affected whether they are male or female. In X-linked dominant disorders, usually twice as many females as males are affected.

MULTIFACTORIAL INHERITANCE

Multifactorial disorders result from an interaction between multiple defective genes and the environment. A thorough analysis of the family pedigree will not reveal a distinctive mode of inheritance as with mendelian patterns of inheritance. However, the increased incidence rate for such disorders in relatives of affected persons, especially in identical twins, yields evidence of a genetic factor. The recurrence risk for the disorder depends upon the number of affected persons within a family, how closely related they are to the person seeking genetic counseling, and the sex of the affected individuals. It has been established that certain multifactorial disorders are more likely to occur in one sex than the other. A pedigree will demonstrate which people within a family are affected so that the recurrence risk may be established.

CHROMOSOMAL ABNORMALITIES

Recent developments now permit accurate identification of each chromosome by using a special staining technique that produces a characteristic banding pattern for each chromosomal pair. The standard systematized arrangement of chromosomes is called a karyotype. It is an orderly arrangement of an individual's autosomal and sex chromosomes according to size, shape, and banding pattern as they appear in cutouts of photographic enlargements (Fig. 16-4). Chromosomal disorders can be diagnosed in a cytogenetics laboratory by examining the chromosomal pattern of cells derived by culture of any of several body tissues. A leukocyte culture obtained from a blood sample is most often used. Syndromes are now being identified that are associated with specific chromosomal abnormalities. Chromosomal abnormalities result from: (1) various failures in the production of ova and sperm within the two gonads (meiosis), and (2) abnormal segregation of chromosomes during the first several mitotic divisions of body cells (mitosis). This would result in cells with different chromosomal numbers within one individual. This condition is called *mosaicism*.

One kind of chromosomal change that may be inherited involves the transfer of material between two chromosomes, called a *translocation*. In a balanced translocation, all the chromosomal material is present in the cell, although not located in its normal position; an unbalanced translocation occurs when a portion of the chromosomal material has been lost or additional material has been gained. This unbalanced condition usually is associated with serious defects in the individual. A parent carrying a balanced translocation, although normal, is at risk for having offspring with an unbalanced translocation. The pedigree may be used to help identify those persons affected with an unbalanced translocation. It would be recommended that such persons have a chromosome analysis (karyotype) performed. Should they carry the translocation, each pregnancy may be monitored by means of an amniocentesis (see discussion on p. 47). The parents would then have the option of either continuing or terminating the pregnancy if the fetus was found to have an unbalanced chromosomal pattern.

Another chromosomal abnormality is related to

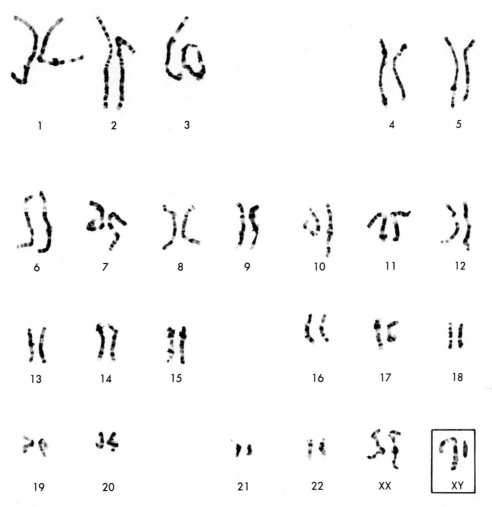

Courtesy of James Mascarello, Ph.D., Director of Genetic Services, Children's Hospital and Health Center, San Diego, Calif.

FIG. 16-4 High resolution G-banded human karyotype (female). The insert box shows the XY pair from a normal male.

nondisjunction of the chromosomes occurring when a chromosomal pair does not separate normally during formation of the sex cells in the ovary or testes (meiosis) or when body cells divide (mitosis). The offspring would then have a total chromosomal count of 47 rather than 46 per cell. This phenomenon is often related to advanced maternal age. The most common disorder resulting from this

process is one type of Down syndrome (trisomy 21). An extra chromosome at the number 21 position produces mental retardation and other physical deviations (see p. 263).

The most common chromosome abnormality is simply a change in total chromosome number. In general, reduction of the total number of autosomal chromosomes is incompatible with life. An increase

TABLE 16-2   PATTERNS OF INHERITANCE AND COMMON DISORDERS

Autosomal dominant inheritance	Achondroplastic dwarfism Huntington's chorea Neurofibromatosis
Autosomal recessive inheritance	Albinism Cystic fibrosis Phenylketonuria Sickle cell disease Tay-Sachs disease
X-linked recessive inheritance	Duchenne's muscular dystrophy Hemophilia Hurler's syndrome
X-linked dominant inheritance	Vitamin D–resistant rickets
Multifactorial inheritance	Cleft lip, cleft palate Clubfoot Congenital heart disease Dislocated hip Pyloric stenosis Spina bifida Anencephaly
Chromosomal abnormalities	Klinefelter's syndrome (XXY) Trisomy 13 Trisomy 18 Trisomy 21 (Down syndrome) Turner's syndrome (XO)

in total number of autosomes results in multiple physical abnormalities, mental retardation, and often a limited life span. Numerical disorders of the sex chromosomes may also be present. One condition characterized by a complete chromosome loss (45 instead of 46) that supports life is Turner's syndrome, coded as 45 XO, indicating that one X chromosome is missing. (See Table 16-2.)

Genetic counseling

Although individual birth defects may seem to be relatively rare (4% to 5% of all births), the total number of families affected is well into the millions. About 250,000 American babies are born each year with mild to severe physical or mental defects. With each passing year more disorders are identified as genetic problems, thereby increasing the known incidence of hereditary disease.

The genetic counselor is one who is capable of communicating to the parents the magnitude of, the implications of, and the alternatives for dealing with the risk of occurrence of hereditary disorders within a family. Unfortunately, most genetic counseling is occasioned by the birth of a defective child. Much care, sympathy, understanding, and insight into human nature are necessary to communicate effectively all the implications and possible options of a genetic disorder.

Using pedigree studies, modern laboratory detection techniques (such as blood tests, enzyme assays, amniocentesis, and chromosome analysis), and knowledge of basic laws of heredity and incidence statistics, the genetic counselor can often predict the probability of recurrence of a given abnormality in a family. The primary aim is to prevent genetic defects or, when that is impossible, at least to reduce their damaging effects to the minimum. Genetic counseling is a form of preventive medicine. It stresses genetic information: diagnosis, prognosis, presentation of odds for recurrence, and the effect of genetic diseases on the family. It is a field with its own body of knowledge and requiring its own expertise. Because a wide range of laboratory resources and consultative skills are frequently required, genetic counseling is best organized on a group basis in large medical centers. A list of genetic counseling centers throughout the United States is sent to physicians or to the general public free on request to the Professional Educational Department of the National Foundation–March of Dimes (see also p. 33).

Environmental influences

Although the impact of a child's genetic background is great, another modifying force exerts an important influence on growth and development—environment. Examples of environmental factors include the family composition, interrelationships, culture and life-styles, the degree and type of accessibility and stimulation offered by the primary caretakers to the inquisitive infant and young child, health habits, nutrition, and the presence of malformation or disease. A child not only interprets his environment in terms of inherited tendencies and mental ability but also in terms of health and emotional balance. A strong, happy child will make the best use of his environment and will be most able to deal with obstacles or defects in his surroundings.

Home and family. To develop naturally and wholesomely, the child needs devoted care and a family setting that is loving, accepting, and understanding. Such a home ideally supplies the growing child with more than the physical necessities. It provides positive, helpful, broad maternal and paternal role models. It fosters respect for the individual not on the basis of beauty or intelligence (over which the child may have little control) but according to the child's attitudes, behavior, and willingness to accept and complete appropriate responsibilities. It increases the sense of personal esteem in ways that allow the child to seek experiences and enjoy new opportunities and challenges. The psychologic nurture given in the home is as important as its physical support. Lack of real affection alone will result in little or no smiling, loss of appetite, poor sleep, failure to gain weight, and persistent respiratory tract infections. Numerous studies indicate that children deprived of love and the kindly stimulation of the home fail to thrive.*

Nutrition. The growing child is vulnerable to many nutritional inadequacies. Disturbed patterns of skeletal development caused by the lack or overabundance of one nutrient exemplify the need for balance. Lack of protein during the prenatal period and early infancy may limit the number and size of brain cells. A well-balanced diet is essential for the development of bones and teeth, good skin, resistance to disease caused by dietary deficiency and infections, and general physical well-being. Clarifi-

cation of the nutritional needs of children and the general abundance of high-quality foods have simplified the feeding of infants and children. Despite this, nutritional inadequacies may occur in the midst of plenty through faulty dietary habits, food fads, or psychic tensions centering around mealtime and the feeding situation.

Overnutrition rather than undernutrition seems to present more problems in the United States. However, a severe form of protein deprivation, kwashiorkor, is common in underdeveloped countries of South America and Africa. Kwashiorkor is found among children under 4 years of age. It typically manifests itself after a child is weaned because of the birth of a younger sibling. Characteristically these children lag in growth and in skeletal development. (For more information regarding nutritional needs see pp. 364 to 373.)

Disease. Illness is both a physical and a psychologic hazard for the young child. Arrested growth is the obvious effect of fever and anorexia. Prolonged illness causes a definite decrease in the rate of growth and height as well as decreased ability to function. Any disease that interferes with physical activity and metabolic processes over a long period will deter normal progress. Although some growth loss may occur during a minor illness, a subsequent growth spurt will compensate for the temporary setback.

Uncontrolled diabetes always results in retarded growth in both height and weight. Chronic heart disability associated with hypoxia hampers growth, as do malabsorption syndromes such as cystic fibrosis and celiac disease.

Growth and development depend on each other and represent a continuous process of interactions between genetic potential on one hand and environment on the other. The kind of environment children live in will determine whether or not they will realize all their inborn capacities for physical, social, mental, and emotional growth. Although nothing can make children do more than their inborn capacities permit, they must have a favorable environment to develop and learn as fast as their growth patterns allow.

---

*Brady, S: Patterns of mothering, New York, 1956, International Universities Press, Inc., p. 97.

PHYSICAL GROWTH

Although all phases of growth are continuous and take place concurrently, for convenience and clarity discussions of the main aspects of growth and development will be presented separately. Since physical growth is most obvious, it shall be discussed first.

Physical growth may be divided into four well-defined periods:

1. The period of very rapid growth during babyhood
2. The period of slow, steady growth during childhood years
3. The period of the growth spurt during puberty
4. The period of decreasing growth and attainment of maximum height

The greatest increase in extrauterine growth occurs during the early part of babyhood. Small, steady gains continue during the slow periods. This general pattern of growth is characteristic of all the body systems with two exceptions. The nervous system grows rapidly during infancy, then decelerates, and after puberty ceases growing; the reproductive organs, however, grow very slowly until sexual maturation, which occurs during the pubertal spurt.

Tables of average height and weight are commonly used to show that a boy or girl of a particular age should approximate a certain height and weight within a certain number of pounds. In the course of development, observable trends in height and weight imply that one can draw certain conclusions regarding these aspects of growth. Regarding growth, norms can be successfully determined for a group of children and may serve as a point of reference for making comparisons. However, any table of averages should be interpreted with caution. Although these tables may accurately state averages, they do not necessarily state what is desirable for individuals. The National Center for Health Statistics (NCHS) has constructed some growth charts for infants and children in the United States showing weight, length, weight for various lengths, and head circumference (Fig. 16-5). Clinical use of the charts can immediately show how the growth of any child ranks in comparison with the rest of the United States' child population of the same age and sex. Their primary use is to detect nutritional and growth disturbances clinically.

The best method of evaluating a child's general growth progress is by comparing the child with himself from time to time. A large number of observations and measurements recorded periodically demonstrates the individuality of the child's own progress.

Height

Infants average about 20 inches in length at birth. During the first year of life the child grows about 10 inches. Five inches are added during the second year, and the child grows 3 inches a year during the preschool period. From the sixth to the tenth year of life the annual gain is reduced to approximately 2 inches. The maximum growth in height occurs during the pubertal period at the approximate time of sexual maturity. Growth in height reaches a peak for boys at about 14 years of age and a year or so earlier for girls. It ceases sometime before the twenties.

Puberty occurs at widely different ages. An early pubertal growth spurt is associated with an early cessation of growth. Individuals who mature late tend to grow for a longer period of time and ultimately become tall adults.

Weight

At birth the infant weighs about 7½ pounds. This weight doubles by the end of the fifth month of life, and by 1 year the birth weight has approximately tripled. A sharp drop in the rate of gain occurs after the first year. The child characteristically appears lanky and even skinny. During the preschool years the weight rises slowly, averaging about 5 pounds each year. *Text continued on p. 315.*

GIRLS: BIRTH TO 36 MONTHS
PHYSICAL GROWTH
NCHS PERCENTILES*

NAME ______________________ RECORD # ____________

A

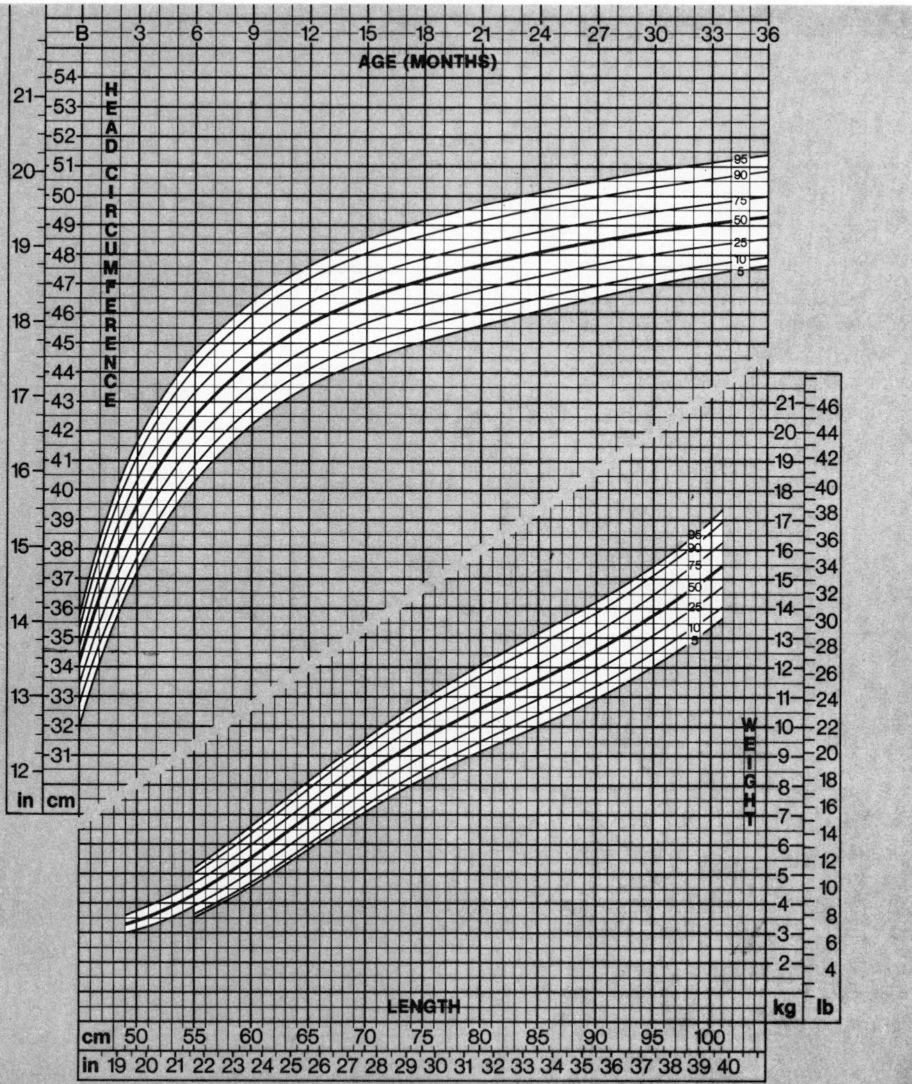

*Adapted from: National Center for Health Statistics: NCHS Growth Charts, 1976. Monthly Vital Statistics Report. Vol. 25, No. 3, Supp. (HRA) 76-1120. Health Resources Administration, Rockville, Maryland, June, 1976. Data from The Fels Research Institute, Yellow Springs, Ohio.

DATE	AGE	LENGTH	WEIGHT	HEAD C.
	BIRTH			

DATE	AGE	LENGTH	WEIGHT	HEAD C.

Continued.

FIG. 16-5 **A** to **D,** These charts were constructed with data from the National Center for Health Statistics, U.S. Public Health Service. The data on these charts are considered representative of the general United States population.

Reproduced with permission from Ross Laboratories.

GIRLS: BIRTH TO 36 MONTHS
PHYSICAL GROWTH
NCHS PERCENTILES*

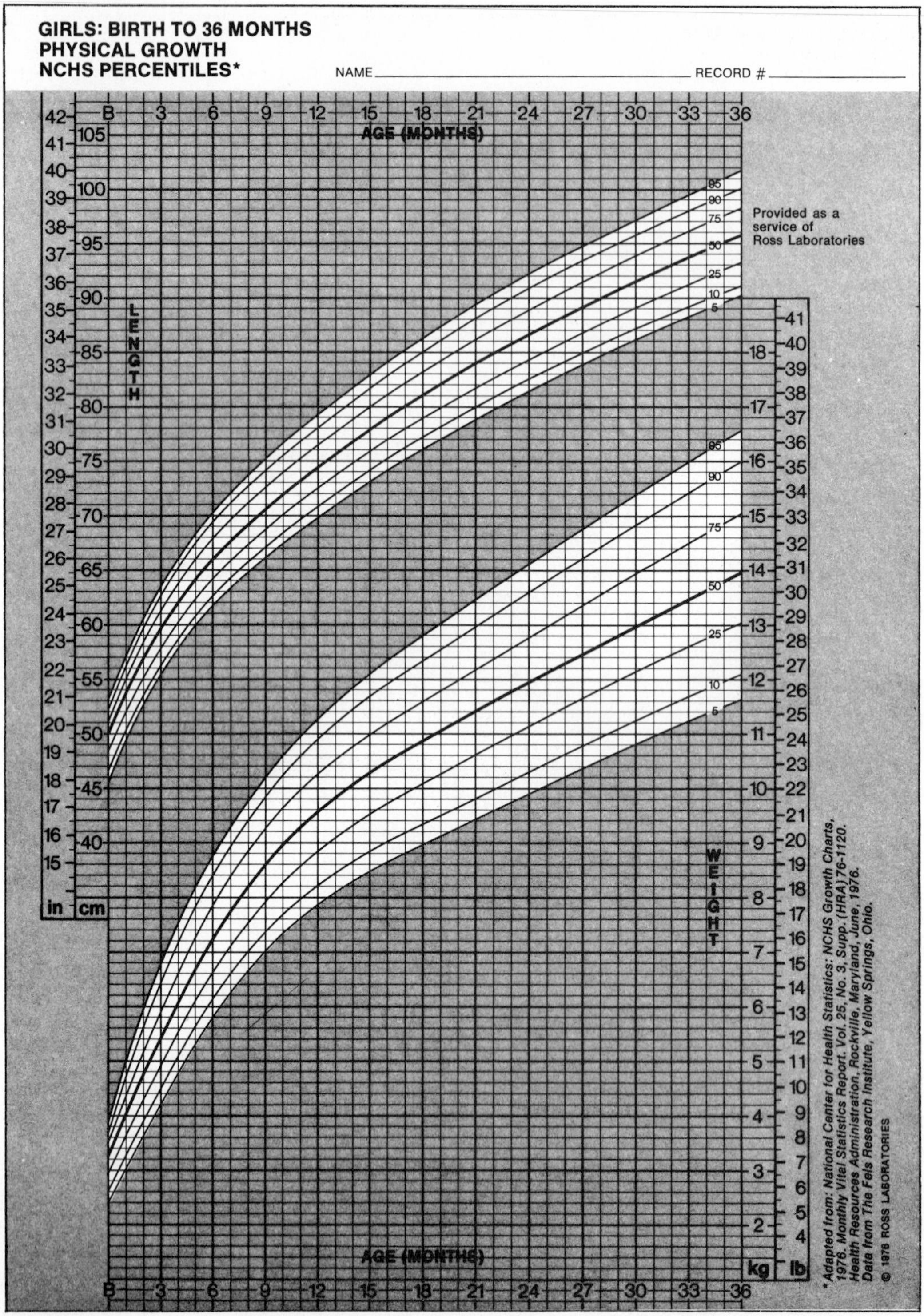

FIG. 16-5,
cont'd

For legend see p. 311.

C

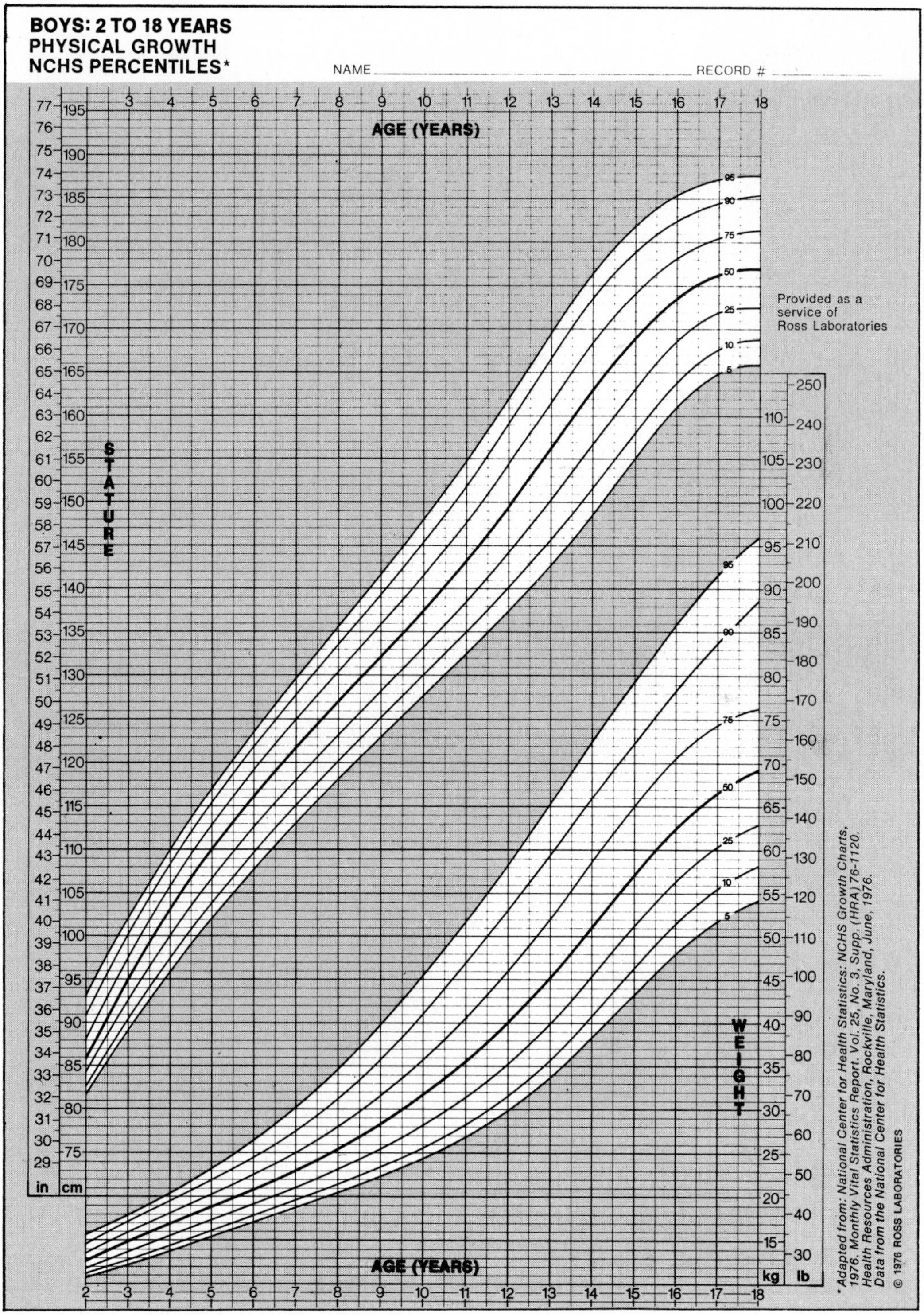

BOYS: 2 TO 18 YEARS
PHYSICAL GROWTH
NCHS PERCENTILES*
NAME
RECORD #
AGE (YEARS)
STATURE
WEIGHT
in
cm
kg
lb
95
90
75
50
25
10
5
Provided as a service of Ross Laboratories
*Adapted from: National Center for Health Statistics: NCHS Growth Charts, 1976. Monthly Vital Statistics Report. Vol. 25, No. 3, Supp. (HRA) 76-1120. Health Resources Administration, Rockville, Maryland, June, 1976. Data from the National Center for Health Statistics.
© 1976 ROSS LABORATORIES

Continued.

FIG. 16-5, cont'd

For legend see p. 311.

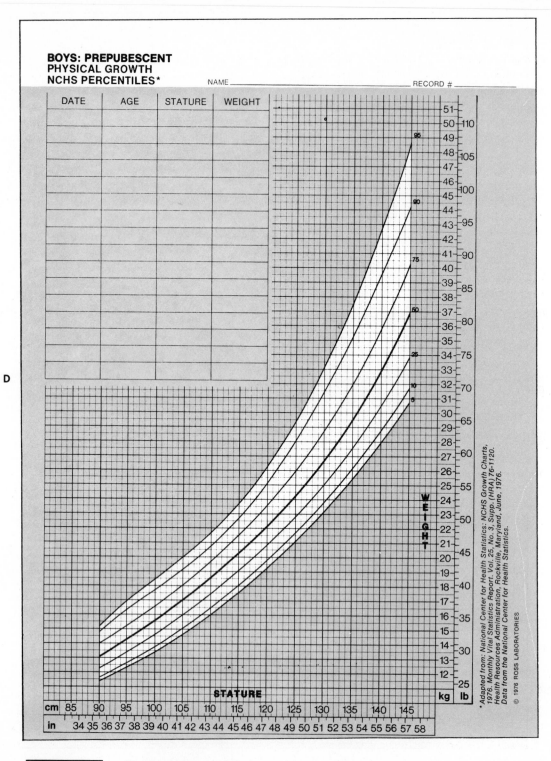

BOYS: PREPUBESCENT
PHYSICAL GROWTH
NCHS PERCENTILES*

NAME _____ RECORD # _____

D

* Adapted from: National Center for Health Statistics: NCHS Growth Charts, 1976. Monthly Vital Statistics Report. Vol. 25, No. 3, Supp. (HRA) 76-1120. Health Resources Administration, Rockville, Maryland, June, 1976. Data from the National Center for Health Statistics.

FIG. 16-5, cont'd

For legend see p. 311.

During the school years the weight gain is slightly increased. Weight varies more than height, since it is readily susceptible to external factors such as dietary intake.

Generally boys are taller and heavier than girls except in the years preceding puberty. A rapid gain in weight usually occurs in both sexes during puberty, corresponding closely with the gain in height. Girls begin their preadolescent growth spurt at about 10 to 12 years of age, 2 years earlier than boys. Girls also reach their adult proportions sooner than boys.

Body proportions (Fig. 16-6)

Distinct changes in body proportions occur between birth and maturity. The small child not only differs from the adult in size but also in body form. At birth the head is relatively large, about one fourth of the total body length, whereas in the adult it is about one eighth to one tenth of the body length. An infant's arms and legs are relatively short. During infancy the trunk is longer than the extremities. The midpoint of the total length of the infant is at the umbilicus, whereas in the adult it is at the symphysis pubis.

During puberty, adult proportions are attained, and the characteristic mature body shape for each sex becomes differentiated. The straight leg lines of the young girl become curved by 15 years of age. Her hips grow wider, but her shoulders remain narrow. The boy's shoulders become broader, whereas his hips remain narrow.

Body proportion and build, or physique, is unique to the individual. Within the individual's own general pattern—slender, stocky, muscular— each child's body seems to be constant.

Bone formation

During the early days of fetal development, bones begin as simple connective tissue. Later this tissue becomes cartilage. By the end of the fifth month of gestation, certain mineral salts, especially calcium phosphate, are deposited in the cartilage, causing it to harden. Cartilage is gradually replaced by bone; this process is called *ossification*. During the early years of life, cartilage persists between the diaphysis (shaft) and epiphyses (ends) of long bones. Bones grow in length by a continual thickening of the epiphyseal cartilage.

As the child grows, changes occur in the texture, size, and shape of the "old" bones, and new bones appear. The process of skeletal maturation is perhaps the best evidence of general growth. Bone development continues in an orderly sequence and is completed by the third decade of life.

Bone age can be determined by x-ray examination of certain joints. The information gained is compared with a standard. The x-ray films are studied to detect the following:

1. The appearance of new bones
2. Changes in the contour of the ends of bones
3. The union of the epiphyses with the bone shaft

Growth of the long bones is complete when the epiphyses and diaphysis are fused.

Bone development of the hand and wrist is a good index of the individual's progress in skeletal growth. Since boys lag behind girls in bone development at all ages, separate standards are used.

At birth the ends of the arm bones (epiphyses) are not developed, and the carpal bones are not present (Fig. 16-7). Shortly after, the carpal bones and epiphyses gradually appear, and changes in the size and contour of the ends of bones continue through the school years. Bone development of the wrist and hand is complete at the seventeenth year of life for girls and 2 years later for boys.

Tooth formation (Fig. 16-8)

The foundation of a child's tooth structure is formed early in fetal life. At birth all the primary (deciduous or baby) teeth and the first permanent teeth (6-year molars) are developing in the child's jaw. Dentition is widely varied.

It is not always possible to predict exactly when

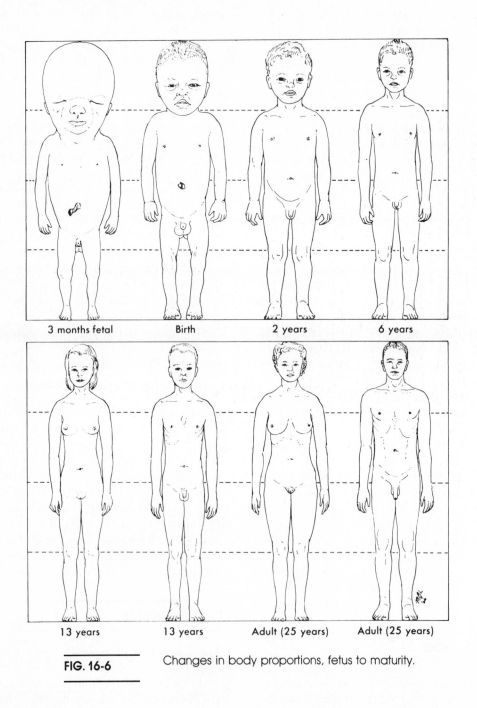

3 months fetal   Birth   2 years   6 years

13 years   13 years   Adult (25 years)   Adult (25 years)

FIG. 16-6   Changes in body proportions, fetus to maturity.

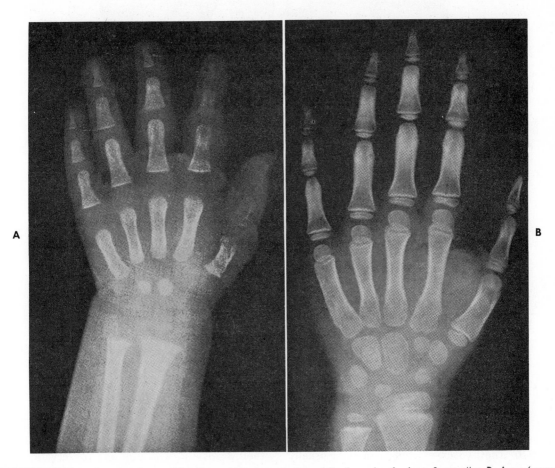

FIG. 16-7   Progressive ossification of the hand of a white female. **A,** Age 3 months. **B,** Age 6 years 3 months.

From Todd, T.W.: Atlas of skeletal maturation, St. Louis, 1937, The C.V. Mosby Co.

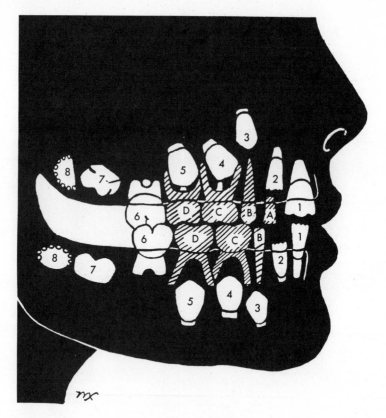

FIG. 16-8   Illustration of 7-year-old child with good occlusion. Primary teeth: *A,* lateral incisors; *B,* cuspids; *C,* first molars; *D,* second molars. Permanent teeth; *1,* central incisors; *2,* lateral incisors; *3,* cuspids; *4,* first bicuspids; *5,* second bicuspids; *6,* first molars; *7,* second molars; *8,* site of wisdom teeth.

the first tooth will erupt, but it is possible to predict with some accuracy which teeth will erupt first (Table 16-3). The two lower central incisors usually appear first, between 5 and 7 months of age. The upper central incisors appear next. Most children have six teeth at 1 year of age and all 20 primary teeth by 2½ years of age.

Wide variation occurs in the pattern of tooth shedding and permanent tooth eruption. Before the appearance of the first molars (6-year molars), all the permanent teeth are growing and maturing. During this time the roots of the primary teeth are disappearing by the process of resorption. Only the crown of the primary tooth is left when the permanent tooth below is ready to erupt. The loose crown then drops out. The care and preservation of the primary teeth are important. Unless they are beyond repair, primary teeth should not be pulled out. They contribute in large measure to proper alignment and good health of the permanent teeth.

Tetracycline antibiotics have an adverse effect on newly formed bones. The drug stains developing teeth with a yellow-brown material. Tetracyclines also cross the placenta. After the fourth month of gestation, the primary teeth of the developing fetus

TABLE 16-3 USUAL PATTERN OF DENTITION

Teeth	Lower (mandibular) appear at age	Upper (maxillary) appear at age
PRIMARY		
Central incisors	5 to 7 months	6 to 8 months
Lateral incisors	12 to 15 months	8 to 11 months
Cuspids (canines)	16 to 20 months	16 to 20 months
First molars	10 to 16 months	10 to 16 months
Second molars	20 to 30 months	20 to 30 months
Total per jaw—10		
Total—20		
PERMANENT		
Central incisors	6 to 7 years	6 to 7 years
Lateral incisors	7 to 9 years	8 to 9 years
Cuspids (canines)	8 to 11 years	11 to 12 years
First bicuspids	10 to 12 years	10 to 11 years
Second bicuspids	11 to 13 years	10 to 12 years
First molars (6-year molars)	6 to 7 years	6 to 7 years
Second molars (12-year molars)	12 to 13 years	12 to 13 years
Third molars (wisdom teeth)	17 to 22 years	17 to 22 years
Total set—32		

are also affected. Such discoloration of the teeth may be avoided by *not using* the drugs during pregnancy and the first 10 years of life.

MOTOR DEVELOPMENT

As children's bodies grow they acquire the ability to function in increasingly complex ways. Motor changes accompany physical growth. Motor abilities involve various types of body movements that result from the coordinated activity of nerves and muscles. Maturation of the nervous system and learning are interrelated in the acquisition of motor abilities.

Motor development is the process of learning, controlling, and integrating muscular responses.

Great advances in body control and locomotion are accomplished during the first 2 years of life. At first an uncoordinated, helpless infant, the child is soon able to sit, stand, walk, reach, and grasp.

Like other phases of growth, motor development unfolds in an orderly sequence that is closely related to the maturation of the nervous system. It follows a definite sequence. Characteristically motor development begins in the head region of the individual and moves downward toward the feet (cephalocaudal). Development also tends to proceed from the center of the body toward the extremities (proximodistal). At first motor response to stimulation (such as an ice cube touching the foot) is diffuse, involving the whole body. As maturation proceeds, the response becomes more specific and may involve only the withdrawal of the foot. The sequence of motor development is similar for all children, but the rate at which the development progresses varies with each individual child.

Prehension and locomotion provide examples of the usual sequences in the course of motor development.

Prehension

The development of the ability to oppose the thumb to the fingers in picking up an object is preceded by reaching, grasping, and raking movements. Early attempts in reaching also involve eye-hand coordination. Effective use of the hands for picking up small objects or for grasping is called prehension. The developmental sequence proceeds from eye-hand coordination in grasping to reaching without looking, from large muscle activity of the arms and shoulders to fine muscle activity of the fingers, and from a crude pawing closure to a closure of the fingertips in a refined fashion.

Gesell tested prehension by placing a little red cube before a baby. He described the grasping sequence as follows. (See Fig. 16-9.)

Development progression in grasping

12 weeks	Looks at cube
20 weeks	Looks and approaches
24 weeks	Looks and crudely grasps with whole hand
36 weeks	Looks and deftly grasps with fingers
52 weeks	Looks, grasps with forefinger and thumb, and deftly releases
15 months	Looks, grasps, and releases to build a tower of two cubes*

Locomotion

The ability to walk alone is also attained gradually after a sequence of developments that can be traced to the first days of life. Moving from place to place and walking are examples of gross motor skills. Complete establishment of this control usu-

*From Gesell, A., and Ilg, L.B.: The child from five to ten, New York, 1946, Harper & Row, Publishers.

ally takes most of the first year for early walkers and about 15 months for those who mature later.

The walking sequence begins when the baby is able to hold his head up, and it is half accomplished when the baby can sit alone. When an infant is able to change from a prone to a sitting position, he tends to begin to creep. The infant usually creeps to an object or person and pulls up to a standing position. Gradually the baby stands alone and finally walks independently.

The motor sequence (Fig. 16-10)

½	to 1	month	Lifts head
2	to 3	months	Raises chest
3	to 4	months	Turns from side to back
5	to 6	months	Sits with support
6	to 7	months	Rolls from back to abdomen
6½	to 7½	months	Sits alone
8	to 9	months	Creeps
9	to 11	months	Pulls self up
11	to 12	months	Walks with help
12	to 14	months	Walks alone

Prehension and locomotion develop independent of any teaching. Knowledge of these motor abilities "just comes." Each skill follows an orderly sequential course whose rate may be affected by environmental factors.

As each skill develops, opportunity to use and practice it is necessary. This means that the child needs plenty of space for walking, objects to pick up and handle, and most of all the child needs health, vigor, freedom, and encouragement to venture. The nurse who understands the development of motor skills will not restrict the child to his crib but will encourage the child's full capacity for motor growth.

INTELLECTUAL DEVELOPMENT

Of all the factors influencing the overall development of the child, intelligence seems to be the most important. Superior intelligence is associated with superior development, whereas inferior intelligence is associated with retarded development.

Intelligence, defined as the ability to solve prob-

FIG. 16-9

Developmental progression of prehensory behavior.

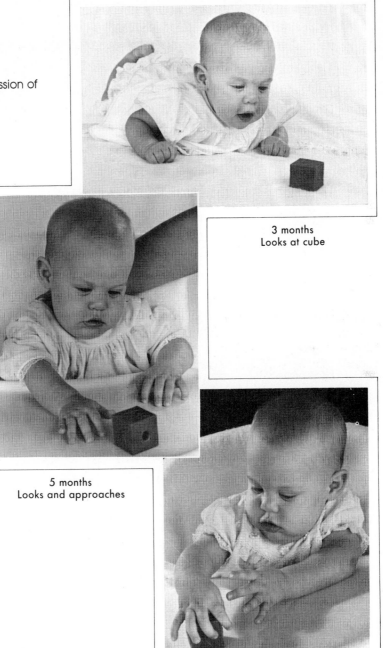

3 months
Looks at cube

5 months
Looks and approaches

6 months
Looks and crudely grasps with whole hand

Continued.

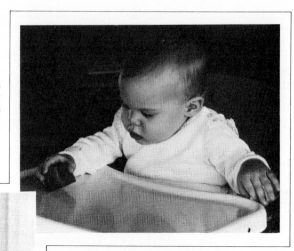

9 months
Looks and deftly
grasps with fingers

12 months
Looks, grasps with
forefinger and thumb,
and deftly releases

15 months
Looks, grasps, and releases,
to build a tower of two blocks

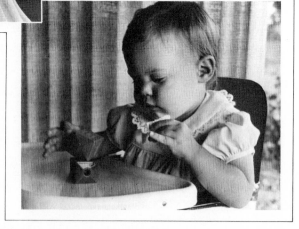

**FIG. 16-9,
cont'd**

See p. 321 for legend.

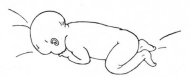

Birth
Keeps his legs tucked up under him and bears his weight on his knees, abdomen, chest, and head.

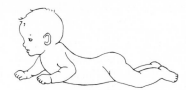

2-3 months
Extends his legs and lifts his chest and head to look around.

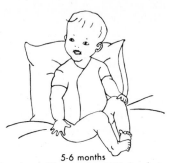

5-6 months
Can sit up with support, hold his head up, and is alert to surroundings.

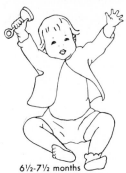

6½-7½ months
Sits up alone and steadily without support. Legs are bowed to help balance.

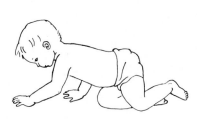

8-9 months
Creeping; the trunk is carried free from floor. With practice, rhythm appears and only one limb moves at a time.

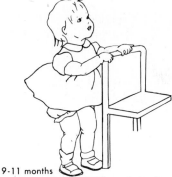

9-11 months
Pulls himself up and stands holding onto furniture. Feet far apart, head and upper trunk carried forward.

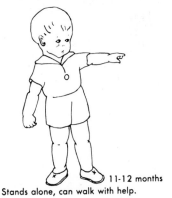

11-12 months
Stands alone, can walk with help.

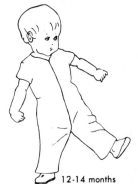

12-14 months
Walks alone on wide base with legs far apart.

FIG. 16-10   Guideposts in motor development, emphasizing the average child.

lems or achieve a goal, will affect the child's observation, thought, and understanding. It strongly influences the level of difficulty at which the child is able to function efficiently and the scope of his activities.

Many changes take place in the intellectual life of children as they develop from infancy to adulthood. At birth the centers of higher intellectual activity in the brain are not fully developed. Furthermore, the sensory acuity necessary for these higher intellectual functions is likewise immature. The mental world of the newborn infant seems to consist primarily of experiences arising through direct physical contact with the environment and through the sensations that originate within the child's own body. New experiences expand the individual's mental world and are interpreted in the light of previous learning. Although it is not readily detected by casual observers, the length of a behavior labeled "habituation" has been said to be predictive of an infant's intelligence. Habituation is defined as the period of time that elapses between the infant's initial response and the cessation of that response to a repeated stimulus. The duration of a child's response is measured by skin electrode and an assessment of motor activity. The shorter the habituation, the higher the intellectual potential. Do infants who demonstrate rapid habituation investigate more? No one knows. Watching intently is an important primary skill.

Beginning very early, children exhibit the ability to imagine and to engage in make-believe activities, which aid in exploring the real world, organizing experiences, and solving problems. Through make-believe, children are able to participate in a wider range of experiences and partially overcome their own limitations. Such fantasies are a necessary and normal part of learning.

As growth proceeds, the ability to concentrate develops. Children's attention spans are likely to be longer during activities that they have chosen or that are at least related to their own desires.

The development of a child's ability to reason is gradual and continuous. Young children are concerned with events related to their own immediate experience and well-being. As they grow, they become increasingly able to occupy themselves with more remote issues and deal with abstractions. Such changes can be noted in connection with the enlargement of the meanings associated with various terms in the language individual children use, the interest and ability they eventually display in facing social issues, and their ability to relate to events in the world beyond their immediate experience.

EMOTIONAL GROWTH

Every infant, child, and adult possesses the drive to express himself in some way. The reaction that accompanies either the satisfaction or frustration of a basic need may be termed an "emotion." Another way of describing an emotional response is to define it as a psychological reaction caused by internal or external stimuli. Although emotions are not identical to basic drives, they are related. The basic drives can be physical, social, intellectual, or personal. Emotional experience includes feelings, impulses, and physical and physiological reactions. For example, if a baby's needs are fulfilled, he is happy, joyful, contented, or loving; if a baby's drives are frustrated, he is anxious, fretful, frightened, or angry. Physiologic changes initiated by emotions may stimulate a person to violent action.

All emotions cause a physical response. But just as no two persons think or act alike, no two react to the same emotion in the same way. For example, because of fear one person may feel belligerent, another anxious, or still another depressed. As soon as one begins to experience emotion, physiologic changes take place. Manifestations of these changes include facial expressions, laughter, and crying.

Emotions appear early in life. Even during the first days of life the infant's need to satisfy his physical needs is accompanied by emotional response. The infant usually reacts by crying or kicking. Soon the baby finds a given stimulation pleasant or unpleasant. When the infant is hungry or uncomfortable, an unpleasant state results, which he makes known by crying or restlessness. When the infant's wants are satisfied, a pleasant state of well-being ensues, which is evidenced by cooing, gurgling, or sleep. Thus the emotional responses of the infant are initially stimulated by physiologic needs.

Through a combination of maturation and learning, more specialized responses soon occur. By the end of the first year, emotions of fear, rage, excitement, anger, and joy become recognizable, and facial expression, vocalization, and body movement become part of the child's emotional equipment. Changes in the expression of the emotions continue progressively throughout the childhood years.

Love. Love is the most important of all the emotions, because it is the foundation on which all positive relationships are built. Children's first love is centered on their mothers, since she usually is the one who initially loves and serves an infant. The child's capacity for affection and love develops gradually from this early association. During the normal course of development children transfer a part of their affection to other individuals who share their pleasures and achievements. Eventually this love will grow to form the nucleus of another family—the child's own. A child who receives loving and considerate care is prepared to give as well as receive love. For such children security is not simply a passive thing but a safe feeling that allows them to be venturesome in the belief that people will be good to them.

Fear. Fear is aroused naturally when infants experience any startling, sudden occurrence such as a loud noise, an unexpected jar, or a fall. They characteristically respond to these threats to their security with crying and general body distress. The young child acquires other fears that are associated with objects and persons in the immediate environment. As children become older, fearful responses become increasingly specific; they are expressed by withdrawal from the fearful situation. Later, children learn to avoid situations that cause anxiety.

Once a child becomes afraid in a certain situation, any repetition of the same or similar situation will reproduce fear. However, if the boy or girl learns that the situation is not truly hazardous, the fear diminishes or disappears. Parents and other adults should not laugh at or ridicule a child's fears—identified or unnamed as they may be—but help the child to understand the situation or thing that is frightening. Reasonable fear is a valuable safeguard against many dangers. Fear acts as a check on behavior. A person may be driven to action by anger, hate, or jealousy, but his conduct is held within reasonable bounds through the fear of consequences. In other words, fear may act as a negative guide to more orderly behavior.

Anger. Anger denotes a variety of emotional states that range from turbulent rage to milder forms of resentment. In infancy, anger arises primarily through interference with body movement or gratification of basic needs such as feeding. Crying, screaming, biting, hitting, and kicking are expressions of anger. In early childhood, anger may take the form of numerous acts of disobedience and resistance. When children learn to talk they gain command of new ways to express their anger. Children may find outbursts of anger useful for attracting attention to themselves and for obtaining a desired end. Children are even more likely to give vent to anger when suffering from lack of sleep, hunger, or fatigue.

Anger may be controlled in small children by guarding the child's general health and physical condition and by providing regular meals, sleep, and time with mother and father for pleasurable experiences. Feelings of anger may be frightening. Young children need to be reassured that these feelings are very common. However, they also need to be guided toward more appropriate means for expressing anger. They are likely to feel more secure when behavior such as "acting out," hitting, and biting are firmly limited by adults. Parents can also aid by maintaining poise and self-control, refusing to be manipulated by theatrical displays of emotion (temper tantrums), and encouraging a friendly home atmosphere.

Jealousy. Jealousy is an emotional response compounded of anger, fear, and love. It is an emotion that, in general, seems to arise when persons or objects threaten to take away something, share something, or interfere with that which is felt to belong to oneself. In the young child, jealousy tends to develop when the child is threatened by possible loss of love as a result of the presence of a newborn brother or sister. Because of the mother's preoccupation with the infant, the older child may equate loss of time and attention with loss of love. This child may see the younger sibling as a rival and become jealous. The reaction of the child may be positive and result in either aggression toward or competition with the new baby. Thus the jealous child may resort to hitting the baby or may turn to infantile habits to gain the desired attention. A negative reaction may consist of withdrawal from competition or repression. For example, a child may sulk or refuse meals. The expression of jealousy varies with age. Behavior caused by such personal envy gradually becomes less direct and less openly violent; it is more subtle but no less real.

The factors precipitating emotions and the reaction patterns they initiate have typical stages of development and can be traced just as the other stages of growth and development. The emotional responses of individuals not only vary in form and intensity from person to person but also from age to age. The emotions identified and the reactions they stimulate are closely related to the individual's maturity and life experience. Emotions always find an outlet; if the most desired expression is blocked, another, perhaps less desirable, is substituted. This observation has many practical applications and is basic to the understanding of many behavior problems and the concept of psychosomatic illness. Talking out problems and learning to communicate rather than "acting out" one's feelings or burying them in the subconscious, where they can cause physical and emotional problems, is extremely important.

SOCIAL BEHAVIOR AND MORAL VALUES

An individual's characteristic response to social situations is a useful way of describing personal-social behavior. Personal-social behavior includes all the modes of behavior that characterize the child's own individuality.

The dynamic interaction of a child's thoughts and feelings that produces a characteristic respose to the environment is called "personality." Personality includes one's intelligence, physique, habits, and appeal to others. As children grow older, their ways of responding become more and more characteristic of themselves. The first social group for a child is the family, a group that plays an important role in establishing attitudes and habits.

The major source of personality growth for the child resides in the maturity and harmony of the parents. The parents provide the models that the child consciously and unconsciously emulates. Home is the place where the child learns, even as a tiny infant, what people and life are like. At home children learn friendliness, confidence, security, belonging, loving, and sharing as these are reflected in the people in their immediate environment.

The awakening of social behavior manifests itself as the baby grows alert to its surroundings and is able to distinguish between persons and objects. During the first weeks of life infants react instinctively to their immediate surroundings and those persons, particularly their mothers, who care for them. Infants, who are primarily concerned with satisfying their basic needs, do not readily make distinctions between people and things. Soon, however, babies begin to respond to the presence of others and their behavior toward them. Babies' awareness of persons around them grows out of the simple responses they give as they care for the baby and supply his wants. For example, if a baby is handled gently and lovingly, its natural response will be a happy one such as cooing, smiling, or tranquil rest. If a baby is treated roughly with impatience, agitation, and frustration, he will respond accordingly, perhaps with fretful crying, kicking, or enraged screaming. Thus certain forms of social behavior begin to develop as children respond to those in contact with them.

Early in babyhood children learn to imitate adults, children, and other babies around them to become a part of the family or social group. At about 6 weeks of age the baby first imitates facial expressions, such as smiling and wincing. Gestures and movements such as waving "bye-bye," shaking the head, or throwing a kiss develop at approximately 6 months of age.

Happy, smiling children are a good indication that their social development is progressing well; the framework for this positive, outgoing nature is built most firmly by parents who have made their child feel loved in the early months and years of life. The way people work and play, their ability to enjoy other people, and how they feel about tackling new things (even the foods they prefer or will not touch) have had beginnings early in life's experience. People can change, but the effects of early childhood experiences are likely to persist throughout life.

Probably the most important medium of socialization is language. Socrates said, "Speak that I may see thee." The early vocalizations of the infant quickly develop from throaty noises at 4 weeks of age to three-word sentences at 2 years of age. Young babies rapidly recognize the urgency to verbalize as they become part of the social group. Although language at first consists of object naming and identification, it soon becomes a vehicle for the transportation of ideas. Hence hand in hand with language development goes the development of understanding.

In the first few weeks of life infants have no understanding of their environment. Gradually, as language ability increases as a result of maturation and learning, children become more able to understand what they observe. It is important to note, however, that no two children can be expected to have the same understanding of an object or situation, since no one has exactly the same intellectual abilities or experiences. If an infant is handicapped in sensory development through deafness or blindness, he will be handicapped in language growth and understanding. To the extent that a child is deprived of such sensory stimulation, that child's personal and social behavior is proportionately delayed or impaired.

Children learn the values and expectations of their culture through the examples and teachings that are provided by the key adults in their lives. One of the important functions of the family is to help provide the appropriate learning experiences for the child during the first few years, whereby the primary drives will bring forth socially acceptable behavior. Children must learn to satisfy their needs in a culturally conforming manner. The hazards involved in this learning are great. Effective training helps build secure personalities whose capacities for adjustment to the needs of others is sufficient to assure wholesome and mutually satisfying relationships throughout life. The style of social interaction, guidance, and discipline displayed by the parents does not appear to be as important as its consistency or reliability.

It is largely in the home that the child's basic moral and spiritual concepts are developed. Community agencies, school, and church make significant contributions, but they seldom occupy the primary position in the child's esteem. It is the parents' behavior and not their words that influences the child. To reword an old saying, "What they are speaks so loud that the child does not hear what they say."

Physical growth, psychologic development, and moral sensitivity should not proceed independently of one another. They are like branches of the same tree, which, when mature, provide strength, protection, meaning, and beauty to both the individual and the community.

CHAPTER 17   Ages and stages of childhood and youth

In caring for children, one must have an awareness of the approximate ages at which the child is capable of various activities and functions and the different types of behavior that are likely to emerge at each stage of development. This information will assist the nurse in fostering the child's growth and development while caring for him in illness and in health. Many books have been written to describe the physical, motor, and psychologic changes that take place as an individual goes through the process called "growing up." Table 17-1 is designed to aid the student in the rapid identification of some of the outstanding characteristics of certain ages and the basic psychosocial challenges of that stage of development as identified by Erik Erikson. It also offers anticipatory guidance for the various stages of growth to help provide for the needs of the child and the development of parenting skills by the mother and father. The nurse must remember as she observes and teaches that a parent's understanding is influenced by his or her previous experiences and intellectual and educational levels. The performance times noted are averages only, and allowance must always be made for individual differences. The reader is referred to pp. 361 to 373 for more detailed nutritional expectations.

At the end of the chapter is a description of the Denver Developmental Screening Test, a device that is commonly used to detect developmental delays in young children. This standardized test is easily administered and evaluates the child's functioning in four areas of development: gross motor, fine motor-adaptive, language, and personal-social.

DENVER DEVELOPMENTAL SCREENING TEST (REVISED)*

The Denver Developmental Screening Test (DDST), a device for detecting developmental delays in infancy and the preschool years, has been standardized on a large cross section of the Denver population. The test is administered with ease and speed and lends itself to serial evaluations on the same test sheet. A simpler test, designed to identify those children who require screening with the DDST, is known as the Denver Prescreening Developmental Questionnaire (PDQ). The test is composed of 10 questions to be answered by the parent. It is not necessary for the child to be present.

Test materials

Assemble a skein of red wool, a box of raisins, a rattle with a narrow handle, a small glass bottle

Text continued on p. 357.

*Prepared by William K. Frankenburg and Josiah B. Dodds, University of Colorado Medical Center, Denver, Colorado; reprinted with permission of the authors.

TABLE 17-1   AGES AND STAGES OF MATURATION

	Physical growth	Motor development	Language development	Anticipatory guidance	Basic psychosocial challenges
Infancy (0 to 1 yr)					
Newborn (birth to 1 mo)	Average weight 7½ pounds (3.4 kg) Gains 1 oz/day (5 to 7 oz weekly for first 6 mo) Average height 20 inches (grows 10 inches during first year) Head circumference 13.2 to 14.8 inches (33 to 37 cm) Head measures one fourth total length Pulse 110 to 150 beats/min Respiration 30 to 50 breaths/min	Readily assumes fetal position Rooting, sucking, tonic neck, grasp, plantar, and Moro reflex present Raises head but not stable Turns head from side to side		Development Early evening crying Sneezing normal Sleeps 20 hr/day Regards faces Will eat every 2½ to 4 hr Breast-fed infants may eat more often Safety Bubble well Prevent suffocation in crib Car safety restraint Stimulation Colorful hanging toys Talk to infant Use of touch Feeding practices Hold while feeding Diaper care Avoiding diarrhea or constipation Bathing	In each stage of child development a central problem has to be solved, temporarily at least, if child is to proceed with vigor and confidence to next stage; each type of challenge appears in its purest form at a particular stage of child development Trust vs. mistrust: As infants grow older, they acquire increasing awareness of themselves as individuals who can be happy and satisfied or frustrated and anxious; when they sense they are loved (i.e., needs are gratified), they are happy, content; they begin to develop a basic sense of trust, which is fostered by a warm and loving mother-child and father-child relationship; discontinuities in care bring frustration and pain; child may then develop basic mistrust that may last throughout life Significant person: mother

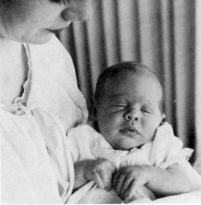
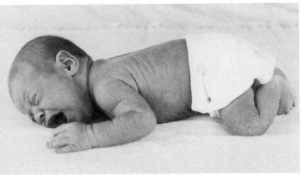

FIG. 17-1   Newborn infant: **A,** grasp reflex is strong; **B,** sleeps 20 hours a day; **C,** readily assumes fetal position.

TABLE 17-1   AGES AND STAGES OF MATURATION—cont'd

	Physical growth	Motor development	Language development	Anticipatory guidance	Basic psychosocial challenges

1 to 3 mo	Posterior fontanel closes at 1½ to 3 mo
	Grows in height about 1 inch/mo
	Head circumference increases ⅓ to ¾ inch (1 or 2 cm)/mo
		Activity diffuse and random
		Specific reflex activities
		May imitate facial expressions
		Cries with tears
		2 mo—can hold rattle; coos, laughs, squeals
		Raises head 45 degrees
		3 mo—raises head 90 degrees
		Will attempt to roll over
			Cooing	Development
				  Head control increasing, alert, likes to look around
				  Follows objects 180 degrees
				5 wk—may sleep 6 to 8 hr through night
				Safety
				  See Newborn
				  Prevent falls
				  Car safety restraint
				  Pacifier
				Stimulation
				  Infant seat
				  Mobile
				  Talk to and touch infant
				  Musical toys
				Feeding practices
				  May "spit up" approximately 1 tbsp
				Other
				  Thumbsucking
				  Immunizations
				  Fever instructions	

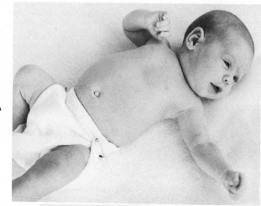

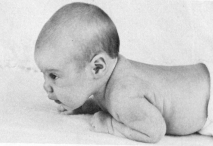

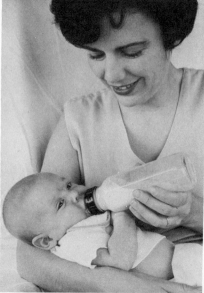

FIG. 17-2   Infant at 1 month: **A,** tonic neck posture is readily assumed; **B,** lifts and turns head when prone; **C,** hold while feeding.

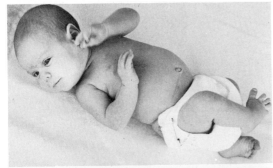

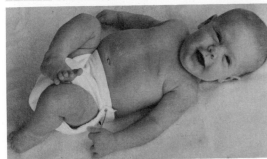

 FIG. 17-3   Infant at 2 months: **A,** activity is diffuse and random; **B,** a sociable smile appears; **C,** raises head 45 degrees; **D,** eyes follow objects.

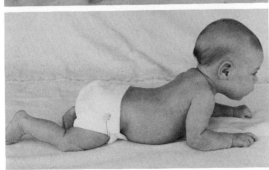

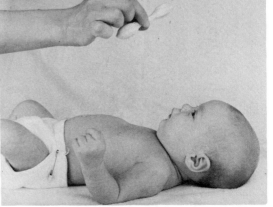

TABLE 17-1   AGES AND STAGES OF MATURATION—cont'd

	Physical growth	Motor development	Language development	Anticipatory guidance	Basic psychosocial challenges
3 to 6 mo	Birth weight doubled by 5 mo Head circumference increases ⅓ inch (1 cm)/mo until age 12 mo	3 to 4 mo—purposefully turns from side to back Reaches out at objects 4 mo—rooting and Moro reflex absent 5 mo—asymmetric tonic neck reflex absent 5 mo—rolls from abdomen to back 6 mo—sits with support Palmar grasp absent	Sociable smile, squeals, coos Imitates several tones 5 mo—understands name and babbles vowel-like sounds Responds to human sound more definitively	Sleeps 8 to 10 hr through night Development Spitting up Teething Safety Prevent falls and burns Car safety restraint Stimulation Play-yard observation Vocal interaction Games Toys to mouth, grab and touch Feeding practices Introduce cereal and cup at 5 to 6 mo (see diagram, p. 363) Immunization	

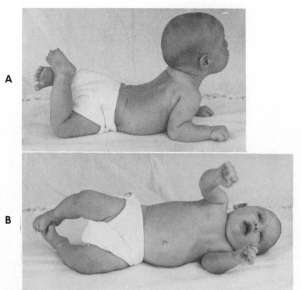

FIG. 17-4   Infant at 3 months: **A,** raises head when prone, supported on forearms; **B,** turns from back to side.

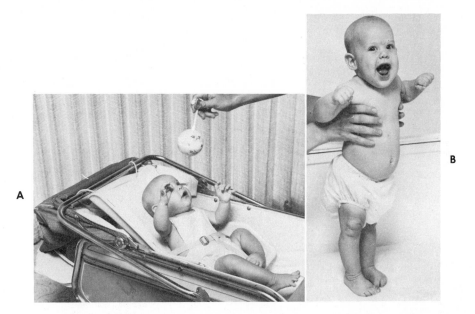

FIG. 17-5 Infant at 4 months: **A,** reaches and grasps at objects; **B,** pushes with feet when held erect.

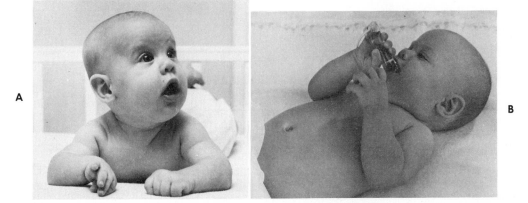

FIG. 17-6 Infant at 5 months: **A,** understands name and babbles; **B,** manipulates and chews small objects.

TABLE 17-1   AGES AND STAGES OF MATURATION—cont'd

	Physical growth	Motor development	Language development	Anticipatory guidance	Basic psychosocial challenges

6 to 11 mo	First primary teeth appear
	6 mo—lower central incisors
	7½ mo—upper central incisors
	10 mo—upper lateral incisors
	Pulse 110 to 120 beats/min
	Respirations 30 to 40 breaths/min
	Blood pressure 90/60 mm Hg
		6 mo—rolls from back to abdomen
		6½ to 7½ mo—sits alone
		9 mo—creeps
		10 mo—pulls self to stand
		Crude pincer grasp, picks up small object using thumb and finger in opposition
		9 to 12 mo—may begin cruising, walking
		Rejects confinement or restraint
			Can grunt, growl, and gurgle; says "da-da" or "ma-ma"	Development
				  Puts everything in mouth
				  7 to 9 mo—fear of strangers
				  Special blanket or toy
				  Dentition and dental care
				Safety
				  Discipline—begin setting limits
				  Prevent burns, poisoning, ingestion of small objects, falls, drowning
				  Child-proof home
				  Car safety restraint
				Stimulation
				  Motion, nesting and cuddle type of toys
				  Peek-a-boo; pat-a-cake
				  Kitchen utensils
				Feeding practices
				  Finger foods, cup
				  9 mo—wean from bottle, no bottles in bed, breast-feeding ad lib	

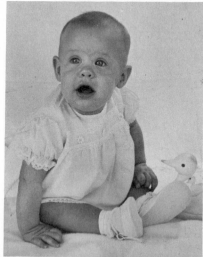

A

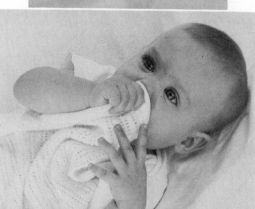

B

FIG. 17-7

Infant at 6 months: **A,** sits alone, leaning forward on one hand; **B,** sleeps with favorite blanket and thumb in mouth.

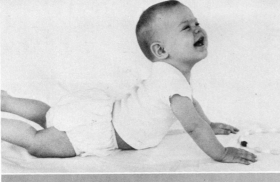

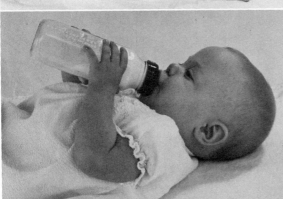

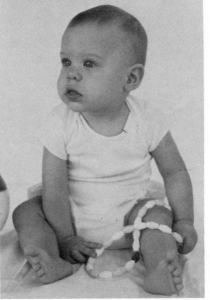

FIG. 17-8   Infant at 7 months: **A,** propels self forward on abdomen (crawling); **B,** can hold bottle; **C,** sits alone without support.

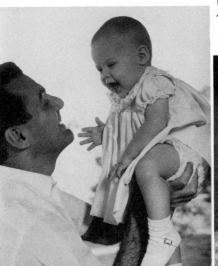

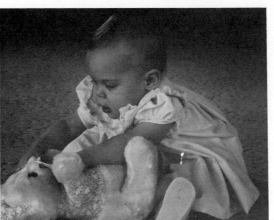

FIG. 17-9   Infant at 8 months: **A,** bubbles, gurgles, loves to play with adults; **B,** can lean forward and straighten up.

A 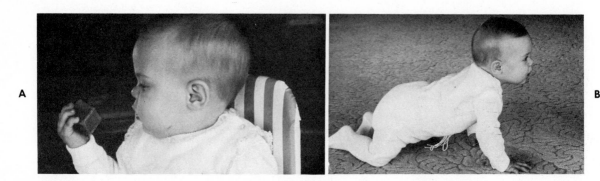 **B**

FIG. 17-10	Infant at 9 months: **A,** grasps small objects; **B,** propels self forward on all fours, trunk above and parallel to floor (creeping).

A   **B**   **C**

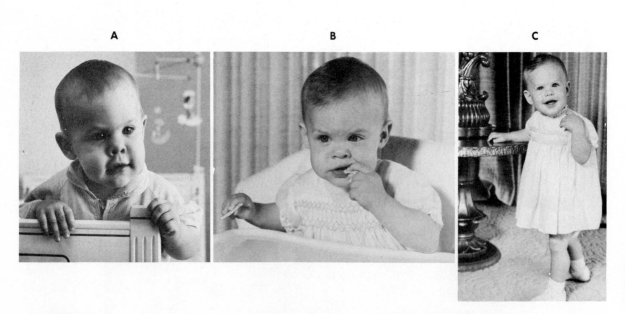

FIG. 17-11	Infant at 10 to 11 months: **A,** can pull self to standing position; **B,** enjoys finger foods, using thumb and finger in opposition; **C,** cruises around, holding on to furniture.

TABLE 17-1   AGES AND STAGES OF MATURATION—cont'd

	Physical growth	Motor development	Language development	Anticipatory guidance	Basic psychosocial challenges

12 mo	Birth weight tripled; height 29 to 30 inches
	6 teeth
	Pulse 100 to 110 beats/min
	Respirations 20 to 34 breaths/min
	Blood pressure 96/66 mm Hg
		Walks alone with wide stance and short steps
		Picks up small objects with forefinger and thumb
		Drinks from cup with ease
			Says "ma-ma" and "da-da" plus two other small words such as "no-no" and "bye-bye"	Development
				  Negativism begins
				  Likes to explore
				  Plays spontaneously
				  1 nap/day
				  Cooperates in dressing
				  Gives a kiss
				Safety
				  See precautions for 6 to 11 mo
				Stimulation
				  Push and pull toys
				  Read to child
				Feeding practices
				  3 meals/day
					Trust, cornerstone of a healthy personality, usually established by end of first year

A	B	C

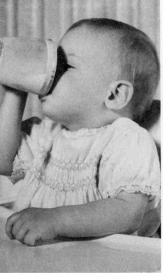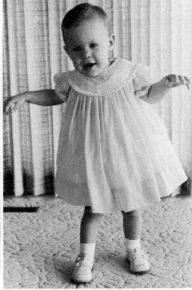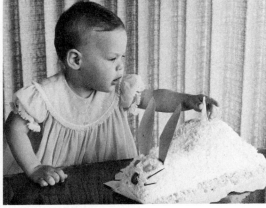

FIG. 17-12   Infant at 12 months: **A,** drinks from a cup with ease; **B,** walks alone with wide stance and short steps; **C,** good finger-thumb opposition.

TABLE 17-1 AGES AND STAGES OF MATURATION—cont'd

	Physical growth	Motor development	Language development	Anticipatory guidance	Basic psychosocial challenges
Toddler (1 to 3 yr)					

15 to 18 mo	Growth rate slows
	Abdomen protrudes
	8 to 12 teeth
	Anterior fontanel closed
		Walks well without support
		Builds a tower of 2 blocks
		Uses spoon but spills
		Can throw object
		Ceaseless activity
		Walks upstairs holding on
		Need for active mastery of new-found motor skills
			Vocabulary of 6 to 10 words; follows simple commands
			Uses jargon that will develop into sentences
				Development
				  Toilet training—may show signs of readiness
				  May be assertive and independent
				  Anger and temper tantrums
				  Ritualistic behavior
				  Takes off shoes and socks
				Safety
				  Lock medications
				  Can climb into everything
				Toddler immunizations
				Stimulation
				  Enjoys coloring, spontaneous scribbling
				  Moves from solitary to parallel play
				  Turns pages of book
				Feeding practices
				  Small servings
				  Decrease in appetite
					Self-esteem (autonomy) vs. shame and doubt: Children's energies now centered around asserting that they are individuals with their own minds and wills; they must have right to choose; they want to do more and more for themselves; feelings of self-esteem, pride, and independence develop; with guidance from parents and others, they learn to make decisions and to become more self-reliant; those who guide growing children wisely will be firm, will avoid shaming them and causing them to doubt their sense of worth
					Significant persons: parents

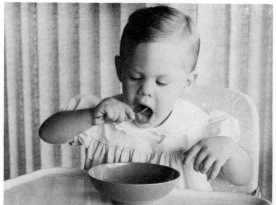

A

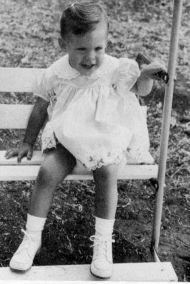

B　　　**C**

FIG. 17-13

Toddler at 15 months: **A,** uses spoon but spills; **B,** walks upstairs holding on; **C,** plays outside.

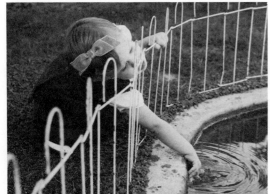

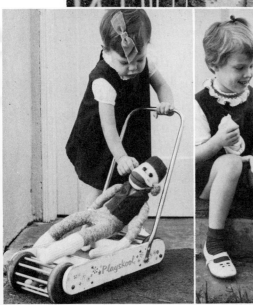

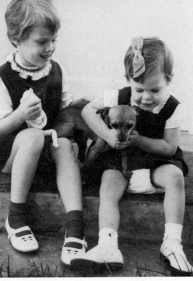

FIG. 17-14

Toddler at 18 months: **A,** needs independence but supervision, too; **B,** loves to push and pull toys; **C,** moves from solitary to parallel play.

TABLE 17-1   AGES AND STAGES OF MATURATION—cont'd

	Physical growth	Motor development	Language development	Anticipatory guidance	Basic psychosocial challenges

24 mo	Grows 3 to 4 inches in second year
	Gains 5 pounds in second year
	Weighs 26 to 28 pounds
	16 teeth
	Pulse 90 to 120 beats/min
	Respirations 20 to 35 breaths/min
		Walks up and down stairs alone
		Runs without falling
		Opens door
		Kicks ball
		Throws ball overhand
		Overestimates own capabilities
			Names familiar objects; says simple phrases; has vocabulary of 300 words; "me" and "mine" dominate	Development
				  May be toilet trained during day
				  Has difficulty sharing
				  Dressing ability increases
				  Thumbsucking and temper tantrums decrease
				  Bedtime rituals important
				  Discipline—limits must be set; define unacceptable behavior
				Safety
				  Set limits
				  See previous precautions
				  Continue to child-proof
				  Avoid foods that may be aspirated
				Stimulation
				  Will advance to cooperative play in next 12 mo
				  Picture books, stories
				  Begins to imitate doing household tasks
				Feeding practices
				  Dexterity increases
				  Appetite fluctuates
				  Feeds self	

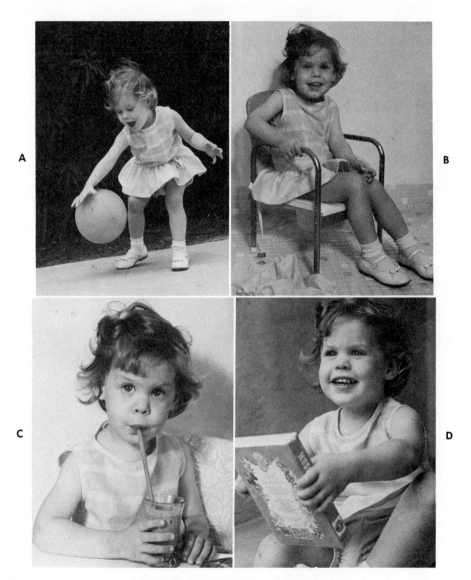

FIG. 17-15 Toddler at 24 months: **A,** muscular coordination greatly advanced; **B,** verbalizes toilet needs; **C,** drinks from straw; **D,** enjoys picture books.

TABLE 17-1 AGES AND STAGES OF MATURATION—cont'd

	Physical growth	Motor development	Language development	Anticipatory guidance	Basic psychosocial challenges

30 mo	Complete set of 20 primary teeth	Builds tower of 8 blocks
		Jumps with both feet
		Walks on tiptoes
		Undresses self easily
			Says full name; sings
			Begins to express needs
				Development
				  Loves routine
				  Magical thinking
				  Bowel training established
				  Bladder training improves
				  Washes and dries hands
				  Make first dental appointment
				Safety
				  Prevent burns, falls, drownings, ingestions
				  Provide stimulation in car seat to help keep content, secure
				Stimulation
				  Exposure to other children
				  Coloring, finger-painting, games, cooking group
				  Short attention span
				Feeding practices
				  Definite likes and dislikes
				Sexual curiosity continues	

FIG. 17-16 Toddler at 30 months: **A,** can put shoes on; **B,** attempts to sing simple songs; **C,** enjoys playing with others.

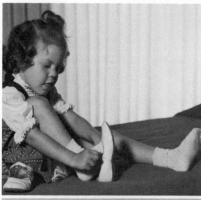

A

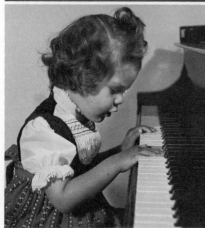

B

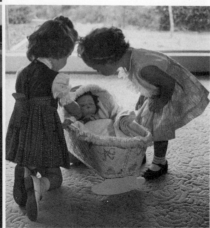

C

TABLE 17-1 AGES AND STAGES OF MATURATION—cont'd

	Physical growth	Motor development	Language development	Anticipatory guidance	Basic psychosocial challenges

3 yr	Relatively slow growth; gains about 5 pounds; height increases average of 3 inches/yr	Uses stairs with alternate feet
		Strings large beads
		Hops on one foot
		Rides tricycle
			Has vocabulary of 900 words or more
			Knows 2 colors
			May talk with imaginary playmate
				Development
				  Can brush teeth
				  May display sibling rivalry
				  Toilet habits well established
				  Interest in sexuality
				  Needs 12 hr sleep a day
				  Allow independence within limits of safety
				Safety
				  Child overestimates capabilities—set limits
				Stimulation
				  Will soon enjoy cooperative play
				  Desires constant activity
				  Resents interference with play or possessions
				  Climbing activities essential
				  Wagons, kiddie cars, tricycles, and boats enjoyed
				Feeding habits
				  Food "jags" common; may not like "mixtures," i.e., casseroles
				  Regularity of mealtime important
					Initiative vs. guilt: Knowing that they are persons in their own right, children of 4 or 5 yr want to find out what kind of persons they can be; they imagine what it is like to be grown up; little girls want to be like "mama" and boys like "daddy"; they imitate parents and yearn to share in their activities; by this age, conscience has developed; an age of avid curiosity and consuming fantasies, which lead to feelings of guilt and anxiety; initiative must be fostered and care taken that young children do not feel guilty because they dared to dream
					Significant persons: basic family

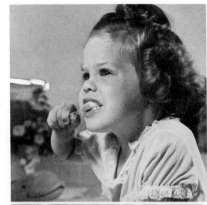

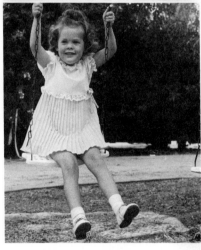

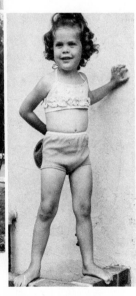

FIG. 17-17 Preschooler at 3 years: **A,** can brush teeth and wash hands; **B,** can pump swing with legs; **C,** knows own age and sex and has good balance.

TABLE 17-1   AGES AND STAGES OF MATURATION—cont'd

	Physical growth	Motor development	Language development	Anticipatory guidance	Basic psychosocial challenges
Preschool (4 and 5 yr)					

4 yr	Height 39 to 41 inches
	Weight 35 to 37 pounds
	Continued relatively slow growth at rate of 3-year-old
	Pulse 100 beats/min
	Respirations 20 to 25 breaths/min
	Blood pressure 100/68 mm Hg
		Uses one foot per step when going down stairs
		Climbs and jumps well
		Increasing finger dexterity
		Buttons and unbuttons clothes
			Vocabulary of 1,500 words
			Can explain own drawing; knows several colors; repeats rhymes and songs
			Asks many questions
				Development
				  Magical thinking
				  Sexual curiosity
				  Continues becoming more self-sufficient
				  Knows own age
				Safety
				  May use seat belt when weight reaches 40 to 50 pounds
				  Teach safety precautions, i.e., cross streets on signals
				  Avoid hot radiator and stove
				  Preschool immunization
				Stimulation
				  Moves from cooperative play with one child to small group play—plan projects accordingly
				  Prepare for school
				Feeding practices
				  Avoid between-meal snacks	

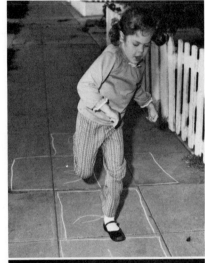

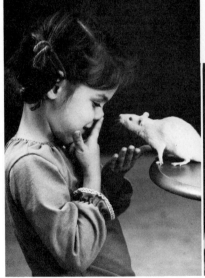

FIG. 17-18

Preschooler at 4 years: **A,** hops on one leg; **B,** enjoys playing with animals; **C,** has increasing finger dexterity with crayons.

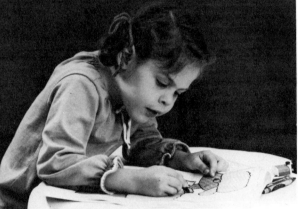

TABLE 17-1   AGES AND STAGES OF MATURATION—cont'd

	Physical growth	Motor development	Language development	Anticipatory guidance	Basic psychosocial challenges
5 yr	Height 43 to 44 inches Weight 40 pounds May lose lower central incisors Pulse 100 beats/min Respirations 20 to 25 breaths/min Blood pressure 94/55 mm Hg	Good muscular coordination; can hop, skip, run, and catch ball Climbs on jungle gym Handles tricycle well Needs rest periods	Names all primary colors and coins Talks in sentences; talks constantly	Development Prints Dresses and undresses without assistance Sensitive to praise Safety Reinforce safety precautions Stimulation Enjoys group activities, conformity, rules Feeding practices Likes finger foods, i.e., carrot sticks, peeled apples, bananas Teach importance of preventing caries	

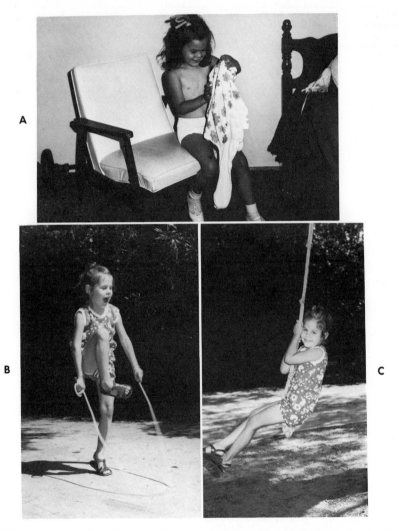

FIG. 17-19 Preschooler at 5 years: **A,** dresses and undresses without help; **B,** can jump rope; **C,** has good muscular coordination.

TABLE 17-1   AGES AND STAGES OF MATURATION—cont'd

	Physical growth	Motor development	Language development	Anticipatory guidance	Basic psychosocial challenges
School age (6 to 10 yr)					
6 yr	6 yr molars; first permanent teeth Annual growth of 2 inches	Good balance Increased dexterity Advanced throwing Roller skates Swims Ties shoes	Vocabulary of 2,500 words Reads and writes Counts May tell time	Development Can bathe self Modest; curious Conscious of rules Household chores important	Industry vs. inferiority: Preoccupation with fantasy subsides; children want to be engaged in real tasks that they can carry through; in learning to accept instruction and win recognition by producing "things," they develop sense of adequacy and accomplishment; when children do not receive recognition for their efforts, they develop sense of inadequacy and inferiority Significant persons: school and neighborhood friends
7 yr	Height 47 to 48 inches Weight 50 to 51 pounds Loses upper incisors	Enjoys outdoor sports; can ride bicycle, swim, jump rope, walk straight line		Begins to write Allow independence Safety Clubs, gangs, hero worship pronounced— may cause problems	

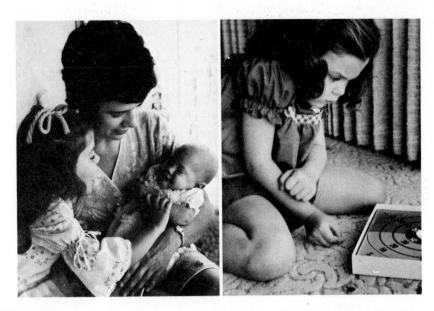

FIG. 17-20 School age—6 years: helps with younger children and has increased interest in games.

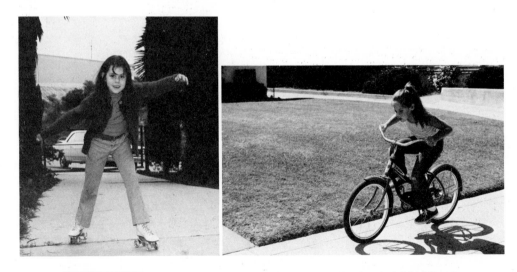

FIG. 17-21 School age—7 years: can roller skate and ride bicycle.

TABLE 17-1 AGES AND STAGES OF MATURATION—cont'd

	Physical growth	Motor development	Language development	Anticipatory guidance	Basic psychosocial challenges
8 and 9 yr	Gradual increase in size—steady growth Pulse 90 beats/min Respirations 16 to 20 breaths/min Blood pressure 106/56 mm Hg	Movements more graceful; able to accomplish more Complex manual skills	8 yr—tells days of week 9 yr—tells months of year Enjoys puns, jokes, stories Reading a useful tool and may be enjoyable pastime	Stimulation Enjoys solitary and group play Bicycles and skates are enjoyed Competitive sports valued Prefers own sex; peer group important Favorite television shows Continues to enjoy stories May enjoy collections Feeding practices Desires afternoon snacks Teach importance of good nutrition; allow time for adequate breakfast May have problems with manners and mealtime punctuality Good eaters from 8 years on	

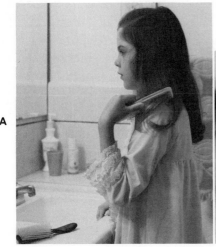
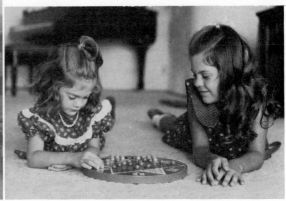

FIG. 17-22   School age—8 years: **A,** personal hygiene important; **B,** satisfaction gained helping younger sister to learn.

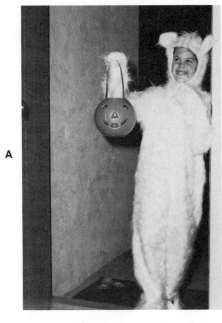
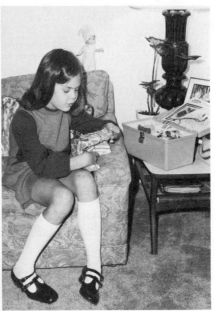

FIG. 17-23   School age—9 years: **A,** Halloween—enjoy puns; **B,** engages in real task, with recognition important.

TABLE 17-1 AGES AND STAGES OF MATURATION—cont'd

	Physical growth	Motor development	Language development	Anticipatory guidance	Basic psychosocial challenges
Preadolescence or puberty (10 to 12 yr)					
	Appearance and development of secondary sexual characteristics Pubescent growth spurt; 2 years earlier for girls Girls may show widening of hips, budding breasts, pubic hair, and occasionally menses Boys ahead of girls in physical strength and endurance; boys increase in muscle mass and bone size especially shoulder girdle and ribs; penis and scrotum enlarge	Poor control will ensue if body framework and muscular development are out of proportion in their rate of growth Posture may be poor	Vocabulary increases; language reflects increasing ability to think introspectively and abstractly	Development Four basic tasks of preadolescence and adolescence: 1. Emancipation from parents and other adults 2. Development of healthy self-concept 3. Beginning acquisition of skills for future 4. Understanding psychosexual differences Possible problems 1. Obesity caused by inactivity and ravenous appetite 2. Poor nutrition (fad diets); needs increased protein 3. Acne associated with hormonal changes 4. Poor self-image (changing body image) 5. Peer pressure; ambivalence toward parents and other adults 6. Lack of sexual identity 7. Adolescent pregnancy 8. Venereal disease 9. Accidents	

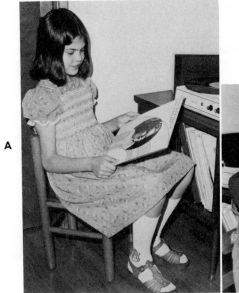

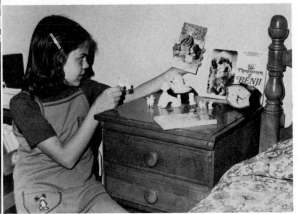

FIG. 17-24   Preadolescence—10 years: **A,** Listening to records is common pastime; **B,** has many collections.

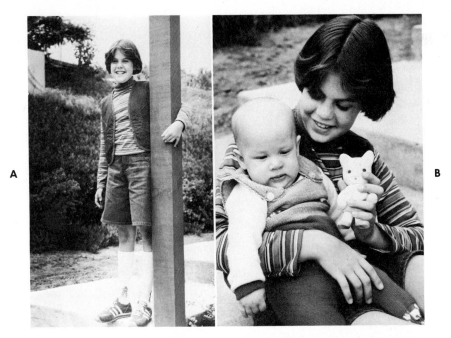

FIG. 17-25   Preadolescence—11 years: **A,** growing up fast; **B,** baby-sitting is favorite pastime.

TABLE 17-1   AGES AND STAGES OF MATURATION—cont'd

	Physical growth	Motor development	Language development	Anticipatory guidance	Basic psychosocial challenges
Adolescence (12 to 19 yr)					
Early adolescence (12 to 16 yr)	Wide individual variability as to onset and rate of growth Girls: growth spurt between 10 and 14 years, gain 2 to 8 inches (5 to 20 cm) in height, 15 to 55 lb (7 to 25 kg) in weight; menarche occurs 2 years after pubescent changes Boys: growth spurt at 12 to 16 years, gain 4 to 12 inches (10 to 30 cm) in height and 15 to 65 lb (7 to 30 kg) in weight Growth of pubic, axillary, and upper lip hair; facial hair appears 2 years after pubic hair	Wide individual variability Hands and feet out of proportion; self-conscious, awkward	Increased vocabulary influenced by attainment of intellectual maturity Talkative, but not communicative; giggly	Development See preadolescent section Needs parental respect and acceptance Preparing for difficult decisions of late adolescence, i.e., continuing education, work, military service, courtship, marriage plans, financial responsibilities, political and religious affiliations	Identity vs. diffusion: Adolescents seek to establish a sense of identity; if a good foundation has been laid (including building blocks of trust, autonomy, sexual identification, initiative, and learning), they will be able to integrate childhood identifications, basic biologic drives, native endowment, and opportunities offered in social roles to feel secure regarding their part in society; self-diffusion or lack of a feeling of identity may be temporarily unavoidable because of physiologic changes and psychologic upheavals in this period Significant persons: peer group

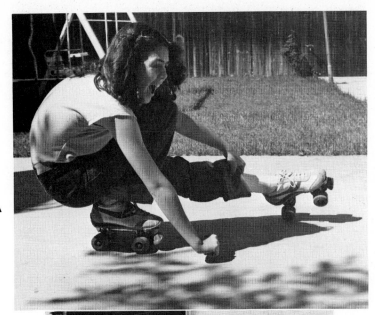

A

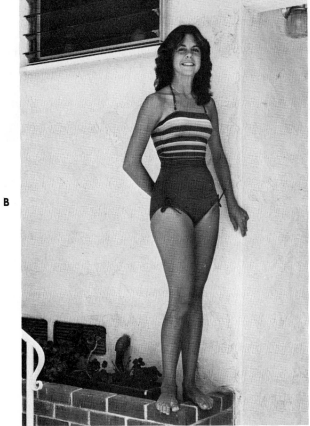

B

FIG. 17-26 Early adolescence—12 to 19 years: **A,** good coordination; **B,** moving toward maturity— 13 years. (See Fig. 17-17, **C,** p. 343: same pose—10 years before.)

A   B

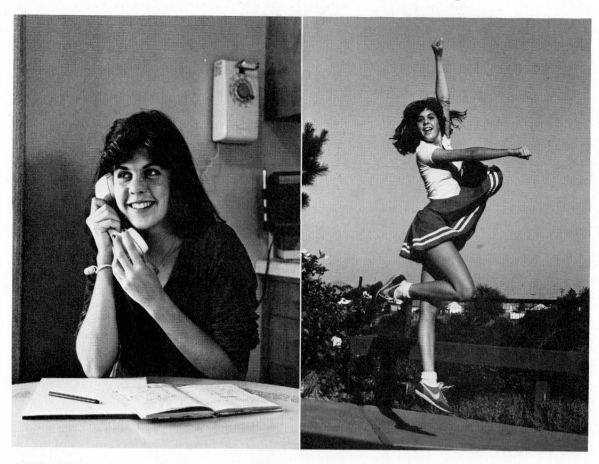

FIG. 17-27   Adolescence—14 years: **A,** talkative—many hours spent on telephone; **B,** Athletic ability highly prized.

TABLE 17-1   AGES AND STAGES OF MATURATION—cont'd

	Physical growth	Motor development	Language development	Anticipatory guidance	Basic psychosocial challenges
Late adolescence (16 to 19 yr)	Adult size and proportion usually attained Spermatogenesis established by 17 years; slow, continuous growth in height ceases at 18 to 20 years in boys and at 16 to 17 years in girls Pulse 70 to 86 beats/min Respirations 14 to 16 breaths/min Blood pressure 118/60 mm Hg	Improvement in coordination; strength and athletic ability highly prized		Dominant developmental thrust Establishment of ego identity: "Where do I fit in this world?" Increased concern for philosophic and religious questions	Intimacy vs. isolation: When young persons feel secure in their identity, they are then able to establish warm, meaningful, constructive relationships with others and eventually a love-based, mutually satisfying sexual relationship with a member of the opposite sex; when individuals are unable to relate to others, they may develop a deep sense of isolation Significant person: opposite sex partner

with ⅝ inch opening, a bell, a tennis ball, the test form, a pencil, and eight 1-inch cubical counting blocks.

General administration instructions

The mother should be told that this is a developmental screening device to obtain an estimate of the child's level of development. This test relies on observations of what the child can do and on report by a parent who knows the child. Direct observation should be used whenever possible. Since the test requires active participation by the child, every effort should be made to put the child at ease. The child above 6 months of age may be tested while sitting on the mother's lap. This should be done in such a way that the child can comfortably reach the test materials on the table. The test should be administered before any frightening or painful procedures. A child will often withdraw if the examiner rushes demands on the child. One may start by laying out one or two test items in front of the child while asking the mother whether the youngster performs some of the personal-social items. It is best to administer the first few test items well below the child's age level to assure him of an initial successful experience. All test materials should be removed from the table, except the item that is being administered, to avoid distractions.

Steps in administering the test

1. Draw a vertical line on the examination sheet through the four sectors (gross motor, fine motor-adaptive, language, and personal-social) to represent the child's chronologic age. Place the date of the examination at the top of the age line. For premature children, subtract the months of prematurity from the chronologic age. After 2 years of age it is no longer necessary to compensate for prematurity.

2. The items to be administered are those through which the child's chronologic age line passes unless there are obvious deviations. In each

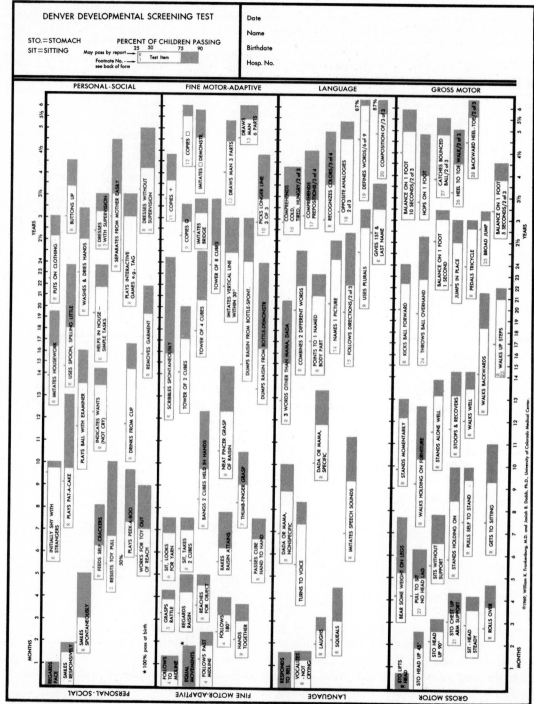

FIG. 17-28 **A,** Denver Developmental Screening Test sheet.

DIRECTIONS

DATE

NAME

BIRTHDATE

HOSP. NO.

1. Try to get child to smile by smiling, talking or waving to him. Do not touch him.
2. When child is playing with toy, pull it away from him. Pass if he resists.
3. Child does not have to be able to tie shoes or button in the back.
4. Move yarn slowly in an arc from one side to the other, about 6" above child's face. Pass if eyes follow 90° to midline. (Past midline; 180°)
5. Pass if child grasps rattle when it is touched to the backs or tips of fingers.
6. Pass if child continues to look where yarn disappeared or tries to see where it went. Yarn should be dropped quickly from sight from tester's hand without arm movement.
7. Pass if child picks up raisin with any part of thumb and a finger.
8. Pass if child picks up raisin with the ends of thumb and index finger using an over hand approach.

9. Pass any enclosed form. Fail continuous round motions.
10. Which line is longer? (Not bigger.) Turn paper upside down and repeat. (3/3 or 5/6)
11. Pass any crossing lines.
12. Have child copy first. If failed, demonstrate

When giving items 9, 11 and 12, do not name the forms. Do not demonstrate 9 and 11.

13. When scoring, each pair (2 arms, 2 legs, etc.) counts as one part.
14. Point to picture and have child name it. (No credit is given for sounds only.)

15. Tell child to: Give block to Mommie; put block on table; put block on floor. Pass 2 of 3. (Do not help child by pointing, moving head or eyes.)
16. Ask child: What do you do when you are cold? ..hungry? ..tired? Pass 2 of 3.
17. Tell child to: Put block on table; under table; in front of chair, behind chair. Pass 3 of 4. (Do not help child by pointing, moving head or eyes.)
18. Ask child: If fire is hot, ice is ?; Mother is a woman, Dad is a ?; a horse is big, a mouse is ?. Pass 2 of 3.
19. Ask child: What is a ball? ..lake? ..desk? ..house? ..banana? ..curtain? ..ceiling? ..hedge? ..pavement? Pass if defined in terms of use, shape, what it is made of or general category (such as banana is fruit, not just yellow). Pass 6 of 9.
20. Ask child: What is a spoon made of? ..a shoe made of? ..a door made of? (No other objects may be substituted.) Pass 3 of 3.
21. When placed on stomach, child lifts chest off table with support of forearms and/or hands.
22. When child is on back, grasp his hands and pull him to sitting. Pass if head does not hang back.
23. Child may use wall or rail only, not person. May not crawl.
24. Child must throw ball overhand 3 feet to within arm's reach of tester.
25. Child must perform standing broad jump over width of test sheet. (8-1/2 inches)
26. Tell child to walk forward, ⌐⊃⌐⊃⌐⊃⌐⊃➔ heel within 1 inch of toe. Tester may demonstrate. Child must walk 4 consecutive steps, 2 out of 3 trials.
27. Bounce ball to child who should stand 3 feet away from tester. Child must catch ball with hands, not arms, 2 out of 3 trials.
28. Tell child to walk backward, ←⊂⊃⌐⊃⌐⊃⌐⊃ toe within 1 inch of heel. Tester may demonstrate. Child must walk 4 consecutive steps, 2 out of 3 trials.

DATE AND BEHAVIORAL OBSERVATIONS (how child feels at time of test, relation to tester, attention span, verbal behavior, self-confidence, etc,):

B

FIG. 17-28 cont'd

B, Reverse side of Denver Developmental Screening Test Sheet. Footnotes correspond to numbered tasks on other side of test sheet.

sector one should establish the area where the child passes all of the items and the point at which the child fails all of the items.

3. In the event that a child refuses to do some of the items requested by the examiner, it is suggested that the parent administer the item, provided she does so in the prescribed manner.

4. If a child passes an item, a large letter "P" is written on the bar at the 50% passing point. "F" designates a failure, and "R" designates a refusal.

5. Note how the child adjusted to the examination; that is, cooperation, attention span, self-confidence, and how the child related to the mother, the examiner, and the test materials.

6. Ask the parent if the child's performance was typical of performance at other times.

7. To retest the child on the same form, use a different color pencil for the scoring and age line.

8. Instructions for administering footnoted items are on the back of the test form.

Interpretations

The test items are placed in four categories: gross motor, fine motor-adaptive, language, and personal-social. Each of the test items is designated by a bar, which is so located under the age scale as to indicate clearly the ages at which 25%, 50%, 75%, and 90% of the standardization population could perform the particular test item. The left end of the bar designates the age at which 25% of the standardization population could perform the item; the hatch mark at the top of the bar, 50%; the left end of the shaded area, 75%; and the right end of the bar, the age at which 90% of the standardization population could perform the items.

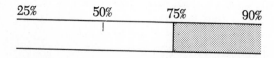

Failure to pass an item passed by 90% of children should be considered significant. Such a failure

may be emphasized by coloring the right end of the bar of the failed item. Several failures in one sector are considered to be developmental delays. These delays may be caused by the following:

1. The unwillingness of the child to use own ability
   a. Temporary phenomena, such as fatigue, illness, hospitalization, separation from the parent, fear, and so forth
   b. General unwillingness to do most things that are asked of the child—such a condition may be just as detrimental as an inability to perform

2. An inability to perform the item because of
   a. General retardation
   b. Pathologic factors such as deafness or neurologic impairment
   c. Familial pattern of slow development in one or more areas

If unexplained developmental delays are noted and are a valid reflection of a child's abilities, the child should be rescreened one month later. If the delays persist, the child should be further evaluated with more detailed diagnostic studies.

CAUTION

1. Fig. 17-28 is an overview of the test and is not complete.

2. The DDST is not an intelligence test. It is intended as a screening instrument for use in clinical practice to note whether the development of a particular child is within the normal range.

3. The training materials and test materials are available through LADOCA Foundation, East 51st Avenue and Lincoln Street, Denver, Colorado 80216.

Nurses should counsel parents that they cannot prevent or hurry growth, nor can they "do the growing" for their children. Adults can provide a healthy and happy environment in which children can grow, develop, and reach their optimum potential. Adults can provide the right equipment, abundant space, encouragement, and tender loving care.

The valuable "ounce of prevention" that everyone has heard mentioned so often is frequently measured in milliliters, drops, or minutes spent with the physician and nurse for regular health supervision. Maintenance of an individual's optimal physical and mental health is a major goal of the physician and nurse.

Child health supervision is an extension of the prenatal care received by the mother and the developing fetus. Such supervision is designed to detect the presence of deformity or disease, to provide help in interpreting nutritional requirements and assuring proper food intake, to protect against certain preventable infectious diseases, and to offer appropriate counseling regarding child-rearing practices and commonly encountered child behavior patterns. Records of the child's individual health history are maintained, and height, weight, and blood pressure are plotted in graph form. Health supervision may be carried on by the private physician, nurse practitioner, a public facility, or a child health conference.

Infants are usually scheduled to visit the physician monthly for the first 6 months and then every other month until their first birthdays. Two to four visits should be made during the second year, and visits should be at least yearly thereafter. Special attention should be directed toward detection of any hearing impairment, visual defect, or orthopedic difficulty. Professional dental supervision should be started before any real problem is apparent, before the child's third birthday. Dental care at home should begin when dentition occurs.

School-age children in U.S. society, because of their multiple community contacts and the activities of the school nurse or public health nurses in some schools, usually receive more consistent health supervision than do preschool children. Even so, school-age children should have annual physical examinations and appropriate help and counseling as their growth and development levels require.

The following topics of study are fundamental to the consideration of preventive pediatrics. It is hoped that these introductory discussions of basic nutrition, immunization, and child safety will encourage the student to continue investigation of the positive approach to health with increasing interest and reward.

SELF-FEEDING AND BASIC NUTRITION

Feeding and eating can be very natural. One should remember that a number of studies have indicated that infants and children select food of the right type at the right time and in the right amounts if it is available to them from the beginning of the self-feeding process. Babies accept solid foods and feed themselves when their neuromuscular progress permits them to do so.

Physiologic guides

HUNGER VS. APPETITE

Babies have a rhythmic pattern of hunger contractions characterized by discomfort, restlessness, and crying. The rhythm of hunger contractions differs in each baby, but they usually reappear every 3 to 4 hours and more frequently in breast-fed babies. Babies should be fed according to their hunger rhythms, since rigidly prescribed feeding schedules ignore these hunger patterns. The normal infant's nutritional needs can be met adequately for the first 6 months by breast-feeding or formula plus vitamins. The Committee on Nutrition of the American Academy of Pediatrics urges that "all bottle-fed infants be given an iron fortified formula for at least the first 12 months of life." The amount of breast milk or formula consumed varies from day to day, but in general most infants take 2 or 3 ounces of formula per pound of body weight, distributed over a 24-hour period. When sucking stops and the healthy infant falls asleep, the hunger-appetite mechanism has been satisfied. The infant should not be coaxed or forced to take more milk, regardless of the amount remaining in the bottle.

During infancy, hunger prompted by physiologic needs chiefly controls food intake. Before 6 months of age an infant will take almost any liquid consistently. However, in the latter half of the first year, preferences related to taste, appearance, and custom (that is, appetite) become important. Maternal diet, likes, and dislikes begin to condition the child's eating habits. By 1 year the baby shows definite preferences and dislikes. If the conditioning process has not been adverse, appetite may be trusted as a physiologic index of the infant's nutritional needs. It is believed that if babies refuse an essential food item, they should not be forced to take it, since they will accept it later when they need it.

Breast or formula feeding should be continued through the first year of life. Whole milk may be introduced in the second year of life. Skim milk should be avoided until after the second birthday, unless prescribed by the pediatrician; skim milk is not nutritionally sound for infants. It provides an inadequate intake of fat, fatty acids, and calories, and protein in excess of four times the estimated requirements.

Developmental guides

PROTRUSION REFLEX

The protrusion reflex manifests itself when the infant pushes out solid food placed on the anterior third of the tongue. This response, common during the first 9 weeks, disappears by the fourth month of life. It does not interfere with the baby's bottle- or breast-feeding, because any nipple empties into the back of the mouth. However, it makes early feeding of solids difficult. The disappearance of the protrusion reflex and the development of the ability to sit with minimal support is the neuromuscular indication for the introduction of semisolid food. There appears to be no advantage in introducing solids (baby foods) during the first 6 months of life.

Getting the baby to accept the spoon willingly is an important learning process that proceeds slowly. Usually new food should be offered first while the baby is hungry. However, *very* hungry babies may refuse new foods because of their urgent desire for milk and their low frustration tolerance. (See Table 18-1.)

SELF-FEEDING

Hand-to-mouth self-feeding begins before 1 year of age. If babies are prevented from feeding themselves when they are neuromuscularly ready, the acquisition of this skill may be delayed for weeks or months. A 6-month-old child can usually put its hands around a supported bottle and guide it to its lips. By 6 months of age, it is a good idea to begin offering juice, formula, or breast milk from a cup, regardless of whether the mother is still nursing or bottle-feeding. If permitted, 7-month-olds may hold the bottle or cup by themselves. At 8 months babies can feed themselves crackers. Chewing motions appear at about 8 or 9 months and are the neuromuscular indications that lumpy foods can be introduced whether the teeth are present or not. Chopped foods should be introduced gradually. If undigested food appears in the stool, one should wait a week and try again. By 6 to 8 months an

TABLE 18-1   CHRONOLOGY FOR INTRODUCTION OF NEW FOODS

Time sequence	Liquids (amount)*	Solids†
Birth to 5 mo	24 to 32 oz/24 hr‡	No beikost (solid food)
5 to 6 mo	24 to 28 oz/24 hr	During first 2 weeks: *Iron-fortified rice cereal*—additional source of calories iron, and fiber, if tolerated well, introduce barley next; avoid wheat first 12 mo (possible allergen) After 2 weeks: *Strained or pureed fruits*—additional source of calories, fiber, vitamin C, and minerals; provides new color and taste; will offset possible constipating effect of cereal
6 to 8 mo	24 oz/24 hr	During first 2 weeks: *Strained or pureed vegetables*—source of calories, fiber, vitamins A and B, and minerals; introduce yellow vegetable prior to green After 2 weeks: *Finger foods*—assists in teething and fine motor coordination
8 mo	24 oz/24 hr	During first 2 weeks: *Strained meats*—source of protein, iron, calories, vitamins; new color and taste
8 to 12 mo	24 to 32 oz/24 hr	*Table foods*—for information and ideas concerning table foods, see *Feed Me! I'm Yours* by Vicki Lanksy§

*Breast milk: Believed to provide immunity, facilitates a close mother-baby relationship, minimizes allergy, is nutritionally sound, provides increased resistance to dental caries, decreases incidence of malocclusion; supplement with vitamin D. *Iron-fortified formula:* Well tolerated when breast milk not available. If community water supply is not fluoridated, both formula and breast milk should be supplemented with fluoride after 6 months of age.
†Introduce solid foods gradually, one at a time.
‡Milk in excess of 32 oz/24 hr may lead to inadequate intake of other vital nutrients and excessive weight gain.
§Lansky, V., et al: Feed me! I'm yours, Wayzata, Minn., 1974, Meadowbrook Press, Inc.

empty plastic or metal cup may be placed on the baby's tray for practice. At 10 months of age babies can begin to practice with a spoon. Shortly after 12 months they can use a cup well, and by 18 months they can use a spoon skillfully. Self-feeding is usually accomplished between 12 and 18 months and combines feeding skills using the spoon, hand, or cup. Several foods are not recommended for children 12 to 24 months of age because of possible aspiration or poor digestibility. These include nuts, popcorn, corn, leafy vegetables, cucumbers, chocolate, olives, peanut butter, uncooked onions, and baked beans.

NURSING BOTTLE CARIES

"Nursing bottle caries," or "nursing bottle syndrome," refers to the rampant decay of the upper anterior primary teeth resulting from bottle feeding of high carbohydrate fluids beyond 12 months (Fig. 18-1). This devastating condition, which may occur as early as 9 to 10 months, is attributed to bottle propping at night and at nap times. When the fluid-filled nipple with a sugar-sweetened beverage remains in the child's mouth, the flow of saliva is minimized and therefore cannot neutralize juice acidity or the acidity developed in the bacteria-laden plaque, both of which promote decalcification of tooth enamel. The result is painful, unattractive, and severely damaged carious teeth. Any child with caries of the anterior teeth, especially the maxillary anterior teeth, should be referred immediately for pediatric dental evaluation and treatment. (See Figs. 18-1 and 18-2.)

Nursing bottle caries can be prevented. Well-

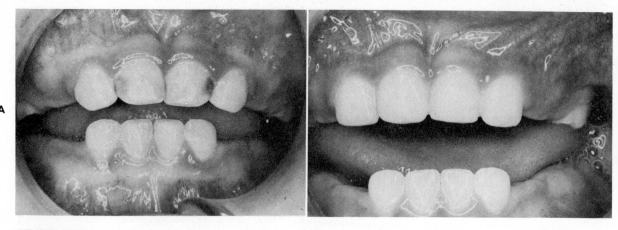

FIG. 18-1   **A,** Decayed teeth. Nursing bottle caries evidenced at 9 months of age. **B,** Teeth returned to normal health and function through aesthetic restoration.

Courtesy Barry H. Gruer, D.D.S., M.S., San Diego, Calif.

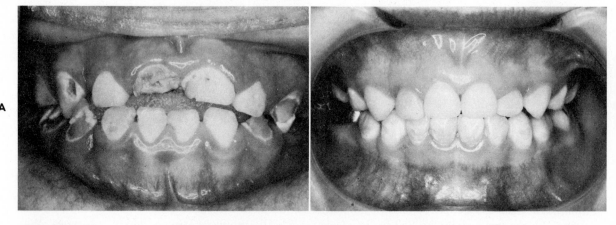

FIG. 18-2   **A,** Extreme rampant caries that began with the overretention of a bottle. **B,** Complete restoration of primary teeth, providing the child a means for mastication and speech and an aesthetic appearance.

Courtesy Barry H. Gruer, D.D.S., M.S., San Diego, Calif.

baby assessments should include appropriate counseling regarding adverse effects of using the bottle at naptime or night time beyond the age of 9 to 12 months. Proper techniques of tooth brushing, restricting intake of sucrose-containing carbohydrates especially between meals, and maintaining desirable fluoride intakes should be encouraged.

Basic nutrition concepts (Table 18-2)

A happy child with good health reflects good eating habits. Good nutrition is like a good insurance policy. During the course of a lifetime it pays dividends in the form of a well-developed body with good muscles, smooth skin, glossy hair, and clear,

TABLE 18-2   CLINICAL SIGNS OF NUTRITIONAL STATUS

	Good	Poor
General appearance	Alert, responsive	Listless, apathetic, cachexic
Hair	Shiny, lustrous; healthy scalp	Stringy, dull, brittle, dry, depigmented
Neck (glands)	No enlargement	Thyroid enlargement
Skin (face and neck)	Smooth, slightly moist; good color, reddish pink mucous membranes	Greasy, discolored, scaly
Eyes	Bright, clear, no fatigue circles beneath	Dryness, signs of infection, increased vascularity, glassiness, thickened conjunctiva
Lips	Good color, moist	Dry, scaly, swollen, angular lesions (stomatitis)
Tongue	Good pink color, surface papillae present, no lesions	Papillary atrophy, smooth appearance; swollen, red, beefy (glossitis)
Gums	Good pink color; no swelling or bleeding, firm	Marginal redness or swelling, receding, spongy
Teeth	Straight, no crowding, well-shaped jaw, clean, no discoloration	Unfilled caries, absent teeth, worn surfaces, mottled, malpositioned
Skin (general)	Smooth, slightly moist, good color	Rough, dry, scaly, pale, pigmented, irritated, petechiae, bruises
Abdomen	Flat	Swollen
Legs, feet	No tenderness, weakness or swelling; good color	Edema, tender calf, tingling, weakness
Skeleton	No malformation	Bowlegs, knock-knees, chest deformity at diaphragm, beaded ribs, prominent scapulae
Weight	Normal for height, age, body build	Overweight or underweight
Posture	Erect, arms and legs straight, abdomen in, chest out	Sagging shoulders, sunken chest, humped back
Muscles	Well developed, firm	Flaccid, poor tone; undeveloped, tender
Nervous control	Good attention span for age, does not cry easily, not irritable or restless	Inattentive, irritable
Gastrointestinal function	Good appetite and digestion; normal, regular elimination	Anorexia, indigestion, constipation or diarrhea
General vitality	Good endurance, energetic, sleeps well at night, vigorous	Easily fatigued, no energy, falls asleep in school, looks tired, apathetic

From Williams, S.R.: Nutrition and diet therapy, ed. 4, St. Louis, 1981, The C.V. Mosby Co., p. 399.

bright eyes. What children eat and how they eat is established in their earliest years. Studies have shown that obesity may be associated with an increase in adipose fat *cell number* (hyperplasia) and in cell size (hypertrophy) or with only an increase in the size of the cell. The number of adipose cells in children who became obese in the first year of life is higher than in those who became obese in later childhood. Dieting in later life can reduce cell size but not the cell number that was laid down in childhood. Thus early feeding practices are of utmost importance.

All systems and tissues in the body depend on proper nourishment for their existence and maintenance; this nourishment is obtained from the foods each individual eats and drinks. Food must perform three functions within the body:

1. Provide heat and energy
2. Build and repair body tissues
3. Regulate body processes

Substances essential to perform these vital functions are the following:

1. Oxygen
2. Water
3. Carbohydrates
4. Proteins
5. Fats
6. Minerals
7. Vitamins
8. Fiber

OXYGEN

Oxygen is so vital to the activity of the body cells that without it, life would cease immediately. The natural source of oxygen is fresh air. Through the activity of the respiratory system, oxygen enters the circulating blood, which carries it to every living cell. An abundance of fresh air is desirable at all ages.

WATER

Second only to oxygen, water is necessary for life. Without water, death ensues in just a few days. Water comprises about 70% of the body weight. It is a basic constituent of all cells and is a major component in blood, lymph, spinal fluid, and the various body excretions such as urine and sweat. During infancy, considerable water is lost through the kidneys and skin. To keep pace with normal fluid losses, the infant must receive an equal fluid intake. The infant is subject to conditions causing water loss, notably fever, vomiting, and diarrhea. Unless water intake is increased during these abnormal states, symptoms of dehydration and its grave consequences appear rapidly. (See p. 454.)

CARBOHYDRATES

Carbohydrates serve as the body's primary source of heat and energy. Examples of carbohydrate-rich foods include grains, fruits, vegetables, and sweets. (Pure sugar is 100% carbohydrate.) Carbohydrates not used for heat and energy are stored in many of the body's organs (especially in the liver and muscles as glycogen), or they are converted in the liver to glucose when carbohydrate is not available in the food consumed. Since immediate heat and energy requirements have priority over tissue growth and repair, the body is also capable of using tissue fat and protein to furnish its energy needs. It is therefore important to have sufficient carbohydrates in the diet to meet these needs adequately, thus sparing protein for its primary use of building and maintaining tissues.

The waste products of carbohydrate metabolism are excreted from the body in the form of carbon dioxide and water.

PROTEIN

Every living cell and almost all body fluids contain protein. Protein is necessary for the growth, repair, and maintenance of all body tissues. Immune bodies, which help the body resist infection, contain protein. Enzymes and hormones also include protein in their composition.

The end products of protein digestion are amino acids—small units, which, when properly reassembled, form the needed body protein. Of the many amino acids known, nine are essential for normal growth and body maintenance. Amino acids are found in varying amounts in various forms in foods.

Proteins are divided into three groups: complete, partially complete, and incomplete. The complete proteins contain all nine essential amino acids. A dietary supply of these amino acids is necessary because they cannot be synthesized by the body. Proteins from animal sources such as meats, poultry, fresh eggs, milk, and cheese provide the essential amino acids. Gelatin is 100% protein from an animal source but is not a complete protein.

Partially complete proteins are found in cereal products and vegetables. They contain many amino acids but not all the essential ones. When protein intake is insufficient, the result is a slow rate of growth and increased susceptibility to bacterial infections.

Incomplete proteins such as corn and gelatin can neither maintain nor support life. When an incomplete protein is the only source of protein, malnutrition, or marasmus, results.

Children will receive adequate amounts of protein in meat, milk, and eggs. The overall protein value may be improved when both animal and vegetable protein are eaten together. Since no amino acids are stored in the body, it is essential that food contain sufficient amounts. Amino acids not needed by the body tissues are returned to the liver, where approximately half are converted into urea, a waste product excreted by the kidney, and half are changed into glycogen or fatty tissue and stored to meet future energy requirements.

Finally, it is important to note that all nine essential amino acids work together. New tissue cannot be formed unless all the essential amino acids are present in the bloodstream simultaneously. Therefore it is imperative that some form of complete protein be included at each meal.

FATS

Certain fatty acids found in dietary fats are necessary to maintain good nutrition. These essential fatty acids permit normal growth and the health and maintenance of normal skin. Fat also provides the vehicle of absorption of the fat-soluble vitamins, A, D, E, and K. Unless dissolved in fats, these vitamins cannot be retained in the body in adequate amounts.

Fats are found in both animal and vegetable foods. Egg yolks, butter, meat, soybean oil, cottonseed oil, corn oil, and olive oil are good sources of the essential fatty acids. One of these sources must be included in the daily diet, since the essential fatty acids cannot be synthesized from other fats. The waste products of fat metabolism, like those of carbohydrate metabolism, are carbon dioxide and water.

If fat intake is inadequate, the child may not receive the essential fatty acids required to prevent the formation of certain types of skin lesions or to promote optimal myelinization of the brain. Brain cells reach adult numbers by approximately 18 months of age.

ENERGY REQUIREMENTS

Whenever work is to be performed by the body, energy is needed. The body must be supplied with fuel in the form of food in sufficient amounts to meet the energy requirements of that individual. To determine how much food a child needs, it is necessary to know the child's metabolic rate, or "rate of heat production." The unit of heat in metabolism is called a *calorie*. (It may be defined as the amount of heat needed to raise the temperature of 1 liter of water 1° C.) A person's *basal* metabolic rate (BMR) is described as the minimal amount of heat produced by body cells when the body is at rest with only vital processes such as circulation and respiration functioning. Several factors—size, age, sex, hormonal levels, and body temperature—influence the BMR. The *total* metabolic rate of a person represents the total amount of heat produced by the body in a given time (usually 24 hours) under normal conditions. The total metabolic rate of a child represents the amount of food the body must burn not only to keep alive and awake but also to continue physical activity, to support growth, to supply specific dynamic action (ingestion and assimilation of food), and to replace calories lost (Fig. 18-3).

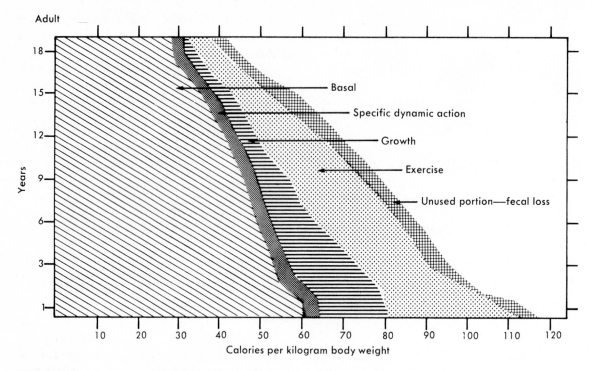

FIG. 18-3   To determine total caloric requirements of a child, multiply weight in kilograms by the number of calories for age.

Total energy expended determines the need for calories. The fuel values of energy-producing foods are as follows:

Carbohydrates	4 cal/g
Protein	4 cal/g
Fats	9 cal/g

The average distribution of calories in a well-balanced diet is as follows:

	Infant	Child
Carbohydrates	29% to 58%	50%
Protein	7% to 16%	15%
Fat	35% to 55%	35% (or less)

If the number of grams of carbohydrate, protein, and fat in a food is known, the caloric value can be determined by multiplying each by the appropriate fuel value.

When food is not available, the body's nutritional reserves and tissues are used to meet its need for caloric energy. Carbohydrates stored as glycogen in different body organs are used first; fat deposits are next. Usually, fat in the extremities is used before fat located in the trunk. Fat in the cheek pads disappears last. Recessed cheeks in young children usually indicate severe malnutrition.

MINERALS

Calcium	Phosphorus
Magnesium	Manganese
Sodium	Chloride
Potassium	Molybdenum
Iron	Selenium
Iodine	Fluoride
Copper	Arsenic
Zinc	Cobalt

The preceding list indicates minerals that are essential to many body structures and functions. The action of minerals are interrelated in the body,

TABLE 18-3   CURRENT FLUORIDE DOSAGE RECOMMENDATIONS

Fluoride content of drinking water (ppm)	Daily dosage (F ion)		
	Birth to age 2-3 (mg)	Age 2-3 (mg)	Age 3-14 (mg)
Less than 0.3	0.25	0.50	1.00
0.3 to 0.7	0	0.25	0.50
Over 0.7	Fluoride dietary supplements unnecessary		

Approved by the Council on Dental Therapeutics of the American Dental Association.

and often one mineral is combined with another to complete the reaction. (For example, in the bones, calcium and phosphorus function together, and sufficient vitamin D is necessary for the proper use of calcium.) Most of these minerals are readily obtained from a well-balanced diet. Calcium and iron require special attention. Deficits of the other minerals do not ordinarily arise from inadequate intake. However, large amounts of minerals may be lost through vomiting and diarrhea.

Fluoride. Fluoride is an essential mineral found in minute quantities in many foods. The main role of fluoride in the body lies in its ability to reduce the incidence of dental caries. Public water fluoridation is the most economical and effective preventive measure against dental caries. Fluorides act to inhibit the demineralization of tooth enamel and its ultimate carious destruction. Fluoridated drinking water, which contains one part per million (1 ppm), will reduce caries by 50% to 60%. The additional use of topical fluoride can contribute to a further decline by 20% to 30%. Since municipal water fluoridation is not available to all, various dietary alternatives are suggested. Tablets, lozenges, or drops should be prescribed when drinking water contains less than 0.8 ppm fluoride (see Table 18-3). If community water is not sufficiently fluoridated naturally, fluoridated water or supplemental fluoride should be prescribed and given on a daily basis from birth until eruption of all perma-

nent teeth. Precaution should be taken to prevent an excessive intake of fluoride, which produces mottling of tooth enamel (dental fluorosis). Continuous, systemic concentrations of fluoride greater than 2 ppm may produce a brown stain on teeth, which is of aesthetic concern, although the strength of the teeth is not diminished.

Iron. One of the most vital elements in the body is iron. It is a component of hemoglobin, the oxygen-bearing element in the blood. Iron is required for growth, and the need for iron varies with the rapidity of growth at different periods of infancy and childhood.

In the United States 30% of children between the ages of 6 and 30 months from lower socio-economic backgrounds and 5% from upper middle-class families of the same age group suffer from iron-deficiency anemia. Iron deficiency leads to the development of anemia, or insufficient hemoglobin for the needs of the body. Anemia causes few deaths but contributes seriously to the weakness, ill health, and substandard performance of many children throughout the world. The greatest incidence of iron-deficiency anemia occurs in infants and young children. Cow's milk does not contain sufficient iron. When the stores present at birth become depleted (at about 3 to 4 months of age), iron-deficiency anemia develops unless a supplement is given. Iron-fortified formula prevents this anemia, and supplementation of iron-fortified cereal after 4 months will help ensure an adequate iron status in both breast-fed and bottle-fed infants. Foods rich in iron are liver, meat, and egg yolk.

Calcium. Relatively large amounts of calcium are required to perform many vital functions in the body. Calcium is essential for normal heart action and is an important element in the blood-clotting mechanism. Calcium builds bones and teeth and is necessary for normal musculoskeletal action. When the diet is calcium deficient, the blood will use the calcium in the bones to maintain its normal composition. Bowed legs and rickets may result. Hypocalcemia may cause neonatal tetany, crying, muscle twitching, and convulsions. Unrelieved, it may end in death. Milk products are good calcium sources.

TABLE 18-4   SIGNIFICANT VITAMINS

Vitamin	Function	Effects of deficiency
A	Promotes good eyesight	Night blindness
	Aids in maintaining resistance to infections	Frequent infections
	Maintains skin integrity	Dry, rough skin, papular eruptions
	Helps form and maintain mucous membrane	Burning, itching eyes
	Helps in formation of bone and teeth	Retarded growth; thin and defective tooth enamel
B complex		
B_1 (thiamin)	Aids in maintenance and function of nervous system	Beriberi
		Listlessness, fatigue, and irritability
	Regulates appetite, normal digestion	Anorexia, vomiting, and diarrhea
	Promotes feeling of general well-being	Generalized weakness; gross symptoms of neuromuscular, digestive, and cardiovascular impairment
B_2 (riboflavin)	Aids in eye adaptation to light	Photophobia; impairment of visual acuity; cataracts
	Provides essentials for metabolism of carbohydrate, fat, and protein	Impaired formation of blood cells
	Necessary for normal growth	Anemia
Niacin (nicotinic acid)	Essential for normal function of digestive tract and nervous system	General poor health
		Gastrointestinal changes—loss of appetite, nausea, vomiting, abdominal pain, red tongue, ulcers and fissures of tongue
		Dermatitis
		Nervous system manifestations—headaches and dizziness, impairment of memory, and neurotic symptoms
C (ascorbic acid)	Important role in formation, maintenance, and repair of teeth, bones, and blood vessels	Scurvy
		Loose teeth; faulty bones; slow growth
	Facilitates absorption of dietary iron	Weakness and irritability
		Delayed healing of wounds
	Maintenance of normal blood hemoglobin levels	Cutaneous hemorrhages
D	Enhances absorption of calcium and phosphorus	Rickets
		Retarded growth and lack of vigor
	Plays a vital role in formation of normal bone	Variety of bone deformities—large head, pigeon chest, kyphosis, and curved long bones
	Promotes tooth development	Teeth erupt late and decay early

TABLE 18-5 FOOD INTAKE FOR GOOD NUTRITION ACCORDING TO FOOD GROUPS AND THE AVERAGE SIZE OF SERVINGS AT DIFFERENT AGE LEVELS

Food group	Servings per day	Average size of servings					
		1 yr	2-3 yr	4-5 yr	6-9 yr	10-12 yr	13-15 yr
MILK AND CHEESE	4	½ cup	½-¾ cup	¾ cup	¾-1 cup	1 cup	1 cup
(1½ oz cheese = 1 cup milk)							
MEAT GROUP (PROTEIN FOODS)	At least 3						
Egg		1 egg	1 egg	1 egg	1 egg	1 egg	1 or more
Lean meat, fish, poultry (liver once a week)		2 tbsp	2 tbsp	4 tbsp	2-3 oz (4-6 tbsp)	3-4 oz	4 oz or more
Peanut butter			1 tbsp	2 tbsp	2-3 tbsp	3 tbsp	3 tbsp
FRUITS AND VEGETABLES	At least 4, including:						
Vitamin C source (citrus fruits, berries, tomato, cabbage, cantaloupe)	1 or more (twice as much tomato as citrus)	⅓ cup citrus	½ cup	½ cup	1 medium orange	1 medium or- ange	1 medium orange
Vitamin A source (green or yellow fruits and vegetables)	1 or more	2 tbsp	3 tbsp	4 tbsp (¼ cup)	¼ cup	⅓ cup	½ cup
Other vegetables (potato, legumes, etc.) or	2 or more	2 tbsp	3 tbsp	4 tbsp (¼ cup)	⅓ cup	½ cup	¾ cup
Other fruits (apple, banana, etc.)		¼ cup	⅓ cup	½ cup	1 medium	1 medium	1 medium
CEREALS (WHOLE GRAIN OR ENRICHED)	At least 4						
Bread		½ slice	1 slice	1½ slices	1-2 slices	2 slices	2 slices
Ready-to-eat cereals		½ oz	¾ oz	1 oz	1 oz	1 oz	1 oz
Cooked cereal (including macaroni, spaghetti, rice, etc.)		¼ cup	⅓ cup	½ cup	½ cup	¾ cup	1 cup or more
FATS AND CARBOHYDRATES	To meet caloric needs						
Butter, margarine, mayonnaise, oils: 1 tbsp = 100 calories		1 tbsp	1 tbsp	1 tbsp	2 tbsp	2 tbsp	2-4 tbsp
Desserts and sweets: 100-calorie portions as follows: ⅓ cup pudding or ice cream, 2- to 3-inch cookies, 1 oz cake, ⅓ oz pie, 2 tbsp jelly, jam, honey, sugar		1 portion	1½ portions	1½ portions	3 portions	3 portions	3-6 portions

Adapted by Bennett, M.J. and Hansen, A.E. from Four groups of the daily food guide, Institute of Home Economics, U.S. Department of Agriculture, Publication No. 30, Children's Bureau, U.S. Department of Health, Education, and Welfare, Washington, D.C.

TABLE 18-6 RECOMMENDED DAILY DIETARY ALLOWANCES, REVISED 1980 (DESIGNED FOR THE

	Age (years)	Weight		Height		Protein (g)	Fat-soluble vitamins			Water-soluble vitamins	
		kg	lb	cm	in		Vitamin A (μg RE)[a]	Vitamin D (μg)[b]	Vitamin E (mg α-TE)[c]	Vitamin C (mg)	Thiamin (mg)
Infants	0.0-0.5	6	13	60	24	kg × 2.2	420	10	3	35	0.3
	0.5-1.0	9	20	71	28	kg × 2.0	400	10	4	35	0.5
Children	1-3	13	29	90	35	23	400	10	5	45	0.7
	4-6	20	44	112	44	30	500	10	6	45	0.9
	7-10	28	62	132	52	34	700	10	7	45	1.2
Males	11-14	45	99	157	62	45	1000	10	8	50	1.4
	15-18	66	145	176	69	56	1000	10	10	60	1.4
	19-22	70	154	177	70	56	1000	7.5	10	60	1.5
Females	11-14	46	101	157	62	46	800	10	8	50	1.1
	15-18	55	120	163	64	46	800	10	8	60	1.1
	19-22	55	120	163	64	44	800	7.5	8	60	1.1

From Food and Nutrition Board, National Academy of Sciences–National Research Council, Washington, D.C., 1980.
*The allowances are intended to provide for individual variations among most normal persons as they live in the United States under usual environmental stresses. Diets should be based on a variety of common foods in order to provide other nutrients for which human requirements have been less well defined.
[a]Retinol equivalents 1 Retinol equivalent = 1 μg retinol or 6 μgβ carotene.
[b]As cholecalciferol. 10 μg cholecalciferol = 400 IU vitamin D.

VITAMINS

Fat-soluble	Water-soluble
A	C
D	B Complex
E	Thiamin (B$_1$)
K	Riboflavin (B$_s$)
	Niacin
	Folic acid
	Pyridoxine (B$_6$)
	Biotin
	Pantothenic acid
	Cyanocobalamin (B$_{12}$)

Vitamins are organic compounds found in minute quantities in foods. They participate as catalysts in almost all metabolic processes and are vital to growth and good health. Vitamins A and D are the only two vitamins stored in the body. Excessive intake of these two vitamins will result in toxic manifestations such as skin lesions, liver enlargement, and bone spurs. Any vitamin may be lacking, causing disturbances in the pattern of growth, metabolism, and development of the child.

The best sources of vitamins are found in the natural foods. A well-balanced diet containing the Basic Four Food Groups (see Fig. 5-2) will ensure an adequate supply of vitamins. Six vitamins merit special consideration (Tables 18-4 and 18-5). The foods that supply these vitamins also supply all other vitamin needs.

SUMMARY

Digestion refers to those processes that prepare food for assimilation into the bloodstream or lymphatics of the body, but metabolism refers to all the changes that occur in the use of those nutrients by the cells and the generation of heat and energy. Amino acids, essential fatty acids, vitamins, and minerals are used primarily for cell growth and repair. They are also used in the formation of enzymes, hormones, and other body substances.

MAINTENANCE OF GOOD NUTRITION OF PRACTICALLY ALL HEALTHY PEOPLE IN THE UNITED STATES)*

Water-soluble vitamins					Minerals					
Riboflavin (mg)	Niacin (mg NE)[d]	Vitamin B$_6$ (mg)	Folacin[e] (μg)	Vitamin B$_{12}$ (μg)	Calcium (mg)	Phosphorus (mg)	Magnesium (mg)	Iron (mg)	Zinc (mg)	Iodine (μg)
0.4	6	0.3	30	0.5[f]	360	240	50	10	3	40
0.6	8	0.6	45	1.5	540	360	70	15	5	50
0.8	9	0.9	100	2.0	800	800	150	15	10	70
1.0	11	1.3	200	2.5	800	800	200	10	10	90
1.4	16	1.6	300	3.0	800	800	250	10	10	120
1.6	18	1.8	400	3.0	1200	1200	350	18	15	150
1.7	18	2.0	400	3.0	1200	1200	400	18	15	150
1.7	19	2.2	400	3.0	800	800	350	10	15	150
1.3	15	1.8	400	3.0	1200	1200	300	18	15	150
1.3	14	2.0	400	3.0	1200	1200	300	18	15	150
1.3	14	2.0	400	3.0	800	800	300	18	15	150

[c] α tocopherol equivalents. 1 mg d-α-tocopherol = 1 α TE.
[d] 1 NE (niacin equivalent) is equal to 1 mg of niacin or 60 mg of dietary tryptophan.
[e] The folacin allowances refer to dietary sources as determined by *Lactobacillus casei* assay after treatment with enzymes ("conjugates") to make polyglutamyl forms of the vitamin available for the test organism.
[f] The RDA for vitamin B$_{12}$ in infants based on average concentration of the vitamin in human milk. The allowances after weaning are based on energy intake (as recommended by the American Academy of Pediatrics) and consideration of other factors such as intestinal absorption.

Carbohydrates and fats are used primarily for caloric energy (that is, to supply fuel to keep the body warm) and mechanical energy for performing the body's work. When caloric needs are not met by fats and carbohydrates, protein is then used for energy. Adequate intake of carbohydrates and fats will spare protein for cell growth. Thus the diet must contain a balance of all six substances—carbohydrate, fat, protein, vitamins, minerals, and water; each one plays a vital role in the processes of growth and development (Table 18-6).

IMMUNIZATION

The brilliant success achieved in conquering the classic contagious diseases of childhood is attributed to immunization through which a person is able to build up defenses against certain infectious diseases. When individuals can resist a certain disease, they are said to be immune. They are immune because antibodies are present that injure or destroy the disease-producing agent or neutralize its toxins. Active immunization (artificial) is achieved when certain substances called *antigens* are injected into the body to stimulate the production of antibodies. Immunization is the best and cheapest method of preventing illness. In fact, it is the most routine procedure in preventive pediatrics.

Because the mechanisms for developing immunity are immature in infants, they are highly susceptible to some infections. The protection they have against infection is obtained from the mother, if she is immune. Any passive immunity acquired from the mother lasts about 4 to 6 months and may protect the child against diphtheria, tetanus, measles, and poliomyelitis. Since such passive protection varies greatly among infants and no passive immunity exists against pertussis (whooping

TABLE 18-7   RECOMMENDED SCHEDULE FOR ACTIVE IMMUNIZATION OF NORMAL INFANTS AND CHILDREN

Recommended age	Vaccines	Comments
2 mo	DTP,* OPV†	Can be initiated earlier in areas of high endemicity
4 mo	DTP, OPV	2-mo interval desired for OPV to avoid interference
6 mo	DTP (OPV)	OPV optional for areas where polio might be imported (e.g., Southwest United States)
12 mo	Tuberculin test‡	May be given simultaneously with MMR at 15 mo (see text)
15 mo	Measles, mumps, rubella (MMR)§	MMR preferred
18 mo	DTP, OPV	Consider as part of primary series—DTP essential
4-7 yr	DTP, OPV	
14-16 yr	Td‖	Repeat every 10 years for lifetime

From Report of the Committee on Infectious Diseases, Red Book, Evanston, Ill., 1982, American Academy of Pediatrics, p. 7.

*DTP—Diphtheria and tetanus toxoids with pertussis vaccine.

†OPV—Oral, attenuated poliovirus vaccine contains poliovirus types 1, 2, and 3.

‡Tuberculin test—Mantoux (intradermal PPD) preferred. Frequency of tests depends on local epidemiology. The committee recommends annual or biennial testing unless local circumstances dictate less frequent or no testing (see Tuberculosis for complete discussion).

§MMR—Live measles, mumps, and rubella viruses in a combined vaccine (see text for discussion of single vaccines versus combination).

‖Td—Adult tetanus toxoid (full dose) and diphtheria toxoid (reduced dose) in combination.

For all products used, consult manufacturer's brochure for instructions for storage, handling, and administration. Biologics prepared by different manufacturers may vary, and those of the same manufacturer may change from time to time. The package insert should be followed for a specific product.

cough), immunization should be initiated as early as possible. Combined antigens reduce the number of injections, enhance the action of each, and establish a desired immunity within the first 6 months of life.

Current practice begins immunization when the infant is between 8 and 12 weeks of age (Tables 18-7 to 18-9). A "triple toxoid" of diphtheria, tetanus, and pertussis antigens in one injection and a concurrent feeding of oral polio vaccine are given. The "triple toxoid" DTP is repeated three times at intervals of not less than 1 month. The necessity of

preventing the high mortality from pertussis (whooping cough) in infancy is the main reason for the early start in basic DTP immunization. However, pertussis vaccine is not considered to be as satisfactory as diphtheria and tetanus toxoids. It does not provide absolute protection.

After the initial series of immunizations, "recall" or "booster" doses are given to stimulate high antibody levels and maintain maximum immunity. Children who have received three doses of triple toxoid (DTP) and two or three doses of oral polio vaccine (TOPV) should be given a booster dose at

TABLE 18-8 RECOMMENDED IMMUNIZATION SCHEDULES FOR INFANTS AND CHILDREN NOT INITIALLY IMMUNIZED AT USUAL RECOMMENDED TIMES IN EARLY INFANCY

Timing	Recommended schedules				Comments
	Preferred schedule	Alternatives			
		#1	#2	#3	
First visit	DTP #1, OPV #1, Tuberculin test (PPD)	MMR, PPD	DTP #1, OPV #1, PPD	DTP #1, OPV #1, MMR, PPD	MMR should be given no younger than 15 mo old
1 mo after first visit	MMR	DTP #1, OPV #1	MMR, DTP #2	DTP #2	
2 mo after first visit	DTP #2, OPV #2	—	DTP #3, OPV #2	DTP #3, OPV #2	—
3 mo after first visit	(DTP #3)	DTP #2, OPV #2	—	—	In preferred schedule, DTP #3 can be given if OPV #3 is not to be given until 10-16 mo
4 mo after first visit	DTP #3 (OPV #3)	—	(OPV #3)	(OPV #3)	OPV #3 optional for areas for likely importation of polio (e.g., some southwestern states)
5 mo after first visit	—	DTP #3 (OPV #3)	—	—	
10-16 mo after last dose	DTP #4, OPV #3 or OPV #4	DTP #4, OPV #3 or OPV #4	DTP #4, OPV #3 or OPV #4	DTP #4, OPV #3 or OPV #4	—
Preschool	DTP #5, OPV #4 or OPV #5	DTP #5, OPV #4 or OPV #5	DTP #5, OPV #4 or OPV #5	DTP #5, OPV #4 or OPV #5	Preschool dose not necessary if DTP #4 or #5 given after fourth birthday
14-16 yr old	Td	Td	Td	Td	Repeat every 10 yr

From Report of the Committee on Infectious Diseases, Red Book, Evanston, Ill., 1982, American Academy of Pediatrics, pp. 18-19.

Alternative #1 can be used in those more than 15 months old if measles is occurring in the community.

Alternative #2 allows for more rapid DTP immunization.

Alternative #3 should be reserved for those whose access to medical care is compromised by poor compliance.

DTP = Diphtheria and tetanus toxoids with pertussis vaccine.

OPV = Oral, attenuated poliovirus vaccine contains types 1, 2, and 3.

Tuberculin test = Mantoux (intradermal PPD) preferred. Frequency of tests depends on local epidemiology. The Committee recommends annual or biennial testing unless local circumstances dictate less frequent or no testing (see Tuberculosis for complete discussion).

MMR = Live measles, mumps, and rubella viruses in a combined vaccine (see text for discussion of single vaccines).

Td = Adult tetanus toxoid (full dose) and diphtheria toxoid (reduced dose) in combination.

For all products used, consult manufacturer's brochure for instructions for storage, handling, and administration. Biologics prepared by different manufacturers may vary, and those of the same manufacturer may change from time to time. The package insert should be followed for a specific product.

TABLE 18-9   GUIDE TO TETANUS PROPHYLAXIS IN WOUND MANAGEMENT

History of tetanus immunization (doses)	Clean, minor wounds		All other wounds	
	Td*	TIG†	Td	TIG
Uncertain	Yes	No	Yes	Yes
0-1	Yes	No	Yes	Yes
2	Yes	No	Yes	No‡
3 or more	No§	No	No‖	No

From Report of the Committee on Infectious Diseases, Red Book, Evanston III., 1982, American Academy of Pediatrics.
*Tetanus and diphtheria toxoids.
†Tetanus immune globulin.
‡Unless wound is more than 24 hours old.
§Unless more than 10 years since the last dose.
‖Unless more than 5 years since the last dose.

18 months of age. Subsequent booster doses are recommended between 4 and 7 years of age. Active, up-to-date immunization produces a degree of resistance in children comparable to that which follows the natural infection.

Precautions

1. A separate sterile needle and syringe, preferably disposable, should be used for each immunization.
2. Preferred sites for subcutaneous and intramuscular injections include the anterolateral aspect of the upper thigh and the deltoid muscle of the upper arm. Each injection should be given at a different site.
3. Injection site and rubber stopper should be cleaned with an antiseptic solution such as 2% tincture of iodine.
4. Toxoids and vaccines (antigens) containing alum are given intramuscularly, preferably into the midlateral thigh or deltoid muscles.
5. The package insert should be read before administering the immunization.

6. Patients and parents should be informed of any possible side effect or adverse reaction. They should be counseled in relation to the benefits of the vaccine and the risks of the disease.
7. Systemic reactions such as fever, rashes, and arthralgia subside within 48 hours and are controlled by symptomatic measures and antipyretics.
8. Aspirin, 1 grain per year of age (up to 5 grains), may be given 2 hours after the injection. This dosage may be repeated as needed *not more than five times at 4-hour intervals* without medical consultation.

Contraindications*

1. Acute febrile illness; *minor infections* not associated with fever (such as the common cold) are *not* contraindications. Interruption of the recommended schedule, with a delay between doses, does not interfere with the final immunity achieved.
2. Pertussis immunization should not be repeated if a history of fever of 105° F (40.5° C) or over, severe screaming episodes, collapse, symptoms of central nervous system disorders, or platelet destruction (such as petechiae or bruising) has been noted after a DTP injection. DT should be used instead.
3. Nonprogressive neurologic disorders *do not* constitute a valid reason for deferring or withholding routine immunization. However, if the child has an evolving neuropathic process, it may be necessary to avoid all immunizations.
4. Immunization procedures are deferred during the administration of steroids, irradiation, and anticancer drug therapy because antibody response is depressed or abnormal. Immunizations should also be deferred if the

*For a more detailed discussion refer to the Red Book, pp. 15-33. See footnote to Table 18-9.

child has recently received (within 8 weeks) immune serum globulin, plasma, or blood.

5. Infants, children, and other household contacts of individuals with an immunologic deficiency should not receive oral poliovirus vaccine, because the polio viruses are transmissible to the immunocompromised individual.

6. Live attenuated vaccines against measles, rubella, and mumps are *not* given to pregnant women or patients with generalized malignancy.

7. If allergic reactions were experienced after immunization, the same or related vaccine should be avoided.

Rubella virus vaccine

The principal objective of rubella (German measles) control is preventing infection of the fetus. This can best be achieved by eliminating the transmission of the virus among children, who are the major source of infection for pregnant women. All children between 15 months of age and puberty should receive the live rubella virus vaccine. It is not recommended for younger infants because of possible interference in active antibody formation by persisting maternal rubella antibody. Children of pregnant women may be given rubella vaccine, since the vaccine virus is not communicable. However, immunization with live virus vaccine during pregnancy should be avoided because of possible risk to the fetus.

Mumps virus vaccine

The principal objective is prevention of mumps in preadolescent males and young male adults. Live attenuated mumps virus vaccine is recommended for all susceptible children over 15 months of age and especially for preadolescent males and men who have not had the disease. The vaccine should not be given to pregnant women.

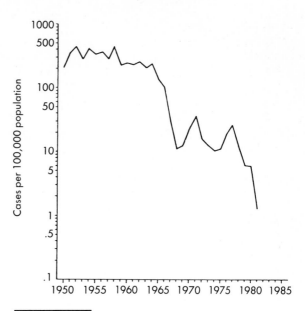

FIG. 18-4

Incidence of reported measles, United States 1950-1981.

From Morbidity and Mortality Weekly Report 31:37, HHS Publ. No. (CDC) 82-8017, February 5, 1982.

Measles (rubeola) vaccine

One successful inoculation with live attenuated measles virus vaccine confers lifelong protection against the disease. Live measles virus vaccine should be given to: all children over 15 months of age unless documented evidence of the disease exists; children who have been immunized against measles with either gamma globulin or inactivated measles vaccines; and children who were immunized before 15 months of age with the live measles virus vaccine. Because measles is often a severe disease with frequent complications, live measles vaccine may be given as early as 6 to 9 months of age if exposure of the infant is probable. A second dose is given after 15 months of age.

School-entrance laws require documentation of measles immunity at the time of entry into kindergarten or first grade. The existence of regulations requiring documented immunity to measles before children are allowed to enter kindergarten or first grade has been shown to correlate with reduced incidence of measles (Fig. 18-4).

Smallpox vaccine

Global eradication of smallpox has been achieved, and the World Health Organization (WHO) by resolution amended the International Health Regulations to eliminate the requirement of smallpox vaccination of international travelers. Because of the risk of complications of vaccination to both those vaccinated and their contacts, physicians should give a signed statement that vaccination is medically contraindicated to persons who plan to travel to any country in which a certificate may be required. Smallpox vaccine is ineffective in the treatment of any disease and should only be administered to laboratory workers directly in contact with smallpox viruses.

Passive immunity

Human immune globulin (IG), formerly called immune serum globulin or gamma globulin, is an antibody-rich fraction of pooled plasma from normal donors. It confers temporary immunity that is attained in approximately 2 days and lasts from 1 to 6 weeks. The large, viscous dose should be divided and given intramuscularly in two different sites with an 18- or 20-gauge needle. IG is limited in supply and has been clearly documented to be helpful in prevention or modification of measles

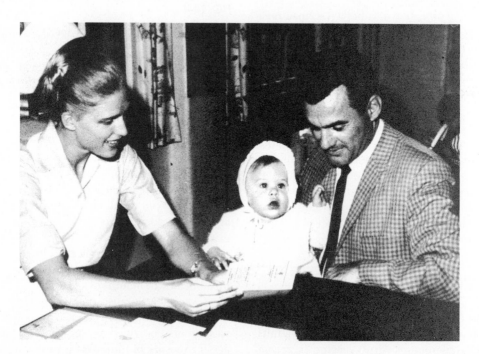

FIG. 18-5   Immunizations should not be given without follow-up instructions to the parents. This nurse is explaining the World Health Organization immunization record and what to do if certain signs and symptoms develop after Mary Ann's inoculation.

Courtesy U.S. Naval Regional Medical Center, San Diego, Calif.

and viral hepatitis A (HAV) and treatment of certain antibody deficiencies.

Nursing responsibilities

Every child should be immunized against the preventable contagious diseases. The office nurse can do a great deal by her efficient, yet kindly manner to help parents realize the importance of continuing the immunization program. She should be sure that the parent knows what type of injections the child is receiving. She should be aware of any allergies that the child has demonstrated and learn if there have been any noteworthy reactions to previous immunizations.

The nurse's good-humored recognition that the medicine does sting a bit and that a sincere "ouch" is not out of place may help wary youngsters. A matter-of-fact, positive attitude rather than an overly solicitous manner seems to offer more support to the parent and child. A continuous written record of the type of protection the child has received and the dates of administration should be given to the parents. The date and time of the next appointment should be clearly understood (Fig. 18-5). In addition the American Academy of Pediatrics also recommends that the following information be recorded: the manufacturer, lot number, and expiration date of the immunization product and the site and route of administration.

It is also important to record all immunizations received on the patient's hospital record or clinic folder. Immunization status is reviewed at the time of each health assessment, illness, or injury.

It is equally worthwhile to inquire about the current status of the parents' immunizations. The proverbial daily apple really is not too successful in preventing illness, but regular immunization is a proved and necessary protection for both young and old.

• • •

Immunization is so important that information about the procedure should be given in prenatal classes. New parents are very concerned about "doing what is right" for their child. Before going home from the hospital, the mother and father should be reminded again about the immunization program. Although immunizations are usually given by the private practitioner or the nurse as part of the baby's regular health checkups, parents should be told of community resources where free immunization services are available.

CHILD SAFETY

Successful prevention and treatment of infectious diseases and nutritional disorders have resulted in a significant decrease in child mortality. The greatest threat to the health and well-being of the child today is accidents. An estimated 15,000 to 16,000 children under 15 years of age die annually in the United States from accidents. Accidents kill more children than the next six leading causes of childhood death combined.

	Death rates* Ages 1 to 14
Accidents	20.2
Cancer	4.4
Congenital anomalies	3.5
Homicide	1.6
Heart disease	1.3
Pneumonia	1.3
Stroke	0.6

The magnitude of the accident problem is further stressed by the fact that 17 million children suffer nonfatal injuries every year. Many of these children are crippled or permanently disabled for life. Of course, not all childhood accidents are brought to the attention of medical personnel. Perhaps an additional 25% of children up to 14 years of age have significant but unreported injuries. Thus the conservative figure of 17 million childhood injuries indicates that a serious national problem exists.

---

*Deaths per 100,000 population, National Center for Health Statistics, 1978.

TABLE 18-10   ALL ACCIDENTAL DEATHS* IN 1978 TO CHILDREN UNDER 14 YEARS BY TYPE AND AGE

	0 to 4 years	5 to 14 years	Total
Motor vehicle	1,551	3,130	4,681
Drowning	630†	1,010†	1,640
Fires, burns	896	586	1,482
Ingestion of food, objects	463		463
Firearms		297	297
Mechanical suffocation	242		242
Falls	121		121
Other	863	1,095	1,958
TOTAL	4,766	6,118	10,884

*Approximations by National Safety Council based on data from National Center for Health Statistics, Public Health Service, U.S. Department of Health and Human Services.
†Partly estimated.

Accidents

An accident is defined as "an unpremeditated event resulting in a recognizable injury." The most common accidents that injure children consist mainly of cuts, piercings with instruments, blows from objects, animal bites, and injuries related to motor vehicles. Motor vehicles are the major cause of accidental death. Also ranked among the leading causes of fatal accidents are drownings, fires, and falls. (See Table 18-10.)

Certain factors seem to be influential in causing childhood accidents: (1) approximately one half of all fatalities occur in children under 5 years of age; (2) boys at all ages have more accidents than girls; (3) the nonwhite population has a considerably higher incidence of accidents than does the white population; (4) most accidents occur during the spring and summer months; (5) a higher percentage of accidents occur in the home, especially during the preschool period; (6) the child between 1 and 2 years of age is most vulnerable to accidents of all sorts; and (7) some children are accident prone. Combinations of certain personality characteristics and environmental influences predispose a child toward repetitive accidents.

Prevention. Accidents do not just happen; there is always a cause. Good safety habits could eliminate many of these causes. Gains in safeguarding the lives of children depend on accident prevention. (See Figs. 18-6 to 18-12.)

Continued emphasis has been placed on two particular approaches to accident prevention: (1) elimination of specific environmental hazards peculiar to different age groups, and (2) supervision of small children by adults, to be gradually replaced by training for safety. A glance at the data of the past years shows a continued increase in the actual number of accidents.

Vital statistics in the United States indicate the number of children injured and the kinds of accidents causing the injuries. However, they do not provide sufficient detail about each individual case to fully describe the complete situation of each accident. This prevents making valid conclusions concerning accident causation and prevention in childhood. Often vital information is not recorded. This is undoubtedly why specific recommendations for the prevention of certain injuries have not always been effective.

To date no single approach to accident prevention has been formulated. "Accidents" are the

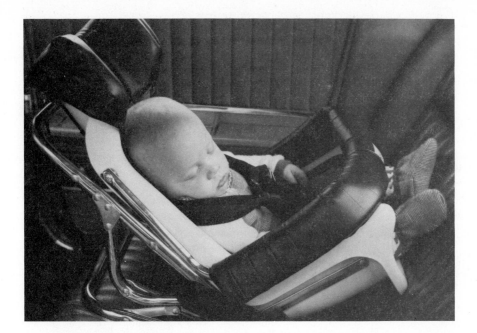

FIG. 18-6　Correct use of an infant car carrier. Children weighing less than 40 to 50 pounds (18.8 to 22.7 kg) need special safety restraints designed to distribute crash forces over a large body area. All car occupants should ride restrained. Purchasing and properly using crash-safe automotive restraints are the keys to prevention or reduction of severe injuries. For information and evaluation of restraints, contact Physicians for Automotive Safety, 50 Union Avenue, Irvington, N.J. 07111.

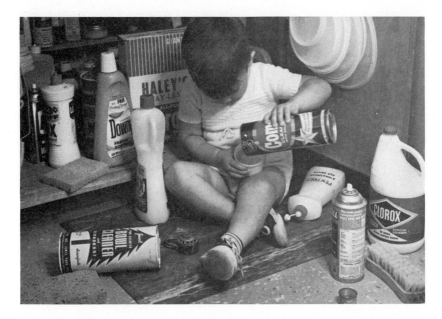

FIG. 18-7　Young children will eat and drink anything regardless of taste. Keep household poisons in a *locked* cupboard.

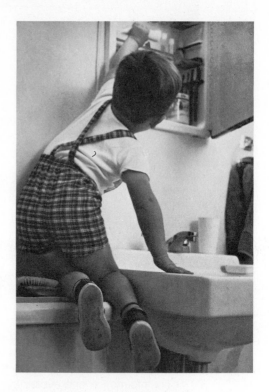

FIG. 18-8

Pink pills are *not* candy. Keep medicine in a locked cabinet.

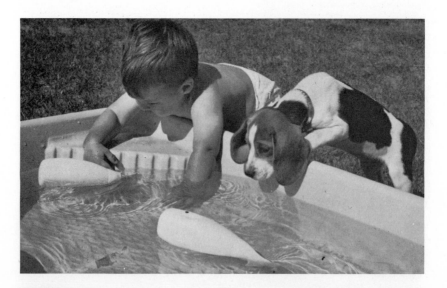

FIG. 18-9   Even shallow water is dangerous for the unattended child.

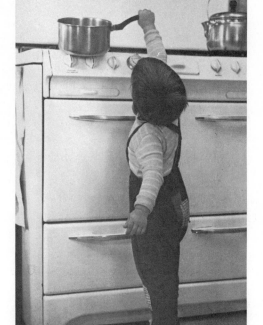

FIG. 18-10

Always turn handles of pots and pans to the back of the stove.

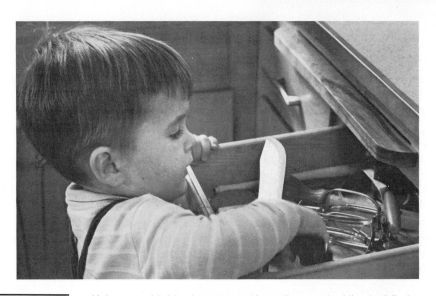

FIG. 18-11   Knives are highly dangerous. Keep them out of the toddler's reach.

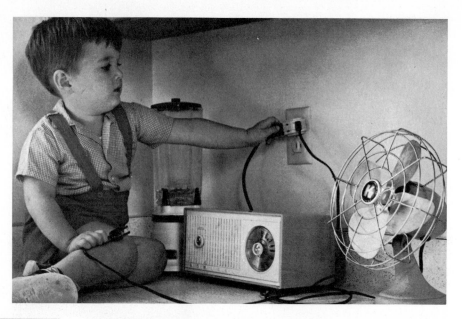

FIG. 18-12   Disconnect appliances not in use. Plug outlets and avoid hurts and burns.

result of a large number of complex mechanisms. Like other illnesses they can be conquered only through systematic investigation. To understand the nature and cause of accidents, several factors must be considered simultaneously: the host (the child who is affected), the agent (the object that is the direct cause), and the environment (the situation in which the accident takes place). This is known as the epidemiologic approach to the study of accidents.

Although a great deal remains to be learned about the interaction of these major factors, the existing knowledge has led to the following new principles aimed at accident prevention:

1. Control of the agent whenever possible (for example, use of child-protective caps on medicine-bottles and household products)
2. Recognition and protection of a vulnerable host (young, inquisitive children, especially those with a history of accidents)
3. Control of the environment, or milieu by offering consistent love and discipline

Alerting and instructing parents. All parents should be made aware of the dangers confronting children at each stage of their development, particularly the toddler and preschooler (Table 18-11). Parents need to fully realize that normal children search for adventure and are ignorant of consequences. Parents should know that fatigue, hunger, family discord, and anxiety increase the likelihood of an accident. A wise and loving parent will know that discipline is a fundamental prerequisite for accident prevention. This discipline of obedience rapidly becomes the only reliable method for ensuring protection of the school-age child.

All children and families should be instructed in safety. Community educational efforts aimed at accident prevention should include information on fire and burn prevention, including flame-retardant clothing, smoke detectors, fire escapes and drills; water and play safety; approved automobile restraint devices; and use and proper storage of potentially toxic household chemicals, medicines, cosmetics, tools, and equipment. Individual re-

TABLE 18-11 ACCIDENTS COMMON AT VARIOUS STAGES OF DEVELOPMENT

Typical behavior	Type of accident	Precaution and safety education
INFANT		
Sleeps most of time	Suffocation	Use a firm mattress, no pillow; destroy plastic covers and filmy bags
Wiggles and rolls	Falls	Never leave child unattended on a surface such as a table or sofa; keep crib bars up
Helpless in water	Drowning	Never leave alone in bathtub or near pools
Sucks on objects	Choking; ingestion of foreign objects	Keep small objects out of reach, especially pins or other sharp objects; buy toys too large to swallow
	Poisoning	Keep medicines and poisons in a locked cabinet
TODDLER		
Roams all over house Climbs into things	Falls	Use gates on stairways; keep windows and doors locked; fence yard
Takes things apart	Cuts	Provide large, sturdy toys without sharp edges or small removable parts; keep sharp instruments and knives out of reach
Curious about everything	Burns	Needs constant supervision; never leave hot coffeepot or running water unattended; turn pot handles inward; keep matches locked up; treat flimsy clothing with fire-retardant (7 oz borax, 3 oz boric acid, 2 qt hot water)
Pokes and probes with fingers	Electric shock	Keep electrical appliances out of reach; cap unused light sockets with safety plugs
Chews everything	Poisoning	Keep medicines, cosmetics, and household poisons out of reach
	Ingestion of foreign objects and aspiration	Keep small objects such as coins, beans, needles, pins, jewelry, and doll's eyes out of reach
Enjoys playing in water	Drowning	Keep away from unattended pools and ponds; stay with child while in bathtub; fence in bodies of water
Rides tricycle	Motor vehicle accidents	Be firm and instruct child to keep clear of driveways and out of streets
Likes to ride in car and wants to go everywhere with mother		Instruct child in proper car safety; keep car doors locked and use safety belts or other approved restraints; never allow child to sit or stand in front seat of a car or allow child to put hands or head out of window
PRESCHOOLER		
Ventures out into neighborhood		Teach child safety rules and demonstrate principles by good example; enforce obedience Do not overprotect—preschoolers can begin to protect themselves, and overprotection deprives them of experience they need in growing up and learning independence

Continued.

TABLE 18-11 ACCIDENTS COMMON AT VARIOUS STAGES OF DEVELOPMENT—cont'd

Typical behavior	Type of accident	Precaution and safety education
PRESCHOOLER—cont'd		
Inquisitive	Burns	Teach children danger of open flames and hot objects
Rides bicycle Plays ball	Motor vehicle accidents	Instruct them in proper traffic safety rules—look both ways before crossing street, walk, never run across street, go with traffic light and walk in crosswalk, and never dart into street to go after a ball
Climbs trees and fences	Falls	Teach them good footing and proper handholds when climbing
Enjoys playing in water	Drowning	Begin swimming instruction; never let child play around unsupervised pools
Plays tough; runs up and down stairs	Blows; cuts	Check play areas for hazards Store dangerous tools and equipment in a locked cupboard
	Poisoning	Teach child not to taste unidentified foods, especially berries Lock up poisons; store in labeled bottles Discard old medicines down drain before putting containers in trash
EARLY SCHOOL AGE, 6 TO 9 YR		
Adventurous	Motor vehicle accidents	Needs intensive instruction in safety rules
Will try anything	Drowning	Encourage swimming safety
Loyal to friends	Falls	Point out importance of fun and not getting hurt Needs to know consequences for failing to follow rules
	Burns	Teach child to avoid smoldering fires; bottles and cans may explode and cause fatal injuries Teach child danger of matches and fires Teach proper use of chemistry sets
	Firearms	Point out serious consequences of playing with dry ice, fireworks, and other hazardous materials
LATE SCHOOL AGE, 10 TO 14 YEAR		
Rides bicycle constantly	Motor vehicle accidents	Enforce safety rules; explain reasons for them
Plays away from home, often in hazardous places	Drowning; burns; explosions	Know where child is at all times
Has lots of energy and enjoys strenuous play	Sprains; concussions	Point out importance of safe play
Enjoys working with power tools	Lacerations	Show children how to work around house safely (they should not use power tools unless tools are in good condition and they have knowledge of their use and safety); use proper equipment and keep it in good condition
Curious about firearms	Gunshot wounds	Lock up firearms and ammunition in separate locations

sponsibility and alertness multiplied to assure intelligent community involvement is needed.

Poison ingestion

Children have been known to swallow a fantastic variety and number of toxic substances (Fig. 18-7). The most frequent poisons are found in the medicine cabinet and under the kitchen sink. Often parental negligence has been directly responsible for the loss of a child's life. The majority of accidental poisonings in childhood are preventable.

Each year several hundred children die as the result of accidental poisoning, and an estimated 500,000 to 2 million children are involved in poisoning accidents. A major number of accidental poisonings occur in children under 4 years of age. This is the "age of curiosity," and these children are not selective about what they ingest. A number of nonfatal poisoning victims are left with permanent disabilities such as esophageal stricture or hepatic or renal damage.

Precautions. The following suggestions must be repeated until parents learn:

1. Keep all drugs, poisonous substances, and household chemicals in a locked cupboard out of the reach of little hands.
2. Do not transfer to or store poisons or flammable materials in food containers or bottles.
3. Never tell children that flavored medicine is candy (not even vitamins). Always refer to medicine as medicine!
4. Discard old medicines in drain before throwing away container.
5. Always read label before giving medicine.
6. Always return medicine to its proper place.
7. Do not underestimate the curiosity and abilities of children.
8. Medications should not be carried in purses; they are objects of interest to many toddlers and preschoolers. If it is imperative for medical reasons to have them (for example, cardiac medications), special precautions must be taken.

Emergency treatment. All accidental poisonings in young children are treated as an urgent emergency. Call the physician or poison control center immediately and bring the child and the poisonous substance to a hospital emergency room. Supportive and symptomatic treatment should be initiated immediately, even though the specific poison substance may not be known. (See section on poison control centers.)

Immediate management. The following immediate action should be taken in the case of poisoning:

1. Identify and remove the poison
2. Administer the antidote
3. Administer other supportive treatment

Removal of poison. In most cases the immediate necessity is to empty the child's stomach, even if hours have passed since the ingestion. *If not contraindicated,* emesis should be induced if possible. Removal (after prevention) is the most important aspect of poison management. However, emesis should *not* be induced in the event of the ingestion of corrosives (lye or strong acids), strychnine, or and hydrocarbons (kerosene, gasoline, fuel oil, paint thinner, and cleaning fluid). Emesis also should not be initiated if the child is unconscious or convulsing.

1. Administration of 15 ml of *syrup of ipecac* followed by 1 cup of water is the most effective way to induce emesis in a child over 12 months of age. The dose may be repeated once in 20 minutes if vomiting has not occurred. The child's head and shoulders should be lowered to prevent aspiration of the vomitus. An injection of apomorphine is sometimes used in the hospital in lieu of syrup of ipecac. An antidote such as naloxone (Narcan) must be given after vomiting has occurred to counteract the depressant effects of the apomorphine. Packaged in 1 fluid ounce containers, syrup of ipecac may be sold without a prescription. Parents should be carefully counseled at the 1-year, well-child visit concerning poison prevention. Information regarding syrup of ipecac should be

emphasized so that parents may have it available for use if necessary.

2. Gastric lavage is usually reserved for use when emesis is contraindicated or for the child who has not vomited after two doses of syrup of ipecac. A gastric tube with a large lumen is inserted, and the stomach contents are aspirated first and then irrigated with copious amounts of physiologic saline. Because of the time lapse in getting to the hospital and because the stomach normally traps material inaccessible to the lumen of the tube, chemical emesis is favored over gastric lavage.

Specific measures can be instituted as soon as the particular poison is identified. In most cases of acute poisoning, the physician can identify the agent by a quick history of the incident or by the label on the container. The poison container should always be brought to the hospital with the child.

Poison control centers. Information about poisons and emergency treatment of poison ingestion may be obtained immediately by telephoning the nearest Poison Control Center. More than 250,000 toxic or potentially toxic trade name products are on the consumer market. Federal law requires that the ingredients of drugs, pesticides, and caustic products be clearly stated on labels. However, many household products frequently involved in accidental ingestions are not required to be so labeled. To assist physicians with their very grave problem of identification, Poison Control Centers have been established in key areas of the United States. These centers are usually associated with medical schools or large hospitals equipped with laboratories, library, house staff, and faculty. They are available to dispense information 24 hours a day. They also serve as treatment centers and are actively engaged in programs of public education to prevent accidental poisoning. In some areas the Poison Control Centers give information to physicians only. However, parents should be instructed to keep the Poison Control Center number on their telephone. Other callers receive first-aid instruction and are advised to call the physician at once.

Administration of antidotes. Antidotes should be given immediately after emesis or lavage to render any remaining poison inert or prevent its absorption. Specific antidotes are not available for all poisons. Among the few available antidotes is dimercaprol (BAL, British antilewisite). Dimercaprol is a good antidote for arsenic, mercury, antimony, and lead poisoning. Activated charcoal is a powerful physical antidote that absorbs most poisons to itself. It should *not* be used with other substances that may interfere with its adsorptive capacity or with which it may interfere (syrup of ipecac). Large doses of the adsorbent should be used, especially when a large dose of poison has been ingested.

An antidote should be put in the Levin tube before the tube is removed from the stomach. The specific antidote is given if one is available.

In the event of caustic ingestion, immediate administration of water or milk to dilute the poison has been advised. Both emesis and lavage are contraindicated because of possible further tissue injury.

Supportive treatment. Check the child's breathing immediately. Assure a clear airway and fresh air. Mouth-to-mouth resuscitation may be lifesaving. Overtreatment by emetics, sedatives, and stimulants is dangerous and should be avoided. Overtreatment may result in more harm than the ingestion of the poison. Keep the patient comfortable, warm, and dry.

ACUTE SALICYLATE (ASPIRIN) POISONING

Until recently, salicylate intoxication was the most frequent cause of accidental poisoning in children. The decreased incidence of salicylate poisoning is attributed to safety packaging of aspirin (including a limited number, 36, of baby aspirins per bottle) and increased public awareness of the dangers of aspirin. Currently about 50% of all hospitalizations for salicylate poisonings are due to therapeutic misuse of aspirin, usually by a poorly informed parent.

The widespread use and availability of salicylates are prime factors in overdosage. The use of salicylates is so commonplace that parents and sometimes physicians underestimate the toxicity of the drug. Salicylates act rapidly but are excreted slowly. A small dose repeated frequently may accumulate to cause a severe state of salicylate poisoning.

Candy-flavored aspirin was invented to obtain an accurate, small dosage and improve the taste, but children should never to told that medicine is candy; flavored aspirin should *never* be left within a child's reach (Fig. 18-8).

A common but grave error occurs when the parent mistakenly gives the child a teaspoon of oil of wintergreen instead of cough medicine. One teaspoon of oil of wintergreen contains as much salicylate as 60 grains of aspirin. It represents a *lethal* dose in most cases.

Ingestion of acetaminophen, birth control pills, iron, and cosmetics is on the rise.

Clinical signs. There are many clinical signs of salicylate poisoning in children. In acute poisoning the first manifestation is hyperpnea with an increase in respiration depth. Severe acidosis, electrolyte imbalance, and dehydration follow. Other common symptoms include restlessness, extreme thirst, high temperature (usually 103° F or higher), profuse sweating, tremors, bleeding, delirium, convulsions, pulmonary edema, and coma. Cerebral hemorrhage may occur.

Treatment. The treatment of acute salicylate poisoning is always immediate emesis. Parents should attempt to induce vomiting as soon as the discovery is made. The physician or nearest Poison Control Center should be called for emergency instructions. The child is usually ordered to the hospital. The parents are requested to bring with the child any implicated container, loose pills, and sometimes the material vomited.

Emesis is induced with syrup of ipecac in the hospital emergency room. After evacuation of the stomach, activated charcoal is administered. A blood specimen is ordered immediately to determine the level of salicylate intoxication (30 mg/100 ml invariably is associated with symptoms). Peak levels are usually reached about 90 minutes after ingestion. Treatment of salicylate intoxication is aimed at correcting electrolyte imbalance. Measures are instituted to promote the rapid excretion of salicylates in the urine. Parenteral fluids are given both to combat dehydration and to facilitate prompt excretion of salicylates from the body.

Nursing care. Nursing care for salicylate poisoning is supportive. Fever is reduced by cool sponges; hourly urinary output is recorded, and pH of the urine is tested with Nitrazine paper. Accurate hourly output notations will help determine amounts of parenteral fluids necessary. Temperature, pulse, and respiration are checked every 15 minutes until stable; oxygen is given as necessary. Exchange transfusions or dialysis may be considered in severe, life-threatening intoxication.

Poisoning is one of the most common pediatric emergencies. It is always difficult to treat. In more than half the cases, the poisonous substances have been carelessly handled and stored by adults. The child often was improperly supervised. As part of the growing-up process, children investigate their environment. This investigation includes feeling and tasting, and these activities are always dangerous. However, supervised opportunities for investigation must be available.

Parents must take time to answer questions, show their children how things work, and help them learn to do things safely for themselves. Patience and supervision will teach children what they want to know and show them the way to safety, too.

Misuse of drugs

Abuse of drugs by youth in society is a major and growing social and personal problem in the United States. The average age level of drug users is dropping steadily. Many junior-high and grade-school children are now frequent offenders.

The word "drug" is used widely to mean a substance taken for pleasurable purposes, usually with the implications of illicitness and danger. The term drug dependence includes *addiction* (which implies tissue dependence, tolerance, and withdrawal symptoms) and *habituation* (which specifies the continuing nature of the drug-taking and implies psychologic rather than physiologic dependence). One may become addicted to heroin and other opium derivatives (narcotics), habituated to barbiturates, or dependent on any of these or on psychedelic drugs (for example, lysergic acid diethylamide [LSD] or mescaline), amphetamines, alcohol, or marijuana.

The subject of drug abuse cannot be treated in any detail in this text, but students are encouraged to learn more about the causes, prevention, and treatment of this problem. Because of the severity and widespread nature of the difficulty, it is likely that pediatric nurses will encounter a variety of different situations related to drug abuse. One usually thinks of teen-age involvement with hallucinogenic drugs, but recently two toddlers were admitted to a pediatric emergency room after ingesting an unknown number of "LSD pills." Treated with chlorpromazine (Thorazine), they did respond favorably.

Drug reactions vary. A heroin overdose produces a severe depression, whereas an amphetamine overdose will result in hyperactivity and overstimulation. Violent psychological reactions, varying from hallucinations to severe psychoses (paranoia) may result from LSD use. In recent years, the use of LSD (Acid) has declined. Unfortunately, phencyclidine (PCP or Angel Dust) abuse has become more common. Nurses should be alert for any unusual behavior not typical of the individual or age group. Such signs include abnormal dilatation of the pupils, excitability, talkativeness, profuse perspiration, staggering, mental confusion, disturbances in perception, and general personality changes. The nurse can best assist these patients by a calm, supportive manner and a quiet atmosphere, carefully attempting through conversation to make the patient aware of reality.

Sincere concern by the nurse for the substance abuser can, in some cases, help build a communication bridge back to society that will help rehabilitate the individual. Unfortunately, such successes have been less frequent than the failures.

Child abuse (nonaccidental injury)

The term "child abuse" includes many types of physical, sexual, mental, and emotional molestation, injury, or neglect. Hundreds of children are killed annually, and thousands of others are permanently harmed at the hands of adults, usually their parents.

Affected children commonly manifest abrasions, lacerations, burns, skull fractures, intracranial bleeding, and multiple long bone fractures in various stages of healing, as well as personality disturbances and mental impairment. One type of child abuse in which the victim is characterized by severe physical injury and neglect was in the past called the *battered child syndrome*. Neglected, nonaccidentally injured children brought to the hospital are typically under 3 years of age, frequently boys. They are many times born out of wedlock, unwanted, mentally retarded, or physically malformed. The children are often too young or too afraid to talk.

Parents of such children are described as emotionally immature and unready to accept the responsibilities of parenthood. Child abuse occurs in families of all socioeconomic levels, but often parents are burdened by adverse social conditions, financial strain, social isolation, and personal frustration. Some have reversed roles with their children, expecting them to provide love, gratification, and fulfillment to meet their own needs. Many of these parents were abused themselves. They are repeating familiar parental behavior experienced in childhood and have not learned different coping mechanisms.

Recognition. When first admitted to the hospital, neglected and nonaccidentally injured children typically shut their eyes, turn their heads away, and cry irritably, in contrast to well-nurtured children who characteristically cry loudly and reach out for their parents. The skillful observer may recognize the difficulty when parents offer no reasonable explanation regarding the character, circumstances, or nature of the trauma sustained.

One 2½-year-old boy entered the hospital to have his leg "checked." He weighed 19 pounds, one front tooth was missing, a fingernail was pulled off, his head and face were covered with skin lesions, and his right femur was broken (Fig. 31-3). The only information offered by his mother was, "He was very clumsy and stumbled in the yard." Two weeks passed before he would turn to look at anyone. His parents visited once in a period of 2 months. Suspicion should always be aroused when any of the following are noted: abnormal uncleanliness, malnutrition, multiple soft tissue injuries or burns in various stages of healing, and illness obviously caused by a lack of medical attention. Often the behavior of the child indicates that he has no real expectation of being comforted or helped.

Reporting. Because parental neglect and abuse are difficult to understand, they may go unrecognized. Children may recover from their injuries and go home, only to be battered again. The alert nurse is usually the first to suspect that a child has been abused. She should carefully chart what she observes and *report* the situation to the physician at once! Every state requires that nurses and physicians report suspicions to the police department or to the appropriate child protection service in the community. After a written report has been submitted, the case is carefully investigated. The person participating in good faith in making a report is immune from civil or criminal liability. Willful refusal to report child neglect or abuse is a violation of the law.

Protection. As part of public comprehensive child welfare services, most communities have established "protective services" for neglected and abused children. The purpose of a protective service is not only to provide care and protection for the child but also to help parents who "want to be good" but for some reason are unable to assume their role. Why else do parents bring their neglected and battered children to the hospital? They always run the risk of punishment. Could an abused or neglected child be their way of actually asking for help? The emergence of self-help parent groups such as Parents Anonymous, as well as "hot lines" nationwide, are a direct outgrowth of parents' need for help and anonymity.

Management of this serious problem may range from professional counseling and the introduction and explanation of various community services involved in chid care—for example, crisis nurseries and lay therapists (parent aides who may serve as role models and friends), to criminal court action. Juvenile courts have power over "neglected children," but do not employ criminal sanctions against the parents. However, when the case is reported, prosecuting agencies may institute criminal charges. According to recent studies, criminal prosecution is a poor means of preventing child abuse. Usually, criminal proceedings divide the family and cause parents to hate their children. Legal action is only advisable when all other means of protection and prevention have failed.

Perinatal nurses are in an ideal position for identifying potential child abusers.

SUGGESTED SELECTED READINGS AND REFERENCES

GENERAL

Boyle, M.P., et al: Assessment and management of anorexia nervosa, Am. J. Mat. Child Nurs. 6:412-418, Nov.-Dec. 1981.

Child health maintenance: focus on health, Nurs. Pract. 5:33-43, Jan.-Feb. 1980.

Ciseaux, A: Anorexia nervosa: the view from the mirror, Am. J. Nurs. 80:1468-1470.

Claggett, M.S.: A behavioral approach, Am. J. Nurs. 80:1471-1472, Aug. 1980.

Cormier, J.F., and Frammel, H.: Fighting tooth decay: the fluoride plan, Pediatr. Nurs. 5:18-22, May-June 1979.

Deal, A.W.: The phenomenon of SIDS, Pediatr. Nurs. 5:48-50, Jan.-Feb. 1980.

Dewhurst, Sir J.: Breast disorders in children and adolescents, Pediatr. Clin. North Am. 28:287-308, May 1981.

Pickwell, S.M.: Primary health care for Indochinese refugee children, Pediatr. Nurs. 8:104-107, Mar.-Apr. 1982.

Post, C.W., and Robinson, J.G.: A "good beginning" for families, Pediatr. Nurs. 6:32-36, July-Aug. 1980.

Richardson, T.E.: Anorexia nervosa: an overview, Am. J. Nurs. 80:1470-1471, Aug. 1981.

Spadaro, D.C.: Factors involved with patient compliance, Pediatr. Nurs. 6:27-29, July-Aug. 1980.

Wei, S.H.V., guest editor: Pediatric dental care: an update for the dentist and for the pediatrician, New York, 1978, Medcom Inc.

Wilson, J.L.: Health problems in Indochinese immigrants, Family Practice 12:551-557, March 1981.

ABUSE AND NEGLECT

Besharov, D.J.: The Third International Congress on Child Abuse and Neglect: Conference highlights, Children Today 10:12-15, 36, Sept.-Oct. 1981.

Dean, D.: Emotional abuse of children, Children Today 8:18-20, July-Aug. 1979.

Fultz, J.M., Jr., et al: When a narcotic addict is hospitalized, Am. J. Nurs. 80:478-481, Mar. 1980.

Funk, J.B.: Management of sexual molestation in preschoolers, Clin. Pediatr. 19:686-688, Oct. 1980.

Harling, P.R., and Haines, J.K.: Specialized foster homes for severely mistreated children, Child. Today 9:16-18, July-Aug. 1980.

Heindl, M.C.: Child abuse and neglect, Nurs. Clin. North Am. 16:101-179, March 1981.

Iyer, P.W.: The battered wife, Nurs. '80 10:52-55, July 1980.

McFadden, E.M.: Fostering the battered and abused child, Child. Today 9:13-15, Mar.-Apr. 1980.

McMillen-Hall, N.: Group treatment for sexually abused children, Nurs. Clin. North Am. 13:701-705, Dec. 1978.

Mira, M., and Cairns, G.: Intervention in the interaction of a mother and child with nonorganic failure to thrive, Pediatr. Nurs. 7:41-45, Mar.-Apr. 1981.

Orr, D.P.: Management of childhood sexual abuse, Nurse Pract. 11:1057-1064, Dec. 1980.

Ortman, E.: Attachment behavior in abused children, Pediatr. Nurs. 5:25-29, July-Aug. 1979.

Pascoe, D.J., and Duterte, B.O.: The medical diagnosis of sexual abuse in the premenarcheal child, Pediatr. Ann. 10:40, 43-45, May 1981.

Recognizing and helping the abused child, Nurs. '79 9:64-67, Feb. 1979.

Sammons, L.N.: Battered and pregnant, Am. J. Mat. Child Nurs. 6:246-250, July-Aug. 1981.

Scherzer, L.N.: Sexual offenses committed against children: an analysis of 73 cases of child sexual abuse, Clin. Pediatr. 19:679, 683, 685, Oct. 1980.

Sredl, D.R., Klenke, C., and Rojkind, M.: Offering the rape victim real help, Nurs. '79 9:38-43, July 1979.

Thomas, J.N.: Yes, you can help a sexually abused child, RN 43:23-29, Aug. 1980.

Woodling, B.A., and Kossoris, P.D.: Sexual misuse: rape, molestation, and incest, Pediatr. Clin. North Am. 28:481-499, May 1981.

GROWTH AND DEVELOPMENT

Betz, C.L.: Faith development in children, Pediatr. Nurs. 7:22-25, Mar.-Apr. 1981.

Bradshaw, T.W.: Teething, Pediatr. Nurs. 7:41-42, May-June 1981.

Brink, R.E.: How serious is the child's behavioral problem? Am. J. Mat. Child Nurs. 7:33-36, Jan.-Feb. 1982.

Calhoun, J.A.: Developing a family perspective, Child. Today 9:2-8, Mar.-Apr. 1980.

Erickson, E.: Childhood and society, ed. 2., New York, 1963, W.W. Norton & Co., Inc.

Fleming, R.A.: Developing a child's self-esteem, Pediatr. Nurs. **5**:58-60, July-Aug. 1979.

Frasier, S.D.: Growth disorders in children, Pediatr. Clin. North Am. **26**:3-14, Feb. 1979.

Gallo, A.: Early childhood masturbation: a developmental approach, Pediatr. Nurs. **5**:47-49, Sept.-Oct. 1979.

Goldstein, H.S., and Snope, F.C.: Child behavior assessment in family practice, Am. Fam. Physician, **21**:142-145, Apr. 1980.

Hammer, D., and Drabman, R.S.: Child discipline: what we know and what we can recommend, Pediatr. Nurs. **7**:31-35, May-June 1981.

Horner, M.E., and McClellan, M.A.: Toilet training: ready or not? Pediatr. Nurs. **7**:15-18, Jan.-Feb. 1981.

Hyman, I.A., and Lally, D.: Discipline in the 1980s: some alternatives to corporal punishment, Child. Today **11**:10-13, Jan.-Feb. 1982.

Jaworski, A.A.: One boy-girl chart for office use from eight NCHS growth charts, Clin. Pediatr. **19**:546-548, Aug. 1980.

Johnston, M.: Toward a culture of caring: children, their environment and change, Am. J. Mat. Child Nurs. **4**:210-214, July-Aug. 1979.

Klaus, M.H., and Kennell, J.H.: Parent-infant bonding, ed. 2., St. Louis, 1981, The C.V. Mosby Co.

Lanes, R., et al: Are constitutional delay of growth and familial short stature different conditions? Clin. Pediatr. **19**:10-24, Jan. 1980.

Lessick, M.L., Van Putte, A.W., and Rowley, P.T.: Assessment of evaluation of hospitalized pediatric patients with genetic disorders, Clin. Pediatr. **20**:178-183, Mar. 1981.

Linde, D.B., and Engelhardt, K.F.: What do parents know about infant development, Pediatr. Nurs. **5**:32-36, Jan.-Feb. 1979.

Lipsitz, J.S.: Adolescent development: myths and realities, Child. Today **8**:2-7, Sept.-Oct. 1979.

Malinowski, J.S.: Answering a child's questions about sex and a new baby, Am. J. Nurs. **79**:1965-1970, Nov. 1979.

Melichar, M.M.: Using crisis theory to help parents cope with a child's temper tantrums, Am. J. Mat. Child Nurs. **5**:181-185, May-June 1980.

Moss, J.R.: Helping young children cope with the physical examination, Pediatr. Nurs. **7**:17-20, Mar.-Apr. 1981.

Nelms, B.C.: What is a normal adolescent?, Am. J. Mat. Child Nurs. **6**:402-406, Nov.-Dec. 1981.

Novak, J.C.: Children vs. divorce, Pediatr. Nurs. **8**:33-39, Jan.-Feb. 1982.

O'Neil, S.M., McLaughlin, B.N., and Knapp, M.B.: Behavioral approaches to children with developmental delays, St. Louis, 1977, The C.V. Mosby Co.

Powell, M.L.: Assessment and management of developmental changes and problems in children, ed. 2, St. Louis, 1981, The C.V. Mosby Co.

Raiti, S.: Short stature: evaluation and treatment, Pediatr. Ann. **9**:14-23, Apr. 1980.

Reindollar, R.H., and McDonough, P.G.: Delayed sexual development: common causes and basic clinical approach, Pediatr. Ann. **10**:30-39, May 1981.

Sapala, S., and Strokosch, G.: Adolescent sexuality: use of a questionnaire for health teaching and counseling, Pediatr. Nurs. **7**:33-34,52, Nov.-Dec. 1981.

Spanier, G.B.: The changing profile of the American family, J. Fam. Pract. **13**:61-69, July 1981.

Tudor, M.: Child development, New York, 1981, McGraw-Hill Book Co.

Warburton, D.: Current techniques in chromosome analysis, Pediatr. Clin. North Am. **27**:753-769, Nov. 1980.

IMMUNIZATION

American Academy of Pediatrics: Report of the committee on infectious diseases, ed. 19, Evanston, Ill., 1982, The Academy.

Benenson, A.S., editor: Control of communicable diseases in man, ed. 13., Washington, D.C., 1980, American Public Health Association.

Center for Disease Control: General recommendations on immunization, Morbidity and Mortality Weekly Report **29**:76-83, Feb. 22, 1980.

Center for Disease Control: Immune globulins for protection against viral hepatitis, Morbidity and Mortality Weekly Report **30**:423-428, 433-438, 1981.

Center for Disease Control: Measles—U.S. 1981, Morbidity and Mortality Weekly Report **31**:37-39, Feb. 5, 1982.

Center for Disease Control: School immunization requirements for measles—U.S. 1982, Morbidity and Mortality Weekly Report **31**:62-67, Feb. 19, 1982.

Center for Disease Control: Vaccine-associated poliomyelitis—U.S. 1981, Morbidity and Mortality Weekly Report **31**:97-98, Mar. 5, 1982.

Center for Disease Control: Varicella-Zoster immune globulin, Morbidity and Mortality Weekly Report **30**:15-16, 21-23, 1981.

Krugman, S., and Katz, S.L.: Infectious diseases of children, ed. 7., St. Louis, 1981, The C.V. Mosby Co.

Linnemann, C.C., et al: Measles immunity after revaccination, Pediatrics **69**:332-335, Mar. 1982.

McConnell, S.D.: Pneumococcal vaccine, Nurse Pract. 7:18-20, Mar. 1982.

Moffet, H.L.: Pediatric infectious diseases, ed. 2., Philadelphia, 1981, J.B. Lippincott Co.

Mumps vaccine: updated recommendations (editorial), Clin. Pediatr. 19:711-712, Oct. 1980.

Steiner, P., et al: A comparative study of the old tuberculin tine test and the PPD tine test, Clin. Pediatr. 19:389-391, June 1980.

Williams, L.: Childhood immunization, Pediatr. Nurs. 8:18-21,53, Jan.-Feb. 1982.

OBESITY AND NUTRITION

Copeland, T.E., and Baucom-Copeland, S.: Childhood obesity: a family systems review, Am. Fam. Physician 24:153-157, Aug. 1981.

Crummette, B.D., and Munton, M.T.: Mother's decisions about infant nutrition, Pediatr. Nurs. 6:16-19, Nov.-Dec. 1980.

Fomon, S.J.: Nutritional disorders of children: prevention, screening and follow-up. Rockville, Md., 1977, DHEW Publication No. (HSA)77:5104, U.S. Department of Health, Education and Welfare.

Fomon, S.J., et al: Recommendations for feeding normal infants, Pediatrics 63:52-59, Jan. 1979.

Golden, M.P.: An approach to the management of obesity in childhood, Pediatr. Clin. North Am. 26:187-197, Feb. 1979.

Kuhn, J.G., and Fischer, R.G.: Vitamins in pediatrics, Pediatr. Nurs. 5:25-31, Mar.-Apr. 1979.

Langford, R.W.: Teenagers and obesity, Am. J. Nurs. 81:556-559, Mar. 1981.

Markesbery, B.A., and Wong, W.M.: Watching baby's diet: a professional and parental guide, Am. J. Mat. Child Nurs. 4:177-180, May-June 1979.

Mowery, B.D.: Family-oriented approach to childhood obesity, Pediatr. Nurs. 6:40-44, Mar.-Apr. 1980.

Overfield, T.: Obesity: prevention is easier than cure, Nurse Pract. 5:25-26,33,62, Sept.-Oct. 1980.

Pipes, P.L.: Nutrition in infancy and childhood, ed. 2, St. Louis, 1981, The C.V. Mosby Co.

Swanson, J.: The toddler's eating habits, Pediatr. Nurs. 5:52-53, Jan.-Feb. 1979.

Williams, S.R.: Nutrition and diet therapy, ed. 4, St. Louis, 1981, The C.V. Mosby Co.

Winick, M.: Pediatric nutrition: introduction, Pediatr. Ann. 10:17-18, Nov. 1981.

SAFETY AND ACCIDENTS

Accident facts, Chicago, 1981, National Safety Council.

Adams, D.: Children's response to a belt restraint program, Pediatr. Nurs. 8:28-30,67, Jan.-Feb. 1982.

Atwood, S.J.: The laboratory in the diagnosis and management of acetaminophen and salicylate intoxication, Pediatr. Clin. North Am. 27:871-879, Nov. 1980.

Berkowitz, R., et al: Dental trauma in children and adolescents, Clin. Pediatr. 19:166-171, Mar. 1980.

Cohen, G.C.: Lead poisoning: 20 years later, Clin. Pediatr. 19:245-250, Apr. 1980.

Conn, A.W., Edmonds, J.F., and Barker, G.A.: Cerebral resuscitation in near-drowning, Pediatr. Clin. North Am. 26:691-701, Aug. 1979.

Gossel, T.A., and Wuest, J.R.: The *right* first aid for poisoning, RN 44:73-75, Mar. 1981.

Hart, N.A., and Keidel, G.C.: The suicidal adolescent, Am. J. Nurs. 79:80-84, Jan. 1979.

Jones, J.G.: The child accident repeater: a review, Clin. Pediatr. 19:284-288, Apr. 1980.

Kilham, H.A.: Hospital management of severe poisoning, Pediatr. Clin. North Am. 27:603-612, Aug. 1980.

Lin-Fu, J.S.: Lead poisoning in children, Child. Today 8:9-13,36, Jan.-Feb. 1979.

Macy, A.M.: Preventing hepatotoxicity in acetaminophen overdose, Am. J. Nurs. 79:301-303, Feb. 1979.

Marcus, D.F.: Child car seats: a must for safety, Pediatr. Nurs. 7:13-17, May-June 1981.

Nursing care of a suicidal adolescent, Nurs. '80 10:56-59, Apr. 1980.

Paulson, J.A.: The case for mandatory seat restraint laws, Clin. Pediatr. 20:285-290, Apr. 1981.

Paulson, J.A.: Injury prevention in children, J. Fam. Pract. 13:123-124, July 1981.

Piomelli, S., and Graziano, J.: Laboratory diagnosis of lead poisoning, Pediatr. Clin. North. Am. 27:841-853, Nov. 1980.

Randolph, J.G. (editor) et al: The injured child, Chicago, 1979, Year Book Medical Publishers.

Rogers, J.: Recurrent childhood poisoning as a family problem, J. Fam. Pract. 13:337-340, Sept. 1981.

Williams, A.: Children killed in falls from motor vehicles, Pediatrics 68:576-578, Oct. 1981.

THE CHILD, THE FAMILY, AND THE HOSPITAL SETTING

CHAPTER **19**   Hospitalization of the child

For most persons, regardless of age, hospitalization is a necessary but not particularly welcome interruptive interlude in their lives. Often a stay in the hospital is not planned, and suddenly one enters a rather strange world with many of one's normal social defenses changed, such as family and community role, privacy—even clothes. This turn of events is disruptive enough for the adult, but it is potentially even more disruptive for the impressionable young child.

PREPARATION FOR HOSPITALIZATION

Not many years ago the preparation of children and their parents for the experience of hospitalization did not receive much consideration. Emphasis was placed on the child's disease rather than the fact that this was a particular person with certain capabilities and needs who happened to be ill. Typically the parents brought little Mary Lou to the pediatric ward, signed some papers, and said a rather hasty and usually tearful good-bye. Perhaps Mary Lou was placed in a special semi-isolation admission area to be observed for 24 to 48 hours for the possible onset of contagious disease before being transferred to the main pediatric ward. Little was done to prepare her or her parents for this sudden change in their pattern of living.

Today, although a great deal remains to be learned about children their needs, and family relationships, health providers do recognize that the old approach and many of the old methods were incomplete and unnecessarily traumatic for all concerned. Recently attempts have been made to shorten hospitalization or avoid it altogether by more reliance on outpatient departments and surgi-centers designed for minor operations and recovery requiring less than a day. The modern nurse recognizes that the family may have a great deal to offer the hospitalized child, and when properly prepared and supported, the parents will be able to help the child as no others can during a difficult but, it is hoped, also a potentially constructive period in the child's heretofore brief experience with life.

The parents

The heart of the problem is preparing children for hospitalization lies in the preparation of their parents, who are then best able to help their children. It is imperative that parents receive sufficient knowledge of the child's illness so that they readily understand the need for hospitalization. It is also necessary for parents to have some understanding of the tests and treatments to be given and the risk and discomfort involved.

A child's morale will inevitably reflect the parents' outlook. When parents are inadequately prepared, they cannot adequately prepare their child. It is extremely important that the parents have sound information about the child's illness, confidence in their physician's recommendations, and the devoted interest of warm, intelligent, and understanding nurses.

The child

According to their level of understanding, children should be told why it is necessary for them to go to the hospital. Truthful assurance is the best guide. The truth is less frightening to youngsters than the ideas their imaginations can invent. Children who are not given the true reason for hospitalization often believe that they have been punished or sent away because they have been naughty. Of course, if the truth is to be supportive, children must have confidence in their parents and other authority figures based on previous experience of their trustworthiness. Such an attitude cannot be established in a day. Its foundation is laid during the first year and perpetuated through each stage of life.

Telling children about surgery is a highly individual matter. Information about the impending operation will depend on the child's age, level of understanding, and emotional makeup. Usually a brief, simple explanation of what is wrong and what must be done to change it or make it better will help the child develop a sound and healthy attitude. A detailed and accurate explanation of the operation is not necessary; the child needs the truth, but not always the whole truth. The belief that an event has been explained relieves tension.

Pediatric units in hospitals throughout the United States have developed methods to prepare parents and children for hospitalization. Colorful booklets and pamphlets, telephone calls, hospital tours, preadmission or orientation parties, including movies and muppet shows, and the use of television sets all have lessened the trauma of admission to the hospital. Advising parents of procedures and inviting children and their parents to visit the hospital before admission help children to know

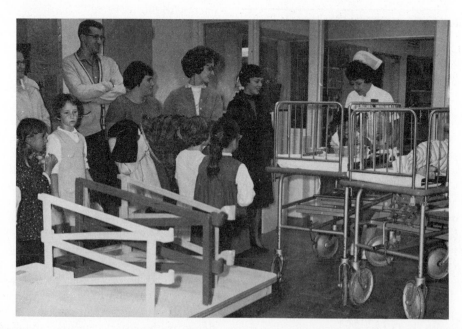

FIG. 19-1   Inviting children and their parents to visit the hospital before admission helps them to know what to expect.

Courtesy Children's Hospital and Health Center, San Diego, Calif.

what to expect (Fig. 19-1). Allowing the child to share in planning for a hospital stay or helping to pack a suitcase is sometimes rewarding.

Children should know in advance what the hospital is like. They should be told simply and in a matter-of-fact manner about such things as the differences between hospital beds and beds at home, use of the bedpan and urinals, baths in bed, special schooling, the playroom, and the food service. If 4-year-old Jimmy knows in advance about the big, wiggly scale that he must stand on to see how heavy

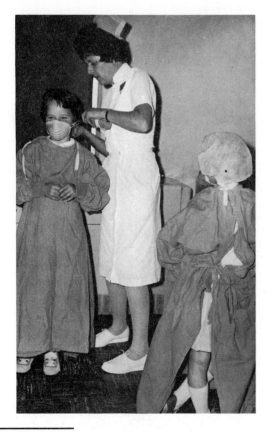

FIG. 19-2

If the child knows in advance what will happen, she is less likely to be shocked when she faces the situation directly.

Courtesy Children's Hospital and Health Center, San Diego, Calif.

he is and some of the other things that will happen at the hospital, he is less likely to be shocked when he faces them directly (Fig. 19-2).

It is not always possible, necessary, or desirable for children to know everything that will happen. All they need to know is enough to assure them that what happens is according to plan and that their parents will be at their side whenever possible. When they cannot be there, kind friends, physicians, and nurses will help care for them until they can go home again.

Printed information sheets to be completed by parents, ideally before admission, are helpful. They request brief background material regarding the health history, habits, skills, likes, dislikes, fears, and family composition of the young patient; this information assists the staff in individualizing care.

Liberal visiting hours that include sibling contacts, rooming-in facilities, and appropriate parent participation in care have made it much easier for the mother and father to continue their supportive role and help counteract any sense of isolation or desertion the child may harbor. However, no matter how well children are prepared for hospitalization, they may still cry at the prospect of treatment, needles, and pain. Explain to the parents that this is a natural reaction and encourage them to stay with their child, since they are best able to comfort the youngster with the thought of feeling better when it is over. Usually the parents' presence helps the child to weather each interference as it comes and greatly reduces the risk of emotional trauma.

SEPARATION ANXIETY

The young child

Considerable evidence has shown that under certain circumstances children may view hospitalization as desertion by their parents and thus may be profoundly affected by their hospital experience. When parents of a young child are unable to come to the hospital for prolonged periods, the

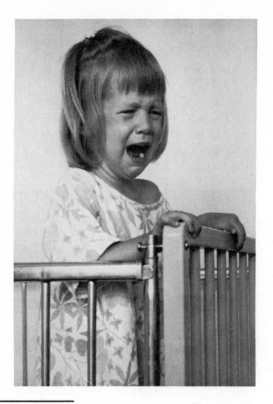

FIG. 19-3

Phase I: Protest. The day after admission, the child (Marie, 2½ years old) cries aloud for "Mama," shakes the crib and is alert for any signs of her mother's return.

Courtesy Children's Hospital and Health Center, San Diego, Calif.

hospitalized child is exposed to numerous traumatic factors resulting in frustration of those inborn needs that are normally met in a family environment. As a result, the child may fail to thrive physically, socially, and psychologically. In extreme situations, maternal deprivation may be manifested as a general marasmus, or wasting away.

The effects of separation do not always manifest themselves immediately. The emotional aftermath of hospitalization may appear in forms such as night terrors, fears, negativism, regressions to earlier, more babylike, clinging behavior, and protracted hostilities. In some cases the effects may not appear until later in life.

Studies have pointed out that in children between 1 and 4 years of age the risks involved with parent-child separation are greatest. These risks taper off beyond 5 years of age but never disappear entirely during childhood.

Separation anxiety is characteristic of all young children who have established a healthy parent-child relationship. The phenomenon of "settling in," or adjustment to hospitalization and separation, is deceptive. Robertson* found that children under 4 years of age experience three phases in the process of settling into the hospital: protest, despair, and denial. These emotional phases may not be as severe when pediatric policies are more enlightened, but they are probably still there.

At first young children *protest* the separation (Fig. 19-3). They cry aloud for "Mama," shake the crib, throw themselves around, and are alert for any signs of mother's return. The nurse may pick up the child and try to quiet him, but this is to no avail. Telling children to stop crying only conveys to them that they are not understood and adds to their feelings of helplessness. This phase may last for a few days or even up to 1 week.

During the phase of *despair* the child becomes apathetic and withdrawn, which is sometimes confused with acceptance (Fig. 19-4). Instead of crying, the child sobs. The hope of mother's return fades, but the wish for her return remains. During this quiet stage, distress seemingly has lessened, and the nurse presumes that the child is "settling in." When the parents arrive, the child may turn away and cry aloud. Children do not understand why they are in the hospital. They reject their parents as the parents seem to have rejected the child. Parents spend most of visiting time trying to get the child to respond to them more normally, and just as the child brightens up, they may leave again. Children's piteous cries on the parents'

*Robertson, J.: Young children in hospitals, New York, 1958, Basic Books, Inc.

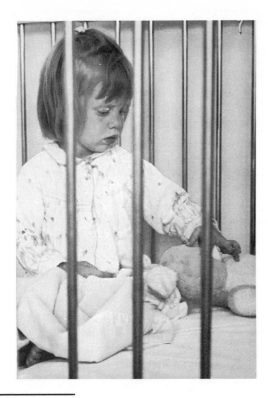

FIG. 19-4

Phase II: Despair. Four days after admission the child has become apathetic and withdrawn. She does not understand why her mother has left her or why she is in the hospital.

Courtesy Children's Hospital and Health Center, San Diego, Calif.

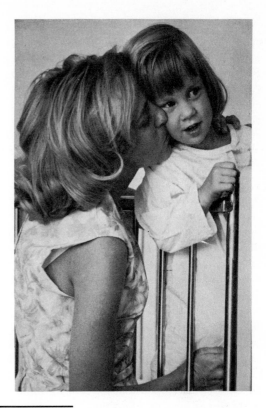

FIG. 19-5

Phase III: Denial. Eight days after admission the little child cannot tolerate the intensity of distress so she represses the need for mother. When her mother comes, she seems hardly to know her, is happy and gay.

Courtesy Children's Hospital and Health Center, San Diego, Calif.

arrival and departure lead the nurse mistakenly to think that the youngsters are better off without their parents. The nurse who understands the reason for this behavior can be of great help to the parents who dread coming back because they anticipate their child's distress. The parents need to realize how much their child needs them, and they should be encouraged to come often. When they leave they should be sure to tell the child when they will come back. It is unfair for a parent to tell their child that he or she is going for a cup of coffee.

Children have lain awake all night waiting for parents to return.

Gradually the stage of *denial* follows despair. Children begin to show more interest in the surroundings, are more responsive to nursing attention, and actually deny the need for their parents. When their mothers come, they may seem hardly to know them, are happy and gay throughout the visit, and may even wave good-bye (Fig. 19-5). Psychologists have explained this phenomenon by theorizing that because young children cannot tolerate the intensity of distress, they repress the need for their mothers. However, after they return home they often demonstrate their disturbed feelings by regressive babylike behavior and are forever clinging to their mothers. This only confirms that the complacency they exhibited in the hospital was a façade.

The school-age child

School-age children are not so susceptible to separation anxiety if their illnesses are short. These children have learned to rely to some extent on adults and other children when away from home. They can understand that hospitalization is a temporary situation and why their parents come only at certain times. School-age children seem more bothered by the disease process and its treatment. Imagination persists strongly throughout these years, and often fantasies and fears of mutilation influence the degree of emotional reaction. Older children worry about the hospital costs. If by chance they feel responsible for causing their illness, their worries are intensified.

Long-term hospitalization imposes numerous anxieties on children of all ages. During a serious illness even older children have a great need for their parents and can tolerate their absence only for short periods. They need to know that their parents will be there when they need them most and that they are loved and missed. (See Chapter 21.)

GROWTH AND DEVELOPMENTAL NEEDS

All children come to the hospital with their own individual makeup and achieved state of development, unique past experiences, and methods of dealing with anxiety. The nurse can encourage emotional growth by accepting these children as they are and by assisting them to continue in their present stage of development. For example, often children are expected to conform to hospital rules by staying in cribs when, in essence, they have had the run of the whole house before hospitalization. Unless acutely ill, a child may refuse to stay in bed. The nurse should not arbitrarily urge the child to "stay there." She should be aware of the dangers of restricting children to cribs when otherwise they could be ambulatory. For the toddler, sustained restriction of movement may lead to a severe state of anxiety and hostility. Whenever the basic motor urge is thwarted, the child becomes frustrated and angry and may regress. This drive is constructively handled by the wise nurse who devises ways to allow the child freedom to move about safely.

• • •

This discussion has highlighted the psychologic risks of hospitalization that are real and well documented. However, it is comforting to note that children usually are able to survive the event of hospitalization without significant emotional scars. It is largely the nurse's function to see that the original trauma is slight and the scars minimal.

CHAPTER **20**   Rehabilitation of the long-term
pediatric patient

For most children the period of hospitalization is brief—a day or two, perhaps a week. Increasingly, the trend is to shorten the treatment period away from home whenever possible; a shorter stay in the hospital has psychological, social, and financial advantages for the child and the family. However, for a few patients, hospitalization is still prolonged. The severely ill child who has a long, complicated convalescence, the child undergoing elaborate orthopedic corrections, and the teenager with a damaged spinal cord who is struggling to recapture skills once considered automatic and to adjust to new expectations and goals are all examples of relatively long-term pediatric patients. The following is a brief discussion of the needs of boys and girls who stay in the hospital for extended periods; it emphasizes the nursing perspectives, challenges, and skills of a relatively new specialty within a specialty—that of pediatric rehabilitation.

In a general sense the definition of rehabilitation is "to restore to a functional state." The families of those patients who have suffered devastating physical disabilities characteristically need a coordinated multidisciplinary team that considers not only the physical but the sociologic, emotional, vocational, and spiritual aspects of the patient's total situation. The rehabilitation of children is made more complex by their continuing need for normal growth and development in the face of disability.

Pediatric rehabilitation is based on at least two concepts: first, that each person is unique and has individual basic worth, and second, that the task involves a committed group of people working together as a team with a common goal. The overall goal of pediatric rehabilitation is to foster maximal growth, development, independence, and personal fulfillment within the limitations of the handicap. Many allied health professionals form the core rehabilitation team: physicians, nurses, physical and occupational therapists, speech and hearing pathologists, medical social service workers, dieticians, financial counselors, recreational therapists, teachers, and educational consultants. Representatives of other specialty areas, such as psychology, psychiatry, psychometric testing, and vocational counseling, as well as community agencies, are available as needed. Team physicians represent each specialty, and the community physician, public health nurse, and teacher are invited to be part of the team for their patient. Each team member evaluates the patient, makes recommendations in writing, and participates in patient planning conferences. The patient and family are, of course, prime members of the team and are included appropriately in conferences where current status and progress are discussed and new goals are set.

The need of the area served by the rehabilitation center should dictate the types of patients seen. Patients with spinal cord injuries, traumatic brain injuries, and incapacitating birth anomalies, such as myelomeningocele (spina bifida), usually make up a large part of the patient load. Those with Guillain-Barré syndrome (a polyneuritis), developmental disabilities, muscular dystrophy, juvenile rheumatoid arthritis, severe scoliosis, osteogenesis imperfecta, and other complex physical problems are also appropriately treated in a rehabilitation setting.

Generally speaking, any patient with a devastating injury or illness that produces lasting or permanent physical disabilities can and should be handled by the rehabilitation team. Nursing principles of rehabilitation must be initiated at the onset of illness or injury to prevent complications and further loss of function. Realistically, many of these children initially require specialized lifesaving care, which can be delivered more effectively in intensive care or medical-surgical units. Ideally the principles of both acute and long-term care will be delivered simultaneously. When the patient's condition has stabilized and the youngster is no longer "ill" as such, it is time to consider transfer to the rehabilitation unit.

A rehabilitation program ideally involves an inpatient unit, an outpatient clinic, and community agencies. They all function to help the patient and family progress smoothly from onset of illness or injury back to the home and community as a functioning, worthwhile member of society.

Throughout the patient's progression from the initial care facility back to the home and community, there must be no surprises. The transition of the patient to units, wards, agencies, and levels of any program must be done smoothly without breaks in continuity. The patient, family, and team members must be kept informed of the patient's status, program, and goals. Continuity in care during and after transfer to the rehabilitation unit takes the coordinated effort and skills of all the persons involved. One person must coordinate the process of admission. Frequently this is the responsibility of the nurse.

Staffing of a rehabilitation unit needs to be 30% to 60% above the usual medical-surgical ratios. Fastidious nursing care, continual teaching, and reinforcement are required. Independence comes with patience, repetition, and allowing the patient or family member to "do" rather than the tradition-al "doing for." The program is expensive, and the cost must be passed on to the patient, insurance companies, and government agencies; but the independence gained may in the end reduce the total financial outlay. Needless to say, the patient, family, and rehabilitation team must expend great amounts of emotional and physical energy as well as monetary resources. Perhaps the former is more difficult to supply.

Before contributing to the formation of an individualized care plan, each team member must assess the patient's current status. A logical, systematic approach will assure the inclusion of all important facts in the nursing assessment. (See the chart on p. 403 for a suggested initial assessment outline.)

Using this evaluation of the patient's current status and pertinent history, one can formulate nursing interventions for existing and potential problems and identify teaching needs. Successful teaching will also include assessment of the cultural values, life-style, and learning capabilities of the child and parents. Teaching needs and nursing intervention must always be discussed with the patient—in a manner appropriate to the child's age—and with the parents to determine the family's readiness to learn. Mutual strategies, goals, and target dates can then be incorporated into a written plan. Visual materials and demonstrations giving clear explanations of the treatment rationale and its importance to the patient will enhance learning.

When the patient's progress is sufficient, as shown on the unit and during progressive home passes, discharge plans are finalized. Discharge should also be coordinated by one person. There should be a home visit before discharge to help plan for program needs or physical changes within the home. These will be evaluated during progressive pass experiences. Before discharge, arrangements for the following must be made: community public health nurse follow-up, admission to a regular or special school, methods of obtaining supplies and medications, return appointments to community physicians, and the sharing of phone numbers of team members with the family.

After discharge, regular visits to a rehabilitation

INITIAL NURSING ASSESSMENT OUTLINE

Introduction	Name, age, chief complaint or problem, circumstances of present injury or illness, referring physician
History	Past injuries, illnesses, hospitalizations
Vital signs	Temperature, pulse, respiration, blood pressure
Allergies	Reactions to drug, food, airborne particles, contact
System check*	
Neurosensory	Level of consciousness, orientation, cranial checks, intellectual level, balance, coordination, sensory abnormalities, emotional stability
Integumentary	Turgor, general condition, complete description of lesions, condition of mouth
Musculoskeletal	Muscle strength, range of motion, motor abnormalities, amputations (follow-up evaluation by PT)
Respiratory	Pattern and sound of respirations, URI? cough? Pulmonary function studies (follow-up evaluation by PT and RT)
Urinary	Vocabulary? Normal voiding or ostomy? Continence? Urinary draining devices, catheter size, date of last change
Gastrointestinal	Vocabulary? Schedule: time, frequency, bowel movement consistency, normal movement or ostomy? Effect of diet?
Diet	Type, likes and dislikes, time and amount; method; bottle, oral, gavage, etc.
Health supervision	Dates of last dental, eye, and hearing exams; performed by? Immunizations? Safety problems?
Growth and development (activities of daily living; motor skills)	Independent, with assistance; dependent: feeding, turning, transfer, bathing, dressing, toileting, standing, walking (follow-up evaluation by OT and PT)
Equipment brought	Cane, crutches, walker, wheelchair, braces, appliances, scooterboards
Current medications and treatments	Medication: dosage, time, route, effects? Treatments: time, duration, specifics
Family composition	Parents, marital status, age, siblings, extended family, resources (follow-up evaluation by MSS)
Social and educational interests	Level of education, special friends, hobbies, security items, community contacts
Understanding of injury or illness	By patient, by family
Specialized care needs	

PT, Physical Therapy; OT, Occupational Therapy; RT, Respiratory Therapy; MSS, Medical Social Service.
*In making this assessment, one should ascertain the status of the patient before his injury or illness.

clinic enable the team to reevaluate each patient with feedback from the school, public health nurse, and other outside agencies.

Because of improved medical care during the last 25 years, increasing numbers of the handicapped have been absorbed into society. As a cohesive group, they are beginning to represent a political force. Through consumer awareness and pressure, legislation for the handicapped has brought about improved wheelchair accessibility in many public buildings and businesses, leading to improved educational and employment opportunities. Additionally, the courts have begun to attack discrimination in the job market, making job performance the sole criterion for employment.

PSYCHOLOGIC SUPPORT OF LONG-TERM PATIENTS AND THEIR FAMILIES

The character and severity of an injury or disease may be sources of considerable stress, but prolonged isolation from normal surroundings, the strange environment of the hospital, and frequent encounters with the many different people involved in patient care make hospitalization particularly difficult. The limited experience and development of the child increase the potential for emotional trauma at this time. Three recommendations seem particularly appropriate for the nursing of children and young people with long-term illnesses: Maintain a sense of trust; protect the child from fear, frustration, and pain; and facilitate social interaction and contact with the community.

A sense of trust is best fostered in children when their parents trust the people working in the facility. This trust is gradually developed as the parents and child learn that the staff, demonstrating forethought, accessibility, and reliability as well as technical skills, cares about them. It may be strengthened through the primary nursing concept or at least the consistent assignment of one or two nurses for each child's care. Trust also increases as the staff helps the family in its grief for the child who is injured or is born with defects. These parents mourn the loss of the well or perfect child they

had expected as though that child had died. Grieving as a result of injury or malformation is similar to that associated with death, although the terminology used may vary (p. 424). The loss is resolved in three stages: (1) shock and denial, (2) developing awareness, and (3) restitution. The immediate response of shock and disbelief is often still present on arrival at the rehabilitation unit. Statements such as, "When will my child walk again?" and "When she is better, things will be like they were before," demonstrate the denial. Each statement does not require refuting but certainly should not be reinforced. The counseling nurse should reinforce reality through an understanding but factual discussion of the patient's status, problems, and required nursing care. Involving the family in this care helps in all three stages and permits the family to feel useful, important, and needed.

The second stage of mourning is demonstrated by increasing awareness and feelings of guilt and anger. Laments of "Why me?" "It's all my fault," "If only I'd looked sooner," or "I shouldn't have let him go," poignantly demonstrate guilt. Anger is often directed toward the child for being careless or disobedient. One parent may accuse the other of being at fault. Often anger is directed at the hospital staff, since this outlet is "safer" than accusing a family member. Criticism of nursing care, the physician, or staff personalities are the most common manifestations. Understanding the causes of these feelings enables the staff to support the family. Reassurance that the accident was unpreventable (if, indeed, it was) will help. Giving the parents information about their child's condition and involving the family care-giving and decision-making are essential. Nonjudgmental listening and prompt attention to problems will help smooth the way toward the third stage of grieving: restitution.

This last stage involves the sharing of grief with others and, it is hoped, the support of relatives and friends. When a loved one dies, a funeral may help a family to accept their loss. In the case of disability, the family frequently substitutes ritualistic behavior such as an exact time for visitation, weekly visits to a special physician, or daily trips to church. Some families seem to adjust to the changes imposed by disability better than others. Unfortunately, the stresses are great, and family dissolution all too often results. Trust helps ease these stresses. Trust through open communication helps the family work through the problems.

The parents and team must realize that as children become aware of their disabilities and limitations, they too will go through a grieving process. They may verbalize anger, quietly withdraw, or become overly cooperative. At times these children may show little motivation or will refuse to learn new skills. The goal during this period should be to assist the child to adjust to a new body image and activities of daily living rather than acceptance of the disability. Psychosocial support can help the child, parents, and team work through this normal process.

It is impossible and probably undesirable to protect a patient completely from fear, pain, or even frustration. However, these unpleasant feelings may be reduced. Since children need to do little to prepare themselves in advance for most procedures, the knowledge that a certain procedure will be done need not be shared until just before its actual performance. Then children should be told in simple, truthful terms how the test or nursing activity will affect them and what they can do to help. If children are told about unpleasant procedures too far in advance, unconscious fantasies and fears may be activated. Opportunities to verbalize and to express themselves through drawings, play acting, story telling, or music should be made available. Feelings that cannot be put into words need to find an outlet before they, in turn, become symptoms.

This need for emotional release ties in with the need to facilitate social interaction and contact with the community. Maintaining friendships is sometimes difficult for a child with flagging energy and extended illness. Yet the knowledge that one still has such relationships encourages stability and incentive and usually makes return to the neighborhood after hospitalization less traumatic. Short, chaperoned trips to recreational areas, cultural centers, or just to visit friends can also be a method

of maintaining one's place in the world outside. These passes should begin as soon as the family has been given necessary instructions and has demonstrated competence in the child's care. Much support and encouragement are often needed, since the hospital often provides a safe, accepting environment of the child's disability, and this acceptance may not exist in the community. The child and parents must be prepared to respond to stares, handle avoidance, and answer questions.

The addition of a recreational therapist to the staff of many hospitals is a welcome event. This specially prepared professional helps patients participate in a wide range of constructive activities either in groups or as individuals. A monthly newspaper planned by the patients, hobby fairs, and picnics on nearby lawns are sample activities.

Whether in the rehabilitation unit or regular hospital area, convalescing long-term patients should be given the opportunity and responsibility of continuing their education. Ideally a classroom for ambulatory patients will be available and provision made for tutors from the public school system. Telephone tutoring is also available in many areas. Education is extremely important to those capable young people whose vocational choices may be somewhat narrowed.

CONDITIONS COMMONLY ENCOUNTERED

Common diagnoses found in rehabilitation units include spinal cord injuries, congenital anomalies of the central nervous system, and traumatic brain injury. Since students working on the rehabilitation unit will frequently meet patients with these problems, they are discussed briefly below.

Spinal cord injury

Children suffer spinal cord injury less frequently than adults do. Other than spinal defects associated with birth anomalies, such as myelomeningocele, spinal cord problems occur almost exclusively in teenagers as a result of automobile or, less frequently, diving accidents and gunshot wounds. Although the spinal cord is partially protected by bone, shearing or torsion forces can destroy or severely damage the cord. The affected portion of the body is determined by the level of spinal injury. The higher the cord injury the greater will be the resulting disability. Paraplegic patients (persons whose paralysis or functional loss involves lower extremities), even though they may experience loss of bowel and bladder control and perineal sensation, can be totally independent; quadriplegic patients (persons whose paralysis or functional loss involves all four extremities) may need supervision or assistance. The more hand function available, the more independent the patient will be. With improved emergency care and quicker retrieval, increased numbers of patients with high spinal cord injuries (C1, C2, and C3 level) are surviving. These patients have no function below shoulder level. Their basic care remains the same as that required by other quadriplegic patients, but the nurse must become familiar with ventilatory equipment and be prepared for more intense psychologic and adjustment problems. Eventual resocialization requires sophisticated electronic equipment such as electric wheelchairs with tongue switches, as well as environmental control systems to operate a television, radio, telephone, or intercom.

The application of lifesaving measures is, of course, of initial importance in the management of the patient with spinal cord injury. Immobilization and stabilization of the spine is paramount. This is often accomplished with a "halo" apparatus that may be worn for a period of 10 to 12 weeks until the spine is stabilized. This apparatus consists of a halo ring to immobilize the head and metal bars that attach the ring to a vest that encompasses the chest and supports the apparatus weight. Plastic vests are often used, but a plaster vest may be needed for the irregularly shaped chest or back. The halo apparatus allows the child to have extra mobility to sit, stand, walk, or lie prone. Respiratory, circulatory, and muscular atrophy problems are also diminished.

Orders for the child in a halo apparatus include

administration of a mild analgesic for initial discomfort. The nurse should especially report swallowing problems, difficulty in opening the mouth, and loosened pins. The pins holding the halo barely penetrate the skull. Therefore, these pin sites must be meticulously cleaned twice a day with half-strength peroxide or Betadine solution. Separate sterile applicators should be used for each pin. Some serosanguineous drainage is expected initially, but one must observe for any change or increase in drainage, redness, swelling, or pain that would indicate development of infection. Although the vests have a protective inner lining, pressure sores often develop over the scapulae and shoulders. These sores may be prevented with proper body positioning and by bridging the vest with foam cutouts. The vest's resistance tends to inhibit respiratory function; therefore, deep breathing and coughing exercises must be encouraged. Observation for spinal cord trauma by performance of daily upper extremity neurologic assessments is required. Any changes should be reported immediately to the physician. Finally, the nurse must teach the child some general safety rules to prevent falls that may inflict greater damage. During the time of bony healing the complications of bed rest must be prevented. This involves meticulous skin care, periodic range-of-motion exercises, adequate fluid intake, venous-support stockings, bowel and bladder programs, and special respiratory care. The patient with injury at midtrunk level or above requires more than position changes and coughing. Because the respiratory muscles have been affected, incentive spirometers and intermittent positive pressure breathing (IPPB) are valuable. An upper respiratory tract infection is a serious threat to this patient.

The higher the level of the cord injury the less tolerance the patient displays for an upright position. The application of elastic hose from toes to groin or of a snug-fitting corset before the patient sits helps prevent pooling of blood in the lower extremities. Gradually (over a period of days), increasing the angle of the wheelchair back and lowering the legs helps prevent dizziness, vertigo, perspiration, fainting, and other signs of hypotension. When these symptoms occur, tipping the wheelchair back to lower the patient's head relieves the symptoms.

Below the level of injury, temperature regulation is affected in these patients, since skin nerve endings that combine with the central nervous system are not functioning to control temperature. The skin does not perspire to aid cooling, nor do the muscles shiver to produce heat. Therefore the skin may be injured by extremes of heat or cold that the patient cannot perceive, and the patient must be made aware of this possibility. In addition, the patient's response to an inflammatory process may register a higher body temperature than is usual for that type of problem. Control is usually obtained by uncovering the patient or using aspirin suppositories. Tepid sponges will generally help lower the most difficult fever.

In the patient with an injury above midtrunk, or T6, a complication known as autonomic dysreflexia may arise. This is a very serious rise in the blood pressure that can lead to a cerebrovascular accident (CVA) or seizures. Signs and symptoms include flushing, headache, sweating, feelings of nasal stuffiness, goose bumps, bradycardia, and a rapid increase in blood pressure. These result from sympathetic system activity and are usually related to physical stimuli, such as bladder and bowel distention, severe pressure sores, or urinary tract infection. Less frequently, external stimuli may trigger autonomic dysreflexia. It should be treated by elevating the patient's head and removing the stimulus. A distended bladder is drained. However, Nupercainal ointment is introduced into the rectum for fecal impaction. If the patient does not improve, hydralazine hydrochloride can be given. Patients who are subject to such episodes should be fully instructed in self-care before discharge.

Spina bifida with myelomeningocele

Myelomeningocele, the protrusion of spinal cord fibers through an abnormal vertebral opening into a meningeal sac on the back of the infant, occurs in approximately two or three of every 1,000 births.

These children require initial habilitation rather than rehabilitation in the strict sense of the term. The physical problems of these boys and girls are similar to those experienced by children with low spinal cord injury. Treatment begins with excision of the protruding sac shortly after birth. Preventive skin care, range of motion, and bowel and bladder programs are taught to the families first; then the children learn to care for themselves as they grow older. The development of hydrocephalus may be a complication of myelomeningocele. Close observation for signs of abnormal head growth is needed. (For discussion of types of ventricular shunts used to help control head enlargement as well as other nursing considerations, see pp. 259 and 267.)

In these patients the effects of gravity, the lack of supportive muscles, and occasionally, uneven growth make a straight spine difficult to achieve. Without the use of external support and possible surgery, a patient may literally sit with the rib cage resting on his thighs. The lower extremities may also be affected; hips often are subluxed or dislocated, and the feet may be clubbed. Urinary tract complications are frequently seen. Urinary tract diversion (Bricker procedure) may be done if there is upper urinary tract destruction caused by infection (Fig. 20-5). With increased acceptance of intermittent catheterization, fewer Bricker procedures are being performed. Indeed, some urinary diversions are being reversed, and catheterization is being taught.

Patients with myelomeningocele face a series of potential threats to the development of healthy, functioning adult personalities. These children are often treated differently by caretakers, who frequently limit the child's developmental experiences more than necessary because of the handicap. Concerns regarding body image, passivity concerning self-care skills, low motivation for achievement-related tasks, and saddened mood have been common features of many patients. Manifestation of any emotional problems, of course, depends on many factors. However, it is safe to assume that the child with myelomeningocele faces an increased risk of psychologic difficulties. Understanding and meeting the needs of these children is particularly complex, since their changing developmental characteristics may demand a different focus at each stage in their lives.

The family must realize that, generally, no mental retardation is present. These children should be treated normally with the realization that they require a certain amount of preventive physical care. In U.S. society, value is placed on youth and athletics, and the loss of physical abilities does not enhance a child's self-image. The value of the person, as opposed to the body itself, should be taught.

For the patient to obtain a satisfying job in adulthood, education is a necessity, and guidance may be helpful. A regular school and college are preferred for their psychosocial value. Psychometric and vocational testing may help in the selection of a school.

By the time a child reaches puberty, the problems of sexual awareness will be complicated by questions regarding sexual performance in relation to the disability. The male patient with myelomeningocele is probably unable to have an erection or any sensation in the genital area. The male patient with spinal cord injury has no sensation but may have erections. Although procreation is possible, only a small number have had children. The female patient with spinal cord injury or myelomeningocele may conceive and bear children without sensation. However, patients with spinal cord injuries who are seeking reassurance regarding sexual relationships should appreciate that the most important aspect of sexual intimacy is a caring relationship and that coitus is only one of many "normal" alternatives to satisfaction. The patient can be an adequate sexual partner through oral and manual stimulation.

Brain injury

The symptoms of patients who have received brain injury from automobile accidents, tumors, or other causes vary according to the severity of the injury and the areas of the brain affected. The minimally injured child may virtually recover or have only a limp or speech defect; another child may be severely damaged and nonfunctional. Patients who make progress and are likely to regain function are seen in the rehabilitation unit.

Initial lifesaving management seeks to prevent complications. Tracheostomy and ventilation equipment are frequently indicated, and careful suctioning techniques and tracheostomy care are required. Positioning may be modified to accommodate the tracheostomy. If placed in a prone position, the patient may need thick padding for chest and head with an open area at the neck to allow adequate space to prevent tracheostomy obstruction. The use of IPPB in addition to turning and positioning helps prevent pneumonia.

The physical needs of the patient may be considerable and in many ways not unlike those of the patient with spinal cord injury. However, this patient typically regains awareness and orientation slowly. Sensory stimulation is carefully planned by the team and is introduced slowly. The physical and occupational therapists work with the patient in developing both fine and gross motor coordination. Although strong, such patients may be unable to feed or dress themselves. Activities of daily living (ADLs) are introduced early in therapy so that, ideally, the patient can begin to achieve some degree of independence. Speech, intellect, and emotional stability are typically affected. Psychomotor testing and educational counseling are helpful. The more severely affected children usually attend special schools for the handicapped.

A child with an impaired intellect and a functional body may ultimately be happy and satisfied. A child with a reasonable intellect and severe physical dysfunction, such as aphasia (loss of normal speech) or ataxia (loss of normal gait), understands the condition and frequently has much difficulty adjusting.

At puberty the person with brain injury also has awakened sexual interest. Parents must be cautioned that as a result of their injury, some patients may be overly friendly and invite unwanted sexual encounters. The problems of marriage and possible child rearing are difficult and must be considered on an individual basis.

Developmental disabilities

Several studies have indicated that about 15% of all babies manifest developmental handicaps or demonstrate a potential for difficulties of this type. This number of children demands attention. Developmental disabilities include problems such as prematurity, cerebral palsy, phenylketonuria, mental retardation of undefined origin, and slow achievement of skill and growth milestones.

Emphasis is on early identification to minimize problems and to foster growth and development. Some programs are federally or state supported, such as Head Start or the Regional Centers for the Developmentally Disabled. State institutionalization of patients is being reduced by home or local placement and "mainstreaming." In mainstreaming, educational and health care opportunities are provided through regular nonisolated community systems. Health care personnel are learning to enhance the progress and adaptation of the handicapped. The nurse assumes a primary role in the assessment and support of family coping mechanisms.

Dressing, ambulating, and feeding the severely disabled child are complex skills, and many books have been written about possible techniques. It is suggested that the student wishing to understand them better should begin with the book *Handling the Young Cerebral Palsied Child at Home* by Nancy Finnie.

PHYSICAL ASPECTS OF REHABILITATION

The complications of prolonged bed rest and immobility represent the greatest dangers to the

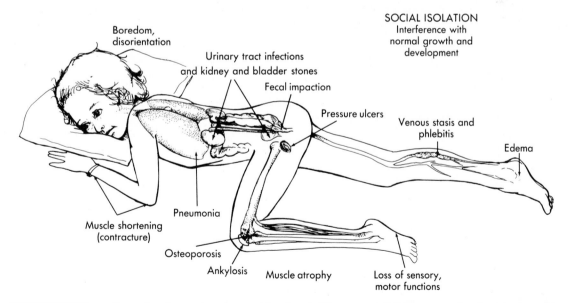

Boredom, disorientation

Urinary tract infections and kidney and bladder stones

Fecal impaction

Pressure ulcers

SOCIAL ISOLATION
Interference with normal growth and development

Venous stasis and phlebitis

Edema

Muscle shortening (contracture)

Pneumonia

Osteoporosis

Ankylosis   Muscle atrophy

Loss of sensory, motor functions

FIG. 20-1   Complications of prolonged bed rest. Of course, all these complications may not be seen in every patient.

life of the long-term patient (Fig. 20-1). Examples of such complications are as follows:

1. Motor and sensory loss involving superficial nerves, skin ulcers, and skeletal deformities due to pressure
2. Muscle wasting and shortening (contractures), bone calcium loss, ankylosis of joints, edema, venous stasis, and thrombosis from disuse atrophy
3. Urinary tract infection, stones, constipation, and fecal impaction related to poor fluid intake and positioning
4. Hypostatic pneumonia from pooling of secretions in the lungs
5. Depression and psychologic disorders resulting from the isolation and interference in normal activities
6. Disturbance in normal growth and development

The meticulous application of a few basic nursing principles can prevent many of these complications from occurring. These principles are discussed in the following sections.

Routine skin care

An adequate blood supply keeps the skin functioning and in repair. A lack of blood to an area will cause deprived cells to die. The small vessels in the

FIG. 20-2

Skin signals.

Response to pressure: the sequence of events	What you see
Caution signs	
1. Area pinkness, leaving area in a few minutes.*	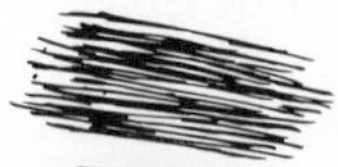
2. Discrete darker reddish spot persisting up to 1 hour.*	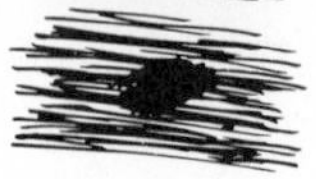
3. Discrete darker reddish spot persisting over 1 hour to several days. The more time needed for the area to regain color after a finger blanching test, the more time needed for return to normal.	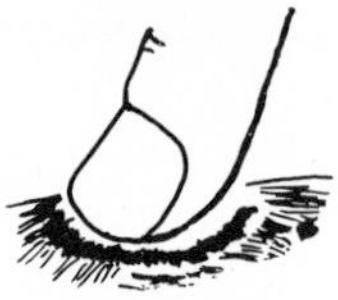
Pressure sores or decubitus ulcers	
4. An unbroken or open blister, sometimes with no color change. May be confused with burn; takes days to heal.	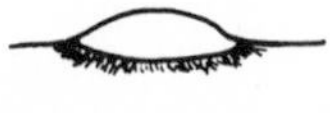
5. A partial-thickness ulcer, damaging part of epidermis; heals from bottom and edges; takes days to heal.	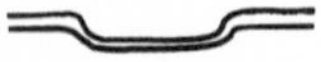
6. A full-thickness ulcer, damaging full depth of epidermis; heals only from edges; takes days to weeks.	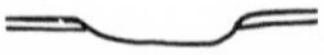
7. A penetrating ulcer, involving bone and connective tissue; takes perhaps months to heal.	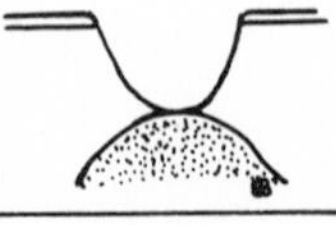
*Best time to treat to prevent sequence. Practice prevention: total body inspections twice daily; pressure point inspections with each position change.	

skin form a network that supplies the skin from all directions. Any pressure, such as that from sitting, standing, lying, braces, shoes, or appliances, causes compression of these small vessels and does not allow blood to the cells. Where bony prominences (such as the hips, sacrum, and knees) are close to the surface, there is no muscle tissue to pad or distribute the pressure evenly, and considerable pressure, which can cause great damage to the skin, develops. The sequence of events leading to skin breakdown and the sores or lesions that result are described in Fig. 20-2.

When red marks are seen, the child must not bear pressure on that area until the skin has returned to normal. Any surface that comes into contact with the skin must be suspect. Soft, moldable surfaces distribute pressure over a larger area, and any one spot receives less pressure, with less damage resulting. If you recall the difference between sitting on a concrete step and a well-upholstered chair, you will appreciate why items such as foam rubber mattresses, wheelchair cushions, and soft leather shoes are encouraged.

For the patient who is wheelchair bound and who lacks sensation over the buttocks area, it is imperative that pressure be relieved over the bony ischial prominences. The method for relieving pressure is called a chair "raise." For the paraplegic patient it consists of lifting the buttocks by using the arms of the wheelchair to raise oneself or alternately shifting from side to side. Recommended frequency for the paraplegic patient is every 20 or 30 minutes for 30 seconds. This activity should soon become automatic so that the paraplegic does it without having to think about it. The quadraplegic patient must have assistance to relieve this ischial pressure.

The use of new braces, shoes, or different positions or postures must always be instituted gradually and frequently evaluated. (See the chart below for suggested schedule.)

In addition to pressure-caused skin problems, one must be aware of the danger of burns, bumps, scratches, and even pimples. Burns can be caused by hot car upholstery, electric blankets, sunburn, hot sand at the beach, spilled hot drinks, and other accidents. Although they may appear to be minor, these can be very serious and must be seen by the physician. Any abrasion or scratch that involves a pressure-bearing surface must be completely

---

SUGGESTED SCHEDULE FOR SKIN TOLERANCE CHECK

Trial periods	Observations of pressure areas (red marks)
1. Beginning periods—15 minutes Increase by 15-minute periods according to tolerance until 2-hour level is reached	Clearing in 15 minutes or no pressure area seen, increase trial period by 15 minutes Clearing in 30 minutes, repeat trial period Clearing in 45 minutes, reduce trial by 15 minutes Persists 60 minutes or more, keep patient off area
2. After 2-hour level is reached, trial periods may be increased to 30 minutes	Use same clearing time evaluation, but substitute 30-minute trial periods

NOTE: Any interruption in the use of a brace, appliance, or position may require a reevaluation period. Prolonged intervals between their use may mean starting again at the beginning of the schedule. When any pressure area is detected, check methods of positioning. Cocoa butter applied daily to bony prominences helps keep skin supple.

healed before pressure bearing is resumed. Diaper rashes and irritations that do not quickly respond to the application of Desitin ointment or zinc oxide should be examined immediately before a severe problem results. Pimples on weight-bearing surfaces should be cleaned gently with mild soap and water and observed closely for increasing size and severity. Because of poor blood supply to scar tissue, healed sores may leave scars that are susceptible to future breakdown and may interfere with children's ability to live a normal life and hold a job as they grow into responsible adults. A small amount of time spent daily in prevention will save a great deal of time, trouble, and money later. Remember the following: (1) never permit any pressure on reddened areas, blisters, or sores; (2) increase positioning times according to the guidelines; and (3) regularly check total body skin, using mirrors as necessary. Teach the child and the family these precautions. By the age of 10 or 11 years children, with supervision, should be assuming responsibility for their own skin care.

If a patient with an existing pressure sore is admitted, some treatment must be undertaken. Many theories exist regarding what to put on a pressure sore. The fact is that one can almost say, "Put anything on it but the patient!" No weight bearing should be allowed, It may be possible to avoid the one position that causes pressure; however, if there are ulcers in several different places, the nurse may have no alternative but to position the patient carefully on the affected side. If this must be done, pressure must be relieved from the ulcer by bridging either side of the ulcer with foam rubber pads or pillows, thus freeing the lesion itself from pressure. But circular or doughnut-shaped supports are not recommended.

Pressure sores must be kept clean. Whatever agent is used, cleaning must be done gently to preserve the new delicate epithelium being formed. Half-strength hydrogen peroxide on applicator sticks effectively cleans away drainage. If the ulcer is infected, a topical enzyme, such as Travase or Elase, and hydrotherapy will debride the sore. A small pressure sore may be left open to the air to dry. Covered sores should be taped loosely to allow air circulation. Op-Site is effective in areas where incontinence is a problem, because it prevents moisture from entering the wound, but allows passage of air and gases. Debrisan (hydrophilic wound-cleaning beads) absorbs excess drainage from clean sores. However, it should not be used in tracts.

Large ulcers are better managed by moist dressings. A fine-mesh gauze pad, such as any eye pad, is cut of the exact size of the crater and moistened with physiologic saline solution. This should be covered with a dry dressing taped down with paper tape to prevent drying. The dressing is changed every 4 to 6 hours, depending on the drainage present and how long it stays moist. If it is allowed to dry, the gauze should be soaked off to preserve the new epithelium. As the ulcer heals, the gauze is reduced in size until finally one can leave the shrunken ulcer open to the air.

Positioning

In the discussion of skin care we have underlined the importance of relieving pressure by turning and changing position. Proper anatomic positioning can help prevent skeletal deformities, muscle shortening (contractures), and venous stasis. Six basic positions may be used: back (supine), abdominal (prone), either side, sitting, or standing. These can all be modified to a certain degree. Positioning problems vary according to the diagnosis and individual needs of the patient. Fig. 20-3, *A* and *B*, illustrates good prone positioning to prevent pressure areas and contractures and to protect catheter drainage when necessary.

Venous pooling and the danger of thrombosis can be decreased by thigh-high, closed-toe support stockings to help collapse the superficial leg veins. To further prevent venous stasis, as well as muscle shortening and contractures, a full range of motion should be carried out. The nurse is responsible for ranging joints *without* stretching muscles. The bywords are gentleness and patience. The hands

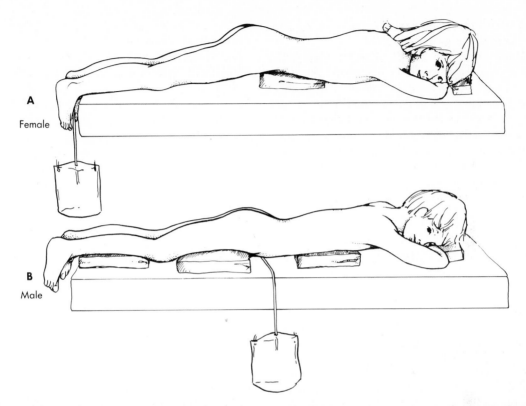

FIG. 20-3 **A,** Prone position with pillow below breast level and small foam rubber support under forehead. Note position of Foley catheter between legs. **B,** Prone position with pillows under chest, thighs and shins to leave hips, knees and feet free from pressure. Note position of Foley catheter.

and fingers are exceptionally delicate, and specific instructions about appropriate range should be obtained from the physician or the physical or occupational therapist. Overzealous range of the fingers could make the hand less functional later.

Position changes also lessen stasis of fluid in the lungs. With regular deep breathing, an incentive spirometer, and coughing (if necessary, stimulated by a suction catheter), pneumonia may be prevented. Changing position and forcing fluids will also help prevent urinary stones and constipation.

Naturally, as soon as patients are physically able to tolerate a wheelchair, they should be placed in a more normal sitting position, even if they are still comatose. This maneuver adds a position to the patients' repertoires and lets them see people and their environment from the more customary vertical perspective, which helps to prevent disorientation.

Depression, disorientation, and hallucinations can result from prolonged horizontal positioning and social isolation of the normal individual. This, added to the physical and emotional trauma of an injury, is a tremendous problem. Anything that will stimulate and orient the mind—people, predictable routines, a clock or calendar—is helpful. Frequent visits by the nurse (just to say "hello") help. Conversation with the patient while in the room or delivering care is essential. The presence of parents and siblings and the friendship of another patient who has experienced a similar injury and made progress helps tremendously.

Interference with growth and development, manifested by disrupted bone growth, delay in reaching skill or functional milestones, or inability to play normally, occurs too frequently in young disabled children. They must have the chance to explore and move about the floor and, if possible, to achieve the vertical position. Their environment should be as "homey" as possible and include measured amounts of supervised responsibility and freedom appropriate for their age, abilities, and general condition.

Urinary bladder care

Based on the neurologic involvement, neurogenic bladder can be classed as uninhibited neurogenic bladder, reflex or spastic bladder, and autonomous neurogenic bladder.

Uninhibited neurogenic bladder. Uninhibited neurogenic bladder results from an upper motor neuron lesion that may be a residual of traumatic brain injury, brain tumors, or multiple sclerosis. The patient may be aware of a full bladder but, like the small child, unable to prevent voiding. The preferred program consists of bladder retraining—sitting the patient on the toilet on a regular schedule (for example, every 2 hours) and limiting fluids in the evening. The patient is not intentionally incontinent. Criticism and scolding are always inappropriate. Praise for appropriate voiding and matter-of-fact dressing after incontinence encourage success and desired behavior.

Reflex or spastic bladder. A spinal cord destroyed above the reflex arc results in a reflex bladder that may be a residual of traumatic spinal cord injury, tumors within the canal, or multiple sclerosis. The patient is unaware of a full bladder and has no voluntary control of voiding. In these patients the sphincter is contracted, and the bladder usually incontinently empties, leaving a large amount of residual urine.

Although some urologists are now *beginning* bladder management with intermittent catheter-

ization, management of this type of patient has characteristically been by continuous closed sterile internal catheter drainage during the acute phase of the illness. After this phase the patient then has a "catheter freedom trial." The catheter is removed, and a regular fluid intake is maintained. After approximately 4 hours, the patient sits up in bed and attempts to initiate voiding. This can be stimulated by: (1) tapping sharply over the fundus of the full bladder, (2) straining, (3) pulling pubic hair, (4) stroking the inner thigh, or (5) lifting the buttocks off the bed, using an overhead frame. If the voiding attempt is successful, the patient should be instructed to note the presence of any sensation or aura of a full bladder before voiding, such as a feeling of fullness, flushing, pressure, or any unusual sign. This would become the signal for the patient to stimulate or "trigger" the bladder and void in a urinal, an external urinary collection device, or on a toilet. Sometimes the patient's bladder will empty when full but will not respond to triggering. In this instance an external collection device would be most helpful unless the times between voiding are consistent or the patient has a predictable aura and time to reach a toilet.

If the patient successfully voids, a residual urine is obtained after each voiding. When the amount of urine obtained by catheterization directly after voiding is 10% or less than the amount of urine in the full bladder, the patient is termed "balanced." When a patient is balanced, the likelihood of infection is small. If the patient is unsuccessful in voiding, intermittent catheterization is instituted. Compared with the use of a long-term indwelling catheter, intermittent catheterization is preferred because it lowers the incidence of infection and increases the chance of a balanced reflex bladder. The passing of a small-gauge, straight catheter on a regular schedule (for example, every 4 hours) can be taught to family members or in some cases to the patient. The aim is to empty the bladder when full without permitting distention. By keeping a regular fluid intake and limiting fluid before bedtime, the patient can sleep through the night and establish a regular daytime schedule.

Clean intermittent catheterization, introduced

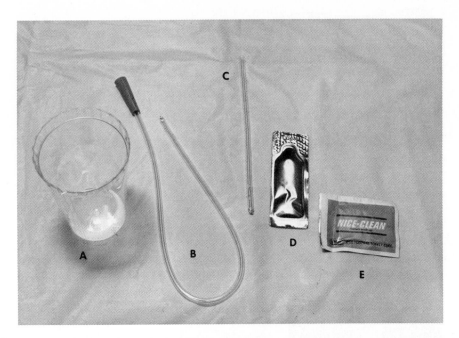

FIG. 20-4   Supplies for clean catheterization technique: **A,** Calibrated plastic container; **B,** catheter for male; **C,** catheter for female; **D,** lubricant; and **E,** cleansing wipe.

by Jack Lapides, a University of Michigan urologist, is now widely practiced. Dr. Lapides theorized that an overdistended bladder has decreased blood flow through its wall. Thus it is susceptible to bacterial infection. Several studies have now shown that frequent emptying of the bladder by catheterization, using clean technique, will decrease the probability of a urinary tract infection.

A urologic workup, fine motor skills, and the ability to tell time and keep simple records are prerequisites for learning clean self-catheterization. Children who are allowed by the urologist or physician to do the clean catheterization procedure enjoy greater freedom, for they need to carry only a few supplies with them (see Fig. 20-4) and may use almost any facility for urinary elimination.

Autonomous bladder. A lack of functional nerve connections between the bladder and the spinal cord creates an autonomous bladder. It is seen in patients with myelomeningocele, with cauda equina injuries, or in those who have had radical pelvic surgery. Their bladder and sphincter are flaccid.

The patient has no sensation and has continuous overflow incontinence. Some believe management can be obtained by Credé's maneuver (the application of pressure above the fundus of the bladder downward toward the perineum). Some attempt intermittent catheterization, whereas others simply let the urine drain. Residual urine, infection, urinary backflow (reflux), and eventual destruction of the upper urinary tracts may follow. The patient may have a urinary tract diversion to preserve the upper tracts.

Such a diversion is also called an ileal conduit, ileal loop diversion, or a Bricker procedure. A urinary tract conduit is constructed from a separated loop of ileum. The ureters are transplanted into this loop, and a permanent opening on the abdominal wall is constructed (Fig. 20-5). Urine is then collected by means of bag affixed over the draining stoma by adhesive. Many bags of this type are available. They should be fitted individually to each patient. The enterostomal therapist has received special training in the selection, fitting,

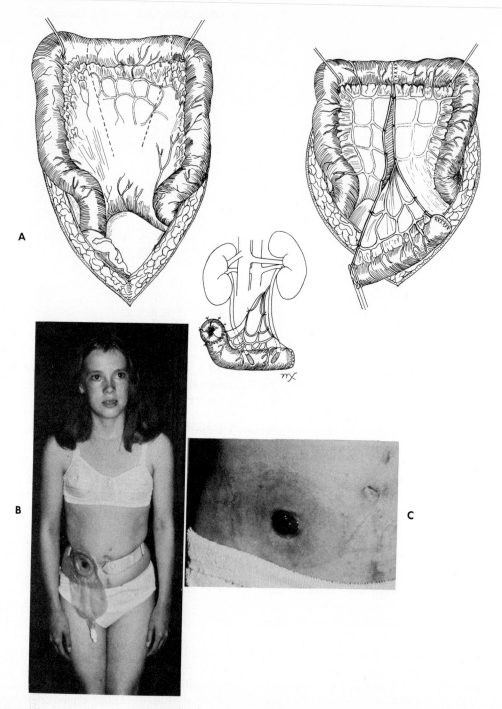

FIG. 20-5 **A,** Ileal conduit, ileal loop diversion, or Bricker procedure. A segment of ileum is removed maintaining its mesenteric attachment. The ureters are transplanted into an open pouch constructed from the ileum. The ileal pouch is brought to the surface of the abdomen and drains urine continuously. **B,** A type of urinary drainage collection bag for daytime use **C,** Close-up of uncovered ileoconduit stoma.

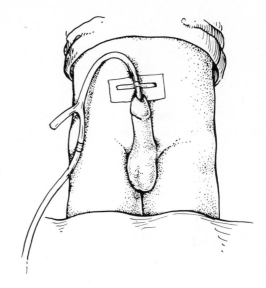

FIG. 20-6

Tape the penis on the abdomen as shown to reduce urethral curve and prevent pressure on the penoscrotal angle, which may cause infection, periurethral abscess, or urethral fistula formation.

application, and maintenance of ostomy bags. Since the appliance is a highly important personal item and many parts are reusable, the nurse should never discard any part unless so directed by the patient or responsible family member. The loss of one part may render the appliance useless until replacement is made.

Catheter care. Indwelling catheter drainage is by suprapubic or Foley catheter. Proper catheter care can prevent abscesses and periurethral fistulas and can reduce infections. The male patient with a Foley catheter usually has more problems. The smallest catheter that will drain without clogging is desired. This will permit exudate to pass around the catheter and out the urethra. The catheter must be taped to the abdomen so that the penis and catheter are directed toward the upper body (see Fig. 20-6). This prevents the catheter from being accidentally pulled, causing damage to the sphincter or urethra. It also eliminates the constant movement of the catheter and penis and irritation and destruction of urethral mucosa. This position prevents excessive pressure against the inside of the urethra by the elimination of the normal S-curve from the penis to the bladder. The meatal-catheter junction is usually cleansed twice daily with mild soap and water.

Foley catheters in girls should be taped to the thigh. The catheter and periurethral area may be cleaned with mild soap and water. The patient should be taught the importance of maintaining straight gravity drainage.

The suprapubic catheter should be cleaned of crusting as described earlier. Some units apply a water-soluble ointment, such as Betadine or polymixin B. A split gauze pad is usually placed at the site of the catheter's entry into the abdomen.

Bladder irrigations are no longer recommended. However, it is important to maintain an acid urine to inhibit growth of urea splitter organisms, such as *Proteus* and *Klebsiella*. Urinary acidification can be accomplished with large intakes of cranberry juice, prunes, plums, or vitamin C tablets. Citrus juices and carbonated beverages make urine alkaline. Maintaining a sterile closed system, the use of urine acidifiers and forcing fluids will help prevent infections, stone formation, periurethral abscess, and fistulas. Feeling "sand" encrustations when rolling the catheter between the fingers is a signal for catheter change (usually at intervals of 4 to 6 weeks).

External urinary collection devices. For the child who does not require an indwelling Foley catheter, an external device is desired. Unfortunately, no successful device exists for girls, and diapers must be used. As the child grows, custom-fitted plastic pants may be purchased or made from patterns. Since urine may contribute to skin break-down, a protecting ointment should be applied with each diaper change.

There are many collection devices available for boys. For those from 6 to 9 years of age, small, medium, or large finger cots can usually be connected to rubber tubing and a leg bag to make a highly satisfactory, inexpensive collection device. The modified finger cot is attached to the penis with nontoxic ostomy cement and a narrow ring of elastoplast that does not touch the skin itself. This can remain on for several days without leaking, but it must be removed daily for penile skin inspection. Those devices that combine a penile sheath and a truss or athletic supporter are available and sometimes useful. However, the extra elastic straps may cause chafing, and pressure points can be hazardous to hyposensitive or anesthetic skin.

Bowel care

Neurogenic bowel may be classified in the same way as neurogenic bladder. Uninhibited neurogenic bowel results in defecation without volitional control when the rectum fills. The reflex, or spastic, bowel exhibits above-normal rectal sphincter tone. When the rectum fills, frequent automatic, partial emptying results. In autonomous neurogenic bowel the rectal sphincter is flaccid and frequent small stools may result.

When the patient has lost normal control, a bowel program should be established early. This helps protect already vulnerable skin from rashes and breakdown. Then, too, the socialization of the older child can be drastically affected by soiling, obnoxious odors, and diapers. Most regular schools will not enroll these children. Furthermore, as an adult, tolerant friends are few and accepting employers are essentially nonexistent.

An adequate program consists of (1) keeping the stool normal or slightly firmer than normal (as soiling is more likely to occur if it is soft or liquid) and

(2) scheduling evacuation time. All children are individuals and their programs must be tailored precisely to their needs. Therefore one child's program may not be identical to that of another child with a similar problem.

Many factors influence bowel patterns: Diet has a very great effect; disruption of eating patterns—skipping meals, eating extra meals, changing meal times, amounts, or types of food eaten—may disturb the program by causing constipation or diarrhea. By trial and error one learns exactly what foods constipate or loosen the stool for each patient. Generally, citrus juices, prune juice, and bulk (or roughage) items, such as raw vegetables and nuts, tend to loosen the stool. Inadequate fluid intake and foods such as bananas and cheese will constipate. Gas-forming items, such as beans and cabbage, may cause diarrhea. Most of these foods are not a problem unless eaten in larger than normal quantities. A normal, stable diet with sufficient fluid intake will usually keep the stool as desired. If possible, any changes in factors affecting bowel habits should be added singly so that the effect of each change will be known.

Bowel patterns are also affected by physical activity. Inactivity usually constipates, whereas great increases of activity may speed the movement of food through the digestive system and cause accidents. Aging, a change of climate or community, altered living patterns, anxiety, and stress may all have their effect.

A number of reflexes, techniques, and agents can be employed to assist in establishing a sound bowel program free of accidents. These include the gastrocolic reflex, digital stimulation, abdominal straining, stool softeners, and bisacodyl (Dulcolax) suppositories.

The gastrocolic reflex is an increase in the peristaltic muscle activity of the large bowel after the stomach has distended from ingestion of food or warm liquids. Therefore about 30 minutes after a meal is a logical time to carry out a bowel program. If the stool is too hard in spite of fluid and dietary measures, stool softeners, such as dioctyl calcium sulfosuccinate (Colace) or dioctyl sodium sulfosuccinate (Surfak), which retain water in the stool, may be used.

Bisacodyl is a safe means of chemically inducing peristaltic movement of the large bowel. It is more predictable and safer than irritating laxatives or mineral oils that could decrease vitamin absorption. A bisacodyl suppository is inserted high up in the rectum, against the side of the bowel wall so that it will dissolve and be absorbed easily. Bisacodyl usually dissolves in 10 to 15 minutes, reaching peak action in another 10 or 15 minutes. Bisacodyl small-volume enemas may be effective for the paraplegic or meningomyelocele patient.

Digital stimulation does not refer to the digital removal of stool from the rectum. It is a gentle circular motion made by the gloved finger inserted ½ inch (1.25 cm) against the rectal sphincter muscle. The patient may be positioned on the left side or may sit on a raised toilet seat. This gentle motion will both relax and dilate the rectal sphincter and cause peristaltic muscle contractions of the large bowel. This procedure should be continued for 10 to 15 minutes. It can be used in conjunction with suppositories or by itself. As evacuation occurs, one should gently pull the rectum to one side and allow the stool to be eliminated.

Although any number and combination of these techniques and agents may be used in the child's bowel training, the program should start with the least and the simplest. The time of day for evacuation should be chosen with regard to previous bowel habits, daily schedules, time limitations, and personal preferences. A reasonable time seems to be about 30 minutes after the morning or evening meal. Once a time is selected, it must remain consistent within 30 minutes.

For a child with a spinal cord injury, one possible routine might be as follows: (1) immediately after breakfast, insert one half of a Dulcolax suppository as high as possible into the rectum (The amount depends on age and size of the child; too much causes abdominal cramping, too little, no action.); (2) wait 10 to 15 minutes, continuing personal care; (3) place the child on a "potty chair" or toilet with the feet touching the floor so that the hips are flexed into the squat position; (4) have the child lean forward against the thighs (to increase intra-abdominal pressure), and massage the abdominal muscles. Encourage the child to strain at the same time. (Have children who do not understand blow on a toy balloon.) If diarrhea should occur, it is wise to check for impaction because liquid feces can seep around impaction, resulting in false diarrhea.

Consistency in the program is essential. Some young children may require the program twice a day. A bowel program takes time, patience, and attention to detail but in most instances is very rewarding.

BEHAVIORAL ASPECTS OF REHABILITATION

Many problems that are encountered, although based on physiologic disability, are psychologic in content. If undesirable behavior can be changed, the long-term outlook for the patient improves. One method of behavioral change, based on the work of B.F. Skinner and his stimulus response (S-R) techniques, is called *behavior modification*. A behavior is an action—something a person does. It may be desirable or undesirable. To be changed, using this technique, it must be observable, describable, and measurable.

An action can be made to occur more often by following it with a favorable consequence—a *positive reinforcer*. A behavior may be reduced or eliminated by withdrawing its reinforcer or may be influenced less effectively by punishment.

While recovering from head trauma, 4-year-old Joseph became incontinent of urine. By positive reinforcement of an observable, describable target behavior that can be counted, he again learned to void in the toilet. After recording the number and frequency of his voidings, his primary nurse established a toileting schedule. The nurses explained what behavior was expected, then remained with him quietly. When Joseph voided into the toilet, he was immediately reinforced with praise, a smile, and a few minutes of attention. In a short time

Joseph was voiding in the toilet, and as his physical and mental condition improved, by further reinforcement he was able to summon the nurse for assistance to the bathroom. In examining Joseph's problem, his nurse discovered that busy staff members had nagged and cajoled him when he voided incontinently. Because Joseph had valued their attention, their actions had reinforced incontinent voiding. During the modification program, if he voided incontinently, his nurse would change him in a matter-of-fact manner, withholding both positive and negative attention.

A reinforcer must affect the frequency of the behavior. If the rate of behavior does not change, no reinforcement has taken place and a true reinforcer must be found. For Joseph praise was appropriate, although a toy or food might have been successful in another situation. A reinforcer must be delivered promptly only when the target behavior occurs. Joseph was reinforced with praise immediately on voiding in the toilet; otherwise, he was matter-of-factly returned to bed. Early in a program, reinforcement may occur after each desired behavior (continuous). Later it may be intermittent—a more effective and efficient technique.

At times it is inconvenient to deliver reinforcers at the time of target behavior. In this instance a token may be delivered after each desired behavior to be exchanged later for a desired reinforcer. This makes it possible to use a variety of reinforcers for single or multiple behaviors. Adults use this system when they work for money.

As Joseph progressed, he learned to dress himself. Each time he completed a dressing behavior he was praised and a poker chip was placed in a glass by his bed. Each chip was worth 5 minutes of evening television time. When establishing a token trade rate, one should aim for a high rate of success. As the patient progresses, trade rates should be revised to require increased performance for a given amount of reinforcement.

A large task achieved through a series of small, planned successes is called *shaping*. When Joseph learned to dress himself, he began with putting on his socks. In the beginning he was reinforced when he picked up his socks to prepare to put them on.

Later he received reinforcement only when he placed his socks over his toes. Finally, his reward was given only after he pulled his socks over his heels.

Generalization occurs when a behavior learned in one situation occurs in another environment, time, or as a broadened scope of behavior, for example, patients who learn to walk in the hospital, then return home where they walk, dress, and brush their hair. They have generalized in all three aspects. This can be accomplished by direct methods using a trained family member or visiting nurse to reinforce the behavior. An indirect approach is called *trapping*, which ties the desired behavior to a naturally occurring reinforcer. Assuming that the previous patient enjoyed the socialization of school, attendance would involve dressing, grooming, and walking. These target behaviors are reinforced by attending school. Trapping increases the chance that the behavior will continue.

In behavioral terms, punishment is either the withdrawal of a reinforcer or application of an aversive stimulus. We believe that the latter method is rarely appropriate for the health professional. In some instances isolation or loss of privileges may apply; however, aversive stimuli are more often used to reinforce the adult's feelings of power and control. The effect of punishment is relatively temporary and produces reactions of fear, anxiety, frustration, and hostility. Alternative approaches are (1) to change the circumstances that evoke undesirable behavior, (2) to reinforce an incompatible behavior, (3) to permit the behavior in a safe place until the desire is satiated, and (4) to extinguish the behavior through lack of reinforcement. Family and staff attention is perhaps the strongest reinforcer of behavior.

• • •

The broad goal of pediatric rehabilitation—to foster growth and development, independence, and personal fulfillment—represents a tremendous challenge. It requires all the support of the family, patient, and rehabilitation team. Its rewards may be delayed but are definite, nonetheless.

CHAPTER 21 The dying child, the family, and the nurse

Few nursing assignments are more challenging than helping a family with a sick child who is afflicted with an illness that is often fatal. Since the nurse cannot change the reality of the tragic situation, she frequently feels sorrowful. Probably no human experience cuts so deeply into the center of one's heart as the loss of a child.

THE CHALLENGE OF UNCERTAINTY

Although this chapter deals with the dying child, concern for the physical and psychologic support of the child during the chronic phase of a terminal illness cannot be overlooked.

Today, because of great medical and technological advances, children with fatal illnesses typically live longer than ever before. Helping such a child reach his developmental potential, physically, intellectually, psychologically, and socially, has become a multidisciplinary challenge. Frequently the short-term or long-term prognosis may be uncertain. The burden of such uncertainty calls for much time and energy from those who provide the child's care.

The chronicity of terminal illness requires much understanding. One must not only have a working knowledge of the ongoing medical treatment but, more importantly, its psychosocial implications to the child. Psychologic strength is very important if the necessary adaptability is to be sustained during this period of prolonged instability. The nurse can promote this quality by honesty, knowledge, and understanding care.

It is extremely important that the child be prepared for living as long as any possibility remains. Communicating this concept to the child's family, teachers, and other significant persons is essential! For example, the school-age child with a life-threatening illness frequently experiences scholastic difficulties because of absences, psychological problems and fears, and "differentness" caused by amputation, chemotherapy, and other treatment or disease sequelae. These problems must be recognized and addressed as vigorously as possible to maintain the child's own psychologic well-being and rapport with the peer group.

To face the almost overwhelming demands of a long-term, life-threatening illness, the child, parents, and hospital personnel need to recognize and use many supportive measures.

Understanding the child's reactions (influenced by his developmental level and possible concept of death), typical parental reactions, and one's personal feelings and philosophy concerning death help the nurse to provide the sensitive support the family needs.

REACTIONS OF THE CHILD

A child's concept of death

A child's concept of death depends to a considerable extent on his age, intellect, life experience, or cultural background. Young children typically do not perceive death as final or terminal. For children 3 to 5 years of age, death is denied; it is only a change of some kind and is not permanent. Children 5 to 6 years of age recognize death but cannot conceive of it as resulting from chance or a natural happening. Causation is personified. Death to them is like part of a game of cowboys and Indians. Everybody kills each other, and then they resurrect themselves and play another game. Hence, when someone dies, in the child's mind the event is usually thought of not only as a deprivation but also as a personal abandonment. It may be considered a hostile act on the part of the person who died.

From approximately age 6 onward, children seem gradually to be accommodating themselves to the proposition that death is final. Many 6- and 7-year-olds suspect that their parents will die someday and that they too may die, but are comforted by the thought that the death of their parents (and their own death) is still far away.

Children 9 to 10 years of age and older achieve a realistic concept of death as a permanent biologic process. A child over 10 years of age is capable of integrating the concept of "not being" if the parents can do so. As children approach adolescence, they are equipped with the intellectual tools necessary to comprehend time, space, life, and death in a logical manner. At about 10 or 11 years of age, children can understand the universality and the permanence of death.

In spite of the common depiction of violence in the newspapers and on television, children in the United States are often shielded from any real involvement with or explanation of death. Dying is not typically viewed as a normal part of the life cycle. Yet studies have indicated that children often fear—usually in terms of separation and loss of security—their own deaths or those of their loved ones. If life includes death, deliberate, thoughtful education in the observation of nature and daily life would seem appropriate.

Children who are terminally ill rarely manifest an *overt* concern about death, probably because they attempt to repress their anxiety concerning it. Nevertheless, children should be allowed to express their fears verbally if they are capable or through play media (drawing pictures, relating to puppets, playing with doll-house or paper doll families; handling, pounding, and shaping clay) if they are not. Highly susceptible to the attitudes of their parents, terminally ill children will likely sense the gravity of the situation and will need to ventilate their feelings. They pick up many cues from their families and surroundings that something has changed, that something different, important, and probably bad is happening or will occur. These cues may include a change in expectations, less emphasis on discipline, unnatural silences or forced chatter, and unusual gifts. These children should not be deprived of the security of usual behavioral expectations, and they should be allowed to participate in their normal activities as much as medical assessment considers possible. Often the children should be reassured that their illness is not their fault and is not a punishment for anything they did.

What to tell the child

If the older child does ask about dying, a statement such as, "You have a serious illness, but no illness is without hope," is likely to be believed and reassuring. To deprive a person of hope even when the outcome is clouded is unrealistic and unkind. One must also individualize responses according to the child's understanding and circumstances. If the child sees or asks about the death of another child, you might say, "Johnny was very sick and died." This implies that the inquirer is not as ill as was the friend. Answer questions simply and always truthfully. Keep in mind the child's level of comprehension. Opportunities to talk should be given. Many times older children will select one staff member who appears open and accepting of what they might say to share their fears and concerns. Most important is the maintenance of an atmosphere that allows patients to ask as much or as little as they wish. Social workers, psychiatrists, or ministers may be used effectively in this role as well.

Although total candor was a popular view in recent times, and that approach still finds many adherents, others now stress the need for acceptable illusions or denial mechanisms to permit coping with extreme stresses. The death of a child presents one of the most traumatic and unexplainable crises in the human experience. Reasonable and common rationalizations should be treated gently. Sincerity and communication between the individual nurse and child are more important than dogmatic insistence by the nurse on one of several conflicting psychologic or ethical theories proposed by "experts in the field."

Three stresses of terminal illness

In addition to having illnesses that cause considerable distress, these children suffering from terminal illness are subjected to three stresses common to other hospitalized children: separation from parents, traumatic procedures, and isolation. Modification of hospital routine and procedure must be considered.

Separation from parents. Depriving parents and children of each other when permanent separation will soon take place would be particularly unfortunate. Children want their parents. Nurses should encourage parents to touch the child. The warmth of physical contact is the most primitive and basic nonverbal comforting technique humans possess. It can communicate a solace or comfort to the frightened child that words can never produce.

Traumatic procedures. When parents are helped to understand the reasons why tubes are inserted, intravenous feedings are ordered, blood is withdrawn, or other treatments are initiated, they feel better satisfied. Parents are usually best able to console and protect their children from fear.

Remember, the nurse is best able to help children allay their fears through their parents. By helping parents to understand, you will have helped the child.

You can also help older children by transferring their attention and concern from their incurable illness to other *curable* problems or symptoms they may be experiencing. Listen with interest and attention to all their complaints, particularly ones related to intercurrent infections, such as rashes, that can be eliminated. Children can receive enormous reassurance and relief if these complaints are treated intensively. They are not being deserted. Wahl* calls this method of relieving anxiety "trading up."

Isolation. The most dreaded possibility does not seem to be that of dying but that of dying alone. Children feel secure with other children, and they know nothing too terrible can happen when Mom and Dad are there.

In the hospital setting. Do not isolate the dying child from his siblings, friends, other relatives, or staff. Usually you cannot conceal a child's death from other children in the unit. Encourage parents and relatives to say when they will come back. It implies a promise: "I will see you again, and you will have nothing to fear in the interim." Although relatives and staff are encouraged not to isolate the child, the nurse should not permit constant or unduly prolonged visits that the child may interpret as a "death watch." Parents also need respite to attend to other responsibilities, to rest, and to reorganize. They should not be encouraged to stay continuously. Arrangements can usually be made so that the child is not left alone, but yet parents have periods of change.

Dying at home

A recent innovation has been the practice of allowing terminally ill children, when the parents agree and cooperate, to spend their last weeks or

---

*Wahl, C.W.: The dying patient, Consultant, Nov., 1961, Smith, Kline & French.

months at home. Nursing care in these situations must be adapted to the family and to the facilities available. Although home care for the terminally ill is a change from recent methods, it has been the norm during most of human history. With the advent of specialized diagnostic and emergency services available only in hospitals, this significant event was often moved outside the home. Yet for many sick children who can no longer benefit from the sophisticated facilities offered in a hospital, the home may be the place of most comfort and security, if the family is willing and able to provide the care needed.

Impetus for this type of terminal care has come particularly from the work of Ida Marie Martinson and the experiences of nursing and medical personnel and parents who participated in the Home Care for the Dying Child Project, first developed as a research study at the University of Minnesota.* The nurse should refer to the work of Martinson, Spinetta, and others for more detailed perspectives.

Another recent trend has been the organization of volunteer nurses who reside near the affected family and can more easily provide the on-call support essential to the family. Decreased costs associated with this type of support are an important factor. The consulting home-care nurse should be prepared to refer the family to financial and other community resources as part of the total care plan. One should bear in mind that financial disaster for the family added to the loss of the dying child can destroy the entire family unit. Follow-up by the nurse after death is extremely important in aiding family adjustment.

Many families have found the home care method very fulfilling. It helps decrease the parents' feelings of helplessness, although the final result may be unchanged. Researchers report the child's emotional well-being and comfort are much enhanced by being in familiar surroundings and associating with family members. Even if a medical emergency requires rehospitalization, the survivors have expressed great satisfaction in the home experience that was possible.

Specialized centers for the care of the dying (hospices), first developed in Europe, are a relatively new development in the United States. Centers devoted to pediatric patients are even more recent. The team care that is ideally offered in these settings seems to hold much promise.

PARENTAL REACTIONS

One of the nurse's most important roles in the management of the child with a terminal illness is helping the grieving parents. Integrating the tragic event of death into their life experience is most difficult. The parents' reactions to the prospective death of the child may be likened to the mechanism of separation anxiety. However, it has much deeper meaning than most separation anxieties that parents and children face.

The mourning process

In recent years much has been written regarding the reactions of patients who perceive themselves to be facing a terminal illness and of the behaviors of parents and close family members or friends when they mourn the impending death of a child. The descriptions and analyses offered are not to be construed as undeviating or as always applicable to all persons and situations, but they may form guidelines for the interpretation and anticipation of events that will be helpful to all concerned.

John Bowlby* was one of the early writers in the field to describe the mourning process. He identified three phases in the natural mourning process: protest, despair and disorganization, and hope and

---

*Martinson, I.M.: Home care for the dying child: professional and family perspectives, New York, 1976. Appleton-Century-Crofts.

*Bowlby, J.: Process of mourning, Int. J. Psychoanal. **42:**331, 1961.

rebuilding. Bowlby's work oriented the three phases of mourning to the period following death. However, mourning often begins before death occurs and his three phases of mourning have been helpfully utilized to describe parental reactions before the death of the child.

Mourning is the process of healing that helps us face and recover from loss. The normal healing process takes a year or more. The clearest evidence of recovery is the ability to remember comfortably and realistically both the pleasures and disappointments of the lost relationship. The following predictable steps in the mourning process—protest, despair and disorganization, and hope and rebuilding—permit a judgment that healing will occur.

The mourning process may encompass before-death or anticipatory mourning as well as after-death adjustment. Most persons will progress through the basic stages discussed below, whether the child's death occurs before, after, or during the process. But it is very important for nurses to be aware of and sensitive to the different interactions that may occur among family members and nurses themselves depending on the phase of the mourning process being individually experienced when death occurs.

Protest. The first phase is characterized by a general tendency to protest or deny the diagnosis of disease or its fatal outcome. In trying to deny the facts, many strong emotions are brought into play—anxiety, yearning, anger, and guilt. Parents cannot believe that this could happen to their child. Often a parent's attitude is one of suspicion, hostility, and constant criticism. Hope for the child is stressed but in a nonspecific way. Parents tell themselves, "Something will be discovered." They want to try anything that might offer hope for a cure no matter how irrational it may seem.

Anxiety is manifested by an intense need to weep, an empty feeling in the abdomen, loss of appetite, and other body complaints. With anxiety there is yearning, longing for a sign that a cure will be found and the child will get well. Guilt feelings are constantly expressed in tears: "If only I had done this or that, if only I had notified the physician

sooner." It is natural and necessary to cry, to be angry, and to feel guilty. These are all healthy signs of normal grief. It is a stage in the gradual process of accepting a great loss.

Involvement of parents when possible in the physical care of the child is extremely important in facilitating parental adaptation. But although parental participation in the care of the sick child is desirable, it should not be at the expense of the emotional and physical well-being of the rest of the family. Mothers and fathers usually want to be with their sick child and need to feel that they personally have done everything possible for the child. Feelings of guilt are somewhat relieved by the expenditure of personal effort in the care of the child. Parents are encouraged to participate realistically in the physical care of their children by bathing, feeding, or entertaining them and escorting them to the laboratory and x-ray departments. Thus parents become integrated into the hospital routine, and communication with personnel is enhanced.

During the initial period in the hospital, mothers physically cling to their children. They are involved solely in their care. After a while parents want to help as effectively as they can with the care of other children. Assisting them to the playroom and reading to a group rather than just their own child are examples of this desire. Manifestations of the capacity to help other children mark a turning point in parental adjustment that reflects acceptance of the child's illness and ultimate death.

Actually, the phase of protest as described by Bowlby is very similar to the stages noted by Elizabeth Kübler-Ross, in which she describes the ill patient's reaction as "No, not me!" (shock and denial), and "Why me?" "Why now?" (anger, rage, and envy). The parent's mourning, however, also typically includes a destructive guilt factor.

Despair and disorganization. The second phase in Bowlby's mourning process also finds a parallel in the observations of Kübler-Ross. It is similar to her "Yes, me, but . . ." (bargaining), and "Yes, me" (depression) stages.

Facing and accepting the reality of the fatal illness, parents feel helpless. Life is stripped of meaning. Active, realistic efforts to prolong life typify the early part of this phase.

The mother spends most of her time ministering to the needs of her sick child. During this time the nurse must be aware that the mother's attempts to cope with the situation may fluctuate from gentle, assured bedside care to inappropriate, exhausting activity. At one moment she may express exaggerated gratitude to the nurses and medical staff; in the next she is overly critical. Her emotions may range from philosophic resignation to sentimentality. She is emotionally fragile and inconsistent.

The reality of the fatal illness and its meaning begins more and more to penetrate the mother's consciousness. Her denial of the character of the illness may disappear, but hope of a cure persists. Her hope is more specific now, often related to particular scientific efforts. Mothers begin to cling less to their children and encourage them to participate in hospital activities. Parents should be encouraged to express their feelings of depression and defeat during moments away from the child. This helps them move beyond the initial shock and recognize some of the specific things they still have to offer their child. Every attempt must be made to enable parents to see the continuing value of their function as parents, despite their feelings of despair and helplessness in the face of death.

As the child's physical energy begins to diminish, preoccupation with measures that involve treatment of the disease begins to subside, and parents are interested in relieving the child's discomfort and pain. Although they continue to hope that their efforts will save the child, the intensity of the expectation is gradually reduced. They are separating themselves emotionally from the child.

Hope and rebuilding. The third phase is characterized by a calm acceptance of the child's impending death. Separation from the child is no longer an adaptive problem for the parents. The mother or father remains with the child whenever possible but with adequate consideration for the remainder of the family. For the first time the parents express a wish that the child could die so that the suffering would end.

Many parents never reach this third phase of mourning during their child's illness. It may not be until after the child dies that the third phase begins. With the loss acknowledged and the depth of pain plumbed, new people, relationships, and activities become meaningful. Some parents take interest in organizations such as the Cancer Society and the Cystic Fibrosis Association. By so doing, the mourner is able to reduce preoccupation with self and the dead child. This allows the parent to reinvest feelings in other love objects—spouse, remaining children, or close relatives. Again, the last stages as described by Kübler-Ross of "Yes" (acceptance or resignation) appear appropriate.

SIBLING REACTIONS

Brothers and sisters are often disturbed by the continuing illness and may require considerable parental support. Parents should be encouraged to divide their time among the various members of the family as the situation warrants. The importance of communication with siblings must always be borne in mind by the parents and all others in contact with the family during this period. They will need the same type of communication and support that the parents require. However, their needs and understanding will, of course, depend on their ages. Nursing care for the family should include the siblings.

Martinson reports that home care for dying children does not have an adverse effect on siblings, even when they actually witness the death. In fact, the experience of participating in terminal care seems to remove many of the false anxieties and fantasies experienced by the siblings who could not participate in the hospital experience.

THE NURSE'S REACTIONS

Personal concepts of death

Awareness of one's feelings about death is essential to acquiring the ability to give comprehensive nursing care to dying children and their parents. Information about children's concepts of death and their parents' fears is not enough. To give sensitive and supportive care to the dying child, the nurse needs help in understanding her own fears about death. The nurse may find her role particularly frustrating if she feels herself a failure because she cannot cure or rehabilitate the child. Her concept of nursing must be changed to include helping the family "cope"—an extremely valid and worthy goal!

Fear of death is the most inescapable and realistic of human fears. Fear and anxiety lead to convictions of immortality on a conscious or unconscious level that are universal in all humans. Each individual recognizes that other people must die but feels an inward assurance that it need never happen to him or her.

Each person feels or reacts differently to the death experience. If this reality (death) is so painful that one handles it by either immersing oneself in it or utterly denying it, it will be difficult to fulfill one's role as a nurse. Nurses ought to let themselves recognize, at least to a limited degree, the awe and fear that everyone experiences in the face of death. Fear of death is handled in several ways: (1) by a religious belief in immortality, (2) by a denial of the awe felt for death, (3) by withdrawal from the dying child, and (4) by the formation of various phobias or compulsions. As nurses, we are involuntarily influenced by illogical but protective defenses in the presence of impending death. However, if we are to help parents who are experiencing deep grief and distress, we must not ridicule them or isolate ourselves from them. We are not to punish them in this way. We must become aware of our own feelings. We must try to better understand how we ourselves feel about death and nursing a young human being who will probably experience it relatively soon. The entire bedside staff should be given aid by the formation of support groups, appropriate patient conferences, and access to information regarding helpful techniques and approaches.

Nursing the dying child requires courage. The nurse must remember that courage is not the absence of fear but the willingness and ability to function in its presence. Nurses who care for dying children and counsel their parents must preserve a sympathy and empathy and yet be free enough of emotional involvement to do their work commendably well. Nurses should not become so personally involved with the dying child that they neglect the other children who have an equal need for nursing care.

Support groups

There has been a recent trend in university centers to set aside one evening weekly for the staff to meet with the parents of leukemic children. Common problems are shared in these small mutual support groups. Discussions have centered around the nature of leukemia and its treatment, as well as the emotional problems faced by parents, siblings, friends, and staff. Most of the groups intermittently include physicians, nurses, a social worker, and a psychiatrist. As a result parents and staff have shared increased understanding of each other's problems. The meetings provide opportunities for parents to meet unit physicians and nurses in a more relaxed setting with ample time for discussion. Specific benefits from these meetings include mutual support during times of stress and uncertainty, the realization that discipline of the child is still desirable, and the possibility for sharing feelings about death and dying. But perhaps the most important benefit is the opportunity for parents to share and identify with one another on a level common to each. This kind of group interaction can be a meaningful and effective source of emotional support for parents of children with other fatal diseases as well.

Basic concepts of religion

The comfort the nurse can give to the parents of the dying child is important. Knowing their religious beliefs concerning death may be a great help. Often the nurse will observe that parents with deep faith in God find real comfort in their religious beliefs. For Catholics and Protestants who believe in personal immortality, great solace and comfort can be found in the conviction that they will one day rejoin their loved ones.

In the Jewish faith the concept of immortality is not clearly defined. Judaism teaches that perhaps there is a life after death, but the only immortality of which man is certain is the immortality he achieves while he is still alive or through his descendants.

Knowing the basic concepts of the various religious faiths concerning death may be of great assistance to the nurse. The nurse is not expected to be a theologian nor should she attempt to share her religious beliefs concerning death unless she is asked, but the nurse can help the child and the parents by supplying physical and emotional sup-

port and the comfort of spiritual counsel by contacting any clergyman the parents desire. This spiritual advisor, especially one who has added skills in personal counseling to his religious training, can well be the one to whom a parent may turn. He can communicate comfort to parents when friends and relatives are helpless.

CONCLUSION

Death is inevitable but no less difficult because of its inevitability. Just as it may be the nurse's privilege to help parents and their infant at the event of birth, it may also be her privilege to ease and comfort a mother and father and a small human being who has come to life's last hours. May she do so with gentleness, reverence, and skill.

SUGGESTED SELECTED READINGS AND REFERENCES

HOSPITALIZATION

Azarnoff, P., and Hardgrove, C.: The family in child health care, New York, John Wiley & Sons, 1981.

Belmont, H.S.: Hospitalization and its effects on the total child, Clin. Pediatr. 9:483-492, 1970.

Bergmann, T., and Freud, A.: Children in the hospital, New York, 1965, International Universities Press, Inc.

Birchfield, M.E.: Nursing care for hospitalized children based on different stages of illness, Am. J. Mat. Child Nurs. 6:46-52, Jan.-Feb. 1981.

Carty, R.M.: Observed behaviors of preschoolers to intensive care, Pediatr. Nurs. 6:27-29, Jul.-Aug. 1980.

Clark, D.: Helping parents cope with their child's hospitalization, J. Assoc. Child Care Hosp. 8:32-35, Fall 1979.

Eichelberger, K.M.: Self-care nursing plan: helping children to help themselves, Pediatr. Nurs. 6:9-13, May-June 1980

Facteau, L.M.: Self-care concepts and the care of the hospitalized child, Pediatr. Clin. North Am. 15:145-155, Mar. 1980.

Farr, K.S.: Communication pitfalls in routine counseling, Pediatr. Nurs. 5:55-56, Jan.-Feb. 1979.

Ferrald, C.D., and Corry, J.J.: Empathic versus directive preparation of children for needles, Child. Health Care 10:44-47, Fall 1981.

Hansen, B.D., and Evans, M.L.: Preparing a child for procedures, Am. J. Mat. Child Nurs. 6:392-397, Nov.-Dec. 1981.

Hodapp, R.M.: Effects of hospitalization on young children: implications of two theories, Child. Health Care 10:83-86, Winter 1982.

Hymovich, D.P.: How children, mothers and nurses view primary and team nursing, Am. J. Nurs, 80:2041-2045, Nov. 1980.

Johnston, M.: Toward a culture of caring: children, their environment, and change, Am. J. Mat. Child Nurs. 4:210-214, July-Aug. 1979.

Knafl, K.A., Deatrick, J.A., and Kodakek, S.: How parents manage jobs and a child's hospitalization, Am. J. Mat. Child Nurs. 7:125-127, Mar.-Apr. 1982.

Koss, T., and Teter, M.: Welcoming a family when a child is hospitalized, Am. J. Mat. Child Nurs. 5:51-54, Jan.-Feb. 1980.

Langford, W.: The child in the pediatric hospital, Am. J. Orthopsychiatry 31:667-684, Oct. 1961.

Lord, R., and Schowalter, J.E.: A ten-year comparison of fathers' and mothers' reactions toward their hospitalized adolescents, Child. Health Care 10:87-89, Winter 1982.

Meissner, J.E.: How can you improve care of the hospitalized child? Nurs. '80, 10:50-51, Oct. 1980.

Nelson, M.: Identifying the emotional needs of the hospitalized child, Am. J. Mat. Child Nurs. 6:181-183 May-June 1981.

Plank, E.N.: Emotional care as a priority: approaches to implementation, J. Assoc. Child Care Hosp. 3:11-14, July 1974.

Poole, S.R.: The overanxious patient, Clin. Pediatr. 19:557-563, Aug. 1980.

Prugh, D., et al: Study of emotional reactions of children and families to hospital and illness, Am. J. Orthopsychiatry 23:79-106, Jan. 1953.

Robertson, J.: Young children in hospitals, New York, 1958, Basic Books, Inc., Publishers.

Sciarillo, W.G., Jr.: Using Hymovich's framework in the family-oriented approach to nursing care, Am. J. Mat. Child Nurs. 5:242-248, July-Aug. 1980.

Steele, S.: Child health and the family, New York, 1981, Masson Publishing USA, Inc.

Stevens, K.R.: Humanistic nursing care for critically ill children, Nurs. Clin. North Am. 16:611-622, Dec. 1981.

Tackett, J.J. and Hunsberger, M.: Family-centered care of children and adolescents, Philadelphia, 1981, W.B. Saunders Co.

Tesler, M. and Savedra, M.: Coping with hospitalization: a study of school-age children, Pediatr. Nurs. 7:35-38, Mar.-Apr. 1981.

Teyber, E.C., Littlehales, D.E.: Coping with feelings: seriously ill children, their families and hospital staff, Child. Health Care 10:58-62, Fall 1981.

Vesial, K.W., and Richardson, K.: The nature of pediatric critical care nursing: perspectives of patient, family and staff, Nurs. Clin. North Am. 16:605-610, Dec. 1981.

Vipperman, J.F., and Rages, P.M.: Childhood coping: how nurses can help, Pediatr. Nurs. 6:11-18, Mar.-Apr. 1980.

Washington guide to promoting development in the

young child, Seattle, 1970, University of Washington School of Nursing (mimeographed).

Whaley, L.F., and Wong, D.L.: Essentials of pediatric nursing, St. Louis, 1981, The C.V. Mosby Co.

Weiczorek, R.R., and Natapoff, J.N.: A conceptual approach to the nursing of children, Philadelphia, 1981, J.B. Lippincott, Co.

Wu, R.: Explaining treatments to young children, Am. J. Nurs. **65**:71-73, July 1965.

LIVING AND DYING

Amenta, M.: Are you cut out for terminal care? RN **44**:47, July 1981.

Assumptions and principles underlying standards for terminal care, Am. J. Nurs. **79**:296-297, Feb. 1979.

Boiko-Weyrauch, P., et al: A young patient dies: the family physician and the survivors, Fam. Prac. **11**:113-119, Dec. 1980.

Bowlby, J.: Processes of mourning, Int. J. Psychoanal. **42**:317-340 1961.

Chee, C.M.: Professionally speaking, a child's right to die, Am. J. Mat. Child Nurs. **7**:81-88, Mar.-Apr. 1982.

D'Addio, D.: Reach out and touch, Am. J. Nurs. **79**:1081, June 1979.

Evans, A.E.: If a child must die, N. Engl. J. Med. **278**:138-142, 1968.

Fochtman, D., and Foley, G.: Nursing care of the child with cancer, Boston, 1982, Little, Brown & Co.

Hutton, L.M.: Annie is alone: the bereaved child, Am. J. Mat. Child Nurs. **6**:274-279, July-Aug. 1981.

Lascari, A.D.: The family and the dying child: a compassionate approach, Med. Times **97**:207-215, May 1969.

Lindermann, E.: Symptomatology and management of acute grief. In Parad, H., editor: Crisis intervention: selected readings, New York, 1965, Family Service Association of America.

Macrae, J.: Therapeutic touch in practice, Am. J. Nurs. **79**:664-665, Apr. 1979.

Mandel, H.R.: Nurses' feelings about working with the dying, Am. J. Nurs. **81**:1194-1197, June 1981.

Martin, A.: Hospice nursing: walking a fine line, Nurs. '81 **11**:128-130, Feb. 1981.

Martinson, I.M.: Caring for the dying child, Nurs. Clin. North Am. **14**:467-474, Sept. 1979.

Martinson, I.M., editor: Home care for the dying child: professional and family perspectives, New York, 1976, Appleton-Century-Crofts.

Matthews, U.F., editor: Manual of pediatric nursing careplans, Boston, 1979, Little, Brown & Co.

McBride, M.M.: Children's literature on death and dying, Pediatr. Nurs. **5**:31-33, May-June 1979.

Paige, R.L.: Living and dying, Am. J. Nurs. **79**:2171-2172, Dec. 1979.

Putnam, S.T., and others: Home as a place to die, Am. J. Nurs. **80**:1451-1453, Aug. 1980.

Solnit, A.J., and Green, M.: The pediatric management of the dying child: Part II. The child's reaction to the fear of dying. In Solnit, A., and Provence, S., editors: Modern perspectives in child development, New York, 1963, International Universities Press.

Spinetta, J.J., and Deasy-Spinetta, P., editors: Living with childhood cancer, St. Louis, 1981, The C.V. Mosby Co.

Spinetta, J.J.: Psychosocial issues in childhood cancer: how the professional can help. In Ahmed, P., editor, Living and dying with cancer, New York, 1981, Elsinier Publishers.

Stichler, J.F., and Showman, T.: A child drowns: a nursing perspective, Am. J. Mat. Child Nurs. **6**:324-328, Sept.-Oct. 1981.

Stoll, R.I.: Guidelines for spiritual assessment, Am. J. Nurs. **79**:1574-1577, Aug. 1979.

Taylor, S.C.: Siblings need a plan of care too, Pediatr. Nurs. **6**:9-13, Nov.-Dec. 1980.

Williams, H.A., Rivara, F.P., and Rothenberg, M.B.: The child is dying: who helps the family? Am. J. Mat. Child Nurs. **6**:261-265, July-Aug. 1981.

Wooten, B.: Death of an infant, Am. J. Mat. Child Nurs. **6**:257-260, July-Aug. 1981.

PLAY

Azarnoff, P., and Flegal, S.: A pediatric play program, Springfield, Ill, 1975, Charles C Thomas, Publisher.

Elmassian, B.J.: A practical approach to communicating with children through play, Am. J. Mat. Child Nurs. **4**:238-240, July-Aug. 1979.

Erickson, E.H.: Childhood and society, New York, 1960, W.W. Norton & Co., Inc.

Gibbons, M.B.: When parents ask about play, Pediatr. Nurs **2**:19-22, Nov.-Dec. 1977.

Hayes, J.S.: The McCarthy scales of children's abilities: their usefulness in developmental assessment, Pediatr. Nurs. **7**:35-37, July-Aug. 1981.

Irwin, E.C., and Kovacs, A.: Analysis of childrens drawings and stories, J. Assoc. Child Care Hosp. **8**:39-48, Fall 1979.

Maurer, J.A.: Play for the hospitalized child, Point of View/Ethicon **17**:4-5, 1980.

McLeavey, K.A.: Children's art as an assessment tool, Pediatr. Nurs. **5**:9-14, Mar.-Apr. 1979.

Petrillo, M., and Sanger, S.: Emotional care of hospitalized children, ed. 2, Philadelphia, 1980, J.B. Lippincott Co.

Stern, D.: Play and learning in the first year: new insights, Pediatr. Nurs. 5:37-42, 1979.

REHABILITATION/LONG-TERM ILLNESS

Altshuler, A., Meyer, J., and Butz, M.: Even children can learn to do clean self-catheterization, Am. J. Nurs. 77:97-101, Jan. 1977.

Bakke, K. Ethical dilemmas: institutionalizing a severely disabled child, Pediatr. Nurs. 7:27-29, Nov.-Dec. 1981.

Benvenuti, C.S.: Independence for the quadriplegic: the Bantam Respirator (pictorial), Am. J. Nurs. 79:918-920, May 1979.

Berni, R., and Fordyce, W.: Behavior modification and the nursing process, ed. 2, St. Louis, 1977, The C.V. Mosby Co.

Brady, M.H.: Lifelong care of the child with Duchenne muscular dystrophy, Am. J. Mat. Child Nurs. 4:227-230, July-Aug. 1979.

Carlson, C.E.: Psychosocial aspects of neurologic disability, Nurs. Clin. North Am. 15:209-320, June 1980.

Downey, J.A., and Low, N.L., editors: The child with disabling illness: principles of rehabilitation, ed. 2, New York, 1982, Raven Press.

Finnie, N.: Handling the young cerebral palsied child at home, ed. 2, New York, 1975, E.P. Dutton & Co., Inc.

Jelneck, J.J.: The special needs of adolescents with chronic illness, Am. J. Mat. Child Nurs. 2:57-61, Jan.-Feb. 1977.

Johnson, J.H: Rehabilitative aspects of neurologic bladder dysfunction, Nurs. Clin. North Am. 15:293-307, June 1980.

King, R.B., and Dudas, S.: Rehabilitation of the patient with a spinal cord injury, Nurs. Clin. North Am. 15:225-243, June 1980.

Lazure, L.L.: Defusing the dangers of autonomic dysreflexia, Nurs. '80 10:52-53, Sept. 1980.

McKeever, P.T.: Fathering the chronically ill child, Am. J. Mat. Child Nurs. 6:124-128, Mar.-Apr. 1981.

Reinisch, E.S.: Quick assessment of hemiplegics' functioning, Am. J. Nurs. 81:102-104, Jan. 1981.

Rodgers, B.M.: Comprehensive care for the child with a chronic disability, Am. J. Nurs. 79:1106-1108, June 1979.

Rodgers, B.M., et al: Depression in the chronically ill or handicapped school-age child, Am. J. Mat. Child Nurs. 6:266-273, July-Aug. 1981.

Rutechi, B., and Seligson, D.: Caring for the patient in a halo apparatus Nurs. '80 10:73-77, Oct. 1980.

Seidl, A.H., and Altshuler, A: Interventions for adolescents who are chronically ill, Child. Today 8:16-19, Nov.-Dec. 1979.

Stauff, S.: Teaching the patient with spinal cord injury, RN 42:55-60, July 1979.

Vigliarolo, D.: Managing bowel incontinence in children with meningomyelocele, Am. J. Nurs. 80:105-107, Jan. 1980.

Ziegler, J.C.: Physical reconditioning—℞ for the convalescent patient, Nurs. '80 10:67-69, Aug. 1980.

PEDIATRIC PROCEDURES

CHAPTER **22**   Hospital admission and discharge

First impressions are important, especially when parents and their child are involved. At times hospitalization of a child may be planned, and a previsit to the pediatric department may be possible to reassure parents and patient, but for many families hospitalization comes as an abrupt, unscheduled, and frightening experience.

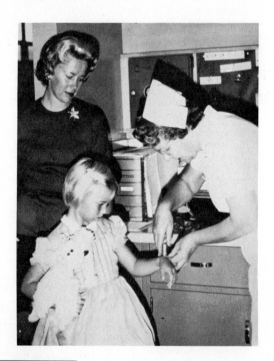

FIG. 22-1

"And here is your bracelet, Mary Lou."

Courtesy Children's Hospital and Health Center, San Diego, Calif.

A cordial, smooth introduction to hospital life extended by a nurse who is sincerely interested in the family involved will do much to ease the anxiety inherent in the situation. All good nurses minister to more than the hospitalized patient's needs. They are alert to the needs, expressed or unspoken, of all family members. However, perhaps nowhere more than in the care of the child is the nurse's response to the entire family so crucial. If the trust of the parent or guardian can be secured initially, the nurse has obtained vital cooperation, a less tense, more relaxed mother and father, and a calmer child. A few more minutes spent at the time of admission may save hours of time later on. (See Fig. 22-1.)

If first impressions are important, so are last contacts. The dismissal may be a most helpful period for the parent, or it may be a confusing "getaway." The following discussion is intended to help the nurse function well in these two eventful situations.

ADMISSION

Identification

The admitting nurse should be introduced or should introduce herself to both the new patient and the parents. In many hospitals identification of the patient is accomplished through use of a bracelet, which should be checked for accuracy. The parent's surname may be different from the child's. This should be clearly and discreetly noted to understand the situation better and avoid embarrassing incidents. To help the staff know their small patients better, many pediatric departments send out questionnaires to the parents of prospective patients requesting helpful information regarding the abilities, habits, likes, and dislikes of the child. Nicknames and special vocabulary used by the child are also investigated. It is good to know that 3-year-old Edmund Atherton Barnstow III responds to "Barney" and loves grape-flavored Popsicles.

Qualifications of a pediatric nurse

The pediatric nurse should feel friendly toward and comfortable with children. She should wish for them the best the future can hold and gain great satisfaction in helping the child become better equipped to meet the demands of life. Her loving concern for children should be expressed through a warm but not "gushy" approach. Children can readily detect people who genuinely care about them. Those nurses who find it difficult to work with children because of inexperience with or isolation from this age group need not feel that they will never function successfully in a pediatric area. But they must really want to learn to know children and think of them as persons and not as *problems*. If nurses are willing to be patient, if they are alert, adaptable, and imaginative, and if they are knowledgeable, kind, and understanding, they possess the potential assets for pediatric nursing.

Nurses frequently find the pediatric area emotionally taxing. It is sad indeed to see a tender, innocent child suffer or a young boy or girl whose life had been bright with promise suddenly struck down by disease or death. Health professionals do not know all the answers to the philosophic questions created by such circumstances, but they do know that these children and young people and their parents need help. There must be those who are willing to try to help them and are especially prepared to do so.

The nature of a pediatric nurse's responsibilities dictates that she possess an ample portion of both fortitude and *discretion*. She must think at least twice before she speaks. Detailed or crucial information about a patient must come from an authoritative source, such as the *head nurse, nursing supervisor,* or *attending physician,* and should only be given to those directly involved, usually attending personnel or parents. Well-meaning but curious casual inquirers should not be given diagnoses or progress reports. Finally, the nurse must develop the capacity for benevolent self-criticism and evaluation of her own actions so that she may constantly improve her ability to meet her patient's needs.

Nurse-parent role

Newer concepts of pediatric care do not picture the pediatric nurse as an authoritarian dispenser of knowledge and skill, who alone has the ability to meet any need of the small patient. She is not a substitute mother, usurping the biological or legal mother's position. However, she is a practitioner who has the advantage of special practical and theoretical education and training not available to most mothers, and she is a person who cares about children, sick or well. The aims of the pediatric nurse and the child's parents should be basically the same—to help develop each child's potential to the optimum level and produce a creative, contributing member of society who finds high purpose in life and a role worth pursuing. The family learns from the nurse, and the wise nurse learns from the family.

The amount of parental participation in the care of hospitalized children depends on the condition of the child and the response and abilities of the parents. To say that they should be allowed to do nothing when they have probably had total responsibility for their children until they were admitted to the hospital is often unrealistic and even unkind. On the other hand, if mothers give their children baths, feed them, and complete their routine hygienic care alone, much valuable observation of the children is lost by nursing personnel. At times, instead of obtaining more relaxed, cooperative parents, an exhausted, worried mother and father may result. Perhaps, when the parent and child seem to gain much from parent participation in hospital care, it is best to carry out such care with the nurse helping the mother and vice versa. Then cooperation is enhanced, observation and reporting are more accurate, and any legal complications of parental care are avoided or minimized.

Some parents are unable to share constructively in the care of their hospitalized children. Others do not wish to participate. Occasionally children may be more relaxed when the mother and father do not participate. Parental anxiety caused by possible feelings of guilt, inadequacy, or frustration may be sensed by children and cause them, in turn, to be anxious. In certain cases the child may be confused about the role of the parent when the mother is at the bedside and the nurse must minister to the small child. In this situation, asking the mother to take a brief rest period until the procedure is completed may benefit both parent and child. For the most part, however, the presence of the parents is a real asset to the child. The mother and father, depending on the condition of the child, can help and be helped by sharing in the admission of the child. They may aid by undressing the child, positioning for temperature readings, helping with feedings, and providing the comfort of their presence. However, no parent should be made to feel that unless he or she is at the bedside the child will not receive complete and loving nursing care. This would cause many anxieties. Parents should not be made to think that they are neglecting their duty to the child unless they are at the bedside almost constantly. The liberal visiting privileges now extended to parents in most pediatric hospitals are designed to ease tensions, not to create them.

To sum up these paragraphs, we would use again the often-repeated comment that is found in many nursing texts: "The modern pediatric nurse is mother's friend and helper—not mother's substitute."

Orientation

If the circumstances of hospital admission and the patient's age and condition permit, the child and parents should be oriented to the unit and be introduced to other children. The parents should be introduced to key personnel and shown where such conveniences as the public telephone, rest rooms, public dining area, and waiting rooms are located. Many children receive a simple toy such as a hand puppet or coloring book at the time of admission, which helps to entertain and to pass the difficult periods of waiting for examination or surgery. The nurse should be sure the child has something appropriate at the bedside for diversion. A specially beloved toy or blanket may be brought from home. The nurse should make sure that any personal toys or clothing left at the hospital are carefully labeled. In most cases the use of the child's own clothes, with the exception of bathrobes and slippers, is discouraged because of the high incidence of loss in the hospital laundry, despite attempts by the staff to avoid such confusion.

When the nurse is speaking to children, it is psychologically good technique to bend or crouch down to their eye level for special introductions, serious talks, or mutual enjoyment. No one likes to talk to knees or stretch to look up all the time!

Nursing procedures

Patients are usually admitted directly to their own units. During the admission, it is customary to secure the following:
1. Pertinent information regarding the child's habits, vocabulary, possible allergies, normal diet, preparation for hospitalization, family structure, history of childhood illnesses, current immunization status, and recent exposure to contagious diseases, especially chicken pox. This type of information may be obtained on a form filled out by the parent while the admis-

sion is in progress if it was not secured before the actual hospitalization.
2. Height, weight, and age.
   a. Babies are routinely weighed without clothes.
   b. Be sure that the scale is covered with a diaper or technique paper and is balanced before weighing!
   c. This information is used to:
      (1) Determine dosages of medications.
      (2) Determine general condition and progress.
      (3) *Note:* All children with diarrhea and vomiting or intake-output problems are routinely weighed every morning before breakfast.
3. Temperature.
   a. Glass or electronic (rectal, axillary, or oral) thermometers may be employed, depending on the policy of the hospital and desire of the physician. The method may be altered depending on the child's age, diagnosis, condition, and tolerance of the method.
   b. Never leave a child alone with a thermometer in place (oral, rectal, or axillary). When rectal temperatures are secured, always have one hand on the thermometer and another on the child to assure safety and accuracy.
   c. Nonoral temperatures should always be taken when:
      (1) The child has seizures or poor muscular control. (There is danger that the child may bite the thermometer, causing self-injury.)
      (2) The child has difficulty keeping the mouth closed because of oral surgery, general condition, or breathing difficulties.
      (3) The child is receiving oxygen by mask, nasal catheter, or cannulae.
   d. Remember, rectal temperatures on the average are 1° F higher than oral temperatures, whereas axillary temperatures are 1° F lower. All rectal temperatures of 100° F or over

TABLE 22-1. APPROXIMATE PULSE AND RESPIRATION RATES AT REST BASED ON AGE*

Age	Pulse	Respiration
Birth-1 mo	110-150	30-45
1 mo-1 yr	100-140	26-34
1-2 yr	90-120	20-30
2-6 yr	90-110	20-30
6-10 yr	80-100	18-26
Over 10 yr	76-90	16-24

*Pulse and respiration rates become slower with age.

and all oral temperatures of 99.0° F and over should be reported to the head nurse or team leader as soon as determined.
   e. In a few instances, rectal temperatures may be contraindicated (rectal surgery, diarrhea, or ulceration).
4. Pulse.
   a. For infants an apical pulse rate is secured by placing a stethoscope between the left nipple and the sternum. It is too difficult to secure an accurate radial pulse rate.
   b. Other pulse points may be used with the older child (the temple, the neck) if there is difficulty keeping the wrist still.
   c. Pulse determinations may usually be made by timing for 30 seconds and multiplying by 2 on the very young child.
   d. Irregularity and quality as well as rate should be noted.
   e. The activity of the child should be taken into account. (For example, the pulse of a sleeping child should be so labeled.)
   f. For rate ranges see Table 22-1.
5. Respirations.
   a. The rate and the character of respirations are important. The nurse should be alert to detect sternal retractions and Cheyne-Stokes respirations.
   b. For rate ranges see Table 22-1.
6. Blood pressure.
   a. The correct-sized cuff is very important. The

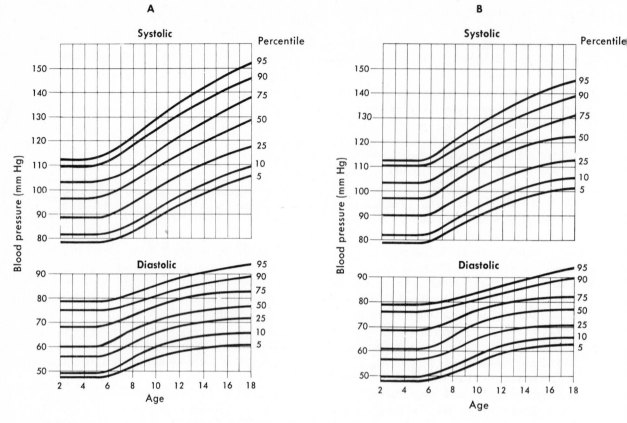

A

B

FIG. 22-2   **A,** Percentiles of blood pressure measurement in boys (right arm, seated). **B,** Percentiles of blood pressure measurement in girls (right arm, seated). (From Blumenthal, S., et al: Report of the Task Force on Blood Pressure Control in Children, Pediatrics **59**:(suppl.):803, 1977; News and Comment **29**:8-13, March, 1978.

Copyright American Academy of Pediatrics, 1977 and 1978.)

cuff should cover two thirds of the upper arm measured from the shoulder to the elbow.

b. It is sometimes difficult to determine the blood pressure of an infant. If regular auscultation is not helpful, the systolic pressure may be secured by palpation of the brachial pulse as the cuff is gradually deflated. In some areas a Doppler or arterial pressure transducer apparatus may be used. Still another technique, called the "flush method," may be employed. The distal portion of an upper or lower limb is made pale by the application of wrappings or manual pressure.

The blood is prevented from entering the blanched hand or foot by an inflated cuff. The cuff is slowly deflated and the systolic reading recorded when a flush, indicating the passage of blood beyond the cuff into the exposed hand or foot, is noted.

c. Any unusual activity of the child just before or during the blood pressure determination must be noted. Try to obtain this reading while the child is quiet.

d. Blood pressure measurements are often taken to determine the onset of shock or increasing intracranial pressure.

e. The average blood pressure at birth is 80/46. For percentile readings for boys and girls ages 2 to 18 years of age, see Fig. 22-2. Most children's blood pressures vary considerably. These charts may be used to evaluate the blood pressure readings obtained, although their real function is to serve as a device for plotting blood pressure over a period of time. Blood pressure measurements should be obtained and plotted at least once yearly.

7. General appearance and behavior as evaluated through observation.
   a. Overall clinical *appearance*.
      (1) In no acute distress.
      (2) Mildly ill.
      (3) Severely ill.
   b. Growth and development.
      (1) Appropriate for age and sex of child.
      (2) Special physical considerations such as orthopedic problems, imperfect vision, deafness, speech or language barriers, malnutrition, obesity, cosmetic defects, prostheses (dentures, glasses, contact lenses, artificial eyes, limbs), surgically created stomas, history of seizures, and general vigor.
      (3) Cultural, intellectual, and emotional considerations, such as cultural heritage (for example, Hispanic-American), mentally retarded or gifted, parent-child-nurse interaction, and initial response to hospitalization.
   c. Skin manifestations.
      (1) Unusual color, flushed, pale, cyanotic, or jaundiced.
      (2) Unusual birthmarks, scars.
      (3) Rashes, bruises, possible boils, blisters, possible infestations (body or head lice, scabies).
      (4) State of cleanliness.
   d. Nervous system manifestations.
      (1) Level of consciousness.
      (2) Abnormally dilated or unequally dilated pupils.
      (3) Tremor, twitching, or periods of blank staring.
      (4) Limp, flaccid extremities.
      (5) Bulging fontanels.
      (6) One-sided or lower extremity weakness or paralysis.
   e. Other signs and symptoms important to note on admission.
      (1) Diarrhea, nausea, vomiting, abdominal distention (type of stool or emesis).
      (2) Nasal drainage, coughing. (Signs of respiratory tract infection noted in a child scheduled for surgery should be reported immediately. Surgery may be cancelled.)
      (3) Difficulty in voiding.

All these observations do not make the nurse a diagnostician. She simply observes as accurately as possible and reports.

COLLECTION OF SPECIMENS

In addition to the preceding measurements and observations, the patient is routinely scheduled for urinalysis and blood examinations.

Urine specimens. The collection of a urine specimen in a child over 2½ years old is seldom difficult. The collection of a specimen from an infant or young toddler poses real problems. Various methods have been recommended. Most pediatric areas use small adhesive-backed plastic bags that adhere to the perineal region or base of the penis (Fig. 22-3). These are usually satisfactory except when the child has a rash or perineal excoriations. The bag must be checked frequently to avoid losing the precious commodity! When a prolonged urine collection is needed, a 24-hour pediatric urine specimen bag with an attached drainage tube may be used, or a small feeding tube may be specially inserted into the top of the routine collection bag and the bag periodically emptied with a syringe. Occasionally the so-called metabolic bed may be employed.

Blood samples. A blood specimen is usually not secured by the nurse, but she may help restrain the child as the physician or laboratory technician obtains the specimen. It may be obtained from a

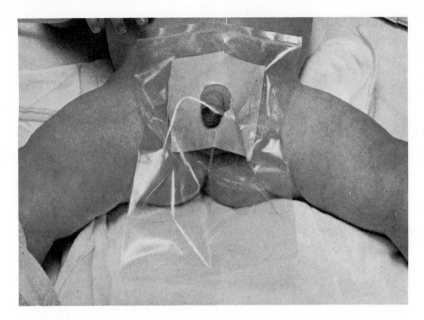

FIG. 22-3   Application of an adhesive-backed plastic bag for collection of a urine specimen. Be sure it is not upside down!

toe, heel, ear, or finger prick, an arterial puncture of the arm, or a venous puncture in the arm or neck. If children must be restrained and if they are old enough to understand, they should be told that the hands, sheets, or other appliances that may be employed are used to help them hold still so that the physician can help them get well. They should not think of the restraints as a means of punishment. Various types of restraints are used during a child's hospitalization. These are discussed in Chapter 23. Common procedures or diagnostic tests that may be ordered at the time of admission (spinal puncture, Clinitest, sweat test) are discussed in Chapter 24.

DIET AND FLUID ORDERS

The diet of a newly admitted child depends, of course, on the reason for the hospitalization, the child's age, food allergies, and general condition. Patients scheduled for pending surgery may be allowed nothing to eat or drink. The diet is ordered by the attending physician. Children may have

many allergies, often involving not only pollens, animal furs, fibers, and dust but also common foods. Chocolate, milk, wheat products, tomatoes, oranges, and strawberries are among the frequent offenders. Nurses should be alerted to these problems and the allergic manifestations they usually cause. The cultural patterns of some patients may cause feeding problems and poor acceptance of the routine hospital diet.

Admission responsibility

The member of the nursing team who has the responsibility of actually admitting a patient will depend on the condition and needs of the child. In certain situations the admission may be made in its entirety by a registered nurse. At other times it may be a joint or delegated responsibility carried out by both the registered nurse and the licensed vocational nurse.

DISCHARGE

Plans for dismissal

The discharge day is usually extremely busy for the parent. Arrangements must be made for transportation (after all, Mary, in a hip spica cast, won't fit in the family Volkswagen). A baby-sitter for the other children in the family may be necessary while Mary's mother takes her home. Maybe her father will have to take time from work to provide transportation. Unless special arrangements are made, the child usually must be dismissed in the morning to avoid a hospital charge for an additional day. If the mother will have little help after her child comes home, she will be busy trying to shop and run errands not immediately possible when the child first returns home. If possible, the nurse should write out any instructions for home care concerning observations to be made or medications and procedures prescribed, rather than rely on oral instructions to the parents. The arrangements for the next follow-up visit to the physician should be clear.

Preparation for home care

NEEDS DURING CONVALESCENCE

If convalescence at home is expected to be prolonged, more preplanning is necessary. The location of the sleeping quarters of the child may need to be changed to save steps and provide greater opportunity for observation. Special equipment may need to be improvised, rented, or purchased. Provisions for help by a visiting nurse may be desirable. Some hospitals now employ a special discharge or "continuity of care" nurse, who helps the parents plan for continued home care and teaches them necessary skills while the child is still hospitalized (for example, gavage, dressing changes, stoma care). She may also go to the home to assess needs and check patient progress.

POSSIBLE BEHAVIOR CHANGES

Parents should be alerted that hospitalization affects children differently. Occasionally, children will have a period of difficulty readjusting to life at home. They may regress developmentally, and activities that they had already mastered before their illness may not be attempted. Irritability and wetting by a previously toilet-trained child are common.

Actual leave-taking

At the time of discharge, every attempt should be made to send all of the child's belongings home with the parent. (Isolation technique may require some restrictions.) Return trips to the hospital to pick up articles left behind are annoying. Bedside stands, closets, cupboards, bedclothes, and flooring must be carefully scrutinized.

Before actually leaving the hospital premises, the parent (or responsible adult) must sign a form indicating who is taking the child. Great care must be taken that the person who is given responsibility for the child at the time of discharge has the legal right to assume that responsibility. At this time a final check is made regarding any medications to be taken home or special instructions to be given.

If at all possible, the child should be taken to the point of actual transfer (usually to a car) in a wheelchair, a rolling bassinette, or on a gurney. The child must always be accompanied by a nurse or hospital employee.

• • •

Admissions and discharges are part of the everyday pattern of hospital routine. The nurse must remember that they are far from routine for most of the patients and parents who find themselves within the sound of her voice and influence of her actions.

daily planning

Every patient has individual needs that, because of their unique combination or background, are particularly personal and special. At the same time, these needs may be said to represent the needs of all people, because they usually fall into broader, more basic categories of care. For this presentation the patient's needs have been grouped to form seven areas of discussion.

BASIC PATIENT NEEDS

The nursing staff is responsible for helping to provide the following:
1. Safety
2. Observation
3. Diagnostic tests
4. Supportive procedures
   a. Aiding respiration and oxygenation
   b. Regulating body temperature
   c. Positioning and appropriate activity
   d. Adequate nourishment and fluid balance
   e. Cleanliness
   f. Rest
   g. Diversion, self-expression, and acceptance
5. Medications and special treatments
6. Rehabilitation
7. Recording of events

Safety

The problem of safety is constant in any hospital. In a pediatric hospital it seems to be constant and compounded. The environment must be continually evaluated to prevent accidents. The patients are often too small to regulate their own surroundings, and they lack the judgment to evaluate their environments properly. Unrestrained or unattended children in high beds or cribs should always have the bed or crib sides securely raised. No nurse should turn her back on an unrestrained child in a crib with the side lowered. Children who have climbing urges should have crib nets properly applied to form a tightly fitting net roof (Fig. 23-1) or be placed in special protective beds unless supervision is constant. Beds of inquisitive boys and girls should be at a "no touch" distance from wall electricity, suction, and oxygen outlets. Toys should be checked for sharp edges, points, or potential danger. Plastic bags should not be used for storage of toys or playthings. Notices of known allergies should be clearly posted in the child's unit. All equipment should be in good working order and used properly. Special precautions should be observed when administering oxygen. When a child is transported in a wheelchair, in most instances a waist or jacket restraint should be used to avoid the possibility of the child's tipping forward or sliding down. Unnecessary traffic and

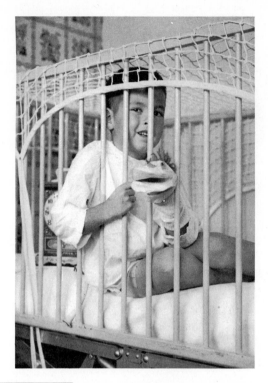

FIG. 23-1

This little boy was a climber at night. A crib net was applied over the top of his bed before lights out.

Courtesy Children's Hospital and Health Center, San Diego, Calif.

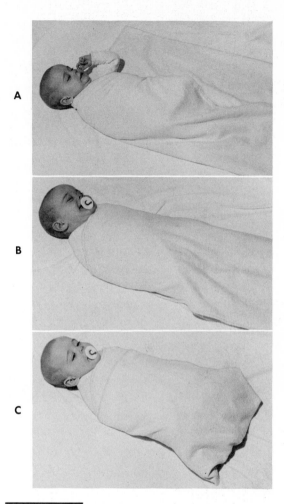

FIG. 23-2

Covered chest mummy wrap. **A,** Center the baby's head at the edge of the "short side" of an open baby blanket or sheet. Place one arm at his side and pull the blanket snugly over his shoulder, arm, and chest and tuck the blanket under the baby. **B,** Position the opposite arm similarly and pull the opposite corner over and around the baby. **C,** Open out the loose end of the blanket and bring it up and around the baby snugly. (We do not generally advocate pacifiers but believe they have a place in certain situations.)

congestion in the halls should be avoided.

An important component of safety is firm but kind discipline. Explaining to the child who is old enough to understand the reason for some rules often works wonders. Good discipline also means realistic expectations and prompt follow-through by the nurse responsible for supervising behavior. It means that nurses must not give choices when no alternatives are possible. It also means offering a choice when the opportunity to choose would bring pleasure, importance, and a sense of self-direction or achievement to the child. Promises kept, a "yes" that means "yes" and a "no" that means "no," and a loving regard for the ultimate welfare of the child

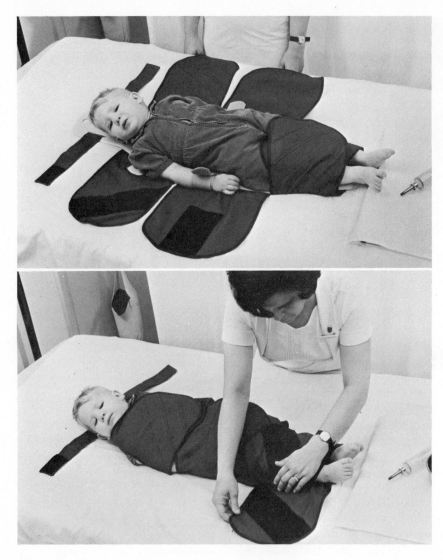

FIG. 23-3   Preparing to restrain a child for gastric lavage using the Olympic papoose board.
Various wraps are possible with the Velcro-lined restraining folds.

Courtesy Olympic-Surgical Co., Inc., Seattle, Wash.

are extremely significant in maintaining good discipline.

Sometimes children must be restrained during treatment to protect them from themselves. Such restraint should never be presented as a punishment but as one way to help children hold themselves still for a little while. An example of such a restraint is the "mummy wrap" (Fig. 23-2). A commercial "mummy restraint" used in many emergency rooms is the Olympic papoose board shown in Fig. 23-3. Another type of control used to prevent children from touching their faces or pulling on gavage tubes is elbow restraints, which are usually fastened to the hospital gown. However, elbow

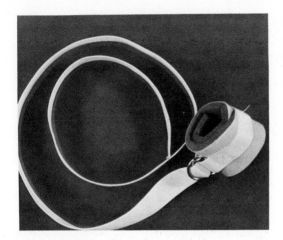

FIG. 23-4

Extremity restraint, incorporating a Velcro fastener.

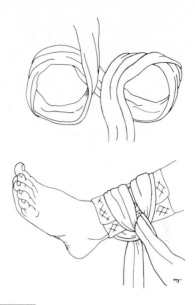

FIG. 23-5

Application of the clove hitch restraint. The formed loops are placed one on top of the other and the body part put through the opening. The body part should always be previously padded.

restraints are not effective if the child can reach the face with a toy or an implement without bending the arms. To control leg and arm motion, specially constructed ankle and wrist restraints (Fig. 23-4) or the timeproven clove hitch tie (Fig. 23-5) may be used. A pediatric Posey belt may be employed sometimes to allow some movement in bed and yet prevent the patient from getting up. A jacket restraint is pictured in Fig. 23-6.

Restraints must be removed periodically to check circulation and exercise the body part involved. They should be so constructed that they will not become tighter with increased tension and impair circulation or endanger the child's respiration.

Observation

Provision for observation is crucial to the welfare of the patient. To plan and pursue the therapy of a patient intelligently, enlightened observation must become an inseparable part of the patient's care. Observation of the patient should be made especially in the light of the diagnosis. If the diagnosis is pneumonia, for example, the fact that the child is pale and has a frequent, loose cough producing thick, white mucus is significant. Sometimes negative observations are important to make. It is important to record that a child admitted because of convulsions has had no seizures for a certain period. The observation that a child hospitalized for vomiting and diarrhea retained a feeding and had no stools for a specific interval may be significant. When observing the patient and recording appearance, activity, and treatment, refer back to the diagnosis. What would be especially important for the physician or supervising nurse to know? A change in the bed placement sometimes may be needed to observe the child more closely.

Diagnostic procedures

The diagnostic procedures ordered must be understood so that adequate preparation, execu-

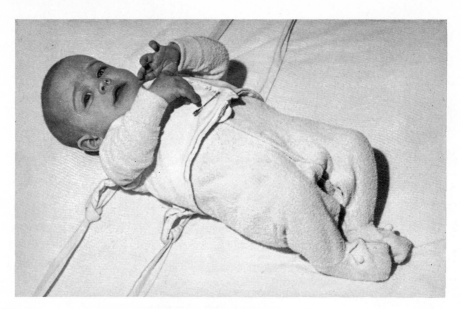

FIG. 23-6   Restraining jacket. The ties are fastened to the bedspring frame, and the pins are placed in front, on top, or underneath, depending on the child's age. It is best if possible to elevate the head of the bed to help avoid problems with aspiration. The ties may be modified to allow some toddlers to sit up in bed. It may also be used as a wheelchair restraint for small children.

tion, and follow-up may be provided. It would be impossible to describe within this brief text all the diagnostic procedures encountered by the nurse in a pediatric setting. But for some of the more common tests and a description of specimen collection, consult Chapter 24 and the hospital procedure manual.

In the morning the nurse must be careful to determine whether any of her patients should not receive anything to eat or drink and are posted NPO. After a test for which a patient has been fasting, the nurse must be sure to inquire *if* the patient may resume his diet. If so, the prescribed foods or liquids must be secured.

Supportive procedures

Various types of supportive procedures and techniques are used to maintain or improve the physi-

cal and emotional resources of the patient. These may include special provisions for aiding respiration or oxygenation, regulating body temperature, positioning and encouraging appropriate activity, maintaining fluid balance or nutrition, relieving pain, or improving body function. They also include the interest and love expressed by parents, family, friends, and nurses and the physical and spiritual serenity promoted by the development of trust. The use of oxygen and humidification equipment is discussed is a separate chapter, as are the methods of regulating body temperature. Positioning of the bed patient, however, is described in the following paragraphs.

SUPERVISION OF POSITION AND ACTIVITY

Even children who are ambulatory and active need to be supervised so that they do not develop poor posture habits that will interfere with the optimum function of their bodies and cause them to

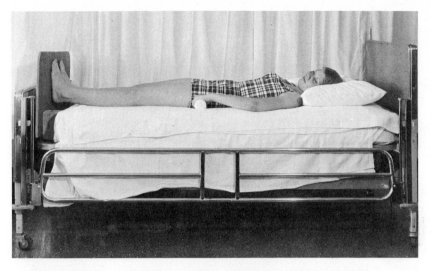

FIG. 23-7   Good body alignment in the supine position.
Courtesy Children's Hospital and Health Center, San Diego, Calif.

feel less than their best. Children in bed, particularly if they must remain fairly quiet for long periods, must be especially helped to maintain good alignment, functional positions, range of motion, and good tissue health for all body parts. (Read also the section on skin care and positioning, pp. 412 to 414.) Barring special treatments involving traction, casting, or specifically ordered body placement, the child in bed should have a posture, when in supine position (on the back) or in prone position (on the abdomen), similar to that which would be considered in good alignment if the child were standing. This is particularly important for those who are not able to change their position easily. Included in this section are some illustrations showing examples of proper positioning.

If patients remain in bed for extended periods without adequate foot support or with tight covers pressing down on their feet, they will develop tightening of the Achilles tendon, or heel cord, causing *foot drop*, which makes walking difficult. One leg may be allowed to fall outward toward the side *(external rotation)*, causing deformity, or it may remain in a common flexed position, which, if not changed often, can result in fixation and *con-*

tracture in a relatively short period. Arms positioned on top of the chest and a partially flexed head position decrease respiratory capacity. Flexed arm and hand positions (very typical of the arthritic patient), if maintained, cause flexion contractures of the shoulder and elbow and *wristdrop*, with loss of function in the hand.

Fig. 23-7 illustrates how good alignment may be achieved with the help of a footboard, pillows, and hand rolls. Incapacitated teenage patients usually need considerable help. It should be noted that a type of foot support is being employed. (However, partially paralyzed patients who exhibit considerable muscle spasticity may be unable to tolerate a hard footboard without tissue damage occurring. They may need a soft boot-type support.) The knees are straight up, rotated neither to the inside nor outside. Sometimes this correct position is maintained in part by a rectangularly folded blanket that has been partially slipped under the buttocks of the patient. The long protruding end is then rolled under tightly toward the thigh to stabilize the leg in neutral position—a trochanter roll. A folded towel or *small* pillow placed under the calves may help relax the knee joints and lift the

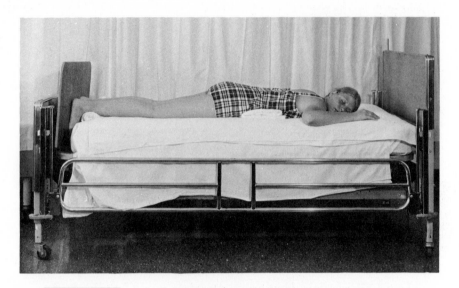

FIG. 23-8   Good body alignment in the prone position.
Courtesy Children's Hospital and Health Center, San Diego, Calif.

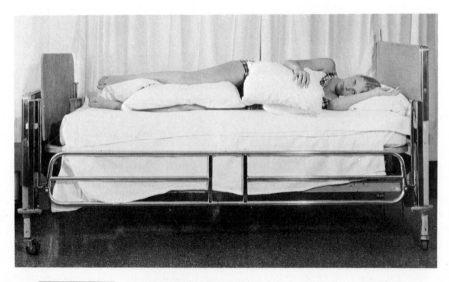

FIG. 23-9   Good body alignment in the side-lying position.
Courtesy Children's Hospital and Health Center, San Diego, Calif.

heels off the bed just enough to relieve pressure. Some patients appreciate a small pillow placed in the small of the back. The arms are alternately rotated for comfort. Soft hand rolls help maintain functional finger-thumb relationships.

When the patient is in the prone, or abdominal, position (Fig. 23-8) the toes should be either over the end of the mattress pointing down between the foot of the bed and the mattress or positioned over the edge of a pillow. A thin pillow support under the abdomen takes pressure off the chest and reduces the lumbar curve. The arms are usually comfortable if abducted and flexed. A pillow may not be required under the head.

The side-lying position is often perferred. The main problem with this position is the strain placed on the hip joint and lower back by the upper leg if it is allowed to fall forward. For a patient who has no back or hip problems and is able to move freely, this is no great difficulty. However, if these problems or conditions exist, this leg position should be avoided by the addition of one or two pillows supporting the upper leg as in Fig. 23-9. Sometimes a pillow tucked lengthwise against the back is comforting. A support for the upper hand relieves the chest.

Good positioning and frequent turning (every 2 hours or less) will do much to comfort the patient; avoid respiratory, circulatory, and urinary complications; reduce deformity; and speed rehabilitation. Infants and toddlers do not require such elaborate supports to maintain alignment and prevent deformity, but they do need to be frequently turned and positioned if they do not move themselves. Older infants or young toddlers often sleep with their heads and chests down on the mattress, faces turned to the side, while their knees are pulled under their abdomens to make their buttocks form the highest point of their sleeping silhouettes. This is a perfectly normal and characteristic posture for this age. A young infant should not be left unattended flat on his back because of the danger of aspiration. A rolled blanket should be placed at the infant's back to maintain a side position.

NOURISHMENT AND FLUID BALANCE

Diet. The diet of a patient does not consist of the type of diet order that the physician writes on the patient's chart. It is not that easy. The diet consists of what a patient eats, drinks, and retains of that which has been sent from the kitchen or prepared by the nursing staff in response to the physician's order. Some diets look beautiful on paper but, infortunately, are not eaten by the person for whom they have been prepared.

Before a tray is served to a patient, it should be carefully checked to see that it is compatible with his diet order, food allergies, abilities, and cultural or religious background. Nuts, raw carrots, and celery should not be served to toddlers who do not know how to handle such "chewy" foods. They sometimes suffer from aspiration. Common diets served in the pediatric area are clear liquid, full liquid, soft, high protein, high carbohydrate, low residue, diabetic, and salt or sodium restricted. Students should review these diets in a diet manual.

A child must often be helped at mealtime. A nurse cannot simply put a tray on a bed or crib table and expect even an older child to eat automatically. The utensils should be appropriate. The food must be easily available and attractive. Toddlers often do well if placed in a high chair for feedings. Some young children prefer to try to feed themselves, but very young children enjoy being held during meals. Bibs and nurse's feeding gown again ease laundry problems.

Infants often drink better if they have a "breathing space" between the time they finish their solids and are offered their formula. Infants and toddlers who need a greater fluid intake may be offered fluids before solid foods when appetites are sharpest to encourage fluid acceptance. Plastic bottles should be used with older infants who enjoy "holding their own." Young children may sometimes be fooled into eating unwelcome vegetables if they are disguised with pureed fruit.

Whether it is necessary to record every bit of food eaten by a child depends on the diagnosis and the child's condition. A diabetic child would require close observation and recording of food intake. Any food left on the tray must be reported in detail so that a replacement may be calculated and prepared by the diet kitchen. Usually, the dietitian wishes all the trays of diabetic patients to be returned separately to the kitchen for evaluation after meals. The true diet of a patient with any metabolic, growth and development, digestive, or feeding problems certainly should be carefully recorded. Some of the trays of these patients will also be returned to the dietitian for evaluation. A continuous "calorie count" or written record of the food item eaten and the amount is often kept at the bedside. Intakes for patients with stabilized conditions could be described as "ate well," "ate fairly well," or "ate poorly." *All* pediatric patients are routinely on a regimen of measured fluid intake, expressed in cubic centimeters (cc) or milliliters (ml). Many are on a measured fluid output regimen.

Hydration. Fluid intake is really of greater immediate importance than solid feeding. The hydration of a child is extremely important. A young child may become dehydrated more rapidly than an adult. An infant is especially vulnerable, having a greater surface area and higher metabolic rate per unit of weight than an adult. Maintaining an adequate fluid intake is one of the very important responsibilities of the bedside nurse. The amount of fluid that is urged depends on the size and condition of the child. Students are reminded that patients who are immobilized in casts or traction apparatus and all those with indwelling urinary catheters must have special attention to assure an abundant fluid intake.

Encouragement. Assuring oral intake often calls for a nurse's ingenuity, patience, and persistence. Small amounts taken frequently are tolerated better by the ill child than copious amounts taken rapidly, no matter how willingly. Fluids taken rapidly are often not retained by children who are ill, upset, or excited.

The kinds of fluids than may be offered to children depend on their diet orders and any allergies they may have. Clear fluids include any liquid

through which one may see the bottom of its container—water, bouillon, strained fruit juices, Popsicles, gelatin, and soft drinks. A full liquid diet would include unstrained fruit juices and milk products such as ice cream, sherbet, milk shakes, and creamed soups.

Learning which fluids the child has accepted well in the past may save time. Offering a choice is often helpful. Sometimes the manner in which fluids are offered is significant. Some older babies seem insulted by a bottle and drink well from a cup. Others regress and will only take fluids well from a bottle with a certain kind of nipple. Some small children are accustomed to warm milk, others like it cold. Older children often reject milk unless it is ice cold. A nurse who is able to sit down with the child beside her or in her lap and offer fluid as part of good companionship is more likely to be successful than the nurse who expresses her frustration in constant verbal harassment. In some cases the use of straws, doll tea-party dishes, colored ice cubes, or a paper star on Johnnie's fluid intake record may help. Popsicles are usually very acceptable. Just plain water should not be forgotten in the search for fluids. With older children, the factual knowledge that other steps (intravenous feedings) will be necessary to assure hydration if oral fluid intake is too low may encourage drinking. For most children a carton of milk and a glass of fruit juice at breakfast, a glass of some other fluid or dish of ice cream or gelatin equaling approximately 200 ml during midmorning, soup and beverage at lunch, and a midafternoon liquid snack fulfill the responsibilities of the day nursing shift.

Restriction. Children with renal disease, central nervous system disease including meningitis, or with heart disease often require restricted fluid intake. Patients scheduled for operative procedures are usually not allowed any oral intake for several hours before their surgeries. After the procedures the amount and type of fluids offered may be restricted. After heart surgery oral liquid intake may be limited to 300 ml during the morning and offered only in small quantities for an extended period. Some postsurgical patients will be allowed nothing by mouth for a considerable period after their procedures, receiving their fluids parenterally (by other routes than oral, such as by vein) until the physician believes that oral administration could be profitable attempted. The child who has had stomach or intestinal surgery initially will be offered very small amounts at a time to ascertain tolerance and to decrease stress on the surgical site. Infants with severe cases of diarrhea and vomiting are usually not allowed anything by mouth or are placed on a limited oral intake to rest the gastrointestinal tract. Fluids for these patients are also administered *parenterally*.

Fluid and electrolyte balance. It has become increasingly apparent in recent years that the content and volume of the body fluid is a key consideration in the maintenance of cellular health and therefore the health of the total individual. The body organs and systems function to maintain the proper internal and external cellular environment and enable the survival of the person. The following brief simplified discussion of fluid and electrolyte balance is included in the belief that an understanding of this area of biology will become more and more necessary for the general public as well as the bedside nurse.

The body functions in sensitive equilibrium. One of the most delicate balances maintained by the body is demonstrated by the composition of body fluid. Major ingredients of this fluid are water and certain chemicals termed *electrolytes*. Electrolytes are so called because they develop electrical charges when they are dissolved in water. Some electrolytes carry a positive charge and are called *cations*. Negatively charged electrolytes are called *anions*. In either case the electrolytes may be referred to as *ions*. A small number of chemical compounds are also found in body fluid that do not ionize or carry electrical charges. Organic compounds such as glucose and urea are the main nonelectrolytes of body fluid. (See Table 23-1.)

Body fluid occupies three permeable compartments (Fig. 23-10): blood vessels, tissue spaces (interstitial areas outside of tissue cells), and the areas inside the cells. *Extracellular* fluid (ECF) is located within the blood vessels and between the tissue cells, and *intracellular* fluid (ICF) lies inside the tissue cells.

Every tissue cell is surrounded by a semipermeable membrane that permits selective passage of certain substances and free passage of water molecules in both directions. Water passes from the side containing the least amount of electrolytes and other dissolved compounds to the side that contains more dissolved compounds. This water movement is called osmosis. In health a dynamic equilibrium of electrolytes and water is maintained between the two areas. Therefore, although each of the fluid compartments of the body contains electrolytes, the concentration and composition of electrolytes in the water of each compartment vary. The electrolytes found in the fluid inside the cells differ greatly in amount from those found in the fluid outside the cells. Interstitial fluid in the tissue spaces is similar to plasma (the fluid portion of the blood), except that it contains very little protein. In interstitial fluid the principal cation is sodium, and the main anions are chlorides and bicarbonates. Intracellular cations are mostly potassium and magnesium, whereas the anions are chiefly phosphates and bicarbonates. Thus chemical differences exist between the extracellular and the intracellular fluids.

Water equalizes quickly in all body compartments. Therefore rapid water intake will not result in edema but will cause swelling of the body's cells and will expand and dilute both the intracellular and extracellular compartments. Salt- and protein-containing solutions will remain primarily in the extracellular compartments. Excessive salt intake may then lead to edema and visible swelling.

Acid-base balance. The acidity or alkalinity of a solution depends on the concentration of hydrogen, or the H ions present. An acid may be simply defined as a compound that has enough H ions to give some away. A base or alkali is a compound possessing few H ions. An increase in H ions makes a solution more acid, and a decrease makes a solution more alkaline. The concentration of hydrogen ions is expressed by pH. A neutral fluid has a pH of

TABLE 23-1 MAJOR ELECTROLYTES AND IMBALANCES

Electrolyte	Deficit	Excess
Sodium (Na^+)—normal value 136-143 mEq/L*	*Hyponatremia* Associated with dehydration; sodium losses from the body in excess of water losses Na^+ below 130 mEq/L Muscular weakness; abdominal cramps; clammy skin; weak, rapid pulse; hypotension; drowsiness; confusion; coma Predisposing factors—excessive sweating and water intake; gastrointestinal suction and excessive oral water intake; glucose water infusion without sodium; diarrhea; renal disease; cystic fibrosis; central nervous system disease	*Hypernatremia* Associated with dehydration; water losses from the body in excess of sodium losses; Na^+ above 150 mEq/L Thirst; dry skin; loss of skin elasticity ("doughy" tissue turgor); fever; weight loss; scanty urine formation; confusion; stupor; seizures; circulatory embarrassment Predisposing factors—sodium chloride infusion; inadequate water intake; watery diarrhea; renal concentrating disease; anorexia; nausea; vomiting; high fever Additional feeding factors—undiluted cow's milk; boiled skim milk; powdered electrolyte mixtures; salt and sugar mixtures; and bouillon soup, etc.
Potassium (K^+)—normal value 4.1-5.6 mEq/L	*Hypokalemia†* K^+ below 3.5 mEq/L Weak pulse; hypotension; muscular weakness; diminished reflexes; loss of peristalsis, cardiac arrest Predisposing factors—diuretics; diarrhea; vomiting; gastric suctioning	*Hyperkalemia* K^+ above 5.7 mEq/L Nausea; apprehension; muscular weakness; confusion; hypotension; cardiac arrest Predisposing factors—burns, excessive tissue damage; excessive infusion of potassium; kidney disease; severe dehydration with scanty urine formation; adrenal insufficiency
Calcium (Ca^{++})—normal value 10-12 mg/100 ml (5-6 mEq/L)	*Hypocalcemia* Ca^{++} below 9 mg/100 ml Tetany; tingling around mouth and fingers; muscular cramps; convulsions Predisposing factors—hypoactive parathyroid; malabsorption syndromes; chronic renal dease; distressed newborns	*Hypercalcemia (rare)* Ca^{++} above 12 mg/100 ml Vomiting; constipation; polyuria; abdominal pains; headache Predisposing factors—prolonged bed rest; overactive parathyroid; overdose of vitamin D
Bicarbonate $(HCO_3)^-$ normal value 19-26 mEq/L	*Metabolic acidosis* $(HCO_3)^-$ below 12 mEq/L Apathy, drowsiness or lethargy; deep, rapid breathing (Kussmaul type) disorientation; stupor; weakness; coma Predisposing factors—diabetes mellitus; starvation; kidney insufficiency; excessive parenteral NaCl; severe diarrhea; salicylate intoxication; respiratory alkalosis	*Metabolic alkalosis* $(HCO_3)^-$ above 30 mEq/L Depressed, shallow respirations; hypertonic muscles; tetany; disorientation Predisposing factors—vomiting (pyloric stenosis); ingestion of alkalies; chloride-deficient diets or formulas; gastric suction; diuretics; respiratory insufficiency

*Milliequivalents per liter (mEq/L).

†Potassium may be given intravenously only after urinary output is well established.

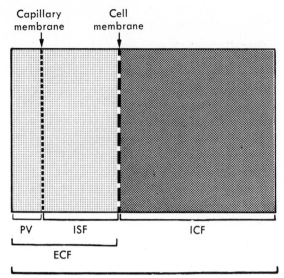

Capillary membrane   Cell membrane

PV   ISF   ICF

ECF

Total body water

FIG. 23-10

Body fluid compartments. *PV,* plasma volume; *ISF,* interstitial fluid; *ECF,* extracellular fluid; *ICF,* intracellular fluid.

7.0 (a lower pH means higher hydrogen ion concentration). An acid solution has a pH value below 7; an alkaline solution has a pH value above 7. The acid-base balance of the blood is maintained in an extremely narrow pH range, normally 7.35 to 7.45. Any slight deviation from this range causes pronounced changes in the cellular functions. This in turn may threaten life. Blood is normally slightly alkaline (pH 7.4). The acid-base balance is maintained by the action of the lungs, kidneys, and buffer systems. The lungs assist in maintaining this equilibrium by varying the rate at which carbon dioxide is blown off, retaining it in acidic form when blood plasma is getting too alkaline or increasing the respiratory rate when the plasma is becoming too acid. When disturbances in blood pH are primarily the result of disease or abnormalities of the respiratory system, the problems resulting are termed either *respiratory alkalosis* or *acidosis.* The kidneys assist in maintaining the normal pH of

blood by regulating the rates of excretion of acids and bases in the urine. Excessive retention of base or loss of acids through diseases of body systems other than the respiratory apparatus results in *metabolic alkalosis;* likewise, excessive retention of acids or loss of base produces *metabolic acidosis.*

Chemical buffer systems protect the acid-base balance of solution by rapidly offsetting changes in its ionized H concentration. Buffer systems defend and maintain the pH of body fluids by protecting against added acid or base.

Fluid volume. The volume of blood plasma, interstitial fluid, and intracellular fluid normally remains relatively constant. Any blood plasma changes that take place during illness usually reflect changes in all the body fluids. Since plasma is relatively easy to obtain from the body and the other fluids are not, it is the chosen fluid for analysis.

Maintenance therapy. Fluid therapy aimed at replacing the patient's daily losses of water, electrolytes, and calories is termed maintenance therapy. The function of maintenance fluid is to keep the body in neutral balance for water, sodium, potassium, and chloride. Water and electrolyte requirements for normal maintenance depend on the child's metabolic rate (calories metabolized), which changes with maturation (Fig. 23-11). Pediatric caloric expenditure can be easily calculated by using the formula on p. 452.

The store of fluid in the body comes from ingested liquid and food. A cardinal principle of fluid balance is that fluid intake must equal fluid output. Under normal conditions the requirement for water is usually derived from the need to replace water lost across the skin and lungs (insensible water losses), which maintain body temperature and dissipate the body's metabolic heat and water lost through urine and stool (Fig. 23-11).

Fluid requirements may be increased in children with increased insensible losses associated with fever, burns, hyperthyroidism, increased respirations or increased urine production (diabetes insipidus). Less fluid is required when insensible losses are reduced (for example, when children are

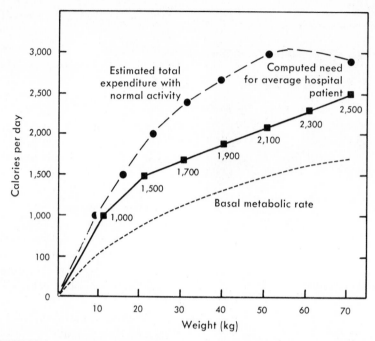

FIG. 23-11   Comparison of energy expenditure in basal and ideal state.

(Modified from Holliday, M.A., and Segar, W.E.: The maintenance need for water in parenteral fluid therapy, Pediatrics **19**:824, 1957.)

CALORIC EXPENDITURE FOR AVERAGE HOSPITALIZED CHILD FOR 24 HOURS

Body weight (kg)	Caloric expenditure
0 to 10	100 Cal/kg
10 to 20	1,000 Cal + 50 Cal/kg for each kg over 10 kg
Over 20	1,500 Cal, + 20 Cal/kg for each kg over 20 kg

Maintenance fluid requirements have been determined to be proportional to caloric expenditure and can be readily calculated when the caloric requirements have been determined as discussed below. The need for water can be estimated to be 100 ml/100 Cal (kcal) or 1 ml/kcal. Therefore the milliliters of water required are equal to the calories as ascertained by the previous method (e.g., a 12 kg child would require 1,000 + (2 × 50) = 1,100 Cal and 1,100 ml of water.

MAINTENANCE WATER REQUIREMENTS

Output	Water required/ expended per day
Insensible water loss*	
Skin	30 ml
Lungs	15 ml
Urine	60 ml
Sweat	0 to 25 ml
Stool water	5 to 10 ml
Hidden intake	
Water of oxidation	Approximately 10 ml (subtract from output)
	100 ml/100 kcal

*Water losses associated with diarrhea or with heavy sweating must be treated as abnormal. Replacement requirements must be computed separately.

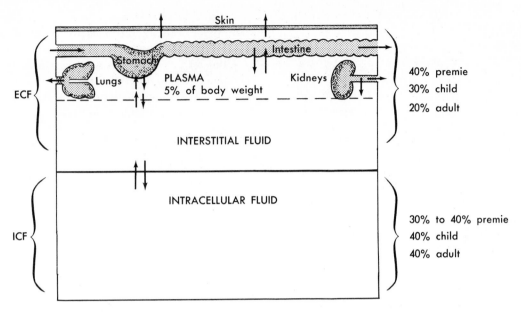

FIG. 23-12 Relative fluid balance in children and adults expressed in percentage of total body weight.

in croup tents or on respirators with increased humidity, or when children have abnormal decreased urine output [renal failure]). Any condition that interferes with an adequate intake of fluid or produces excessive fluid loss threatens the life of the young child.

When fluids are administered parenterally, maintenance electrolytes are necessary to replace urinary, stool, and skin losses of sodium, chloride, and potassium. A child usually needs 3 mEq of sodium, 2 mEq of chloride, and 2 mEq of potassium per 100 kcal expended to meet his maintenance requirements. These electrolyte requirements usually do not need to be altered when maintenance water requirements are varied. It is important to note, however, that sodium is not given to patients in heart or renal failure. Potassium is excreted almost exclusively by the kidneys; therefore replacement of potassium is withheld until the child has demonstrated adequate renal function. Potassium is omitted if the child is oliguric.

To prevent acidosis and ketosis and to lessen pro-

tein breakdown and to provide calories, glucose must also be added to most parenteral fluids. Although full caloric replacement is difficult to accomplish, about 5 g/100 kcal/24 hr of glucose should be given. Fluid maintenance and electrolyte requirements should be administered over the greater part of the 24-hour period for which they were intended.

Fluid compartments. Fig. 23-12 illustrates that plasma is the only portion of body water in contact with the external environment. It is the first fluid storage supply to be tapped in gastrointestinal disturbances (vomiting, diarrhea, rapid respirations, or deficient fluid intake). Interstitial fluid is the reservoir that responds most easily to the shifting fluid conditions present in disease (for example, overhydration may cause edema, and dehydration causes the skin to lose its turgor and become wrinkled). The intracellular compartment represents the largest reservoir and is the least accessible. Here water is lost or gained over a period of days. Without water a well infant in a temperate environment can live about 3 days, and an adult can survive about 10 days.

Several differences between body fluid compartments in the infant and older child must be considered. A newborn infant's weight is approximately 80% water, the older child's is 70% water, and the adult's is 60% water. This percentage varies with the amount of fat. Since fat is essentially water free, a lean individual has a greater proportion of water to total body weight. The proportion of intracellular fluid to body weight remains comparatively constant at all ages. Extracellular fluid constitutes about 40% of the infant's weight as compared with 20% of the adult's body weight. An infant, then, may approach a fluid loss of 10% of body weight before a severe fluid deficit occurs. A weight loss of 5% represents a severe fluid volume deficit in the adult. However, remember, 10% of a baby's body weight is not very much!

Although the infant's body has a relatively greater fluid content per pound, a baby is *more vulnerable* to fluid volume deficit than is the adult. There are several reasons why infants lose a proportionately larger volume of water daily. The baby's body surface in relation to body weight is three times that of the older child. Therefore infants lose a relatively greater amount of fluid through the skin and gastrointestinal tract. Their high metabolic rate produces more waste products, which must be diluted for excretion. Their immature kidneys are less able to concentrate urine, thus adding to the volume of urine. Accumulation of acidic wastes (because of the high metabolic rate and immature kidneys) stimulates respiration, causing greater evaporation through the lungs. Infants may react to infections with higher temperatures, which also result in a higher water loss from evaporation. As the nurse reviews these facts about the infant's body fluid balance, she can more readily understand why the infant, at one-twentieth the adult's weight, requires one third as much water.

Dehydration. Inadequate fluid intake or excessive fluid loss causes dehydration. It is almost always associated with fever, burns, vomiting, diarrhea, hyperventilation, or hemorrhage. Dehydration seldom denotes water loss alone but rather loss of fluid volume, electrolytes, and water. During periods of dehydration, plasma volume is usually maintained at the expense of interstitial volume.

Clinically, dehydration is described by the percentage of body weight that has been lost as water. The most accurate method to assess the child's degree of dehydration is by noting changes in body weight.

Mild	5%
Moderate	7% to 10%
Severe	10% to 15%

Since accurate recorded weight before the child's episode of dehydration is seldom available, clinical signs of dehydration have been defined.

Early signs of dehydration in a patient are dry lips and mucous membranes, diminished urinary output, reduced weight, and lethargy. Moderate dehydration is further characterized by depressed fontanels, sunken eyeballs, loss of skin turgor, and oliguria. As dehydration increases, the child becomes acutely ill, and the circulation may begin to fail. The skin is grayish; the pulse is rapid and weak. Temperature elevation and low blood pressure are characteristic. Recorded output is scant, and weight loss is obvious—10% or higher. Apathy, restlessness, and even convulsions may occur. An infant's condition may require the use of preweighed diapers to determine output. Each gram increase in the weight of a urine-wet diaper is counted as 1 ml of output. Obviously, diapers must be changed and weighed promptly. The blanket under the infant may need to be preweighed as well. It should be next to a waterproof pad.

Intravenous therapy. Because it is often difficult to perform and maintain a conventional intravenous infusion for prolonged periods in the small child, a *cutdown* may be performed (Fig. 23-13). This is a minor but important surgical procedure that is usually completed in the treatment room. The physician "cuts down" to a vein, directly exposing it. A small plastic tubing is inserted into a minute nick in the vein and sutured in place. This tubing is then joined io the intravenous tubing.

Whether fluids are administered through a cutdown or a needle puncture through the skin into a

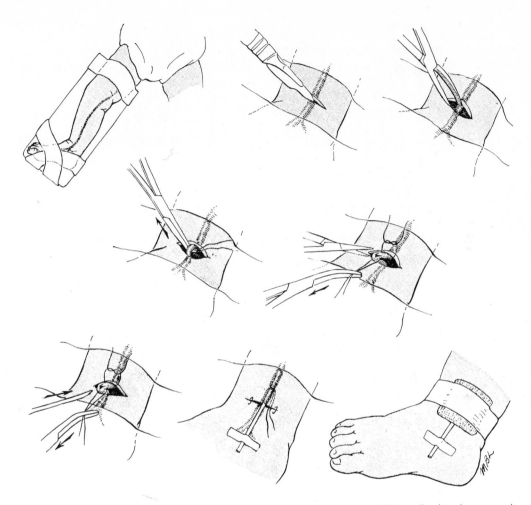

FIG. 23-13   A cutdown procedure. Great care is necessary in immobilizing the leg to prevent impairment of circulation and pressure areas. A cutdown may be used for a number of days to help maintain fluid balance or administer medication. It is used when vein access is difficult or precarious.

vein of the scalp or extremity, it is important that the amount of fluid being given to the child be gauged very carefully to avoid overloading the circulatory system. The rate of flow ordered should be known, marked on the bottle, and meticulously observed. Special pediatric intravenous counting chambers simplify calculation. The usual drop size used is $\frac{1}{60}$ ml or 60 drops/ml. Although a number of semiautomatic infusion sets have added a special margin of safety to administering fluids, the nurse must continue to keep a close watch on the flow rate, the infusion site, and the child's response to the fluid therapy. The infant and small child must be appropriately restrained to avoid dislodging the infusion. The nurse should be aware that changes in the child's position may slow or speed the infusion, and she should frequently observe the rate of flow in the drip chamber (Fig. 23-14). Extreme care should be exercised in moving the patient. The vocational nurse shares responsibility for observa-

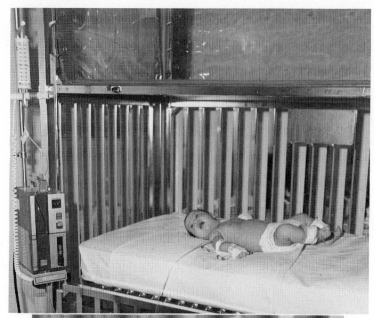

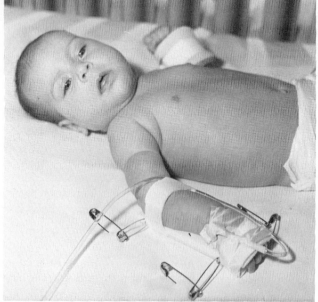

FIG. 23-14   Intravenous fluid with IVAC gravity flow infusion controller that can be set for a specific amount of fluid delivery and is able to detect infiltration. Side rail down for illustration only. The arm board is pinned to the bedding. Inset shows arm immobilization.

Courtesy Naval Regional Medical Center, San Diego, Calif.

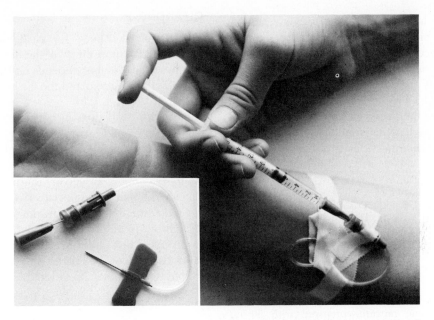

FIG. 23-15 Heparin lock with needle in diaphragm. Child injecting heparinized saline solution into heparin lock on arm.

tion of the intravenous apparatus with the supervising registered nurse. If a vocational nurse observes an infusion running more rapidly than ordered, she may slow it to the known ordered rate, but she must immediately contact the supervising nurse regarding her action. The insertion point of the needle must be checked frequently to detect infiltration or inflammation. Pain and swelling are signs of possible dislocation of the needle.

The responsibility for observation is even greater if the child is receiving blood. There is more danger of circulatory overload, tissue damage, and untoward reactions. Patients receiving blood should be carefully watched and, when necessary and possible, questioned regarding back or chest pain or chills. The temperature, pulse, and respiratory rate should be frequently determined to detect any possible incompatibility. Hives may occur.

Parenteral hyperalimentation. Some children who cannot tolerate oral or nasogastric feeding can now survive by intravenous alimentation. Total

parenteral hyperalimentation may provide glucose, proteins, fats (lipids), minerals, vitamins, and fluid necessary for normal growth and weight gain. Three intravenous methods for total parenteral nutrition (TPN) are currently used: (1) A central venous line may be established by threading a Silastic catheter through an incision on the side of the neck into a jugular vein to the superior vena cava; (2) a multipurpose Hickman catheter may be installed by way of the jugular vein into the right atrium, exiting via a subcutaneous tunnel on the right thorax or sternum, or (3) peripheral or surface veins may be used. The first two approaches may be preferable, since a concentrated life-sustaining solution can be given at a uniform rate into large veins where it will dilute rapidly and thereby prevent thrombosis and phlebitis. However, meticulous sterile technique is required to prevent infection. Hyperalimentation using peripheral veins is also performed, but the risk of tissue damage is considerably greater if infiltration should occur.

Another modification of intravenous therapy is

the so-called heparin lock, for patients receiving intermittent medicines. It allows more mobility without the need for continuous intravenous fluids or frequent venipunctures. The heparin lock (Fig. 23-15) consists of an IV needle attached to plastic tubing sealed by a rubber insert that is maintained in a certain manner to assure patency and sterility. Because selected patients and parents are being taught this technique, it is given here in some detail.

Technique for use of heparin lock

Equipment:
1. Alcohol sponge
2. Tourniquet
3. A special No. 25-gauge butterfly scalp vein needle with associated plastic tubing and rubber cap insert (heparin lock)
4. Heparin-saline mixture—prepared with 30 ml saline solution mixed with 1 ml of 1,000 units/ml heparin (The heparinized saline mixture is kept refrigerated and can be used for 72 hours before being discarded.)
5. 22-gauge, 1-inch needle—to insert into lock initially.
6. Tuberculin syringe—for heparinized saline
7. 35 ml syringe or metriset for administration of medication
8. 25-gauge, ⅝-inch needle for subsequent clearing of the tubing with heparinized saline solution

Procedure:
1. The 22-gauge, 1-inch needle is inserted through the disinfected rubber diaphragm of the heparin lock so that blood will advance into the tubing when the vein is entered.
2. The butterfly needle is then usually inserted into an arm vein and taped into position.
3. Heparinized saline mixture is injected into the tubing with the tuberculin syringe until it replaces the blood (0.5 to 1 ml).
4. The needle is then withdrawn from the rubber diaphragm.

Note: Before and after the administration of intravenous medications or in the event that any blood is seen in the tubing, the tubing of the heparin lock is cleared with 0.5 to 1 ml heparinized saline mixture. Careful instructions and return demonstrations must accompany the outpatient use of this device.

CLEANLINESS

Satisfying the need for cleanliness is almost entirely the responsibility of the nursing staff. The way in which it is met depends on the condition of the individual patient and the facilities of the pediatric unit.

Bed bath. A bath is usually administered each day to prevent skin irritation and provide refreshment, stimulation, and comfort. It also serves as an excellent period for patient observation and evaluation. Bed baths are given routinely to patients who are quite ill, are especially susceptible to chilling and respiratory tract infections, have dressings or incisions to be protected, or who are in traction or casting. Most children with elevated temperatures usually have bed baths, although occasionally a tepid tub bath may be ordered to reduce fever, a treatment that may also be a period of cleansing. Bed baths are carried out in essentially the same manner for children as for adults. A bath blanket or towel should be used for a covering, and, except in the case of an infant, the area should be curtained or screened. Unless contraindicated, a good light should be available for the bath area to aid in the detection of any special changes in skin color, rashes, or other abnormalities.

Perineal care. Children should be helped with the care of their genitalia if they are too young to cleanse the area properly. Any irritation of the penis or labia should be reported. If a little boy is uncircumcised, no extraordinary force should be exerted to retract the foreskin, nor once retracted should it remain so, but observation of the area for cleanliness and possible inflammation should be made. Occasionally, more formal perineal care using an irrigation technique will be desirable to encourage cleanliness, especially in the case of older girls having their menses.

Nails. The nails of young children often need attention. Cleaning the nails when necessary should be part of the daily care. Usually, the nails of children may be cut or filed without an order except when the patient is a diabetic or has peripheral circulatory, sensory, or bleeding disorders.

Oral hygiene. Oral hygiene should also be carried out routinely. However, remember that a child with a recent cleft lip, cleft palate, or dental repair usually is not allowed to have a brush or anything hard in his mouth. For those too young to have more than two or three teeth, oral hygiene may be a simple drink of water, but for older children the essentials of good care of the teeth should be taught. A small toothbrush that can easily fit into the mouth is needed. Massage of the gums and correct brushing and flossing of the teeth are important health habits and often make food and fluid intake more pleasant. Cracked or dry lips may be lubricated with petrolatum.

Bed patients are usually dressed in pajamas or gowns, but sometimes if the child is convalescent, a bright dress or striped tee shirt may be a big lift to the morale of the child and parents.

Unit care. Part of the daily care of the patients is the care of their units. The bath is not technically complete until the unit is clean and orderly. Whether a complete linen change is necessary depends on its condition. Most children's beds need frequent changes, but linen should not be used needlessly!

The patient's bedside stand should be neat (inside and out), and the unit furniture wiped down with a moist paper towel. The aim is not to have each little bed "just so" with a neat and clean but unhappy occupant but to cut down on confusion and reduce safety hazards. Children *need* to have their toys and a certain amount of freedom in their bed activities. But they are not aided by mounds of equipment taking over their beds or cribs. In some hospitals, special bags are available for toy storage. The patient's room should be comfortably warm and well ventilated but free from drafts.

Tub bath. When tub baths are allowed, the amount of supervision required depends on the age and condition of the child. Young children should never be left alone because of danger of burning from the hot water faucet, drowning, or falling while trying to climb out. Teenagers usually resent much observation in the tub room and many times need only a minimum of supervision. Unless a prolonged tub bath is ordered for treatment purposes, the bath should not be too extended. There is greater possibility of chilling, and others may be

waiting in line. When facilities are available, there is a greater tendency than formerly to give hospitalized children tub baths. Be sure to clean the tub well after each child is finished.

Prolonged tub bath. A prolonged tub bath lasts at least 20 minutes. It may be ordered to relax the muscles before physical therapy, to help remove dressings or crusts, or to apply a certain soothing medication to the skin, such as oatmeal or Alpha-Keri. To help the patient relax in the bath and get the whole body in contact with the water, a pillow may be constructed from a rolled bath blanket to raise the head out of the water while the child lies flat in the tub. If a rubber headrest is available, it may be used for this purpose.

Table tub bath. The infant who may have a tub bath is placed in a smaller basin for greater security and easier handling. The following procedure could be used for a newborn infant whose umbilicus has healed or, with modification, for an older infant. It may be carried out at the bedside or at a special table or counter. The instructions are written to help the new mother at home bathe her newborn infant, but the principles are the same. Only the organization of equipment may be different. The older child, who enjoys the bath and is able to sit steadily, may have more freedom in the tub and could be soaped while in the water.

Table tub bath

Materials needed:
1. Baby bathtub, large basin, or bathinette
2. Tray with
   a. Mild soap, dish
   b. Jar of cotton balls and twists
   c. Jar of safety pins
   d. Bottle of baby oil or lotion
   e. Capped 4-ounce (120 ml) baby bottle of sterile water
   f. Small box of tissues
3. Large heavy towel or mat (possibly placed on several thicknesses of newspaper on the surface used for drying and dressing)
4. Newspaper or hamper for dirty clothes discard
5. Paper bag or handy wastebasket to receive waste
6. Two soft towels
   a. One on which to undress and inspect baby
   b. One for drying baby

7. Two soft washcloths or paper mesh squares
8. Baby clothes (clean)
   a. Diaper   c. Kimono
   b. Shirt   d. Receiving blanket
9. Apron

Procedure:

1. Check the temperature of the room (72° to 75° F [22° to 24° C] and free from drafts).
2. Wash hands thoroughly, put on apron.
3. Assemble equipment (the kitchen table is a good place).
   a. Tray of baby supplies
   b. Tub on newspapers on table
   c. Mat or heavy towel for undressing and drying (next to tub)
   d. Wastebasket
   e. Newspaper on seat of chair to receive dirty clothes; clean towel for drying on back of chair
   f. Clean clothes and blanket stacked in order of use
   g. Tub one-third full of water comfortable to your elbow
4. Place the infant still dressed on the mat.
   a. Inspect the eyes, and wash the lids with sterile cotton and water if any discharge is present, proceeding from the inner corner of the eye outward. With older infants, a fresh washcloth or cotton dipped in clear water is sufficient. Inspect the ears.
   b. Wash the face with the washcloth and clear water from the tub. Dry.
   c. Soap the scalp; support the infant, using the football hold, if possible. The infant's head should be over the tub, and if possible the ears should be covered with the nurse's fingers. Rinse the scalp carefully. Dry. Check for cradle cap.
5. Remove the shirt and diaper. If the buttocks are grossly soiled with stool, discard the washcloth used for the cleanup and use another to continue the bath or use tissues for initial cleanup.
6. Quickly soap the infant's entire body, except the head paying special attention to body creases and the area under the chin.
7. Lift the child carefully into the tub, feet first, using appropriate holds.
8. Rinse the soap off the infant quickly.
9. Lift the infant back to the towel on the mat. Pat

dry. Oil or lotion may be used sparingly on the body creases.
10. Inspect and clean the genitalia with cotton balls or tissues p.r.n. Retraction of the foreskin on newborn male infants should not be forced. Many infants have adhesions in the area during the first 4 to 5 months (see also p. 227). Dress the child quickly in clean clothes and wrap him in a receiving blanket.
11. Offer drinking water and inspect his mouth.

Shampoo. The state of the patient's scalp, the patient's general condition, and the length of the hair will determine the need for a shampoo.

Whether a shampoo for an older child must be ordered by the physician depends on hospital policy, the condition of the child, and the type of shampoo contemplated. Many children can easily have their hair shampooed by lying on a gurney with their head extended over the end next to a sink or tub. A trough to guide the water may be constructed of plastic or rubber sheeting. If a wall spray hose is used, great care should be taken in regulating the water temperature before the water touches the child.

If the child is bedfast, a simple head basin and trough may be constructed from two bath blankets rolled together lengthwise (like a snake) and curved into a horseshoe shape with the open end pointing toward the side of the bed. This form is draped by a plastic or rubber sheeting to make a waterproof basin that leads off the side of the bed into a large bath basin or baby tub. Some hospitals use inflated Kelly pads. A few have bed shampoo basins available, similar to those found in beauty salons. The hair must be rinsed of suds until squeaky clean. Some patients like a vinegar or lemon rinse. Hair should be dried quickly to avoid chilling the child.

REST

Personal and environmental cleanliness and order should promote rest, but rest is not automatic. Nap times must be provided and promoted. Most children do best with a rest period after lunch lasting at least an hour. Other nap times should be encouraged, depending on the needs of the child. Shades should be drawn, the television set turned off, the area straightened up, and the child covered comfortably. A reminder of something pleasant that can happen when the child has rested is often helpful in making the nap more acceptable.

DIVERSION, SELF-EXPRESSION, AND ACCEPTANCE
(Table 23-2)

A convalescing child should not be expected to sit or lie quietly all day long without diversion and opportunities for self-expression. Although rest is very important, a child may rest better when allowed moderate activity during the day. To stay perfectly still is impossible and the attempt may be fatiguing in itself. The nurse can help by supplying appropriate toys, providing suitable television programs, setting up controlled group play for patients in the same room when possible, playing with the child herself, or askng for the help of the "play lady" or auxiliary worker. She may enlist the aid of occupational or recreational therapists or child life workers if they are available. A hospital library may be a good resource.

Play is a learning activity that promotes physical, mental, emotional, and social growth. In play children develop new abilities, acquire knowledge about themselves, and explore the feel, look, and taste of the world around them. They use play to express what they are thinking and feeling and to relate and interact with others. Dramatic play is recognized as a form of emotional release.

The nurse can help children choose the play materials that will be fun and satisfying. The following principles should be kept in mind when choosing toys: (1) suitability for a particular age, (2) safety, and (3) durability.

Choosing the right play materials at the right time is not an easy task. However, an understanding of the wide variety of play interests can often give helpful clues.

Every child needs a well-balanced toy selection for all-around development. The choice should be planned to stimulate (1) social play, (2) dramatic play, (3) creative play, (4) manipulation and constructive play, and (5) active physical play.

Play activity is as vital to growth as medicine, food, and sleep. What is the worth of a healed body if the mind is permanently limited from lack of opportunity to grow socially and emotionally?

Medication

The administration of medication to young children entails special skills and knowledge. It is a particularly heavy responsibility because dosages vary so greatly from child to child, as the result of weight, body area, and metabolic differences.

GENERAL PRINCIPLES

Pediatric dosages may be calculated in different ways by physicians. Young's rule uses age as a basis for determination.

Young's rule:

$$\text{Child's dose} = \frac{\text{Age of child in years}}{\text{Age of child in years} + 12} \times \text{Average adult dose}$$

More helpful, since the size of children who are the same age may differ, is Clark's rule, based on weight:

Clark's rule:

$$\text{Child's dose} = \frac{\text{Weight of child in pounds}}{150} \times \text{Average adult dose}$$

Another concept used in computing pediatric dosage is based on the surface area of a child.*

To use this method one must know the weight and height of the child to calculate the surface area in square meters. The average surface area of an adult is calculated to be 1.7 square meters. The final formula used is:

$$\frac{\text{Surface area of child (m}^2)}{1.7} \times \text{Average adult dose}$$

---

*Campbell, J.: The BSA method of calculating pediatric drug dosage, Am. J. Mat. Child Nurs. 3:357-360, Nov.-Dec. 1978.

TABLE 23-2   PLAY-AND-GET-WELL CHART

Age	Interest	Toys	Books
Infant (Birth to 1 yr)	Toys that attract the eye, make little sounds, and tempt grasping hands	Bright hanging objects; large plastic rings; string of gaily colored rings; rubber toys that squeak; tinkling bells	None (enjoys a song or lullaby)
Toddler (1 to 3 yr)	Toys that enable parallel play, provide security and attention, and help development of muscle coordination	Nest of blocks; mallet and wooden pegs; trucks and cars; cuddly toy animals; large dolls; rocking horse; toy telephone; musical toys; kiddie car	Large linen picture books; nursery rhymes; ABC books; farm and zoo animal stories Likes the same story over and over again
Preschooler (3 to 5 yr)	Toys that stimulate child's imagination and develop creative abilities	Nurse and doctor sets; trains and trucks; Tinker Toys; cabin logs; magnets; toy army men; record player; hand puppets; crayons and color books; dolls and clothes; simple puzzles; modeling clay; scrapbooks; cuddly toy animals	Dr. Seuss books; Golden Books; once-upon-a-time stories Enjoys stories about airplanes, trains, and police and fire stations Likes to look at pictures while being read to
Early school age (6 to 9 yr)	Application of mental as well as physical skills Interest and enjoyment in playing with children of same sex Realistic toys that bring child into contact with world outside hospital	Craft sets; models; picture painting; stamp collection; string marionettes; spool knitting; beadwork Games such as Monopoly; checkers, and Clue Paper and pencil games; jigsaw puzzles; paper dolls	Comic books; riddle books; crossword puzzles; fairy tales; adventure stories simple science book; how and why books; who-when-where books; *Highlights*
Middle school age (10 to 12 yr)	Adaptable to group activities Combine companionship and challenge and coordinate work and play in teams	Card games; photoelectric football; science toys; chess; checkers Skill games such as sculptoring and wood carving Walkie-talkie; telescope; transistor radio; camera; television; picture viewer	Comic books; school textbooks; biographies; adventure stories Junior classics such as *Heidi, Little Women, Treasure Island, Robin Hood, Alice in Wonderland, Andersen's Fairy Tales, Aesop's Tales*

Some dosages must be individualized for the specific child by his physician.

Giving medication is sometimes difficult because the child often does not recognize the need for the medicine and may, despite the kindliest approach, resist its administration. However, although the licensed vocational nurse usually is not given major responsibility in the administration of medicines in the pediatric area, she should know the principles involved and receive practice in giving selected medications to children during her pediatric experience.

As with the administration of medication anytime, the following factors must be identified:

1. The right patient
2. The right medication in the right form
3. The right dosage
4. The right method of administration
5. The right time of administration

Before any medication is given, it should be identified on a medicine card or on the medication Kardex. In some hospitals, orders for certain medications must be renewed after a certain time. Common medications that are often automatically stopped unless reordered are broad-spectrum antibiotics and narcotics. Medications that are ordered on an "as necessary," or p.r.n., basis must be checked to see when they were last given to avoid too frequent administration. It also must be determined whether the need for the medication truly exists. The nurse should look up any unfamiliar medication before assuming the responsibility of its administration. She should know its common usages, contraindications, side effects, common dosages, and peculiarities of administration.

COMMON MEASUREMENTS

Before giving medications, the nurse should review the common measurements used in the metric and apothecary systems and frequently used conversions. There should be an easily read table available for her reference. Some of the most common conversions follow:

1 dram or ʒ	= 4 ml
1 teaspoon or tsp	= 5 ml
1 tablespoon or tbsp	= 15 ml
1 ounce or ʒ	= 30 ml
15 or 16 minims or ♏ xv or ♏ xvi	= 1 ml
gr xv	= 1 g
gr i	= 0.06 g or 60 to 65 mg

ORAL MEDICATION

Preparation. If possible, medications for children are prepared as solutions for greater ease in administration. Suspensions must always be shak-

en well before being poured. Most may be diluted, although it is not wise to dilute medicines more than a few milliliters to wash out the measuring container. Children may not take the increased volume easily. Placing a medication in babies' formula is also precarious. If they refuse to take all the formula, how much have they taken? Was the medication evenly distributed throughout? These are difficult questions to answer.

Administration. Before giving any type of medication, the nurse must check the patient's identification. Very young children cannot identify themselves. It is imperative that the nurse check their identification bands.

Always place a bib on a small child before administering oral medications. Such a simple maneuver will save many extra changes and important minutes of the nurse's time, best used in other ways. Remember, if a child is given water or other fluid to wash down a pill, this liquid must be recorded on the intake record.

Fluid medications may be given fairly easily to infants when placed in a nipple fitted in a standard ring (used on ring-and-disc–type baby bottles). The baby sucks out the medication while the nurse supports the head to prevent aspiration. Small medication cups are also employed. Syringes may also be used to administer oral fluids, thus increasing the accuracy of the dose. The medicine is poured slowly with the baby in sitting position or with his head elevated. Rubber-tipped medicine droppers may be helpful too. Pills and capsules usually must be crushed or opened for children under 5 years of age. The medication may be placed in a cherry syrup, honey, or jelly and given from a spoon. Many of these medications are bitter so that a good disguise must be used. However, children must never be told that they are receiving "candy" when they are being medicated.

The child who takes medicine well should be praised for being such a "big boy or girl." If children find it difficult to take medicine, they should be made to feel that the nurse understands some of their distaste and fear and wants to help them during this brief but difficult period. Although a young child may be helped by gentle restraint in the administration of medicines (the nurse may hold the child on her lap with one of the child's hands wedged behind her and the other controlled by her encircling arm and hand), pouring medication down the throat of a struggling, crying youngster is an invitation to aspiration, early emesis of the medication, and subsequent trying periods when medicine time comes again. At times children will respond much better if allowed to hold the cup and drink at their own rate. Many of the small, disposable medicine cups are safe play objects for successful medicine takers, who in turn medicate dolls and stuffed toys.

INTRAMUSCULAR INJECTIONS

When the nurse gives an intramuscular injection to a child, she usually needs a second person to help support, distract, restrain, or comfort the child receiving such an injection. If the child is old enough to understand, the nurse should explain the procedure just before administering the injection. Resistant, tearful children might be told that the medicine will help them get better so that they can go home sooner. The infant or younger child needs to be restrained adequately to assure safe and correct administration of the drug. For most infants and children an injection means simply "hurt" and may establish a lasting fear. To lessen children's fear and to maintain a degree of trust, the nurse should always comfort them by holding them afterward. When dealing with older children she should indicate that she understands why they react the way they do.

In final preparation for intramuscular injection, 0.2 to 0.3 ml of air is drawn into the syringe. When the syringe is inverted, the bubble rises and serves to clear all the solution from the needle into the tissues and prevent backflow.

Equipment
Damp antiseptic sponge
1 or 2 ml syringe
22-gauge, 1-inch needle for infants and children
23-gauge, ¾-inch needle for tiny infants.

Because the gluteal muscle is not well developed in the infant or young child, and permanent sciatic nerve damage is possible, the buttocks are never used for an intramuscular injection. The most desirable sites for pediatric injections are the lateral and anterior aspects of the thighs, the deltoid areas, and the soft tissue inferior to the iliac crests (Fig. 23-16). The medicine and syringe should be completely prepared and ready for use before the nurse enters the child's room.

Method. The site is cleansed with the antiseptic damp sponge, using a circular motion. The skin is pulled taut. In young children who have minimal muscle, the needle is inserted at a slightly oblique angle; if the child is large and well developed, it is inserted perpendicularly. The plunger is pulled back to assure that the needle is not in a blood vessel, and the medicine is injected slowly. When the air bubble leaves the syringe, the sponge is placed over the needle, the needle is quickly withdrawn, and the area is gently wiped with the sponge. A bandage is placed over the site. Many older children seem to be helped a great deal if they can grasp the crib sides with their hands and count during an injection. some gain satisfaction in helping to put on a Band-Aid after the procedure. Afterward a child should be comforted by the nurse administering the injection, if possible. After all, she is not his enemy but a special friend, and everything should be done to help the child recognize this.

SUPPOSITORIES

Aspirin, sedative drugs, and bowel stimulants are often given to children in the form of rectal suppositories. Most of these suppositories may be lubricated with a jellylike material before insertion. Since they are often refrigerated to preserve their shape, warming them, unwrapped, in a clean hand for about a minute may be helpful. The nurse should wear a clean glove or finger cot for the insertion of the suppository. The child should be asked to take a deep breath, if possible, and the medication should be pushed about 2 inches past the rectal sphincter. After insertion, pressure should be

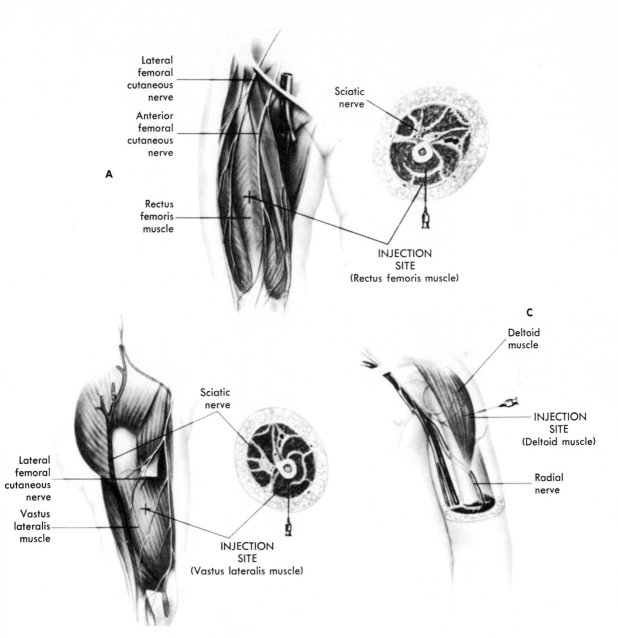

FIG. 23-16   Site of injection chart. The most desirable sites for pediatric intramuscular injections are
A, the rectus femoris muscle, **B,** the vastus lateralis muscle; **C,** the deltoid muscle.

Courtesy Ross Laboratories, Columbus, Ohio.

exerted on the buttocks, holding them together for more than a minute, or the suppository may be ejected and its effect lost.

NOSE DROPS

Nose drops are ordered fairly often for infants and children. They are primarily used to combat nasal congestion and make breathing, eating, and drinking easier. In the case of an infant, nose drops may be ordered 20 minutes before meals to improve sucking and formula intake. If the nose is very congested, gentle suctioning of the nasal passageway may be indicated before the drops are administered. It will do no good if the drops only roll in and out again or do not remain in the nose! Young children do not understand the reason for nose drops and may need to be gently restrained by a second person or with a modified mummy restraint. The child should be lying down with the head tilted back over a folded towel or small pillow. The dropper should be pointed slightly toward the top of the nasal cavity. The child should remain positioned for several seconds after the instillation. Oily nose drops should be avoided because of the possibility of aspiration and lipoid pneumonia.

EARDROPS

Eardrops are still used occasionally in the pediatric area. They should not be cold but close to body temperature or warm. Cold eardrops are painful. The child's head should be resting comfortably on the bed, turned with the ear to be treated exposed. When ear drops are given to children under 3 years of age, the earlobe should be gently pulled down and back to straighten the canal. Older children and adults should have their earlobes pulled up and back for the same reason. After instillation, cotton should not be routinely inserted because it may interfere with drainage of discharge to the exterior or serve to soak up the recently instilled medication.

EYEDROPS

Eyedrops, when ordered, should not be dropped on the cornea but instilled in the lower conjunctival sac while the child, lying flat, tries to look at the hair on top of his head! After instillation of the eyedrops, his eyes should be lightly closed, not squeezed shut, since this may force out the medication. It is a good practice with some toxic medications such as atropine to put a little pressure at the inner angle of the eye after the drop has been placed to prevent drainage into the nose through the tear duct.

TOPICAL MEDICATION

Ointments or creams may be applied to the skin with a finger cot or buttered on gauze with a sterile tongue blade if the area is to be covered with a sterile compress. Liniments and lotions are often applied with clean hands or cotton balls, depending on their contents and the condition of the area to be treated.

Special treatments

Special treatments related to the particular physical problem that the child may be facing are discussed in separate chapters describing procedures involving the various body functions, systems, or diseases.

Provisions for rehabilitation

As convalescence progresses, provisions for rehabilitation may be necessary to recapture skills lost during illness. This usually begins during hospitalization and continues after discharge. In some cases the problem involved is not so much rehabilitation as *habilitation*, or the formation of skills not previously mastered. This is particularly true of patients suffering from neuromusculoskeletal problems. Emphasis is placed on the development of function with the least cosmetic defect and maximum appearance of normalcy. Priority is placed on skills needed for daily tasks. The hospital may have a special rehabilitation unit. (See discussion in Chapter 20.)

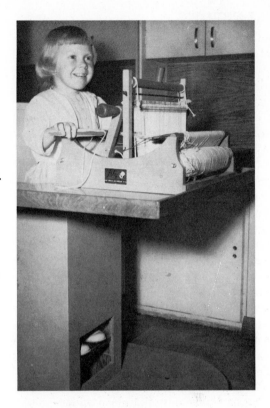

FIG. 23-17

Susan enjoys her weaving in occupational therapy. The stand-up table with a little gate at the back helps her maintain balance. The finger exercise encourages the joint movement that is so necessary for rheumatoid arthritis patients like Susan.

Courtesy Children's Hospital and Health Center, San Diego, Calif.

PHYSICAL THERAPY

Those engaged in the specialty of physical therapy concern themselves primarily with the treatment of disease and injury by physical agents such as heat, cold, electricity, and water. The most common techniques used involve therapeutic exercises in and out of water. These specially prescribed exercises are fundamental to the treatment of delayed motor development and respiratory, orthopedic, and neuromuscular disease. They are designed to prevent and correct deformities, increase muscle strength and function, and establish normal postural reflexes. The physical therapist institutes normal patterns of motion and teaches coordination, balance, walking, and stairclimbing (with and without orthopedic appliances), as well as other activities of daily living (ADLs). Thus through the careful selection of techniques the physical therapist prevents deformity, relieves pain, and promotes functional capacity.

OCCUPATIONAL THERAPY

Occupational therapy is more often concerned with the maintenance or stimulation of small muscle control necessary for the accomplishment of more refined but equally important skills involving finger and wrist manipulation (Fig. 23-17). Occupational therapy uses many crafts to motivate and involve the patient in activites that strengthen muscles or are psychologically stimulating. Weaving, ceramics, shell jewelry manufacturing, woodworking, and painting are usually just means to an end—a better-functioning patient. Often the occupational therapy department can help by locating or fashioning equipment to aid the patient in carrying out necessary ADLs: appliances that help malfunctioning hands to hold combs and toothbrushes, special cups, plate guards, angled spoons and forks to help with eating, and elastic shoestrings and long-handled gadget sticks to aid dressing are just a few of many possibilities (p. 639).

OTHER SPECIALTIES

Speech therapists and hearing specialists may be part of the efforts to better fit the child or youth for life and meet needs for communication and participation. A bedside teacher provided by the public school system may help to make the return transition from hospital to regular school less difficult. Greater provision for socialization, according to the developmental needs of the child, may need to be considered to provide for optimum personality development for children undergoing long-term hospitalization. A sense of individual worth, importance, and purposefulness should be fostered.

• • •

An appreciation of the importance of individuals and the contributions they may make to their world should be part of the nursing perspective of the staff. If the child or youth is personally incapable of making a constructive contribution, society itself may become a source of growth and hope by channeling efforts toward rewarding research and increasing compassion and understanding. A nurse should have a faith that will recognize the tragic realities of life without destroying its sweetness, a philosophy that will allow her to give without becoming empty and brittle, and an outlook that carefully measures minutes in the light of an eternity.

Recording

Although the recording of nursing observations and care may seem to be of minor importance when compared with the proper execution of these responsibilities, clear, concise, and appropriate record keeping is a nursing necessity. It serves as a permanent record of the patient's treatments, medications, and changing condition. It is especially important to have a clear record of pediatric patients who often, because of their ages, lack communication skills. The nurse's notes may help influence therapy, may be important in research studies, and may become of specific legal importance.

The notes should be hand printed in ink. Errors in charting should never be erased. A line should be drawn neatly through the error in such a way that the entry may still be read and the portion labeled "error." All notes should be signed with the first initial, last name, and title of the person making them. In recording, one should always ask oneself, "What is the reason for this child's hospital entry? What signs and symptoms would be significant to record? Is there any change in condition? Is the intake and output record accurate?" If the child has had any bowel movements, they should be described in terms of amount, consistency, and color. Of course, treatments and medications and patient reactions also form part of the record and are recorded after they are completed or administered. The visits of physicians and parents and relatives should be noted.

The nurse should not be too wordy, but she should give an accurate description of the condition of her patient. Good charting for most nurses is not automatic. If it develops, it is the result of concentrated effort and experience. Each hospital will probably have a different form to use, but the principles of charting will remain the same.

DAILY PLANNING FOR PATIENT CARE

After the basic needs of patients have been identified, learning to plan nursing care to meet the needs of patients takes time, ingenuity, and experience. The student requires guidance in executing care so that priorities in need are recognized and work progresses safely and efficiently, benefiting all the patients and staff.

When given her morning assignment and report, a student must plan her individual care to accomplish her goals in the best way possible. To do this, she must be aware of the organization of the nursing unit and the staff utilization pattern. The head nurse, team leader, or student instructor may assist in her planning.

Usually, the best beginning is a *quick* tour of all the patients assigned to check on any immediate needs. The following things could be done during the tour:

1. Introduce the nurse to the child and parent, when appropriate
2. Check the general safety of the patient's environment
   a. Restraints and side rails, crib nets
   b. Intravenous apparatus for rate of flow and possible infiltration and type of solution
   c. Humidification devices for function
   d. Oxygen equipment
   e. Inappropriate toys
3. Help set up and supervise breakfast, when appropriate, checking diet for accuracy
4. Evaluate the need for supplies
   a. Linen
   b. Sizes of underwear, dresses, trousers, shirts, hospital gowns, or pajamas
   c. Procedural supplies
      (1) Dressing supplies
      (2) Solutions—irrigating sets, etc.

After this brief "grand tour" the patient's needs must be evaluated again. In deciding which patient should receive basic care first, one must consider the following:

1. Any prior appointments that have been scheduled for the patients
   a. X-ray examination or therapy
   b. Physical therapy
   c. Speech therapy
   d. Bedside tutoring
   e. Scheduled dressing changes
2. General condition of the patient
   a. As a general rule, the patient who is least comfortable has the priority
   b. Presurgical patients who have had their preoperative medication are usually not disturbed
   c. Patients who are sleeping and need the rest may, at the discretion of the supervising nurse, be left temporarily undisturbed. Sleep may be their most pressing need
3. Types of treatment that are ordered and when they are to be given
   a. Enemas would ordinarily be given before the bath and bed change
   b. Shampoos would ordinarily be given after the bath but before the bed change
   c. A patient's care would preferably be completed before a blood transfusion or other infusions are started
   d. Ideally, sterile dressings are best changed when local movement, bed making, and mopping are at a minimum
4. Hospital routine
   a. Taking the temperature, pulse, respiration and blood pressure is routine for most patients; the time at which it is done depends on the hospital policy and the type of nursing organization pattern followed
   b. Meal schedules: Children usually need more supervision and aid than adults; babies are usually fed their ordered solids, bathed, and then given their formula

A good rule to follow that saves steps and time during the morning is, if possible, never go anywhere empty-handed. Usually something needs to be carried to or from a patient's unit.

An active brain, gentle skill, and good humor should accompany a nurse's many steps.

CHAPTER 24

Common diagnostic tests used in

evaluating maternal and child health

A day does not pass in a busy hospital without many diagnostic tests being performed. The tests may entail the services of the clinical laboratory, the x-ray department, the operating room suite, or other specialized areas. They may be performed in the nursing unit. Although the nurse does not need to know the details of all these procedures, she should know the purpose of the test, whether patient preparation is necessary, the general procedure followed during the test, its effect on the patient, and the follow-up care needed.

For convenience the tests described in this chapter are arranged in table form and grouped as follows: tests of blood specimens, tests of urine specimens, tests of stool specimens, miscellaneous specialized tests, and x-ray tests. Only those tests commonly performed and of special interest in obstetric or pediatric areas are described. The details of each test frequently differ from hospital to hospital. The nurse is advised to consult the procedure manual of the institution where she is employed before participating in any test.

BLOOD SPECIMEN TESTS (Table 24-1)

General considerations

1. Blood specimens are secured by the laboratory technologist, physician, or, occasionally, the nurse.
2. Some blood specimens for chemical analysis are

collected after a period of fasting. Nurses should be aware when food should be withheld before blood is drawn. Water usually may be allowed in normal amounts.
3. Blood specimens are obtained by the following methods:
   a. Prick of the great toe, heel, earlobe, or finger. The blood is collected by pipette, capillary tube, or "Microtainer." Equipment is supplied by the laboratory.
   b. Venipuncture.
      (1) Various sites may be used in children (Fig. 24-1):
         (a) Infants—jugular or scalp vein; occasionally veins of the arm
         (b) Children 2 to 3 years old or more—usually veins of the arm
      (2) Necessary equipment may include the following:
         (a) Tourniquet or blood pressure cuff
         (b) Antiseptic and sponges
         (c) Needles, Nos. 20 to 22 (depends on vessel size), 1-inch or butterfly or scalp vein needles for babies
         (d) Syringes, sterile and dry with excentric tips (size depends on amount of specimen)
         (e) Vacuum collecting containers or tubes, with or without anticoagulants; other special tubes as needed
         (f) Glass slides, as needed
         (g) Band-Aids

Text continued on p. 478.

TABLE 24-1   TESTS OF BLOOD SPECIMENS

Test	Purpose and rationale	Preparation of patient and specimen	Special considerations	Normal value
Albumin, globulin, total protein, and A/G ratio (usually performed together)	To aid in diagnosis or in evaluating treatments of many diseases, including those of liver and kidney Blood may contain excessive globulin when albumin is abnormally displaced or lost, causing change in blood protein and A/G ratio	Fasting patient Specimen—3 ml clotted venous blood		A/G ratio—1.5 to 2.5:1 Total protein—6-8 g/100 ml serum (lower level for newborn infant)
Antistreptolysin O titer	To aid in diagnosis of suspected rheumatic fever (not specific for this disease) Indicates presence of antibodies formed to combat recent streptococcal infection	Nonfasting patient Specimen—3 ml clotted venous blood		50-166 Todd units
Arterial blood gases (children and adults)	To evaluate respiratory exchange and acid-base balance	Specimen—1 ml from arterial puncture or line collected in heparinized syringe	Specimen in syringe placed in ice for transport and immediate exam	Pco_2 35-45 mm Hg Po_2 75-100 mm Hg pH 7.35-7.45
Bleeding time	To determine time needed for constriction of small blood vessels; frequent T and A screen Prolonged bleeding time in thrombocytopenic purpura and other blood disorders	Nonfasting patient Basic procedure—standardized puncture wound made in earlobe; on forearm (Ivy method or Simplate II) drops of blood produced removed with filter paper every 30 sec; time needed for bleeding to end noted		1-7 min, depending on procedure

Continued.

TABLE 24-1   TESTS OF BLOOD SPECIMENS—cont'd

Test	Purpose and rationale	Preparation of patient and specimen	Special considerations	Normal value
Blood counts				
Cell differential	To aid in diagnosis of certain diseases by study of white blood cell percentages and structure Five main types of white blood cells Certain diseases cause alterations in proportions of different cells found in circulating blood as well as individual RBC, WBC and platelet abnormalities	Nonfasting patient Specimen—drop of fresh capillary or venous blood spread on glass slide, stained, and examined under microscope Blood from anticoagulant tube may cause distortion	Usual percentage pattern of type of white blood cells for adults: Neutrophils—50%-65%, increased during infections; eosinophils—0%-6%, increased in allergic conditions and parasitic infections; basophils—0%-1%, increased in some blood disorders; lymphocytes—25%-40%, increased in some viral and bacterial infections; monocytes—0%-10%, increased during some infections Morphology of WBC, RBC, and platelets is also noted	
Platelet count (thrombocytes)	To aid in diagnosis of bleeding tendencies, thrombocytopenic purpura, aplastic anemia, etc. Platelets necessary for coagulation	Nonfasting patient Specimen—drops of capillary or unclotted venous blood (if automated procedures used, larger sample may be necessary)		150,000-450,000/mm^3 methods and thus normals differ
Red blood count (erythrocytes, RBC)	To aid in determination of primary blood disease or effects of secondary disease on blood Red blood cells carry oxygen and carbon dioxide Elevated counts (polycythemia) may indicate dehydration or cardiopulmonary problems; low counts (anemia): hemorrhage, red blood cell destruction, or failure in red blood cell formation	Nonfasting patient Specimen—drops of capillary or unclotted venous blood	Newborn infant has higher red blood count than adult 1 yr: 4.0-5.6 million/mm^3	Adult; 4.5-5 million/mm^3—male, 4-4.5 million/mm^3—female

TABLE 24-1 TESTS OF BLOOD SPECIMENS—cont'd

Test	Purpose and rationale	Preparation of patient and specimen	Special considerations	Normal value
White blood count (leuko- cytes, WBC)	White blood cells help combat in- fectious organisms Blood levels usually elevated in bacte- rial infections, may be elevated in blood diseases (leukemia) Depressed levels may result from blood disease, tox- ic drugs or chemi- cals, or viral infec- tions	Nonfasting patient Specimen—drops of capillary or anticoag- ulated venous blood	White blood count aver- ages 20,000/mm^3 at birth; however, counts as high as 38,000/mm^3 may be considered normal White blood count grad- ually falls with age; ap- proaches that of adult by 3 yr of age	Adult: 5,000- 10,000/mm^3
Blood culture	To identify microor- ganisms that may be circulating in bloodstream Drug sensitivity test usually performed subsequently if or- ganisms found	Nonfasting patient Special venous blood container with culture media Often ordered when high temperature spikes present	Area of blood sample should be cleansed with iodine prep No speaking or air agita- tion during collection of speci- men to avoid con- tamination Preliminary re- ports may be avail- able in 36 hr Final report in 3 wk	Normal blood is sterile
Blood sugar (glucose)	To aid in determina- tion of abnormal glucose metabo- lism Blood sugar level problems are hy- perglycemia,	Fasting or specifically timed specimens may be ordered Timed postprandial (af- ter eating) tests com- mon		65-110 mg/100 ml fasting (Ortho- toluidine meth- od) but normals depend on tim- ing

Continued.

TABLE 24-1   TESTS OF BLOOD SPECIMENS—cont'd

Test	Purpose and rationale	Preparation of patient and specimen	Special considerations	Normal value
Blood sugar —cont'd	caused by diabetes mellitus, liver diseases, or other endocrine overactivity; hypoglycemia, caused by tumor of islets of Langerhans (in pancreas) or other endocrine disturbances; insulin-glucose imbalance, caused by diabetic treatment	Specimen—3-5 ml venous blood in tube with sodium fluoride		
Blood types ABO grouping	To determine blood type for possible transfusion or maternal-newborn blood studies— ABO incompatibility	Nonfasting patient Both unclotted and clotted blood desired for transfusion cross matching		Four main blood types found in U.S. population: A— 38% B— 12% AB— 5% O— 45%
Rh factor (Rh$_o$ [D])	To determine blood type for possible transfusion or maternal-newborn blood studies—Rh incompatibility	Nonfasting patient Both unclotted and clotted blood desired for transfusion cross matching		85% of Americans, Rh+ (positive); 15% of American, Rh− (negative)
Blood urea nitrogen (BUN)	To determine kidney disease or urinary obstruction Urea, a waste product of protein metabolism, normally excreted by kidney; if urinary system fails, blood urea levels will be elevated	Fasting patient Specimen—3 ml clotted venous blood		7-20 mg/100 blood (depending on method)
Clotting (coagulation time)	To determine time needed for blood to clot outside body Many factors necessary for normal clotting; clotting	Nonfasting patient Several methods, using fresh venous or capillary blood		Wide range, depending on method used

TABLE 24-1 TESTS OF BLOOD SPECIMENS—cont'd

Test	Purpose and rationale	Preparation of patient and specimen	Special considerations	Normal value
	may be slow in hemophilia, anticoagulant therapy, etc.			
Coombs' test	To detect weak or incomplete type of antibody reactions Used especially to diagnose erythroblastosis fetalis, caused by Rh incompatiblity or need for $Rh_o(D)$ prophylaxis	Nonfasting patient Specimen—2-5 ml clotted or unclotted blood, depending on laboratory methods and type of test ordered	Direct or indirect Coombs' tests may be ordered Infant cord blood → direct Mother's blood before childbirth → indirect	If direct Coombs' test negative and baby Rh+ or D^u+; Rh− mother is $Rh_o(D)$ immune globulin candidate
C-reactive protein (CRP)	To aid detection of inflammation and tissue breakdown Nonspecific test, often used to aid diagnosis of rheumatic fever and infarctions; to ensure validity of test, patient given high-CHO diet for previous 24 hours	Serum from clotted capillary or venous blood may be used, depending on technique employed		Normally, no C-reactive protein present
Glucose tolerance	To aid in determination of abnormal glucose metabolism More informative than single fasting blood sugar determination	Fasting patient, except for timed dose of glucose and H_2O; oral or IV glucose tolerance tests may be ordered Fasting blood and urine specimen secured; calculated dose of glucose given fasting patient Multiple periodic blood and urine specimens may be ordered during ½-5 hr period Consult hospital manual	Patient's current weight determined to calculate amount of glucose to be given. Drinks commercially prepared for this purpose are calculated with glucose dosage	Normal range: Oral—peak of not more than 150 mg/ 100 ml blood, return to fasting level within 2 hr Intravenous— return to fasting level within 1 hr Comparison to standard curve reveals various metabolic prob-

Continued.

TABLE 24-1   TESTS OF BLOOD SPECIMENS—cont'd

Test	Purpose and rationale	Preparation of patient and specimen	Special considerations	Normal value
Glucose tolerance—cont'd			Testing procedures differ according to basic reason for test (possible hypoglycemia or hyperglycemia)	lems (thyroid, liver, pancreas)
Hematocrit (Hct)	To determine relative proportion of cells and plasma in blood Most reliable screen test for anemia—low in anemia, high in polycythemia and dehydration (usually performed routinely with CBC)	Nonfasting patient Specimen—3 ml anticoagulated venous or heparinized capillary blood Specimen placed into a special hematocrit tube and spun; height of resulting column of packed red blood cells recorded in percent	Newborn 45%-65%; a low of 35% may be seen at about 2-6 mo of age	Adult: Male—40-50 mm red blood cells/100 mm of column height Female—35-45 mm red blood cells/100 mm of column height
Hemoglobin (Hgb)	To determine amount of hemoglobin in blood available for transport of oxygen Hemoglobin levels help determine color of blood; amount of red blood cells and level of hemoglobin in blood are not always parallel	Nonfasting patient Specimen—capillary or venous blood in EDTA or citrated tube	Newborn infants have higher normal levels than older children or adults (14-19 g); low of 11 g may be seen at 3-6 mo of age	Female adult—11.5-15 g/100 ml Male adult—14-17 g/100 ml
PKU (Guthrie inhibition assay)	To identify excessive phenylalamine in the blood and treat to prevent mental retardation	Newborn Capillary blood obtained as close as possible to time of discharge from the nursery	Infants screened before 24 hours of age should be rescreened before the third week of life; phenylalanine present in	1.2-3.4 mg/100 ml Level above 8 mg phenylalanine per 100 ml blood, diagnostic of PKU

TABLE 24-1 TESTS OF BLOOD SPECIMENS—cont'd

Test	Purpose and rationale	Preparation of patient and specimen	Special considerations	Normal value
			urine only after third day of life in milk-fed babies Cord blood cannot be used	
Sedimentation rate	To aid in detection of inflammation and tissue breakdown Nonspecific test, which, when elevated, may point to rheumatic fever activity, arthritis, infections, and infarctions	Nonfasting patient Specimen—3 ml unclotted venous blood Blood measured into a calibrated thin tube, and level of plasma separating from cells is measured	If patient anemic, "corrected sedimentation rates" may be reported	Depends on age and equipment—0-20 mm/hr (Wintrobe), 10-13 mm/hr (Westergren)
Serology test for syphilis (RPR, VDRL, FTA-ABS)	To aid in detection of syphilis Legally required before marriage in most states; routine at prenatal examination; some hospitals require on all admissions	Nonfasting patient Specimen—serum from 3 ml clotted venous blood	Nonspecific tests—false positive and false negative results may be obtained Handle report of positive results discreetly	Negative
T$_4$ (Thyroxine) assay	To identify hypothyroidism and prevent mental retardation and cretinism	Cord or capillary blood may be used	All infants should be screened T$_4$ levels of 4 μg/dl or less are tested for thyroid stimulating hormone; TSH levels greater than 25 μg/ml are diagnostic for congenital hypothyroidism	Cord blood 8-12 μg/dl Birth to 4 days 14-23 μg/dl 5 days-1 month, 14-21 μg/dl After 1 month, 4-11 μg/dl

FIG. 24-1

Suggested restraint and positioning for puncture of a jugular vein.

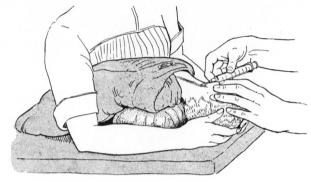

c. Cord blood.
   (1) From the placenta at birth
   (2) From the umbilical cord vessels (artery or vein) of the newborn by means of an umbilical catheter
4. Nursing care during the collection of blood specimens usually consists of explaining the procedure to the young child and helping support or restrain him.
5. Blood specimens must be collected, labeled, transported, and checked into the laboratory properly. Immediately after collection, invert tube containing anticoagulant eight times to assure mixture—do not shake. If an addressing machine is available, stamping the paper tape with the patient's charge-a-plate will easily assure the inclusion of the patient's name, unit, physician's name, and date on the label. A laboratory requisition form should accompany each specimen. The time that the specimen is sent is recorded.

URINE SPECIMEN TESTS (Table 24-2)

General considerations

1. Urine specimens, except for bladder taps, are secured by the nurse.
2. Urine specimens may be obtained in various ways, depending on the physician's orders. Specimens may be ordered regulating the preparation of the patient or the timing of the specimen collection.
   a. Routine voided specimen. No special preparation is usually needed. The patient is asked to void into a clean container.
   (*Note:* Children and some adults do not understand the word "void"; select terminology in accord with the age and education of the patient. Little children may say "pee-pee," "tinkle," "number 1," "pass water," or "urinate.") The patient should be told not to put toilet paper in with the specimen. If the patient is menstruating, a routine voided specimen will be of no diagnostic value. A "clean catch" may be ordered, or the test deferred until later.
   b. Voided "clean catch midstream specimen." Special preparations are made before the specimen is collected.
   (1) Necessary equipment may include the following:
       (a) Six + (?) sterile cotton balls, gauze compresses or four povidone-iodine prep packets if patient is not allergic to iodine
       (b) Povidone-iodine solution in squeeze bottle or bowl, (or four povidone-iodine prep packets), other antiseptic or soap solution
       (c) Sterile water for rinse of area
       (d) Paper bag or other waste recepticle
       (e) Sterile collecting bottle
       (f) Clean gloves

(2) For female patients the perineum is carefully cleansed with povidone-iodine or other appropriate solution. The labia are retracted, and each cotton ball compress or prep is used only once, moving from front to back. Following the cleansing with the antiseptic, the area is rinsed with sterile water using compresses, cotton balls, or an irrigation technique. The labia are kept retracted if possible. After the urinary stream begins, the collecting bottle is positioned to collect an adequate specimen and removed before the stream slows. Older patients may be able to carry out the procedure alone if properly instructed. Younger patients may find it difficult to void when directed. Little girls may be washed off and placed directly on a sterile bedpan if unable to void with the labia retracted. Infants and toddlers must be "taped" for a specimen using a sterile plastic bag that adheres to the perineum with adhesive and tape. If the patient is well hydrated, the request for a specimen is more easily fulfilled. A midstream collection kit includes everything necessary for the collection of sterile specimens. For male patients the glans penis is carefully washed with antiseptic solution, and the foreskin, if present, is retracted to assure proper cleansing (unless the infant is under 5 months of age). When the patient begins to void, the container is positioned to collect an adequate specimen and removed before the stream dwindles. Older boys and young men often carry out this procedure alone or with the assistance of an orderly.

c. Three-glass specimen (for male patients). The glans penis is cleansed. Three sterile urine specimen bottles are labeled No. 1, No. 2, and No. 3. The patient begins the urine stream, voiding approximately 20 ml in bottle No. 1. Without interrupting the urine stream he voids about 100 ml into bottle No. 2. Without interrupting the urine stream he continues to collect the specimen in No. 3 until his bladder is empty. The assistance of the orderly or a male nurse may be needed.

d. Catheterized specimen. This is used much less frequently because of danger of infection. Male catheterizations usually are performed by a male nurse or orderly; female catheterization technique has been described in Chapter 10. The urethra of the female infant curves downward; therefore, the catheter should be inserted in a slightly downward direction.

e. Percutaneous bladder aspiration (bladder tap). This specimen is obtained by a physician. If possible, the patient is given some fluid about 20 minutes before the tap. The patient is placed in a supine position on a firm surface. The abdominal area is cleansed with antiseptic. The puncture is made above the pubis with a No. 22 (1-inch) or No. 21 (1½-inch) needle with a 5 or 10 ml syringe attached to aspirate a specimen in a sterile manner. With female infants the labia are tightly closed, or pressure may be placed on the urethra to prevent voiding before the aspiration. The procedure should be delayed if the infant voids just before it is scheduled. Afterward, pressure is applied digitally with a gauze sponge over the tap site, and then the site is covered with an adhesive bandage.

f. Timed specimen. This specimen usually consists of voided urine, although it may involve drainage from a urinary catheter. To begin the specimen collection, have the patient empty his bladder. Note the time. Discard this first urine specimen. Label a large collection bottle of the type approved by the laboratory with the patient's name, his physician's name, and the time the discarded urine specimen was voided. This is the start of the test. Collect all voided spec-

Text continued on p. 484.

TABLE 24-2   TESTS OF URINE SPECIMENS

Test	Purpose and rationale	Preparation of patient and specimen	Special considerations	Normal value
Routine urinalysis Acetone	To determine presence of ketones in urine, a possible sign of developing acidosis found as a result of diabetes mellitus, starvation, vomiting and diarrhea or prolonged protein diet	Usually done by nurse for diabetic patients; 1 drop of urine placed on Acetest tablet, and after 30 sec color change compared with scale; or dip stick analysis (Diastix) may be performed	Diabetic patients may have urine specimen free from sugar but containing acetone, although this is uncommon	No acetone present normally
Albumin	To detect loss of plasma albumin through kidney May indicate kidney disease, heart failure, drug poisoning, or toxemia of pregnancy	Dip stick analysis		Usually no albumin present; however, orthostatic or postural albuminuria sometimes occurs in absence of disease Albuminuria is common finding in newborn infant
Blood, occult	To determine presence of free hemoglobin (hemolized cells) or intact RBCs	Dip stick analysis		Normally none present; found with hemolytic or urinary tract disease
Glucose	To detect presence and amount of glucose in urine, possibly caused by diabetes mellitus	Clinistix—simple to use; good screening device Clinitest—follow directions issued with Clinitest tablets *carefully;* The "5 drop" and/or "2 drop" method may be ordered	When performing the Clinitest, observe reaction—rapid passage through green, tan, orange, and finally to dark shade of greenish brown indicates amount of glucose is over 2% in "5 drop" method;	No glucose usually present Clinitest sensitive to other simple sugars (lactose, pentose, fructose)

TABLE 24-2 TESTS OF URINE SPECIMENS—cont'd

Test	Purpose and rationale	Preparation of patient and specimen	Special considerations	Normal value
			continue testing with "2 drop" method, which indicates up to 5% glucose Do not touch tablets; store away from heat and sun; watch for "blue color and stickiness"; cap tightly immediately	
Gross appearance (color, clarity)	To aid in estimation of degree of hydration and ability of kidneys to concentrate or dilute urine		Turbidity does not always indicate pathology	Color may depend on amount of hydration—may change greatly from one time to next Smoky urine may indicate hematuria
Microscopic studies Cells	Red blood cells and white blood cells found in urine in urinary tract disease	Need approx. 12 ml specimen of urine placed in centrifuge; sediment examined microscopically	Presence of red blood cells or white blood cells in voided specimen of mature female has little significance, since these results may be caused by vaginal contamination Recheck by midstream clean catch	No red blood cells A few white blood cells (0-5) A moderate number of epithelial cells may be present
Casts	Casts, representing abnormal sediment in urine, may be formed of many substances passing relatively slowly through tubules; presence usually indicates kidney disease	Specimen of urine placed in centrifuge; sediment examined microscopically		Rare hyaline cast may be present; normally other types indicate pathologic condition

Continued.

TABLE 24-2   TESTS OF URINE SPECIMENS—cont'd

Test	Purpose and rationale	Preparation of patient and specimen	Special considerations	Normal value
Bacteria	If large number present in fresh or refrigerated voided specimen, midstream clean catch specimen may be ordered for culture		Freshly voided specimens should be refrigerated within 1 hr	
Specific gravity	To measure density of urine as compared with distilled water High specific gravity may occur in albuminuria, glycosuria, and dehydration Detects presence of many abnormal substances, but does not identify them Test also indicates patient's ability to concentrate or dilute urine	Tested with a urinometer (calibrated float) or refractometer—needs only 2 drops—is more accurate (Fig. 24-2) Be sure to clean and dry the urine chamber of refractometer immediately after use; dip stick now also available		1.003-1.030 (adults) 1.002-1.010 (newborns after ingestion of milk)
pH	To determine acidity or aklalinity of urine To differentiate acid urine from alkaline amniotic fluid and detect ruptured bag of waters	Strip of Nitrazine paper is dipped into urine, placed in a baby's diaper, or dampened by vaginal drainage; color change compared with scale Other dip sticks available	pH should be measured quickly because urine becomes alkaline on standing Sometimes alkaline urine is needed to keep excreted substances soluble (during sulfadiazine therapy or blood or tissue destruction), and therapy is directed to this end	4.5-7.5 (urine is usually acid, but pH may vary, depending on diet, patient's condition, and age of specimen
Vanillylmandelic acid (VMA)	To aid diagnosis of neuroblastoma and follow the response of therapy Urine measurements of vanillylmandelic acid (VMA)	24-hour urine specimen collected in refrigerated brown bottle with preservative hydrochloric acid; 2 days prior to collection diet restricted by elimination of bananas, ice cream, foods containing vanilla flavoring; no vigorous exercise on day before collection	Certain drugs interfere with test Discontinue 2 days prior to test Check hospital manual	0.5-7.0 mg/ 24 hr

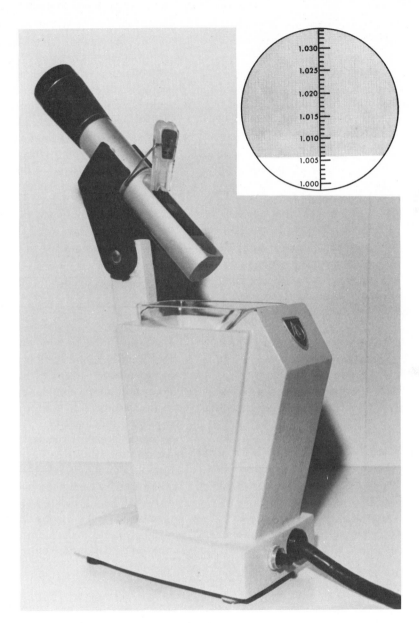

FIG. 24-2   One type of total solids (T.S.) meter or refractometer. Insert shows what is seen on specific gravity scale with specific gravity of 1.006.

imens for the ordered period in this single large collection bottle. Even if a special preservative is used, the bottle must be kept in a refrigerator unless instructed otherwise by the laboratory. At the end of the period have the patient empty his bladder again and add this specimen to the total collection. Send the total specimen to the laboratory. Since this represents the total urine output of a patient within a known period, the collection *must* begin with an empty bladder. Twenty-four–hour urine specimens are notoriously difficult to obtain in pediatrics, especially from little girls. One method employs a modified incubator, crib, or bed in which a nylon screening device is placed above a drainage unit. (This is sometimes called a "metabolic bed.") The child is positioned on the screen. As she voids, the urine is "filtered" through the screen.

3. Urine specimens should be properly collected, free of fecal material, labeled, transported, and checked into the laboratory with proper requisitions. Urine specimens should be sent promptly to the laboratory unless protected from deterioration by refrigeration or a preservative.

STOOL SPECIMEN TESTS (Table 24-3)

General considerations

1. Stool specimens are obtained by the nurse.
2. Stool specimens are obtained by collection from a bedpan or diaper or, occasionally, by rectal swab. They are placed, with tongue blades, into a clean disposable receptacle. They must *not* be contaminated with urine. The entire specimen need not be sent to the laboratory unless a timed specimen is ordered or the reason for the stool collection is the detection of a tapeworm head (scolex). Specimens for ova and parasites should be sent to the laboratory immediately. If transport will be delayed, place about 2 cc of stool specimen in polyvinyl alcohol (PVA) solution and seal container tightly. Balance of specimen can go in a carton to the refrigerator.
3. Stool specimens should be collected, labeled, transported, and checked into the laboratory immediately and properly.

TESTS OF SPUTUM

General considerations

1. Occasionally sputum specimens are requested for culture and sensitivity studies, cell analysis ("Pap" smear), Gram stain, or wet mounts. Sputum specimens are difficult to obtain from young children. Even older children and adults may find it difficult to produce material originating in the bronchial tree.
2. Specimens are best secured from cooperating patients after IPPB treatment or chest therapy (cupping, vibration, and postural drainage).
3. For those who cannot cooperate, the use of a sterile specimen trap connected to a suction apparatus has been helpful. Avoid saliva if possible. It is better to obtain scant material from lower areas than more volume with saliva.

TABLE 24-3   TESTS OF STOOL SPECIMENS

Test	Purpose and rationale	Preparation of patient and specimen	Special considerations	Normal value
Fat determination	To confirm diagnosis of steatorrhea (excess fat in stools), signs of celiac syndrome	Patient on normal diet 2 or 3 days before test Timed specimen usually ordered		Between 15% and 25% of weight of fecal sample
Occult blood	To detect presence of fecal blood, which is changed by process of digestion	Usually random specimen used If positive, patient is on meat-free diet for 3 days and another specimen obtained	Diet containing meat may sometimes cause positive result, depending on method used Hematest tablets or commercially prepared packets with developer are available	No occult blood
Ova and parasites (see p. 484)				
Timed stool specimen	To determine amount of certain substances excreted in feces in given time	Patient should not void or place tissues in bedpan with stool Determine date and approximate time of previous defecations; this will be start of test collection; refrigerate total specimen until complete and then take to laboratory		

TABLE 24-4   MISCELLANEOUS SPECIALIZED TESTS

Test	Purpose and rationale	Preparation of patient and/specimen	Special considerations
Amniocentesis (see p. 47.)			
Electrocardiogram (ECG or EKG)	To aid in determination of irregularities in electrical impulses controlling heart action and to help diagnose heart damage	Usually no special preparation except simple explanation; no pain involved Leads positioned on limbs and chest by technician	
Electroencephalogram (EEG)	To aid in determination of abnormalities in brain waves Useful in diagnosing convulsive disorders, brain tumors; estimating cerebral activity	Simple explanation Young children need to be sedated before test Testing takes approximately 1 hr; no pain involved Electrodes placed on scalp with adhesive substance by special technician in quiet atmosphere May need shampoo before and following	
Fetal lung maturity Foam stability test (Shake test); positive result usually indicative of fetal lung maturity L/S (lecithin/ sphingomyelin) ratio; 2: 1, or 2, usually indicative of fetal lung maturity	To detect presence of surfactants denoting fetal lung maturity or possibility of respiratory distress syndrome	Amniocentesis necessary to secure sample of amniotic fluid for analysis	Used to best advantage to determine time of elective cesarean procedures
Lumbar puncture	To obtain cerebrospinal fluid specimens for cell count, protein and sugar content, culture, or Gram stain Spinal fluid glucose lowered in cases of meningitis	Inform child just before procedure Positioning: place child on side with knees drawn up sufficiently to arch back, or in sitting position with his spine curled forward to increase the space be-	Three specimens properly labeled, transported, and checked into the laboratory immediately Normal value in children: Pressure 70-200 mm of water

TABLE 24-4 MISCELLANEOUS SPECIALIZED TESTS—cont'd

Test	Purpose and rationale	Preparation of patient and specimen	Special considerations
	Spinal fluid protein elevated in meningitis or subarachnoid hemorrhage White blood cell count moderately increased in encephalitis; greatly elevated in most cases of meningitis	tween vertebrae for needle insertion (Fig. 24-3) Child must be supported and maintained in position throughout procedure	Cell count 0-8 WBC (under 5 yr) and 0-5 WBC (over 5 yr), 0 RBC Protein total 15-40 mg/100 ml Glucose 50-90 mg/100 ml

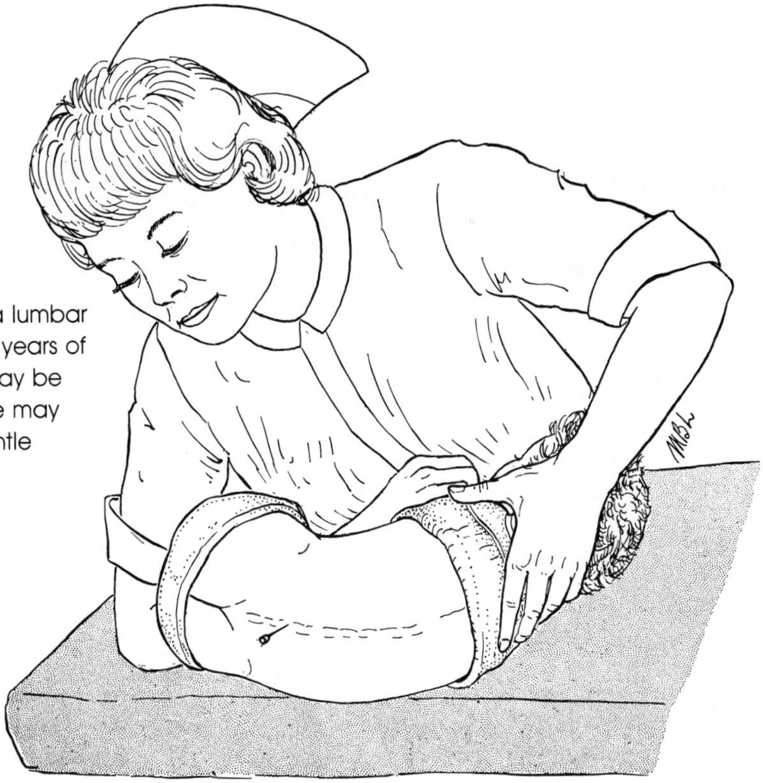

FIG. 24-3

Restraining a small child or infant for a lumbar puncture. When an older child (2 to 3 years of age) is positioned, the child's head may be tucked under an elbow, and the nurse may have to lean over her charge in a gentle but firm fashion to maintain positioning.

Continued.

TABLE 24-4   MISCELLANEOUS SPECIALIZED TESTS—cont'd

Test	Purpose and rationale	Preparation of patient and specimen	Special considerations
Nonstress test (NST)	Purpose same as OCT below but does not employ oxytocin Based on knowledge that FHR accelerates with fetal movement and baseline shows variability in "healthy" *reactive* fetus Effects of any contractions may also be evaluated	Semi-Fowler's position with external fetal and contraction monitors obtain baseline FHR and vital signs Run 20-40 min monitor strip; have mother confirm fetal movement Observe for accelerations with fetal movement and baseline FHR variability	Test done after 28 weeks' gestation; test shorter, less expensive, noninvasive vs. OCT Reactive tests usually indicate fetal health Fetus may demonstrate rest-activity cycle of approximately 40 min, necessitating 40 min strip to observe FHR changes False nonreactive tests may occur as result of maternal sedative medication May be used in conjunction with OCT if test nonreactive
Oxytocin challenge test (OCT) or Contraction stress test (CST)	To determine circulatory-respiratory reserve of utero-placental-fetal unit before labor and evaluate ability of a *high-risk* fetus to withstand the stress of labor by recording the effect of oxytocin-induced contractions on his heart rate	Semi-Fowler's position with external fetal and contraction monitors Obtain a baseline FHR pattern and vital signs If three interpretable contractions with FHR present in 10 min, no oxytocin necessary If insufficient contractions, dilute oxytocic infusion begun Dosage increased to produce three contractions/10 min at not less than 90 sec intervals lasting less than 1 min; usual dosage 5 mμ/min	Test done after 28 weeks' gestation Negative test: no late decelerations with adequate contractions Take blood pressure every 10 min to detect "supine hypotension" Tests may also be *equivocal* (inconsistent results) or unsatisfactory (failure to obtain adequate contraction or monitoring records) Contractions present in 80% of patients by 38 weeks Infusion pump required Average time for test approximately 90 min Avoid overstimulation of uterus Frequency of false positive tests high False negative tests infrequent

TABLE 24-4   MISCELLANEOUS SPECIALIZED TESTS—cont'd

Test	Purpose and rationale	Preparation of patient and specimen	Special considerations
Sweat test	To help detect presence of cystic fibrosis Abnormal amount of sodium chloride present in perspiration of affected persons Positive sweat chloride 60 mEq/L or higher Positive sweat sodium usually 10 mEq/L higher than sweat chloride	Pilocarpine iontophoresis: an electric current via attached electrodes drives pilocarpine into skin of forearm, stimulating local sweat production in about 5 min; a specimen of perspiration is then absorbed into gauze or filter paper; usual time for sweat collection is 30 min; sample is weighed and analyzed	

TABLE 24-5   X-RAY TESTS

Test	Purpose and rationale	Preparation of patient and specimen	Special considerations
*Barium enema	To aid in diagnosis of lower bowel pathology by outlining colon with radiopaque material May be part of treatment for intussusception	Cathartics or cleansing enemas may be ordered on previous day or morning of test Clear liquid diet may be given 1 day before test until test completion Barium enema given in x-ray department when patient is under fluoroscope; examination takes 1 to 2 hr Enema or cathartic may be ordered after radiographs completed	Carefully note and record patient's bowel movements after procedure
*Brain scanning Computerized transaxial tomography (CTT or CAT)	To provide a visual display of abnormal tissue within skull; useful in diagnosing brain tumors	Injection of radioactive isotope (radionuclide pertechnetate [^{99m}Tc] Before scanning, minimum wait of 15 to 60 min after IV injection	If anesthesia used, patient should be NPO
*Cystogram	To aid in diagnosis of urinary obstruction or other abnormality by visualiza-	Urethral catheter inserted prior to procedure Bladder emptied	

*If the nurse is holding or positioning the child during the x-ray procedure, she should wear a lead apron.   *Continued.*

TABLE 24-5   X-RAY TESTS—cont'd

Test	Purpose and rationale	Preparation of patient and specimen	Special considerations
*Cystogram—cont'd	tion of bladder, ureter, and urethra with radiopaque material during filling and emptying of bladder	Radiopaque material injected into bladder and radiograph taken Catheter removed	
*Voiding cystourethrogram		Radiographs taken during voiding process	
Ciné cystourethrogram	To determine whether reflux appears or increases at voiding pressure	Continuous fluoroscopic pictures taken during voiding process	
*Gastrointestinal series (G.I. series)	To aid in diagnosis of stomach and small bowel pathology by outlining areas with radiopaque material	Night before test, patient may have light supper No food, fluids, or medications after midnight until 6 hr radiographs completed X-ray department gives barium under fluoroscope Patient remains NPO until x-ray department gives release after 6 hr studies If 24 hr studies ordered, no enema or cathartic given until studies completed Check for enema or cathartic orders when test completed	
*Intravenous pyelogram (IVP)	To detect kidney or urinary disease by intravenous dye injection followed by abdominal radiographs	Cathartic or enema ordered to clear bowel on day before test Patient may eat light dinner with little fluid Fluids, food, and medications withheld after midnight Radiographs of abdomen taken before and after intravenous injection of dye by physician Fluids usually forced after completion of test	Allergy to iodine is contraindication to routine technique

*If the nurse is holding or positioning the child during the x-ray procedure, she should wear a lead apron.

TABLE 24-5   X-RAY TESTS—cont'd

Test	Purpose and rationale	Preparation of patient and specimen	Special considerations
*Pneumoencephalo-gram	To detect abnormalities of brain by injection of air or oxygen into spinal canal Lumbar puncture done, and some spinal fluid withdrawn and replaced by air, which rises to ventricles of brain, forming characteristic outlines	Patient NPO 6 hr before test; given preoperative sedative and analgesic; may be done under local or general anesthetic in x-ray department After procedure, patient kept flat and observed carefully; headache, nausea, and vomiting fairly common; signs of increasing intracranial pressure should be reported; treated as postoperative patient	
*Ventriculogram			Similar to pneumoencephalogram, except air introduced directly into ventricles through burr holes in skull Performed in operating room

CHAPTER 25   The child surgical patient

Anatomic relationships, physiologic activity, and psychologic responses are greatly influenced by the phenomena of normal growth and development.

This chapter discusses some of the differences that set the child apart from the adult and reviews routines and procedures encountered when nursing the pediatric surgical patient.

CHILD-ADULT DISTINCTIONS

The following list of child-adult distinctions is not complete, but it may prove helpful in the evaluation of the needs of children.

1. The metabolic rate of infants and young children is much greater proportionately than that of adults. Children are growing and need to be fed more frequently.

2. Abnormal fluid loss is more serious in the infant and young child than in the adult. Fluid intake and output must be calculated extremely carefully, including fluid loss from diaphoresis or wound drainage. A 7-pound (3.2 kg) infant who sustains a blood loss of 1 ounce (30 ml) has been compared with a 150-pound (68 kg) man who has lost 600 ml (20 oz) of blood.

3. The child lacks the physical reserves that are available to the adult. The child's general condition may change rapidly, almost without warning.

4. The body tissues of the child heal quickly because of the rapid rate of metabolism and growth.

5. The child usually needs proportionately less analgesic than an adult patient to obtain relative comfort after surgical procedures.

6. The young child lives more in the present than an adult does. This may be both to the child's advantage and disadvantage. "Now" is understood and very important, but "later" is difficult to grasp. On the other hand, children seldom become upset by anticipating unpleasant future problems or prospects or worrying about finances or loss of a job!

PREPARATION FOR SURGERY

When relatively simple surgery is contemplated, the growing trend is toward 1-day hospitalization or the performance of operative procedures at outpatient surgi-centers. However, many youngsters are still formally admitted to a hospital, even for minor surgery.

Preparing a child for surgery must be based on the following factors: age and developmental level; the child's perception of hospitalization and the upcoming surgery; the surgical procedure to be performed; and postoperative care, previous hospitalization experience, expected length of hospitalization, and parental attitudes.

Psychologic preparation

The method of preparation must be geared to the actual developmental level of the child or the regressed level, not merely to chronologic age.

492

Many nurses use puppets, dolls, drawings, and films in conjunction with group and individual discussions as methods of preoperative preparation. Research has demonstrated that children who receive systematic psychologic preparation and continued supportive care demonstrate less disturbed behavior and more cooperation in the postoperative period. Parents are also less anxious and more satisfied with the information and care received.

The nurse should remember that in all contacts with patients, regardless of age, explanations and emotional support should be adapted to the individual's ability to understand and to personal needs. She should also remember that as parents are reassured, the confidence they gain in turn helps support the child. The presence of parents at the bedside immediately before and after surgical and diagnostic procedures is usually very beneficial. Some hospitals admit parents to the recovery room area as well.

Physical preparation

Patients being admitted for surgery should be especially evaluated for the presence of respiratory infection and signs of malnutrition. Occasionally surgery may be delayed until the child's general condition improves.

Except in emergency situations physical preparation for surgery usually begins the night before the procedure. Although some children may be admitted to the hospital early in the morning of the day of minor surgery, most come into the hospital the previous afternoon.

If orthopedic surgery is planned, the child is usually given a povidone-iodine (Betadine) bath as ordered in the evening. The body part to be involved in the surgery is carefully washed and inspected. The fingernails or toenails of any extremity involved are cleansed and trimmed. Frequently any ordered shave of the operative area is delayed until the morning of surgery. If a shave prep is requested, it will often be done in the OR suite just before the procedure to reduce the possibility of infection. For some types of surgery, preparatory enemas may be ordered.

Food, fluids, and oral medications are withheld as ordered, depending on the type of surgery planned, the age of the child, and the time of the procedure. The fact that the child must not receive anything by mouth should be conspicuously posted. Children should be told of this so that they do not think that they have been forgotten when the breakfast trays are passed. Any loose or missing teeth should be noted and recorded on the chart. (It may be easier with babies to record the number of teeth present.)

Sedative and analgesic drugs are given, usually in two stages. Preliminary sedation is usually ordered approximately 2 hours before surgery. Analgesic and atropine compounds, which prepare the patient for general anesthesia, are routinely given "on call." Every effort should be made to see that the child is allowed to rest after receiving the preoperative medications. The room should be dimmed and quiet and the side rails in place.

Children may be taken to surgery in their cribs or on carts, or they may walk or be carried, depending on individual circumstances. Unless they are scheduled to go to an intensive care unit, their units are prepared for their return. The bed, if present, is made up according to the child's postoperative needs, and any special equipment desired is placed conveniently. An orthopedic patient may need bed boards under the mattress, an overbed frame and trapeze, and extra firm pillows. Additional equipment that may be required, depending on the individual, includes a suction machine, intravenous standard, oxygen mist tent, and properly sized restraints.

POSTOPERATIVE CARE

Immediate observation

When patients return to the nursing unit from the recovery room, their general condition must be noted. Periodically pulse, respirations, and blood pressure are determined and recorded. Until patients are responsive and alert, they should be kept on the abdomen or side unless the surgery performed contraindicates these positions. The nurse should note the condition and placement of any dressing and describe any apparent drainage. The presence of a plaster cast or mold should be noted. Arms or legs in casts should be elevated, and frequent checks for circulatory disturbances should be made. Intravenous infusions should be checked for possible infiltration and correct rate of flow. Children should be protected from harming themselves (pulling out needles or tubes or tampering with suture lines) by the use of appropriate restraints, as necessary. If a child is immobilized with restraints for an extended period of time, it is imperative that appropriate range of motion be included in the plan of care and that explanation be given to the child and family. Urinary catheters should be connected to dependent drainage and stabilized properly. The type and amount of urinary drainage should be observed. The patient's skin color and temperature are checked. The nurse must always watch for and quickly report signs of shock: low blood pressure; cold, moist, pale, or cyanotic skin; rapid pulse; dilated pupils; and restlessness.

Diet

Whether oral fluids will be allowed after the child is responsive will depend on the physician's orders and the child's general condition. Sometimes surgical patients are not allowed oral fluids for a considerable period; instead, they are fed intravenously. When oral feedings are introduced, they are begun gradually, and the patient's tolerance is observed. The routine postsurgical diet follows this sequence with modifications for different ages—clear liquid, full liquid, soft, and regular. Rich, spicy, highly seasoned, or gas-forming foods should be avoided. Because of the confusion that may result, oral surgery patients are not served red gelatin products!

Ambulation

Early progressive ambulation for the general surgery patient is the rule in the modern care of patients. In only a few situations will the physician delay ambulation beyond the first postoperative day. The general surgery patient usually has orders to stand at the bedside and take a few steps the day after surgery. The nurse should be sure to follow these orders because judicious ambulation strengthens the patient, aids in the restoration of gastrointestinal function, and helps prevent complications such as pneumonia and the formation of blood clots and pressure areas.

When the patient's condition or young age makes it impossible or inadvisable for the child to get out of bed, the nurse must be sure that the child is turned frequently, receives good skin care, and breathes deeply at intervals. The physician may order the use of incentive spirometers or intermittent positive pressure treatments to aid lung expansion.

After surgery, toddlers and preschoolers usually move about spontaneously in their cribs or beds; ambulation presents few problems for them. However, older children may express the same timidity and fear of pain that most adult patients exhibit when asked to move or get up and may need a great deal of initial support and encouragement from their parents and the nursing staff.

Usually it is not long before these same youngsters are enjoying the freedom of the playroom. Most will recover quickly, gather together their little hoard of treasures, and say their "goodbyes" in a few days. At times some possessions are overlooked; one nursing staff fondly remembers Bobby, who left his turtle in the linen closet!

COMMON PROCEDURES

A few of the common procedures encountered when nursing pediatric surgical patients are described in the following pages. Some of these treatments may also involve medical patients. They will include skin preparation for surgery, cleansing enema, dressing change, gavage feeding, gastrostomy feeding, and irrigation of nasogastric or intestinal tubes.

Skin preparation for surgery

Purposes: To cleanse the area of prospective surgery to help prevent infection, provide a clearly visible operative field, and carefully inspect the skin for possible pustules, lesions, or signs of poor circulation. More skin preps are being done in the operating room just before surgery. Many surgeons are omitting a shave of the operative site.

Materials:
1. Sharp, sterile razor (if shave-prep is ordered)
2. Clean bowl for warm water
3. Prescribed soap or antibacterial solution
4. Waterproof pad or sheeting
5. Towels (2)
6. Washcloth or gauze sponge
7. Clean cotton applicators, if the areas to be "prepared" involve the umbilicus or toes
8. Nail clippers, if extremities are involved
9. Bath blanket or drawsheet
10. Gooseneck lamp or other good light

Procedure:
1. Check the order, the operative permit, and the time preoperative medications will be given.
2. Identify the patient.
3. Explain the procedure to patients according to their level of understanding. Small children usually respond to the explanation, "We're going to wash your tummy to make it very clean." When you are ready, begin by doing just that. Explain as you work. As the child gains confidence, you may show the youngster the tiny hairs on the arm and talk about how adults shave. Run your finger along the child's skin to show how the razor feels. Suggest that it may tickle a little but that being very still will help.
4. Position the lamp and raise the bed to a convenient working level.
5. Wash your hands.
6. Place the waterproof pad and towel under the patient to protect the bed.
7. Prepare and place the warm water and ordered antibacterial agent conveniently. (Some physicians may order a dry shave.)
8. Apply tension to the skin with a washcloth or gauze sponge if you shave. (If the feet or fingernails are very dirty, they may be soaking in a basin of warm

water while the adjacent areas are being shaved.)
9. Crouch down frequently to look *across* the surface of the skin to check for remaining hairs.
10. Retain your "prep setup" until the skin preparation has been checked by the team leader, head nurse, or instructor.
11. Record the procedure. Any skin lesions (for example, pustules) must be reported. Pustules are *not* to be opened. Razor nicks should be treated with direct pressure with a sterile sponge and should be reported. Great care must be used in shaving, especially in areas of old scars, insect bites, or bony prominences, where nicking may easily occur.
12. In some cases a povidone-iodine (Betadine) scrub of 10 minutes may be ordered after the shave is complete. The physician may order the prepared area wrapped in sterile towels until surgery.

Cleansing enema (Fig. 25-1)

Purposes: To cleanse the lower bowel before surgery or diagnostic procedures, relieve constipation or flatulence, and aid in the expulsion of parasites.

Materials:
1. Rectal catheter or tubing and clamps, appropriately sized
   a. For infants, size 12 to 16 French
   b. For young child, size 12 to 20 French
   c. For older child, size 16 to 22 French
2. Container of ordered solution
   a. At 105° F (40.5° C) when given
   b. Suggested total amounts
      (1) Infant—60 to 100 ml
      (2) Toddler to 5 years—250 ml
      (3) School age—250-750 ml
   c. Any infant or young child should not be expected to retain a cleansing enema until the total amount of fluid is given. Small amounts should be instilled and then allowed to return around the catheter. The amount expelled should be measured if possible.
3. Lubricant and wipes
4. Asepto syringe barrel or enema can or bag, depending on the amount of fluid to be given and the size of the child

Note: Disposable enema setups may be easily used for some patients depending on amount of solution needed.

Procedure:
1. Check the order.

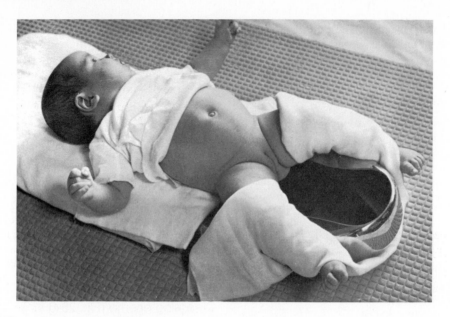

FIG. 25-1   One way of positioning an infant for an enema. The restraining diaper is centered under the tip of the pan and then brought up and over the infant's legs and pinned to itself.

2. Identify the patient.
3. Explain to the child what will be done as you do it according to the level of understanding. In the case of the very young child, understanding will not be complete, of course, but the tone of voice and the socialization such explanation offers can be helpful. Telling a small child that you are "going to put a little water in where we take your temperature to help you go to the bathroom," sometimes helps.
4. Screen the unit and position the child. A number of positions are advocated when giving an infant or toddler an enema.
   a. For most children the side position with the upper leg flexed seems to be the most comfortable. The left side is preferred because this placement puts the descending colon lowest. However, a left-sided position is not absolutely mandatory. In fact, some investigators question the supposed advantages of left-sided placement. Infants and small toddlers often do well if placed on a firm pillow, which has been draped with a lightweight plastic sheet and covered with an absorbent towel, with their hips pulled to the edge. The plastic extends over the side of the pillow into or beside a curved basin or small bedpan, which is placed snugly against the buttocks just below the rectum. For warmth, the child is covered by a bath blanket or towel.
   b. If the infant is very active and a nurse has no one to help maintain the child in a side position, the infant may be gently restrained in supine position over a small bedpan. The back and head are supported by a small pillow or folded bath blanket. The buttocks are placed over the bedpan and the legs gently drawn to either side and secured by a diaper placed under the bedpan and drawn up and over the lower extremities and pinned to itself as illustrated in Fig. 25-1.
   c. Older children with sphincter control are usually positioned on their sides and given enemas in basically the same way as any adult.
5. Place the ordered amount and type of solution in a can or Asepto barrel attached to a clamped rectal tube. Expel the air from the tube and lubricate the tip. Do not occlude the eyes of the catheter.
6. Gently insert the tubing approximately ½ to 3 inches (3.7 to 7.6 cm) depending on the size of the patient into the rectum and observe the flow. Hold the con-

tainer of solution no higher than 12 to 18 inches (30 to 46 cm) above the patient's hips.

7. Observe the patient closely during the procedure for an increase in respiratory and pulse rates and exhaustion.
8. As needed, put the child on a bedpan or potty chair, or allow the child to go to the bathroom.
9. Remove equipment and tidy up the area.
10. Record the procedure and the results obtained.

Sterile dressing change

Purposes: To protect the incision or wound from contamination be replacing wet dressings, allow direct observation of the incision or wound to evaluate the healing process or measure wound drainage, increase the cleanliness and comfort of the patient, and, in some instances, apply local medications or carry out irrigations that assist in treatment.

Materials: Materials vary according to the area to be dressed, whether sutures are to be removed or local debridement attempted, and the wishes of the physician. The following supplies may be needed, although not all the supplies listed are needed every time. Simple dressings may require only sterile compresses, handling forceps, adhesive tape, and a discard bag.

1. Dressing tray containing the following:
   a. Basic instrument kit with sterile
      (1) Suture-remover scissors
      (2) Clip removers
      (3) Sharp-pointed suture scissors
      (4) Tissue forceps
      (5) Smooth forceps
      (6) Small hemostat
      (7) Probe
   b. Wrapped, sterile cotton applicators
   c. Wrapped, sterile dressings of various thicknesses and sizes
      (1) Thick, absorbent pads (ABD or composite pads)
      (2) 4×4-inch and 2×2-inch gauze squares (flats)
      (3) Nonadherent dressings (Telfa)
      (4) Soft gauze dressings that have been fluffed out (fluffs)
   d. Various sizes of gauze roller bandage, Kerlix or Ace tensor bandage
   e. Various sizes and kinds of adhesive tape or Montgomery straps

2. Sterile gloves (used when the area to be dressed is large or difficult to manage)
3. Large paper or plastic bag to receive old dressings
4. Clean kidney basin for antiseptic pour-off overflow
5. Bandage scissors
6. Appropriate antiseptic, irrigating solution, or medication; sterile syringe and basin
7. Clean paper towels

Procedure:

1. Check the order.
2. Select a time when there is little bedmaking or mopping activity in the area. These activities increase the bacteria count in the air.
3. Identify and screen the patient and explain the purpose of the dressing change according to the level of understanding. At times positioning assistance may be needed.
4. Drape the patient appropriately.
5. Adjust the lamp, if needed; position and open discard bag and kidney basin, if needed.
6. Wash your hands.
7. Open only those supplies needed.
8. Place sterile handling forceps on the edge of a sterile wrapper—points on the sterile surface, handles over the edge.
9. Remove bandages or adhesive tape (Always pull tape toward the incision or wound to prevent undue strain or pain.)
10. Lift off the top dressing, your hand protected by a clean, folded paper towel or clean plastic gloves. Contact only the side of the dressing that was exposed to the exterior. Drop dressing and towel or glove into open paper bag.
11. Lift off any remaining inner dressing with the sterile handling forceps or use sterile gloves. Be careful not to pull drains, if present. Dressings that stick to the skin may usually be moistened with a small amount of sterile saline solution to facilitate their removal. Always note the presence of a drain when recording the dressing change.
12. Cleanse the area gently of any old drainage present with mild antiseptic or solution as ordered, using sterile gauze sponges mounted on handling forceps or gloved hands. Pour the solution onto the sponge over the discard kidney basin or use a sterile basin. Dry the area with a sterile compress.
13. Place the new sterile dressing, appropriate for size of the incision and amount of drainage present, using handling forceps or sterile gloves. Remove gloves, if used, before handling tape.

14. Secure with adhesive tape, Elastoplast, or Montgomery tapes. If using adhesive tape, turn back the ends slightly "sticky side against sticky side" to make the tape easier to remove.
15. Discard used dressings, wash your hands, and tidy up the area.
16. Record the procedure and the condition of the wound or incision. Describe the type and amount of any drainage present and report any unusual odor. Note any skin irritation caused by adhesive. Note any drains present.
17. *Note:* If your patient is having the sterile dressings weighed to calculate the amount of wound drainage you may:
    a. Weigh the total amount of dressings to be used in their sterile wrappers using a gram scale and mark their weight on the outside.
    b. Apply the dressings and save the wrappers carefully after marking the time and date of the dressing change next to the weight previously indicated.
    c. At the time of the next dressing change, discard the old dressings on the saved wrappers and weigh them again. The difference in weight expressed in grams will equal (for this purpose) the milliliters of drainage present.

Gavage feeding using an indwelling nasogastric tube or oral feeding tube

Purposes: To avoid mouth and lip motion when it may endanger surgical repair, nourish a child who is too weak to be fed orally in the normal fashion, and supplement oral feeding when nutritional buildup is imperative and sufficient intake by normal means is impossible.

(*Note:* When needed, feeding tubes for premature infants are now usually inserted orally before each feeding. Such an approach keeps the nose unobstructed and untraumatized, helps maintain a sucking reflex, and reduces incidence of bradycardia during insertion.)

Materials:
1. Sterile Asepto or piston-type syringe (If the child is receiving sterilized formula, a sterile syringe will be secured for each feeding. If the child is not receiving sterilized formula, the nurse may wash and store the syringe in a clean manner for use next time.)
2. Container of formula (infants who receive sterilized formula will have the tube feeding sterilized)
3. Glass of water (bottle of sterile water for infants)
4. Towel or napkin
5. Perhaps bib and infant seat

6. Appropriate tube and tape as needed
7. Stethoscope
Procedure:
1. Check the order.
2. Identify the patient and explain the procedure according to his needs and level of understanding.
3. Briefly warm the formula, if necessary, so that it will be tepid at the time of the feeding. (Feeding cold formula, if not given by Barron pump or slow drip, can be upsetting to the patient and may initiate vomiting.) Evaluate the consistency of the feeding: Is it too thick? Will it clog the tube? Many times you cannot dilute a feeding and administer the entire amount to maintain the caloric count ordered without overloading the stomach.
4. Unless contraindicated, raise the backrest of the bed of a child or place a baby on the side, head elevated. This position lets gravity aid the flow of the formula. Restrain as necessary.
5. Protect the area next to the tube opening with a towel.
6. If insertion of an oral tube is indicated:
    a. Measure the tube for insertion from the tip of the nose, to the lobe of the ear, to ½ inch below the xiphoid process; mark with tape.
    b. Gently pull down on the chin and advance the tube over the tongue to the tape marker.
    c. Observe the infant continually for color change, gagging, coughing, or respiratory distress. Withdraw the tube if they occur.
    d. Secure the tube to the face with tape or hold it in place with one hand.
7. Test the position of the end of the tube by each of the following methods:
    a. Observe the length of the tube exposed.
    b. Inject approximately 1 to 5 ml of air (depending on patient) into the tube. Listen with a stethoscope just below the sternum for sound of air passage. Withdraw the air and suction further for evidence of stomach contents, or, if ordered, measure entire aspirate to help determine digestion of previous feedings and current stomach capacity. Measured aspirate is usually returned to the stomach and the amount of the ordered feeding reduced by the amount of the aspirate.
    c. Ask the patient to hum, if possible. If the tube is in the trachea, the patient cannot hum.
8. Continue with the administration of the formula. In most instances allow the formula to flow by gravity. Exerting additional pressure may be dangerous. If

the flow is sluggish, raise the barrel. If it is too fast, lower the barrel or pinch the tube. If the flow has stopped, change position of the patient slightly. If the flow still does not continue, *gentle* pressure with a syringe bulb or piston may *start* the flow. If no response is forthcoming, the tube must be removed and another inserted. If the infant is crying, flow will be slower than when the child is quiet.

9. Add more formula before the barrel is empty to avoid introducing additional air into the stomach. If the tube is to be left in place, when the formula is finished (just before the last few drops leave the barrel), add 5 to 15 ml of water to rinse the tube. (Failure to include this step will cause a clogged tube.) If the tube is to be removed, pinch it tightly before and during its quick removal to prevent drops of formula from entering the airway.
10. Any infant must be bubbled after gavage just as he would be bubbled after routine oral feeding.
11. Record any aspirate obtained, the amount and type of feeding, and the tolerance of the patient.

Gastrostomy feeding

Purpose: To provide nourishment by way of a tube that has been surgically inserted through the abdominal wall into the stomach because of obstruction or surgical repair of the child's oroesophageal tract or to avoid the constant irritation of a nasogastric tube when oral feedings are not possible.

Materials:
1. Tray containing the following:
   a. Syringe barrel (sterile for small infants receiving sterilized formula)
   b. Container of formula (sterile for small infants)
   c. Container of water (sterile for small infants)
2. Towel or napkin

Procedure:
1. Check the order.
2. Identify patient and explain the procedure according to his needs and level of understanding.
3. Evaluate the formula as for a gavage feeding. Position the child either flat with the head raised or elevated in a semisitting position.
4. Attach the syringe barrel to the tube and fill with formula before unclamping the tube. (*Note:* There may be orders to aspirate the contents of the stomach into the barrel. The amount aspirated is noted, and it is allowed to return to the stomach. The feeding to be given is decreased accordingly to prevent overloading.)

5. Unclamp the tube and allow the fluid to flow slowly by gravity. Never use pressure of any kind to start the flow of formula into the gastrostomy tube. This may cause unwanted backflow into the esophagus.
6. Continue to add formula to the barrel before it completely empties to avoid introducing air into the stomach.
7. Finish the feeding by adding 15 to 30 ml of water to rinse the tube. Clamp off the tube before all the water leaves the barrel to avoid introducing air into the stomach. (*Note:* In some cases involving infants, the physician may order that the tube not be clamped but be left opened with the barrel attached and elevated above the baby's body. The formula is allowed to return to the barrel as the child cries or changes position.)
8. Record the amount and type of feeding and the tolerance of the patient.

Irrigation of a nasogastric or intestinal tube attached to suction

Purposes: To prevent the clogging and assure the patency of an indwelling nasogastric or intestinal tube. The tube may have been inserted for the following reasons:
1. To prevent vomiting
2. To relieve postoperative abdominal distention, discomfort, and pressure on surgical repairs

When the tube has been inserted for the reasons cited, it is attached to some type of suction or drainage device. Usually the suction ordered is intermittent; occasionally it may be continuous. High or low negative pressure may be prescribed. Sometimes only gravity drainage is ordered. Most children are placed on low intermittent suction. Irrigation is only carried out when the wishes of the physician concerning the individual case are known. Double lumen or sump-type nasogastric tubes are frequently used. A small tube, or sump, which serves as an "airway," is incorporated into the larger suction tube. As the suction pulls out gastric contents it also pulls in air via the airway; this helps prevent the end of the suction tube from "grabbing" the stomach mucosa and causing tissue damage.

Materials: Unless the type of surgery would make it necessary to employ sterile technique, the materials used to irrigate a tube must be kept meticulously clean but need not be sterile. The type and amount of irrigating fluid to be used is ordered by the physician. Physiologic saline solution is frequently requested. The amount to be used will depend on the size of the child and the type of surgery performed.

A setup would usually include the following:

1. Syringe (10 to 30 ml, depending on amount to be used)
2. Basin or solution reservoir
3. Clamp
4. Towel and emesis basin
5. Ordered solution

   Procedure:

1. Identify the patient.
2. Explain to the child according to the level of understanding. For young children it is usually sufficient to say that you are putting a little "water" in the tube.
3. Draw up the amount and kind of solution ordered in the syringe.
4. Place a folded towel and emesis basin under the junction of the tube leading to the suction apparatus or gravity drainage.
5. Turn off any mechanical suction device.
6. Clamp the tubing that leads to the suction or drainage bag and disconnect the two parts of the tubing; wrap the end of the tubing that leads to the suction machine in a towel, cover it with cap, hang it from a support on the machine or hold it between your last two fingers.
7. Fit the syringe of irrigating fluid into the patient's tube and gently instill the ordered amount. Whether the nurse will be allowed to withdraw any of the irrigating solution with the attached syringe will depend on the preferences of the physician. If a sump-type tube is being irrigated the saline may be installed in either the end of the sump or "airway" or the end of the suction tube. Regardless of the route used for irrigation after the instillation, approximately 10 cc of air should be injected into the sump to clear the tube. The sump tube outlet should never be clamped while the suction is in operation.
8. Detach the syringe, and reconnect the tube either to the suction machine (removing the clamp and restarting the suction) or to the gravity drainage. (Recheck any suction setting.)
9. Remember, this patient is usually not allowed oral fluids except perhaps *small* amounts of ice chips. However, lubrication of the nares, renewal of the tape maintaining the tube's position, and oral hygiene are fairly frequent patient needs.
10. Record in the patient's output record the amount of irrigating fluid used. (*Note:* If a tube is not draining and resistance is encountered during an attempted ordered irrigation, the nurse should notify her supervisor immediately.)

• • •

One of the most satisfying aspects of the role of the pediatric nurse is watching children master their fears and anxieties about impending surgical procedures. A nurse truly fulfills the role of the helping person when she is able to assist children and their families to cope with a potentially traumatic situation.

The process of respiration brings oxygen into the body for circulation to the individual cells by way of the bloodstream and removes waste products, carbon dioxide, and water from the body. In some diseases the transfer of oxygen to the tissue cells is made very difficult by a breakdown in the anatomy or physiology concerned. To aid the handicapped processes, various procedures, apparatuses, and medications have been developed to help clear the airway, enrich the oxygen content of inspired air, stimulate or maintain adequate respiratory effort, or achieve the proper circulation of blood.

Respiratory therapy is a technical specialty devoted to the maintenance of optimal breathing and prevention of respiratory disease. In many hospitals the responsibilities of respiratory therapists will include supervision of gaseous therapy (such as intermittent positive pressure or special tents), performance of chest vibration, clapping, postural drainage (respiratory hygiene), and resuscitation measures. These skilled therapists and nurses working together can do much to maintain and improve the respiratory function of their patients.   .

alveoli, which make up the functional tissue of the lungs, must remain open to assure proper oxygenation. Any obstruction, whether caused by the position of the tongue, aspiration of a foreign body, edema, a tumor, the presence of tenacious secretions in the laryngotracheobronchial "tree," or spasm of the bronchioles, will lead to respiratory difficulty. Any condition such as pneumonia, emphysema, tuberculosis, or a malignancy that causes a depletion in the ability of the lung tissue to receive air and transfer oxygen and carbon dioxide may cause respiratory distress. Any interruption in the mechanisms of breathing will also affect respiration and therefore oxygenation. Of course, in the final analysis the circulatory system must also be adequate to deliver the oxygen to the final destination—the individual microscopic body cells.

The most accurate way to determine the extent of oxygenation of a patient's blood is by chemical analysis of the oxygen and carbon dioxide level in an arterial blood sample. Transcutaneous monitoring of arterial PO_2 levels is now being introduced.

HINDRANCES TO OXYGENATION OF THE BLOOD

To understand the rationale of many of the treatments ordered, the student should review the structure and function of the respiratory system (Figs. 26-1 and 26-2). The passageways from the exterior of the body to the microscopic air sacs, or

SECURING AND MAINTAINING AN AIRWAY

Position

The first concern in aiding breathing always involves the airway. Occasionally it may be obstructed because of the position of the tongue. This may be true especially in the unconscious

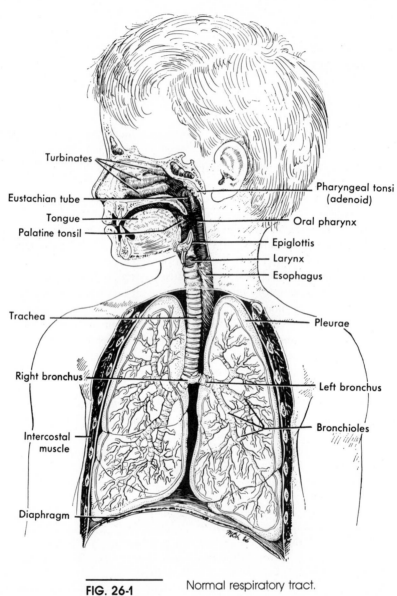

Turbinates

Eustachian tube

Tongue

Palatine tonsil

Pharyngeal tonsi
(adenoid)

Oral pharynx

Epiglottis

Larynx

Esophagus

Trachea

Pleurae

Right bronchus

Left bronchus

Bronchioles

Intercostal
muscle

Diaphragm

FIG. 26-1   Normal respiratory tract.

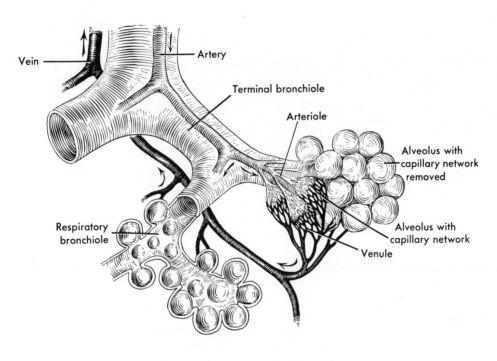

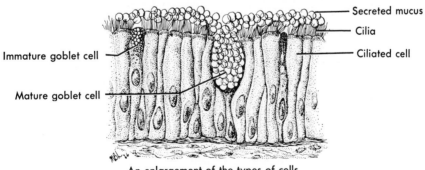

An enlargement of the types of cells
lining the respiratory tract

FIG. 26-2   Microscopic anatomy of the lower respiratory tract.

patient; the tongue is not actually swallowed, but it may fall backward and obstruct the pharynx. An open airway may be obtained by placing the patient on his back with his head in "sniffing" position and his lower jaw held up. This returns the tongue to normal position. At times the insertion of a plastic oropharyngeal airway will be needed.

If the airway is obstructed by a foreign body or secretions, the emergency relief usually attempted *first* involves gravity drainage. However, in cases of choking and inability to breathe, several repeated, controlled, upward thrusts of the thumb side of a fist just below the rib cage that cause the diaphragm to suddenly force air out through the airway to dislodge a *foreign body* have proved life saving in older children and young people. Further evaluation and detailed instruction should be consulted.* Occasionally the bronchi may need to be visualized with a special instrument called a bronchoscope for removal of the foreign body.

To prevent aspiration, a child in danger of vomiting or regurgitating should be maintained on the side or abdomen. If this is impossible because of other more important considerations (such as type of surgery, or administration of an anesthetic), the head should be lowered and turned to the side during episodes of nausea and vomiting. Babies are sometimes placed upright in infant seats to help prevent vomiting.

Suction

Suction of the naso-oropharyngeal passages or even deeper suction may be necessary to clear the airway. Suction may be accomplished by using a bulb syringe, a simple manual suction catheter (DeLee trap), or a catheter setup attached to wall or portable suction. The following points about procedure should be remembered when a catheter is used:

---

*Heimlich, H.J.: A life-saving maneuver to prevent food-choking, J.A.M.A. **234**:398-401, 1975; Richards, N.C.G.: Treatment of choking, Nurs. Times **73**:856-857, 1977.

1. The suction apparatus should be personal for each patient and kept free from contamination. Some hospitals now employ a "use-once-only-and-throw-away" catheter technique.
2. The drainage bottle should contain about 1 inch of disinfectant solution at the outset to thin out the secretions, ease its cleaning, and reduce the number of bacteria in the bottle.
3. Catheters should be lubricated with water or water-soluble gel before use to assure greater ease of insertion.
4. During catheter insertion, the suction should be temporarily discontinued by pinching the catheter or uncovering the Y-tube control to avoid depleting the patient's supply of oxygen or injuring the mucous membranes.
5. The lowest amount of suction necessary should be applied. Suction should not be prolonged (no more than 10 to 15 seconds); suction administered too frequently may aggravate congestion instead of relieve it.
6. The catheter and tubing should be rinsed immediately after use to prevent clogging and stored conveniently in an aseptic manner, unless the catheters are not reused.
7. The child usually will need to be restrained during the procedure.

Humidification

Sometimes secretions are so thick that they are difficult to drain by gravity or suction, and various procedures and agents may be used to thin out the secretions. These may take the form of simple moist inhalations provided by a convenient cool mist humidifier at the bedside or under a canopy or tent. (Warm mist or steam tents have been almost entirely replaced because of the danger of burns.)

A form of aerosol therapy that has been found to be effective in liquefying thick respiratory secretions is that provided by the *ultrasonic nebulizer*

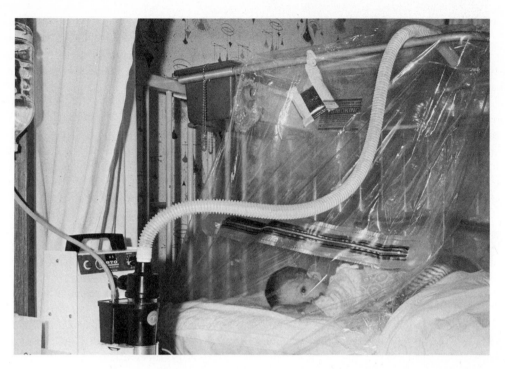

FIG. 26-3   Ultrasonic mist has gained favor because the small mist particles penetrate the respiratory passages better than former misting techniques. The equipment is compact and relatively easy to handle. Side rail down for picture only.

Courtesy Children's Hospital and Health Center, San Diego, Calif.

(Fig. 26-3). This unit, although generally used with a tent, is not dependent on a gas source for mist formation, produces fine penetrating water particles, is quiet, and occupies little space. It employs sterile distilled water. It has been used particularly for cystic fibrosis patients. However, the small infant in such a dense water-aerosol environment must be observed carefully for overhydration, since relatively large amounts of water can be absorbed from the lung into the circulation. Infants may be weighed frequently to assess the amount of such absorption, and fluid intake modifications may be necessary in certain cases. The patient's hair, sleepers, and bedding should be checked often to maintain dryness. Most patients may be removed from tents for feeding and bathing, depending on the physician's orders and the patient's tolerance.

Medications

Medications are frequently ordered to aid in clearing the airway.

Nose drops. Nose drops, such as phenylephrine hydrochloride (Neo-Synephrine), may be ordered to shrink mucous membranes and ease nasal congestion.

Expectorants. Oral expectorants, which increase the bronchial secretions and may help thin mucus, are occasionally ordered. Common medications of this type are potassium iodide and guaifenisin syrup.

Aerosols. Acetylcysteine (Mucomyst) reduces the thickness and tenacity of mucus. If a vial of acetylcysteine is opened and not completely used, it should be stored in the refrigerator and used within 48 hours. In tents a 20% volume solution is usually ordered. It is used primarily for patients with cystic fibrosis.

Isoetharine hydrochloride 1% (Bronkosol) is an effective, rapid bronchodilator that is being used more frequently.

If the airway is impaired because of spasm of the bronchi or bronchioles, as is often the case in asthmatic attacks, the addition of other medications to relax the bronchioles may be needed to relieve wheezing and respiratory distress. Chief among such medications used is the very powerful epinephrine (Adrenalin).

Some anatomic alterations of the respiratory system are difficult to treat and may be of long duration. However, some of the swelling and distortion of lung tissue and bronchioles may respond to the use of antibacterial drugs or medications used for specific chest diseases such as tuberculosis. Abnormal dilatation of the air sacs, or *emphysema*, may be particularly persistent and troublesome in the asthmatic child. Air is typically breathed in and depleted of its oxygen content. The air sacs have lost their normal elasticity, and cannot force the "old air" out of the lungs properly. Another full breath of well-oxygenated air cannot be taken, since the "old air" still occupies some space in the air sacs. Real distress may develop, especially on expiration. Medication such as epinephrine and a calm, reassuring manner on the part of the nurse help, but structural changes may be enduring.

Postural drainage and percussion techniques

Some respiratory diseases (for example, cystic fibrosis and emphysema) produce such exaggerated amounts of tenacious secretions deep in the lungs that it may be difficult for the patient to expel them even with the aid of medications, humidification, and suction techniques. These secretions interfere with proper pulmonary ventilation and set the stage for frequent respiratory tract infections that

further endanger the patient. Another way of promoting drainage of a clogged or potentially obstructed respiratory tree is through the use of breathing exercises and selective postural drainage consisting of positioning, cupping, and vibration, followed by purposeful coughing and possible suctioning.

When respiratory therapists are available, they usually perform these maneuvers and instruct the family if continued treatment is necessary at home. In the event that respiratory therapists are not available, nurses may be asked to learn the techniques. Anyone responsible for performing them should be specially instructed and initially supervised in their use. The following brief explanation is not intended to take the place of such instruction.

The treatment is most effective when preceded by aerosol therapy and is enhanced by diaphragmatic breathing. It may be prescribed as a prophylactic as well as a therapeutic measure.

Various postures assumed by the patient help drain different parts of the lungs. Therefore the position or positions in which the patient is placed depend on the site of the congestion and the general aims of the therapeutic program. In general the placement of the patient enlists the forces of gravity and the sweeping action of the respiratory cilia in clearing the lungs. Any constrictive clothing should be removed. The patient's knees and hips should be flexed in the various positions necessary so that relaxation will be promoted, and less strain will be exerted on the abdominal muscles when coughing is encouraged. When the patient's head must be lowered, usually all that is needed for an infant or young child is a well-positioned, firm pillow. (See Fig 26-4.) Premature infants should *not* be placed in head-down positions because of the increased dange of intracranial hemorrhage. An older child may have to assume a modified jackknife position, lying over an elevated knee-gatch. Teenagers may be able to hold their heads and chests down crosswise over the side of the bed while helping to support themselves by grasping a low stool. However, they should not be left alone

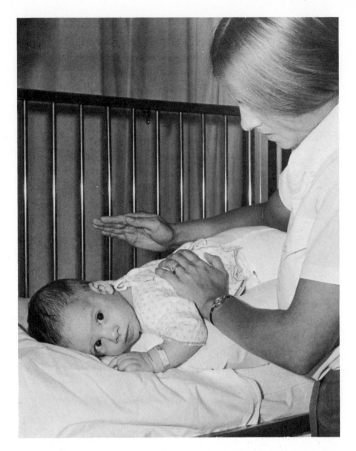

FIG. 26-4 The respiratory therapist is performing the early morning, before breakfast ritual on a small patient with congenital structural weakness of the bronchi. Scheduled cupping and vibrating have proved particularly helpful.

Courtesy Children's Hospital and Health Center, San Diego, Calif.

in this predicament! A baby or toddler may respond best when positioned on the nurse's or therapist's lap. These assisted postural drainage techniques should be done before meals or at least an hour after eating. It is never initiated if the patient is hemorrhaging or in pain. When treating children, the nurse or therapist usually begins percussion with the patient in the upright position and terminates with the head lower than the rest of the body.

Two basic maneuvers are used: (1) cupping, also known as clapping or tapping, and (2) vibrating.

The first is performed with the palm of the hand raised, the fingers and thumb forming the sides of a firm cup (Fig 26-5, *A*). When the cupped hands are gently but abruptly applied to the patient's chest wall, the wrist is alternately flexed and extended. A characteristic hollow sound is produced. The technique is continued for about 30 seconds over the affected area while the patient both inhales and exhales. It is then followed by the vibrating motion, done only while the patient is exhaling slowly. This second maneuver is accomplished by tensing the hands, arms, and shoulders and pro-

Text continued on p. 517.

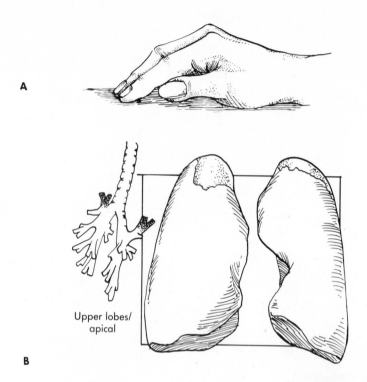

A

Upper lobes/
apical

B

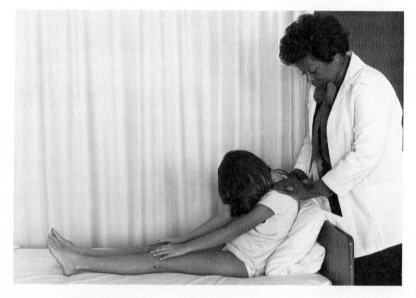

FIG. 26-5   For legend see opposite page.

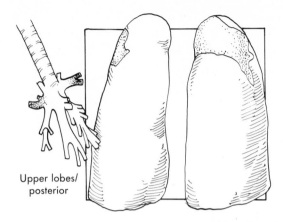

Upper lobes/
posterior

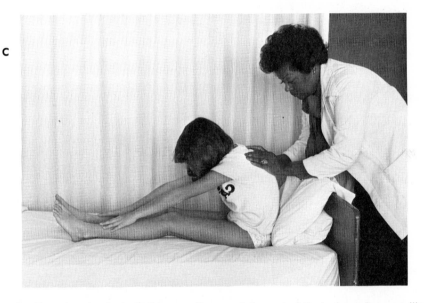

C

FIG. 26-5 cont'd Positions for chest physiotherapy. Figures **A** through **J** illustrate various positions for proper drainage of the upper, middle, and lower lobes of the lungs in children. The procedure may involve any one segment or the entire lung field and usually includes positioning (postural drainage), clapping, vibration, effective coughing, and expectoration or suctioning of secretions. **A,** Clapping is accomplished by striking the cupped hand intermittently against the chest wall, producing a more vigorous impact than if the hands were flat. The hand is cupped with fingers together, which creates an air pocket between the clinician's hand and the chest wall. Clapping should be performed on the chest wall over the segment to be drained. **B,** Upper lobes; apical segment. Cupped hands above scapula on either side of neck. **C,** Upper lobes; posterior segment. Cupped hands over back on both sides.   *Continued.*

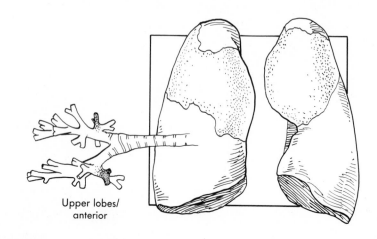

Upper lobes/
anterior

D

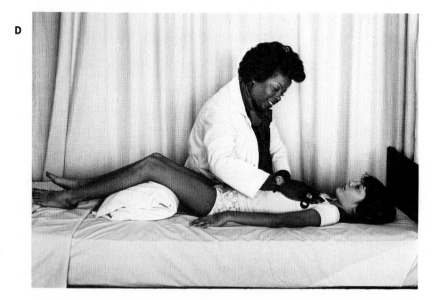

**FIG. 26-5
cont'd**

D, Upper lobes; anterior segment. Cupped hands between clavicle and nipple on each side.

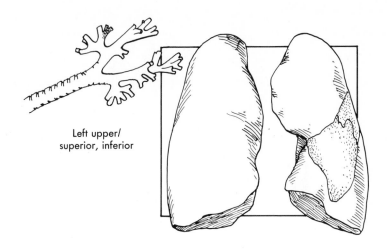

Left upper/
superior, inferior

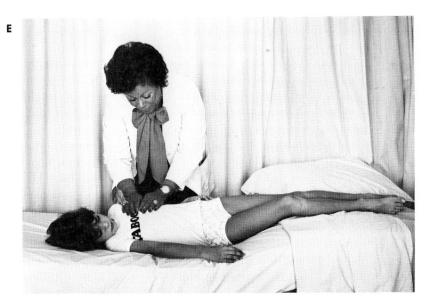

FIG. 26-5
cont'd

E, Left upper lobe; superior segment. Cupped hands over left nipple.

Continued.

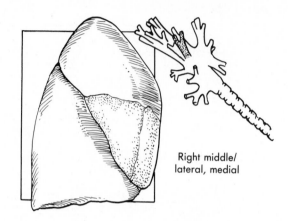

Right middle/
lateral, medial

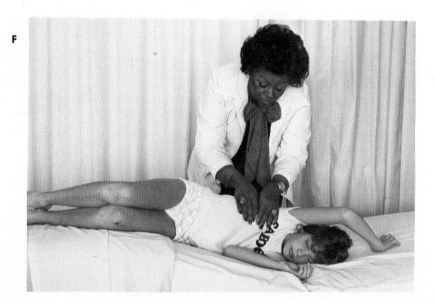

F

**FIG. 26-5
cont'd**

F, Right middle lobe; lateral segment. Cupped hands over right nipple.

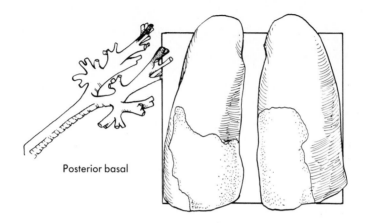

Posterior basal

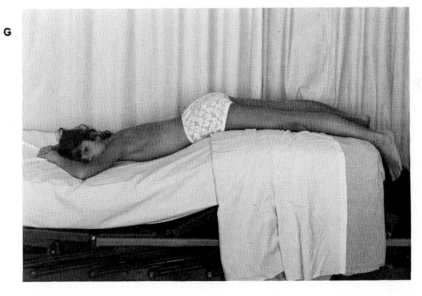

G

**FIG. 26-5
cont'd**
G, Lower lobes; posterior segment. Cupped hands should be placed over the lower ribs close to the spine (foot of bed elevated 18 inches).   *Continued.*

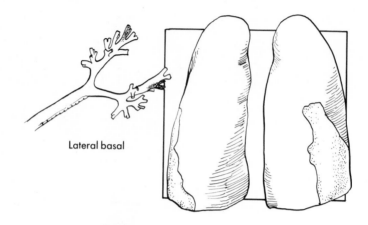

Lateral basal

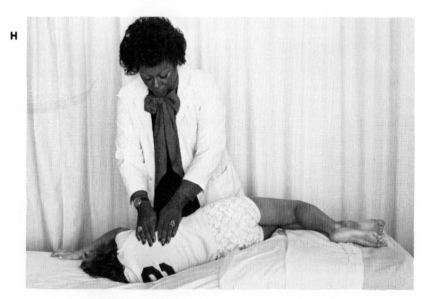

H

**FIG. 26-5
cont'd**

H, Lower lobes; lateral basal segment. Cupped hands over uppermost portion
of lower rib.

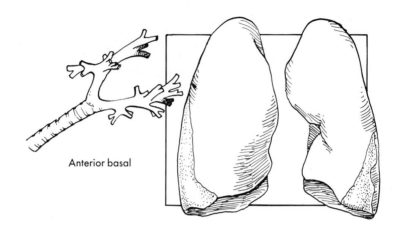

Anterior basal

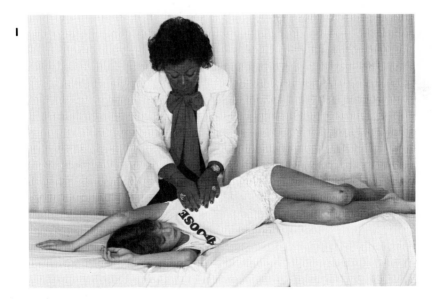

FIG. 26-5
cont'd

I, Left lower lobe; anterior segment. Cupped hands over lower ribs just beneath axilla.

Continued.

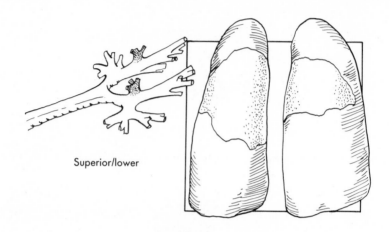

Superior/lower

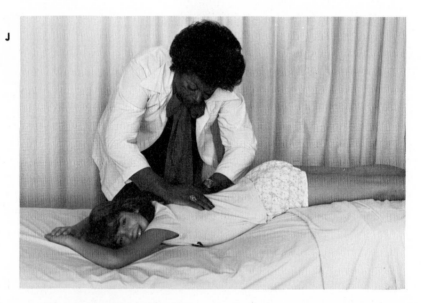

J

FIG. 26-5 cont'd   **J,** Lower lobes; superior segments. Cupped hands over the middle part of back at tip of scapula on both sides

ducing gentle and fine vibratory movements on the chest wall. The two maneuvers are then repeated several times, depending on the tolerance of the patient. Mechanical vibrators or soft percussion aids made from nipples or small face masks may also be employed on infants and small children.

Percussion techniques are performed on top of a light shirt or diaper. They should not be used over the spine, kidney area, abdomen, sternum, or developed breast tissue. Coughing should be encouraged as needed.

Laryngoscope

If a patent airway cannot be maintained through positioning, simple suction, insertion of an oropharyngeal airway, humidification, percussion, or administration of appropriate mucus-thinning or bronchodilatory medications, the larynx may be visualized with a laryngoscope and an endotracheal tube inserted for suction and ventilation.

Tracheostomy

If continued airway obstruction is observed or contemplated, a surgical opening of the trachea (tracheostomy) may be created to provide an artificial airway and allow easier access to the trachea for suction. Care of a patient with a tracheostomy is a very serious responsibility.

The adult or child who has had a tracheostomy usually cannot speak or make any vocal noise unless the opening of the tracheostomy tube, which retracts the surgical incision, is temporarily covered. For persons who have previously been able to communicate well orally and for young children who make their wants known by crying, failure of oral communication, accompanied by respiratory problems, is extremely frightening.

Children with tracheostomies should be placed in areas where they will be under constant observation. When appropriate, signal cords or handbells should always be available. For those able to write, a magic slate or paper and pencil should be near at hand. The method of temporarily closing off the tracheostomy opening with the fingers to speak should be taught to the older child during convalescence. Temporarily obstructing the tube in this way will also aid defecation. A calm, efficient nurse does wonders in alleviating the anxiety of tracheostomy patients.

These children need to be closely observed for signs of unintentional tracheostomy obstruction and need for suctioning as indicated by increased, noisy "bubbling" respirations, restlessness, and cyanosis.

Most tracheostomy tubes available today do not have an inner and outer cannula. A single lumen tube (Fig. 26-6) is thought to be less complex and just as safe. It is fitted with an obturator that is used to ease the tube's insertion into the trachea by helping to keep the tube clear, protecting the mucous membranes from injury, and assisting in the tube placement. The obturator, another tracheostomy tube, a nasal speculum or hemostat (to prevent wound closure), an Ambu bag fitted with a tracheostomy adapter, a sterile suction setup, and a tracheostomy care tray should all be easily available at the bedside to be used in the event of airway obstruction, inadvertent extubation, or respiratory arrest.

The nurse suctions the tracheostomy using meticulous sterile technique. She may suction as deeply as necessary to remove secretions. Often 0.5 to 2.0 ml of sterile physiologic saline solution is injected into the tracheostomy tube to help thin out any secretions before suctioning. If oxygen is being administered, a small humidification unit may be fitted directly over the tube, or a humidifier may be placed in the patient's room to furnish the necessary moisture.

A Y-tube connection or thumb control is recommended on the suction catheter to facilitate its use. Suction is obtained by covering the open end of the Y-tube or special opening with the thumb. It is more gentle to the mucous membranes than a plain catheter that has been pinched to stop suction during insertion. Insertion of the catheter is made with

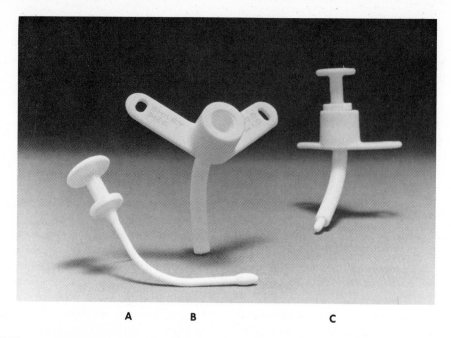

FIG. 26-6   **A,** Shiley pediatric tracheostomy tube obturator; **B,** pediatric tube; **C,** Shiley neonatal tracheostomy tube with obturator in place.

Courtesy Shiley, Inc.

no suction applied. Suction is applied periodically as the tube is rotated on withdrawal. It has been suggested that the nurse hold her breath during suctioning so that she will not suction for too long an interval and inadvertently interfere with respiration. (The catheter may partially block the passage of air or remove necessary air.) If bronchial suction is desired, if possible, the patient's head should be turned first to one side and then the other during the suctioning process. In the child past infancy this assists the catheter to enter both bronchi instead of following the easier pathway to the less-angled entrance of the right bronchus. Too frequent aspiration should be avoided. Very young children usually resist suctioning. Often better results are obtained if they are positioned on their backs with the shoulders raised on a folded bath blanket and the child's head dropped back. Assistance or a modified mummy restraint may be needed.

ENRICHED OXYGEN ENVIRONMENTS

Safety factors

Various methods and devices are used to make inspired air richer in oxygen. The oxygen content of air in a well-ventilated room is about 21%. Therefore any device used to elevate the oxygen content must be capable of administering oxygen of a higher percentage. However, because of the danger of eye damage and loss of sight as a result of retrolental fibroplasia caused by oxygen excesses in the blood, many devices are set to deliver no more than 40% oxygen to a specific area without a special maneuver. Premature infants are especially vulnerable to retrolental fibroplasia; still, there are times when their environmental (ambient) air must contain more than 40% oxygen to meet their needs, which have increased because of respiratory or cardiac problems. The most accurate way of assessing the actual oxygen needs of these infants is by periodic blood gas determinations. The results of these tests are compared with the oxygen concentrations delivered in the hood or incubator, which are monitored at least every 2 hours.

When oxygen is being used, other safety factors involved must be clearly understood to avoid fire. Oxygen readily supports combustion, and all sources of possible ignition of flammable materials should be removed from the environment. Also, safe storage and maintenance of oxygen cylinders, if used, must be carried out to avoid fire and explosion hazards.

Rules for oxygen administration. The following rules should be observed during oxygen administration:

1. No open flames, cigarettes, cigars, matches, cigarette lighters, or candles should be allowed in a room in which oxygen is being used. Signs that read OXYGEN IN USE— NO SMOKING should be clearly posted.
2. No device that is capable of producing a spark should be operated in the oxygen-enriched environment. Any electrical equipment used must be especially grounded to be safe. Therefore most electrical equipment is prohibited; no standard television sets, radios, vaporizers, heat lamps, electrical beds, or call bells (unless particularly prepared) should be used. Occasionally television sets and hospital equipment are elevated high on special shelves. In this position they can be used in a room where oxygen is being administered, since the room is not airtight and the oxygen (which is heavier than air) seeks lower levels.
3. No oil or alcohol rubs should be given in oxygen tents or other closed units.
4. No wool blankets should be used on the bed of a patient receiving oxygen.
5. At no time should an oxygen outlet, tank, regulator, or administering apparatus be oiled, greased, or handled with greasy hands or gloves.
6. All enclosed oxygen units (such as incubators or tents) should be "flushed" with oxygen before the patient is enclosed within them.
7. Because of the potential danger of excess carbon dioxide accumulation, all tents or enclosures should provide some method of ventilation or chemical control that will prevent this problem.

Methods of oxygen enrichment

Oxygen tent. A large oxygen tent may be ordered for an older child. Such a tent is usually a plastic canopy suspended from an overhead rod and attached to a cabinet containing a machine which, when properly adjusted, regulates the tent's ventilation and temperature and may also provide a control for increased humidity along with an orifice for the appropriate oxygen flow (Fig. 26-7). An oxygen tent may be set up in the following manner:

1. If time and the patient's condition permit, place a bath blanket between the bed mattress and the bedspring to prevent snagging the plastic canopy, which can be easily torn. A plastic or rubberized sheet under the sheet covering the mattress will cut down on oxygen loss if the mattress is permeable.
2. Bring the tent canopy and control cabinet to the bedside. Extend the overhead bar, designed to support the tent during use, and expand the tent folds slightly along the bar.
3. Plug in the electrical cord leading to the control cabinet, and turn on the motor.
4. Set the air circulation or ventilation control on the cabinet, if available, halfway between low and high.
5. The temperature control on the cabinet is usually placed at 70° F (21° C). However, even in extremely hot weather the temperature setting should not be more than 10° to 15° F (5.5° to 8.3° C) below the room temperature to prevent shocking the patient when the canopy is lifted and decreasing the working efficiency of the tent.

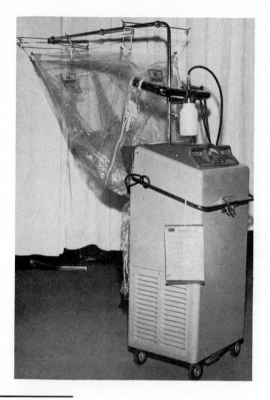

FIG. 26-7

One type of oxygen tent with a temperature control and ventilating humidification units.

Courtesy Children's Hospital and Health Center, San Diego, Calif.

6. If ventilation deflectors are present in the tent, arrange them so that the cool air entering the tent does not blow directly on the patient.

7. Connect the oxygen inlet tube to the wall flowmeter or oxygen cylinder regulator and start the flow at 15 L/min. Maintain this rate for 30 minutes and then analyze the oxygen concentration. If the ordered concentration is attained, the flow is usually reduced to 10 to 12 L/min—the minimum flow required to wash out and dilute exhaled carbon dioxide. Instead of increasing the oxygen flow to 15 L/min for 30 minutes, frequently the same concentration can be achieved by holding a flush valve open for at least 2 minutes after the tent has been placed around the patient. Warn the patient that such a valve opening causes a rushing noise as the tent floods with oxygen.

8. Gently place the canopy over the patient in such a way that its sides (skirts) do not touch the patient's face.

9. Many tents of this type seem drafty to the patients. The amount of protection from cold that is necessary depends on the patient's own body temperature. Scarfs, hoods, and cotton jackets may be desirable.

10. Mold the tent canopy around the child's body to prevent unnecessary oxygen loss. A folded sheet may be placed at the end of the tent, molded around the child's body, and tucked under the mattress with the tent. If the tent is not tucked in properly, much leakage will occur.

11. When lowering or raising the head of the bed, take care not to catch the tent canopy in the mechanism or put the canopy under undue tension. Often the patient in an oxygen tent will feel better with the head of the bed moderately raised, if orders permit this.

12. Plan nursing care so that the tent is opened as little as possible and many of the patient's needs are met during one interval. The motor blower may be shut off before opening the tent to reduce oxygen waste. Be sure to restart the motor after the nursing care has been completed.

High-humidity tents. High humidity concentrations may be achieved with the addition of jet humidifiers on many of the oxygen units (Fig. 26-8). Sterile distilled water alone or additional ordered medications may be used. Tents may also use compressed air rather than oxygen to achieve desired mist.

Patients placed in the cool, high-humidity environments produced by such tents must be checked *frequently* to see if their hair and clothing are damp. If the patients do not have excessively ele-

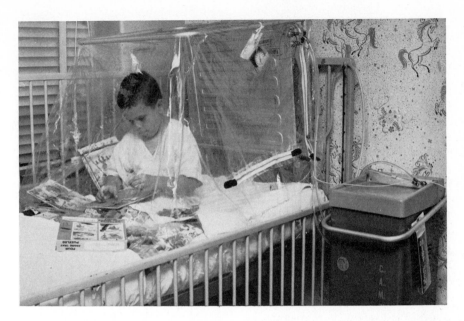

FIG. 26-8   The C.A.M. tent, used for oxygen or mist therapy, is cooled and ventilated electrically. The working apparatus is not near the patient, and more room is available for activity. Side rail down for picture only.

Courtesy Children's Hospital and Health Center, San Diego, Calif.

vated temperatures, they should have undershirts under their cotton gowns. Infants seem to do best when they are dressed in long-sleeved, foot-in sleepers.

Nasal cannula. Oxygen may also be administered by nasal cannula. The cannulas used are generally short, paired, open tubes made of plastic or metal that are attached to a larger tube leading to the oxygen supply. These tubes are placed just inside the nostrils. A nasal cannula should be used when only low concentrations of oxygen—less than 35%—are desired. Oxygen administered by cannula should be passed through a humidifier to prevent uncomfortable drying of the mucous membranes. The cannula should not obstruct the nostrils, and the patient should not breathe through the mouth.

Oxygen mask. Oxygen by mask is usually administered through a tube leading from the oxygen supply to a light plastic face mask. Some of the units available are disposable. Masks are capable of administering high oxygen concentrations quickly and are ideal for emergency use. A rather wide variety of oxygen masks is available; some masks allow rebreathing of the first one third of the air expelled with each expiration (the fraction of an expiration richest in oxygen content) along with oxygen from the tank or wall supply. A well-known partial rebreathing face mask is the BLB, named for the initials of its inventors, Boothby, Lovelace, and Bulbulian. A partial rebreathing mask must fit tightly to the face, but a simple face mask that does not provide for rebreathing and is used for emergency or short-term use should not be applied tightly unless an escape valve or opening for carbon dioxide release is present. Nurses should be well acquainted with the particular oxygen equipment used in their setting and should study the manufacturer's instruction.

Incubators with increased oxygen. Incubators may be employed to provide both increased oxygen and humidity to the infant as well as a controlled environmental temperature. Incubator temperatures and oxygen concentrations (whenever supplementary oxygen is being used) should be recorded at least every 2 hours.

The humidity of the incubator may be regulated by setting a special control that allows varying amounts of air to flow over a water reservoir under the incubator deck. If additional humidity is desired, a jet humidifier may be positioned on the side of the incubator. The amount of relative humidity desired by different physicians may vary. (For more details regarding types of incubators and their use, see p. 554.)

STIMULATION AND MAINTENANCE OF RESPIRATORY EFFORT

If respiratory effort is absent or precarious, various methods may be employed to stimulate or maintain respiration. They all presuppose an *adequate airway*.

In the delivery room or nursery, if a newborn is not breathing regularly, the nurse often stimulates more effective respirations by rubbing the infant's back, snapping the soles of the feet, or jarring the bed or incubator.

Mouth-to-mouth resuscitation

If respiration has actually ceased, mouth-to-mouth resuscitation is an extremely practical prompt source of aid, no matter what the setting, since it requires no additional equipment and can be instituted while other methods are being prepared for use. The following is a description of mouth-to-mouth resuscitation that can be used alone if cardiac function is adequate or with cardiac compression in the absence of heartbeat. (See Table 26-1.) Often children will respond to mouth-to-mouth resuscitation alone.

If the child is found facedown at the scene of a possible accident, the child must be rolled over in a

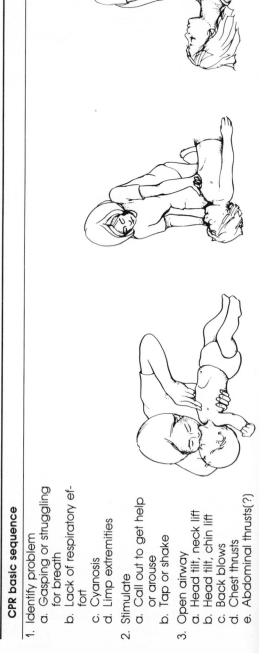

TABLE 26-1 EMERGENCY CARDIOPULMONARY RESUSCITATION (CPR) REMINDERS*

CPR basic sequence

1. Identify problem
   a. Gasping or struggling for breath
   b. Lack of respiratory effort
   c. Cyanosis
   d. Limp extremities
2. Stimulate
   a. Call out to get help or arouse
   b. Tap or shake
3. Open airway
   a. Head tilt, neck lift
   b. Head tilt, chin lift
   c. Back blows
   d. Chest thrusts
   e. Abdominal thrusts(?)

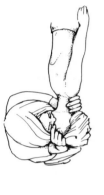

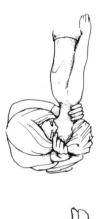

4. Breathing
   a. Look, listen, feel
5. Four breaths
   a. Only enough to make chest rise and fall
6. Pulse
   a. Palpate brachial artery in infants, carotid artery in children and adults
7. Use rescue breathing or CPR as needed

Consideration	Infants (less than 1 year)	Children (1 through 8 years)	Older children and adults
Pressure point	Midsternum—on line with nipples	Slightly below midsternum	Lower half of sternum
Hands	Tips of 2 or 3 fingers	Heel of one hand	Both
Compression distance	½ to 1 inch (1.3 to 2.5 cm)	1 to 1½ inches (2.5 to 3.8 cm)	1½ to 2 inches (4 to 5 cm)
Compression/ventilation C/V ratio	5/1 (3 minute cycle) 100C/20V/minute Use only slight hyperextension of neck; mouth or mask covers nose and mouth; use only small breaths from cheeks	5/1 (4 minute cycle) 80C/15V/minute	Alone—15/2 2 Rescuers—5/1 60C/12V/minute

Victim should be supported on hard surface for best results. Gastric emptying (decompression) is now recommended only if the abdomen is so tense that ventilation is ineffective. Effective CPR is accompanied by improvement in skin color, pupillary constriction, spontaneous movement, and some gasping respirations.

*From Standards and guidelines for cardiopulmonary resuscitation (CPR) and emergency cardiac care (ECC), 1979, J.A.M.A. **244**:453-509, Aug. 1, 1980.

manner that avoids twisting the neck or back. The child is positioned supine on a firm surface with the head in "sniffing" position, which clears the tongue from the airway. Only slight hyperextension is used with infants to avoid collapsing the trachea. *Obvious* foreign material in the mouth should be removed. However, *blind* finger sweeps in the mouth to dislodge material in infants and children are not recommended because a foreign body may easily be pushed back where it will increase an obstruction.

Four breaths in rapid succession are performed (mouth-to-nose-and-mouth with an infant; mouth-to-mouth with the child or youth, with the nose pinched). Controlled puffs of air from the cheeks should be used with an infant and gentle breaths just large enough to make the chest rise and fall with child.

In infants and children relief from continuing foreign body airway obstruction may be achieved by a combination of back blows and chest thrusts. In this age group abdominal thrusts are not recommended because of possible injury to abdominal organs, chiefly the liver. Chest thrusts in the infant are a succession of four external chest compressions similar to those performed during CPR. Four chest thrusts are performed on a child, as external chest compression is applied in the adult.

Once a clear airway is obtained, the circulatory status of the victim is evaluated. In infants it is now advised to feel for the brachial pulse instead of the apical pulse, since some infants may have good cardiac function but a heartbeat that is difficult to palpate. Though the carotid pulse may be less accessible in infants, the carotid pulse is to be sought in young children, as it is in adults.

If the pulse is present, rescue breathing is continued at a rate of 20 ventilations per minute for infants, 15 ventilations per minute for a child, and 12 per minute for children over 8 years of age and for adults.

Resuscitation of some kind is continued until the victim responds spontaneously or is pronounced dead, or until the rescuer is physically unable to continue.

Cardiopulmonary resuscitation

1. See basic procedure on pp. 522-523.
2. External heart massage is not without danger. However, the danger of injury (broken ribs, traumatized liver) is probably less than the danger of circulatory collapse.
3. A precordial thump or blow on the chest *is not used* to initiate heart action in the event of a witnessed arrest involving a child.
4. It is usually not attempted in cases in which such dramatic efforts would only delay a death that will take place minutes or hours after the treatment is terminated (for example, in a child dying of a malignancy or advanced leukemia).

A nurse should make use of every opportunity to secure practice and instruction regarding resuscitation measures during nonemergency situations. She should know where emergency resuscitation and oxygenation equipment is stored in the area in which she works. This would include knowledge of the location of the following items:

1. Resuscitation apparatus
2. Suction setup
3. Oxygen mask and cylinder
4. Emergency drug supply

Mechanical ventilation

A common type of resuscitation apparatus available is the Ambu resuscitator (Fig. 26-9). Use of this resuscitator is much less fatiguing for the operator than mouth-to-mouth resuscitation. The operator may stand or sit behind the supine patient's head with the top of the patient's head stabilized against her body. One hand of the operator holds the mask firmly against the patient's mouth and nose while tilting the head back and maintaining the forward position of the jaw to clear the airway. With her other hand the operator lightly compresses the air bag in a rhythm of *1, 2, 3, 4, 1, 2, 3, 4,* compressing during the count of 1 and taking her

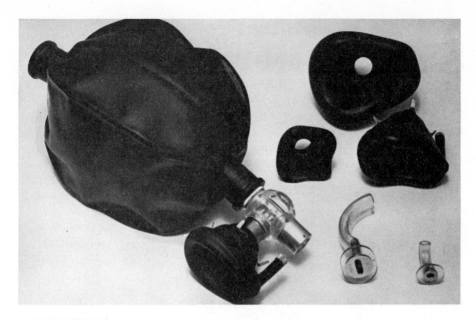

FIG. 26-9   Ambu resuscitator. Various-sized masks and plastic airways.
Courtesy Children's Hospital and Health Center, San Diego, Calif.

hand completely off the bag for 2, 3, 4. Too rapid, excited compression of the bag will cause greater respiratory distress. The operator should observe the chest rise and allow the patient time to exhale adequately. When the patient makes an effort to breathe spontaneously, the treatment may be discontinued while the patient's respiratory attempts are evaluated.

Several mechanical ventilators are available that may, when appropriately "set," sustain respiration artifically for prolonged periods while administering oxygen at predetermined percentages. These various types of ventilators force air into the lungs through masks or endotracheal or tracheostomy tubes. They may be regulated to cycle automatically at a certain rate and depth of respiration.

Intermittent positive pressure

Intermittent positive pressure breathing devices (IPPB) may also be used periodically on patients who are breathing voluntarily in an effort to prevent or reduce respiratory complications by expanding the lungs, administering aerosol medication, and helping to thin respiratory secretions. Orders directing their use should include the number of treatment to be given per day, the length of the treatment, the pressure to be used, the oxygen concentration to be employed, and the type and strength of solution to be used in the nebulizer. A face mask or mouthpiece is used for this type of therapy.

Although a respiratory therapist usually has the responsibility for these treatments, the nurse should familiarize herself with the equipment used in the hospital where she works. She should know when a treatment is ordered. Some children will receive certain morning treatments in a specified order. For example, a child may be given a bronchodilator as a medication to be followed by an aerosol administered by IPPB, to be followed by respiratory hygiene (percussion, vibration, postural drainage, and possibly suctioning). Only after

FIG. 26-10

A, Triflo incentive spirometer; patient inhales and raises the balls. **B,** Spirocare incentive breathing exercises; patient inhales, lighting up various colors as preset goals are achieved.

Photo by Bob Burgin; courtesy Children's Hospital and Health Center, San Diego, Calif.

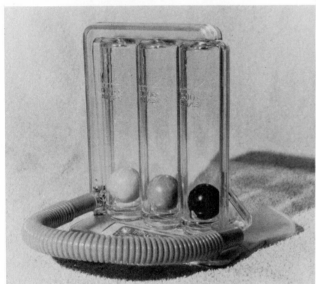

A

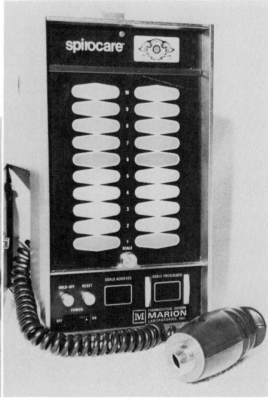

B

this sequence may the patient have breakfast. Respiratory hygiene is not given within an hour following a meal.

Other equipment or techniques used to improve respiratory exchange include various types of incentive breathing devices, which serve to emphasize inhalation rather than exhalation. (It has been found that the use of blow bottles with pronounced exhalation may promote alveolar *deflation*.) Therefore the patient is now encouraged to practice voluntary sustained inspiration. Deep breaths should be held for at least 3 seconds. Two types of incentive devices are pictured in Fig. 26-10.

EVALUATION OF RESPIRATORY DIFFICULTIES

If the signals of respiratory distress are unknown, unobserved, or ignored so that proper methods of instituting aid are not begun promptly, the patient will not benefit. A child may be suffering from lack of ventilation, and proper equipment for the child's aid may be nearby, but unless this aid is given properly, no improvement will result. A nurse should be thoroughly familiar with signs of respiratory difficulty or potential difficulty. Such signs and symptoms of respiratory difficulty may include the following (Fig. 26-11):

1. Depressed or elevated respiratory rate at rest

CHEST MOVEMENT

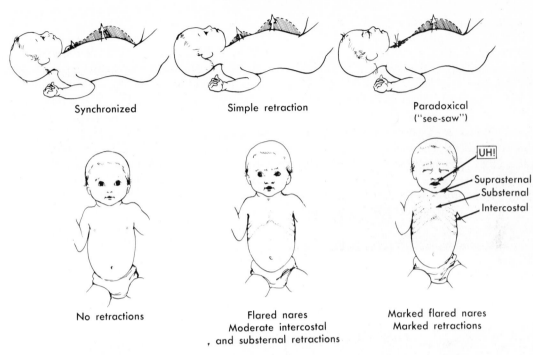

Synchronized Simple retraction Paradoxical ("see-saw")

No retractions

Flared nares
Moderate intercostal
, and substernal retractions

Marked flared nares
Marked retractions

Normal **Moderate distress** **Severe distress**

_____

FIG. 26-11 Types of respiration—visible signs of respiratory distress.

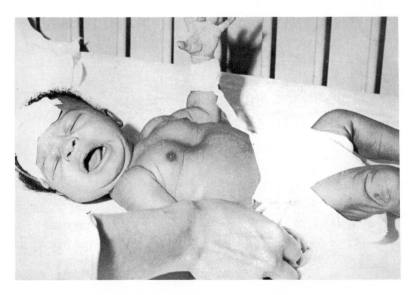

_____

FIG. 26-12 Deep substernal retractions caused by pneumonia (note hollow in chest area).
Courtesy Naval Regional Medical Center, San Diego, Calif.

for the age of the child considered (see p. 435 for a pulse and respiration table)

2. Any retractions present
3. Noisy, labored breathing, grunting
4. Flaring nostrils and the use of facial and neck muscles in attempts to aid respirations
5. Pallor or cyanosis (gray to purple skin coloring), which may be localized or generalized and associated with circulatory problems
6. Restlessness, apprehension, and disorientation
7. Inflamed respiratory tree with thick nasal discharge and intermittent blockage of the nasal passageways
8. Frequent productive or nonproductive coughing

Note: The absence of coughing is not in itself necessarily a sign of respiratory improvement.

The observation of any of the preceding signs and symptoms deserves prompt report and evaluation. If a child becomes cyanotic and a bedside oxygen unit is available, first make sure that the child's airway is open, then start the oxygen and signal the supervising nurse for assistance and further evaluation of the patient. The pulse rate and respirations should be counted. Many children with circulatory and respiratory problems in which fluid tends to collect in the chest or the abdomen breathe more easily when propped in a semi-Fowler's position or supported in an infant seat.

A breath is such a small thing, but so necessary. One who watches and records respirations is a guardian of life.

CHAPTER **27**   Traction, casting, and braces

This chapter presents for initial consideration or review basic nursing procedures and responsibilities involved in the care of patients receiving therapy in traction, casts, or braces. These patients may be hospitalized for various reasons; fractures, musculoskeletal diseases, and neurologic disorders account for most of their diagnoses. For more information regarding specific illnesses in this grouping, the student is referred to Chapter 31, Part 1, which discusses in greater detail some of these problems and the nursing care they require. However, to avoid needless repetition, the orthopedic nursing entailed in the care of such patients is discussed separately in this section.

TRACTION

Traction, or methods of exerting pull, is discussed first because at times it must precede casting. Traction is used for the following reasons:
1. To bring a broken bone back into alignment (reduce a fracture) and provide immobilization for correct union
2. To secure a corrected position to treat a congenital or acquired deformity not involving a fracture (reduce a dislocated hip, scoliosis)
3. To prevent or treat contracture deformities
4. To relieve muscle spasm and pain (back injury)

Basic types

Traction may be exerted manually or by the use of certain appliances. There are two main types of traction—skin and skeletal.

SKIN TRACTION

Skin traction helps position the bone indirectly by pulling on the skin and muscles. It is relatively simple to apply and involves no surgical operation. However, only a limited amount of weight may be added with this type of traction, and occasionally the amount of pull possible is insufficient to produce the desired results. Also, the skin may show signs of irritation—allergic reactions, circulation difficulties, or friction—caused by the supportive wrapping. The weight is usually secured to the skin by running strips of adhesive material, cotton or perforated plastic-backed adhesive tape, or foam rubber up both sides of the extremity and securing the strips with an Ace bandage. The ends of the strips are then attached to a foot spreader, which in turn is connected to the desired weight.

SKELETAL TRACTION

Skeletal traction is secured by inserting some mechanical device directly into or through the bone and attaching the prescribed weight. Wires, pins, or tongs may be used to obtain the bone contact. Considerable weight may be attached to such an arrangement, and no bulky or irritating skin wrappings are necessary. Nevertheless, skeletal traction, too, has its drawbacks. Since the bone is actually pierced, danger of infection is always present, and a surgical procedure is involved in both the insertion and the removal of the mechanical attachment. The areas where the holding devices are inserted through the skin must be frequently inspected for signs of inflammation, infection, and drainage. Special pin care may be ordered, usually involving the cleansing of the skin around the pin with hydrogen peroxide or povidone-iodine (Betadine) solution followed by the application of a protective antimicrobial ointment.

Nursing considerations

The beginning student may express perplexity after viewing her first traction patient. Often there seems to be a surplus of weights, ropes, pulleys, and bars, and she wonders how they all fit in to produce a desired result. The mechanical apparatus used may seem complex at times, but the basic principles of traction that guide their use are neither numerous nor obscure.

MAINTENANCE OF PROPER TRACTION

The maintenance of proper traction depends on the direction and amount of pull exerted through the use of ropes, pulleys, and weights and the positioning or alignment of the patient. Therefore it is important that the nurse understand the orders concerning the care of each individual patient in traction and maintain the correct relationship of the various parts of the traction apparatus to the patient. The following points should be noted:

1. Pulleys increase the amount and change the direction of pull on a body part by a weight. A rope should ride smoothly on a pulley to exert the ordered weight.

2. Weights should not be added or subtracted by the nurse. Too much weight may cause the nonunion of a break; too little weight may cause unwanted overriding and an extremity of unequal length. Weights should always hang freely; they should be frequently observed so that they do not come to rest on a rung of the bed, a poorly placed chair, or the floor.

3. The amount of time that traction is to be applied should be clearly understood. Skin traction may occasionally be removed (but such removal always depends on the physician's order). Skeletal traction is usually continuous.

4. Ropes should be in good condition and frequently inspected for signs of wear. Knots should be taped for additional safety. Multiple weights attached to the same rope should be taped together so that they cannot easily fall or be removed. Some pediatric-orthopedic areas place the foot of the beds over which weights hang next to the wall to discourage tampering by the small fingers of ambulatory patients.

COUNTERTRACTION

Pull in one direction must be balanced by pull in the opposite direction for traction to remain effective. This opposing pull is called *countertraction*, not to be confused with *balanced* traction (p. 535).

Countertraction may be exerted in various ways. If the weights used to create the initial pull are not extremely heavy, it may only be necessary to keep the patient in a certain placement in bed, checking periodically to see that the patient has not slipped past the desired place. The patient's body provides the countertraction. The friction of the patient's body against the bedding may also help prevent the child from slipping out of position.

If the pull is stronger, the end of the bed where the initial traction is applied may need to be elevated to allow gravity to increase the countertraction created by the patient's body weight. Elevation may be achieved through the use of grooved blocks under two legs of the bed, a mechanical bed lift, or special positioning of an electric bed.

If it is very difficult to maintain the child in proper position in bed, sometimes some type of restraint may be used (a restraining jacket or waist restraint). However, the use of such devices may cause other problems—pressure areas, hypostatic pneumonia, and constipation. The use of restraints must be carefully evaluated.

Sometimes the body part being treated is placed in a type of frame or splint that is lifted off the surface of the bed. When this arrangement is used, a counterweight may often be connected to this frame, exerting force in the opposing direction.

In review, countertraction may be created in four basic ways:

1. Maintenance of body placement in bed by constant observation and correction, if needed
2. Elevation of the part of the bed next to the weights
3. Use of restraints
4. Application of a counterweight

The method employed depends on the desires of the physician and the responses of the patient. Failure to maintain correct placement in bed while the patient is in traction may (1) cause the weights, which are supposed to create initial pull, to rest on the floor or some other surface and temporarily stop traction altogether, in some cases allowing possible displacement, or (2) change the angle of pull and distort the result desired.

Both situations are potentially harmful. When a nurse is told "Keep Susie's hips at the level of the tape markers on the bed," or "Be sure that Roger is kept pulled up in bed," the staff is trying to avoid the situations just described.

ACTIVITY AND BODY POSITION

The amount of movement and activity allowed the patient in traction should be understood and promoted, and good body alignment and support should be maintained. Bed boards may be placed under the mattress to prevent sagging.

Some patients are allowed relatively little movement or position change because of their individual musculoskeletal problems or traction arrangements. If the nurse allows these patients to sit up or turn on their sides, the traction may be lost or altered so that no treatment or perhaps even real damage may result. A patient who has a leg in a Thomas splint support raised off the surface of the mattress is allowed considerable movement because such a traction maintains proper alignment when the patient's trunk is raised. Even a slight amount of turning toward the splinted leg is usually possible. Such an arrangement is termed "balanced traction." When balanced traction is used in conjunction with an overhead bar and trapeze, the patient enjoys considerably more activity, and nursing care is greatly simplified (Fig. 27-9).

Although it is important that patients not be moved in a way that will disrupt their traction, it is also important that they be moved to the extent permitted to encourage proper body function, elimination, respiration, and circulation and to avoid pressure areas. Exercise and correct positioning of the uninvolved extremities are very necessary to prevent other problems (stiffness or deformity) from occurring in some patients. As in all cases of prolonged immobilization, a high fluid intake should be encouraged. A diet well supplied with roughage and natural laxatives, such as prunes, helps avoid constipation. Special attention should be given to the prevention of foot drop or undesired internal or external rotation of the lower extremities.

CIRCULATION AND SKIN CONDITION

The circulation and skin condition of a patient in traction or other immobilization devices such as casts should be frequently evaluated.

The skin of any patient who is bedfast for long periods with only limited movement permitted must be meticulously observed and protected. Pressure areas are most likely to develop over bony prominences such as the hips, sacrum, ankles, elbows, scapulae, and shoulders. Areas exposed to continuous friction are also likely spots for skin breakdown. If a Thomas splint is being used, the skin area under the padded ring must be frequently inspected. The heels of both the affected and nonaffected leg should be carefully observed. Often the foot that is not being treated may develop a sore heel because the patient moves up in bed by digging the good heel into the mattress to obtain leverage. To prevent unnecessary pressures, the bed linen must be kept smooth and tight, and crumbs and other irritating small objects must be eliminated from the bed. Skin traction wrappings may cause circulation and nerve interference similar to that occasionally encountered with the casted patient. Inability to dorsiflex the exposed big toe of a wrapped affected lower extremity should be reported to the physician promptly.

Pressure areas are much easier to prevent than to treat. Frequent inspection, cleansing, and massage of susceptible areas and encouragement of as much movement as is allowed, consistent with the patient's well-being, will greatly reduce, if not entirely eliminate, pressure areas. Every complaint of skin tenderness, a burning sensation, or aching should be investigated. It does not take long for a small red area to become an enlarged open sore, particularly in areas where circulation may already be impaired. Any devices that lift a pressure area off a surface must be used with caution and frequently evaluated, since they may sometimes cause circulatory disturbances themselves. Patients who are paralyzed or suffer from sensory loss must receive special care and observation. A child in traction should routinely receive back and skin care during a bath and at least twice more during the day shift. The use of an overhead bar and trapeze can greatly facilitate back and skin care when such aids are feasible. If no such arrangement is possible, a nurse may press down on the mattress with one hand to allow her other hand to massage, or two nurses may work together to lift the child *slightly* to facilitate skin care, depending on the type of traction used.

Sometimes the use of imitation or genuine lamb's-wool mats under the patient is helpful. Tincture of benzoin applications on closed areas of pressure or potential pressure are sometimes prescribed. The benzoin serves to toughen the areas but may stain the sheets.

BEDMAKING

Some hospitals are supplied with special traction linen designed to fit under or around different traction appliances such as the Thomas splint. A special "split" top sheet may be available to use on either side of the splint. More commonly a large sheet is simply pulled to one side over the uninvolved leg and a light baby blanket draped over the splinted leg at night. Another satisfactory and modest arrangement uses two blankets, each contained within a separate folded sheet. One such blanket-sheet combination is placed over the chest and abdomen of the patient, with open edges under the chin; the other is placed on top of the uninvolved leg and below the suspended leg, with open edges toward the foot of the bed where they are tucked in. The upper and lower blanket-sheet combinations are then pinned together around the thigh of the leg in traction. This makes a very neat bed. Traction patients may have special snap-on pajamas (tops and bottoms) to facilitate dressing, or perineal drapes or G-strings may be used.

Types of traction equipment

Traction equipment may vary depending on the individual needs of the patient (see Table 27-1).

PROGRESSIVE ABDUCTION TRACTION

Fig. 27-1 shows a type of traction, called circle or rainbow traction, which is used to achieve progressive reduction of congenital dislocation of the hips. The photograph shows an infant who is almost ready for casting. When this child was first placed in skin traction, her legs were suspended at right angles to the bed. Gradually her legs have been abducted until they are almost flat on the bed. When her legs are properly abducted, she will be placed in a plaster cast for further treatment. Such a patient must be carefully observed for developing circulation problems because the leg wrappings may interfere with the blood flow. Swollen, cool, or "blotchy" looking toes, slow blanching on pressure, or delayed return of skin color after pressure is released from a toenail bed are all signs that should be promptly reported. The pulse at the ankle may be checked to detect circulatory problems. Unexplained restlessness, crying, and complaints or indications of leg pain must be further evaluated and noted as well. This type of patient should be raised slightly during feedings to prevent aspiration. The jacket restraint may be loosened or

TABLE 27-1 COMMON TYPES OF TRACTION

Name	Basic type	Most common indications	Major nursing considerations
Bryant's	Skin—to lower extremities	Fractured femur in child under 30 pounds	Report immediately any signs of neurovascular problems
Buck's	Skin—to lower extremities	Hip or knee contractures or immobilization	Avoid skin breakdown around ankles and heels
Russell's	Skin (may incorporate skeletal)—to lower extremities	Hip contractures or immobilization for fractured femur	Maintain proper alignment with patient flat
90°–90°	Skeletal	Fractured femur—preschool and school age child.	Avoid any movement of bed or traction setup

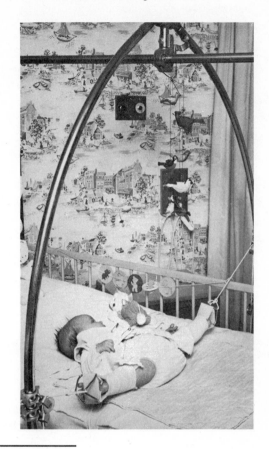

FIG. 27-1

This baby in progressive abduction (circle or rainbow) traction is almost ready for a hip spica cast. Frequent back care is essential.

Courtesy Children's Hospital and Health Center, San Diego, Calif.

removed if a responsible person is *at* the bedside, but it should be in place when the child is alone. To make the bed, one nurse may lift the baby's body just enough to allow another nurse to slide the bed sheets under the hips and back. The weights should not be removed. Frequent back care and diaper changes are a necessity.

BRYANT'S TRACTION

Bryant's traction is often used for the treatment of fractured legs in young children (Fig. 27-2).

FIG. 27-2

Bryant's, or vertical, traction may be used for infants or young children weighing less than 30 pounds. The pelvis is no longer lifted above the mattress by the traction, since this has been found to be associated with circulatory problems in the legs. The knees should be slightly flexed.

Courtesy Children's Hospital and Health Center, San Diego, Calif.

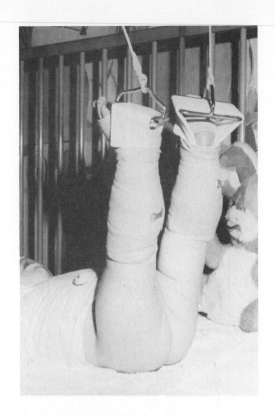

Nursing care of the child in Bryant's traction is similar to that described for children in the traction pictured in Fig. 27-1.

RUSSELL'S TRACTION

Russell's traction, a skin traction using a sling and single rope arrangement attached to one weight supported by multiple pulleys, is used to treat fractures and provide postoperative hip and knee immobilization in older children (Fig. 27-3). Because the extremity is suspended, more patient movement is allowed, and nursing care is considerably easier.

90°–90° TRACTION

90°–90° traction is commonly used to reduce a fractured femur (Fig. 27-4). Both the hip and knee are placed in 90° of flexion. A pin is inserted through the distal femur or proximal tibia, and traction is applied. A sling on the lower leg is used for suspension.

BUCK'S EXTENSION

A rather simple, frequently used skin traction for treatment of the lower extremities or lower back is called Buck's extension (Fig. 27-5). Note the adhesive strips on the sides, the elastic bandage wrapping, the foot spreader (to prevent pressure of the adhesive strips against the ankle), the pulley, and rope leading to the freely hanging weight. Some physicians order a small flattened pillow under the leg just above the Achilles tendon to protect the heel from pressure. In this picture the angle of the pull elevates the heel slightly off the bed.

CERVICAL TRACTION

The patient in cervical traction may have a sling or halter arrangement around the chin and occiput (Fig. 27-6), or the patient may be placed in skeletal traction, which involves the placement of some types of tongs into (but not through!) the cranium (Fig. 27-7). Orders regarding the placement of the patient, the movement allowed, and whether any

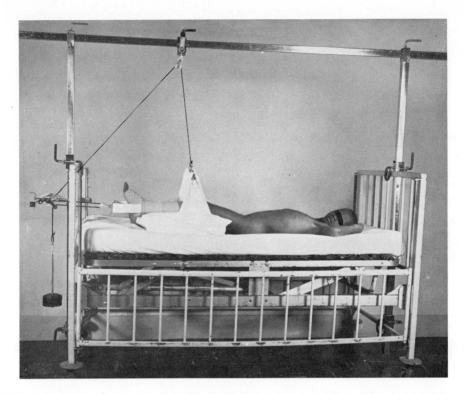

FIG. 27-3   Russell's traction may be used to treat fractures in older children and adults. Split–Russell's traction makes use of two rope, pulley, and weight setups for the two directions of pull. The pillow under the sling is not always present.

From Brashear, H.R., Jr., and Raney, R.B.: Shand's handbook of orthopaedic surgery, ed. 9, St. Louis, 1978, The C.V. Mosby Co.

elevation of the backrest is permitted should be clearly understood. Patients in skeletal-cervical traction are often positioned in slight hyperextension, and flexion of the cervical spine is not permitted. If cervical skin traction is used, foam rubber padding may be necessary in the chin area to prevent skin irritation. Gum chewing may help relieve aching jaw joints.

PELVIC TRACTION

Occasionally pelvic traction may be ordered to relieve lower back pain. Pelvic traction is exerted by use of a pelvic band or girdle attached to a weight or weights. Sometimes a thoracic belt may be used for countertraction. Such an arrangement is designed to relieve muscle spasm and lessen pressure on nerve roots. Pelvic traction may be ordered for continuous or intermittent application. Many patients are given bathroom privileges.

BALANCED TRACTION

As previously mentioned, *balanced traction*, involving the suspension of the affected limb above the surface of the bed, provides the opportunity for more movement or activity by the patient. Patients may raise their hips, have their backrests elevated, or turn slightly toward the side of the splinted lower extremity. An overhead bar and trapeze greatly facilitates lifting. The suspension device takes up the slack created and maintains the line of traction.

Text continued on p. 540.

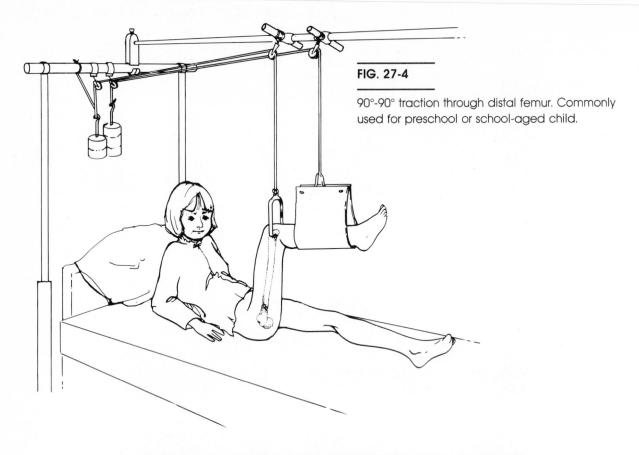

FIG. 27-4

90°-90° traction through distal femur. Commonly used for preschool or school-aged child.

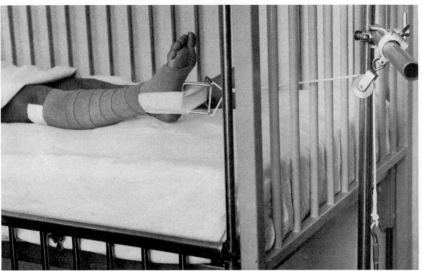

FIG. 27-5
Buck's extension. Note that the heel clears the mattress. Some physicians use a small flat pillow under the leg to provide clearance.

Courtesy Children's Hospital and Health Center, San Diego, Calif.

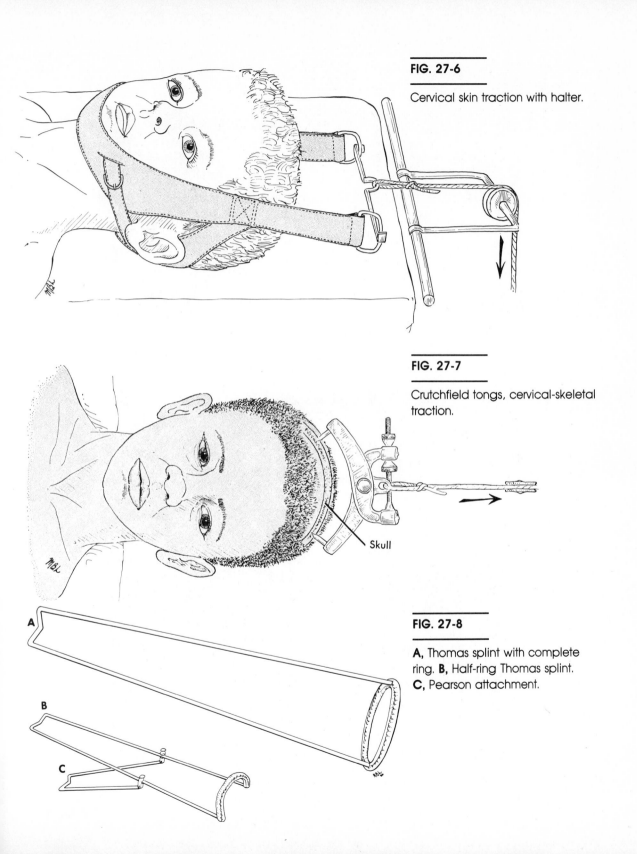

FIG. 27-6

Cervical skin traction with halter.

FIG. 27-7

Crutchfield tongs, cervical-skeletal traction.

Skull

FIG. 27-8

A, Thomas splint with complete ring. **B,** Half-ring Thomas splint. **C,** Pearson attachment.

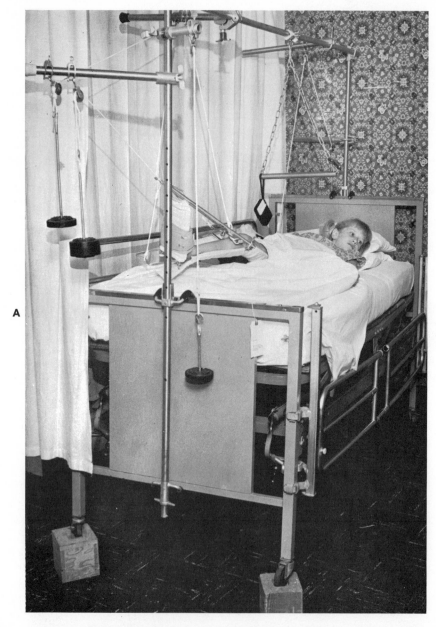

FIG. 27-9 **A,** Patient in balanced traction. **B,** Explanatory drawing. **C,** Close-up view of leg.
Courtesy Children's Hospital and Health Center, San Diego, Calif.

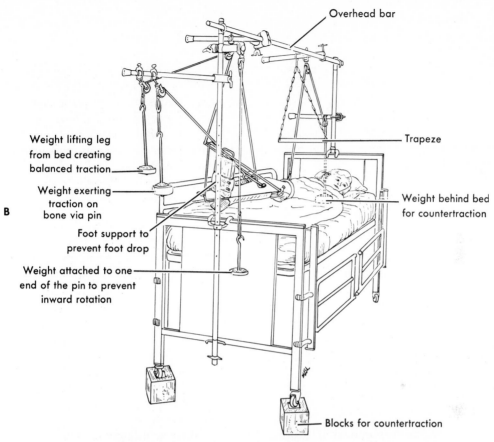

B

Overhead bar

Trapeze

Weight lifting leg from bed creating balanced traction

Weight exerting traction on bone via pin

Foot support to prevent foot drop

Weight attached to one end of the pin to prevent inward rotation

Weight behind bed for countertraction

Blocks for countertraction

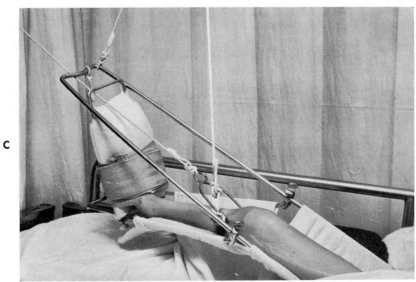

C

FIG. 27-9, cont'd

For legend see opposite page.

It is well to remember that, no matter how much these patients want to stay up, they should intermittently rest flat, without the elevation of the backrest, to prevent hip contractures.

Although suspended traction gives greater liberty of movement and effectively relieves heel pressure, the area where the ring of the Thomas splint rests must be frequently inspected for the development of skin problems. Each day the skin may be gently pulled up or down from under the ring and washed, dried, and massaged. The ring, if leather, may be polished with saddle soap. Fig. 27-8 shows a Thomas splint with a complete ring and a Thomas half-ring splint with a Pearson attachment, which is used to support the extremity. Fig. 27-9 shows a young girl with a balanced skeletal traction, including an extra support to prevent foot drop and an additional weight to correct a tendency toward internal rotation of the leg. Not long after this photograph was taken the girl was sent home in a long leg plaster cast.

CASTS

Casts are often applied subsequent to treatment by traction, supplying a form of external immobilization of a body part. Occasionally, a cast may be applied over a skeletal pin, thus helping to continue traction as well as contributing to immobilization. Such a procedure may be called plaster traction. The ends of the protruding pins should be covered with plaster or some sort of protective device to avoid the snagging of clothing or bed coverings or injury to others. Plaster traction allows greater mobility for the patient (when feasible). In addition to immobilization and possible traction, casts may also be a means of aiding proper positioning or resting a body part.

The most common kind of cast consists of plaster of paris–impregnated crinoline bandages that have been applied and molded while moist over some type of soft, protective layer and allowed to dry to a hard, resistant shell. Dry plaster of paris is a form of calcium sulfate; when mixed with water, it forms the substance known as gypsum. Plastic-type syn-

thetic materials are increasingly being used to form casts. They typically set rapidly and in some instances may be ready for weight bearing as early as 15 minutes after setting. They are durable, lightweight, porous, and, when applied over special nonabsorbant synthetic padding, may be immersed if necessary. But they must be carefully dried. Manufacturers' instructions must be consulted for details of application and care. The exteriors of these casts may be somewhat rough, and they are more expensive.

Application of the cast

Because of the "orderly disorder" that invariably accompanies plaster applications, it is preferable to schedule cast work in a room especially designed for such procedures—a room that is easily cleaned and contains all the equipment and supplies usually needed.

Commonly needed supplies are as follows:
1. Materials that protect the skin, to be wrapped around the body part before application of plaster or synthetics
   a. Sheet wadding (Webril)
   b. Tubular stockinette
2. Various widths of plaster of paris bandages and strips (splints) or synthetic tapes
3. Materials to reinforce or protect areas of the cast or body that are under special pressure or strain
   a. Felt
   b. Yucca board
   c. Wire netting
   d. Rubber heels (for leg casts of ambulatory patients)
4. Special tools
   a. Various types of cast knives
   b. Plaster shears
   c. Cast spreaders and cast benders
   d. Manual and electric cast cutters
   e. A bucket for water to moisten the cast materials (temperatures vary)
5. Other possible needs
   a. Cover gowns

b. Gloves, caps, and masks

c. Special lamps to cure certain synthetic casting materials (Lightcast II)

The furnishings of a cast room need not be elaborate. Usually an examining table, some benches, good lighting, an x-ray view box, and a sink are sufficient. A sink with a plaster trap is convenient because water used to soak the plaster of paris rolls may be discarded into the drain without too much danger of plugging the plumbing. If large body casts or scoliosis jackets are applied, additional supportive frames, tables, or slings will be needed. Newspapers placed on the floor under the working area will aid cleanup.

PREPARATION OF THE PATIENT

Some patients undergoing casting procedures are anesthetized to aid muscle relaxation, relieve pain, and facilitate the entire procedure. Patients who have open reductions of fractures or other operative procedures just before casting are, of course, always anesthetized. Small children are frequently anesthetized for close reduction procedures. Such patients are given nothing by mouth for several hours before the procedure and usually receive preoperative sedation. If a flammable general anesthetic is used, all precautions against explosions should be taken. The staff must be dressed appropriately and all equipment properly grounded. Even if the use of anesthetics is not contemplated and a closed manipulation before casting is the only maneuver scheduled, a preoperative analgesic drug may be ordered and oral feedings temporarily withheld.

The nurse must make certain that the child and the parents have been informed of this procedure beforehand and know what to expect after the cast has been applied. Sometimes meeting another youngster with a cast or seeing a doll with a casted arm or leg is a helpful preparatory experience for the young boy or girl.

DUTIES OF THE NURSE

The nurse helping the physician in the cast room is responsible for making available all the necessary equipment and supplies. When plaster of paris is used, the desired width of plaster of paris bandage is removed from its waxed paper wrapper and immersed on end in tepid water. When air bubbles no longer rise from the roll, the bandage should be lifted from the water. The sides of the closed bandage may be gently squeezed to help remove water and retain plaster. The loose end of the bandage is unrolled slightly, and the roll and its end are handed to the physician for application. The bandage should not be dripping at the time of the transfer. The nurse may also assist by helping to hold the extremity being casted. She may be asked to support part of the newly formed cast. If she does, she should remember to use only the palms of her hands in rendering such support to prevent the formation of pressure areas.

Cast changes and removal (Fig. 27-10)

Sometimes a patient must have one cast removed and another applied. The frequency with which a child must have a cast changed depends on the child's rate of growth, the condition of the cast, and the progress of the desired correction. The plaster cast may be cut manually with a cast knife, which may be shaped like a short kitchen paring knife, and a hand cast cutter. The cut is made along a predetermined line, which may have been dampened by a vinegar solution, hydrogen peroxide, or water from a syringe. A metal strip may be inserted just below the cutting line to protect the body part. An electrical vibrating-blade cast cutter may be used instead. The electric saw makes a great deal of noise, which sometimes frightens the patient. When the cast has been carefully cut, the sections are separated by a cast spreader, and the padding underneath is released with large bandage scissors. The body part that has had the support of the cast must be gently supported and handled and not forced into new, unfamiliar positions. Sudden lack of support or movement will often cause considerable distress.

Professional opinion differs regarding the care of the skin of a patient who has been in a cast for a considerable time and will almost immediately be

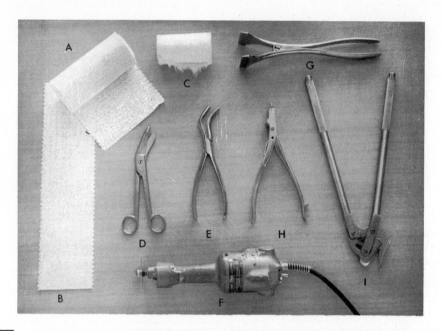

FIG. 27-10   Instruments and materials used in preparing or removing plaster casts. **A,** Plaster roll; **B,** plaster splint; **C,** Webril (sheet wadding); **D,** plaster shears (large bandage scissors); **E,** cast bender; **F,** cast cutter or saw (electric); **G** and **H,** cast spreaders; **I,** cast cutter (manual).

Courtesy Children's Hospital and Health Center, San Diego, Calif.

enclosed in a cast again. Some physicians want their patients to have baths; others believe that the least amount of handling possible is the best choice. All wish to avoid trauma to the skin, which would lead to trouble during the subsequent period of casting. If the use of a cast will be discontinued permanently or for a considerable time, the physician may order a combination of gentle baths and the application of baby oil to help loosen the crust of old skin and sebaceous material that has collected on the body part that was under the cast. With patience and time this crust may be removed with no injury to the underlying epidermis.

Care of the newly casted patient and the cast

A newly casted patient may complain of the heat generated by the plaster as it undergoes physical reaction with the water. This heat of crystallization is transitory; however, in body casts it may cause considerable annoyance. Newly applied casts are soft, damp, and grayish white and have a slightly musty smell. They must be handled carefully.

TRANSFER OF THE PATIENT

When transferring a newly casted patient, the nurse should lift the cast with the palms of the hands rather than grasp it by the fingers. Finger pressure may cause indentations, tissue injury, and disturbances in circulation. If the patient is in a body cast (hip spica) covering the trunk or hips and legs, many hands may be necessary to make an efficient, smooth transfer from cart to bed.

PREPARATION OF THE UNIT

The unit of a patient who is having a new body cast applied requires special preparation. Bed boards should be placed under the mattress to pre-

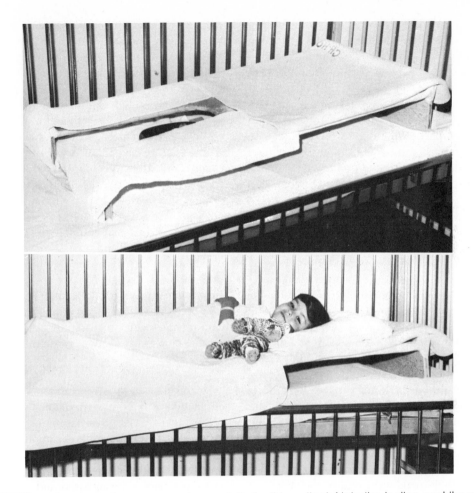

FIG. 27-11 Cast board premeasured especially for this patient. Note the incline and the positioned bedpan.

Courtesy Children's Hospital and Health Center, San Diego, Calif.

vent sagging. Numerous firm pillows should be available to support the contours of the soft cast.

If the child is old enough and able to benefit, an overhead bar and trapeze should be attached to the bed. The room should be well ventilated to assist in the drying of the cast. Occasionally special cast driers may be available, or an undraped heat cradle may be used to help speed drying. A new cast should be exposed to the air. However, for modesty's sake a G-string or diaper may be positioned over the perineal area. A fracture pan should be available in the bedside stand. In many hospitals infants and small children in body casts are measured for so-called cast boards or for a Bradford frame, which holds the child at a slight incline, elevated from the bed mattress (Fig. 27-11). A bedpan is kept positioned under the child at all times, and plastic strips, which are tucked into the perineal area of the cast, guide waste material into the pan below. Very young children who are incontinent may be "taped" with urine collection bags until the cast is dry enough to be protected against accidental soiling. If this is done before cast application, soiling can more effectively be prevented.

For patients with newly casted extremities, often all that is necessary for the nurse to have ready in the patient's unit is a supply of firm pillows to aid in the elevation of the body part to help prevent swelling. Sometimes elevation is best maintained through the use of a Gatch bed, placement of pillows under the end of the mattress, or suspension of the affected part from an intravenous pole. The cast should be left exposed to the air to facilitate drying and the patient should be turned frequently. Most casts dry in approximately 24 hours.

CARE OF THE CAST

When the cast is dry, as indicated by a chalky white finish and a hard, nonmoist surface, it should be protected against accidental wetting in the perineal region. This may be done in several ways. Various types of plastic material may be cut to fit under the perineal edge of the cast and to protect the curved band of the cast just adjacent. It may be held in place by pieces of water-repellent adhesive tape. Plastic adhesive tape may be cut into wedge-shaped pieces and positioned around and under the perineal rim and on the outer surface. Regardless of the method selected to protect the cast, the waterproof material should not be applied until the cast is dry, because the adhesive usually will not stick. When the cast is dry, all rough or potentially rough edges of the cast should be covered. This process is called "petaling" because the pieces of adhesive tape first used for this purpose were cut in the shape of flower petals. However, nurses today may use adhesive tape cut like chevrons, circles, or wedges as well as the traditional "petal" to protect cast edges (Fig. 27-12). Petaling keeps small bits of plaster from the cast edges from falling into the cast, helps prevent skin irritation around the cast, and may waterproof and improve the appearance of the cast. If tubular stockinette is applied before the plaster bandage during the construction of the cast, it may be neatly trimmed and brought up over the cast edge and secured with adhesive or plaster splints to make a smooth, attractive edging when the cast is dry.

Various methods have been employed to enhance the appearance of a cast and help protect it from damage and soil. Some physicians apply shellac, varnish, or plastic spray to a dry cast to increase its longevity and help keep it clean. It is best not to get a cast dirty or stained in the first place but if it does become soiled, the nurse may clean the area with a damp, not wet, cloth and a small amount of white cleanser (such as Bon Ami) or fast-drying white shoe polish. Some dry, dirty areas may be covered by adhesive tape or additional plaster of paris strips. Children should be cautioned against getting their casts damp. Swimming is definitely out if plaster has been used!

The preceding paragraphs have dealt primarily with the cast itself; however, the most important consideration in orthopedic care is not the cast but the patient it encloses. Casts are a great help in correcting various musculoskeletal problems, but they may also cause or accentuate problems. The casted patient must be carefully observed to detect the development of any of these difficulties.

OBSERVATION FOR COMPLICATIONS

A newly casted extremity may suffer impaired circulation. Sometimes circulatory problems compound themselves. Because of injury, operative procedure, or a tight cast application, there may be swelling under the cast. The increasingly tight cast impedes circulation further, and tissue damage may take place. Certain signs and symptoms indicate abnormal pressure and swelling that should be reported long before significant tissue damage occurs. They should be sought frequently after casting and periodically thereafter. (See box on p. 546.)

Excessive bleeding after surgery, as estimated by bloody drainage seeping through the cast layers may be worrisome. One should consider the type of surgical procedure involved. Physicians seem to differ in opinion concerning the advisability of circling with pencil the drainage stains on a cast and marking them with the time noted. One orthopedist was heard to say that he thought that such a practice alarmed patients unduly.

When possible the corresponding unaffected

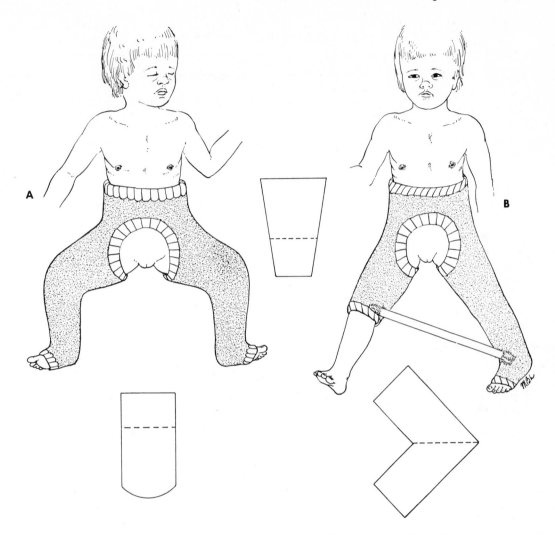

FIG. 27-12 Different types of petaling. **A,** Bilateral hip spica cast. **B,** Unilateral hip spica cast with an abductor bar.

extremity should be compared with the casted arm or leg. Some people have cold hands most of the time, with or without casts. Any complaint of a burning sensation or pain should be promptly reported and investigated. Considerable damage may occur in a relatively short period. If such complaints are neglected, the body part may become numb and no additional complaints may be heard for some time, until tissue damage is significant.

A casted extremity that is swelling must be relieved soon. A nurse should not hesitate to call a physician if circulation is impaired even though the hour may be inconvenient. In the unusual situation in which no physician can be contacted, the nurse should be prepared to cut the cast herself. Certainly such a situation would be extraordinary, but if no help will be available for a considerable period, it is better to have a damaged cast than a gangrenous extremity. The usual emergency procedure involves cutting the cast in half and forming an upper

SIGNS OF NEUROVASCULAR COMPLICATIONS

Pain	Patient feels discomfort or burning sensation, especially when toes or fingers are passively stretched. Very small children are unable to verbalize subjective symptoms; they should be watched for "fussiness."
Puffiness	Toes or fingers are swollen.
Pallor	Toes or fingers are cold (they should be pink and warm). The nurse should compare them with uninvolved extremity if possible.
Purple tint	Toes or fingers are cyanotic or mottled.
Pressure response delay	Blanching sign is absent or delayed. Pressure is made on the nail beds to blanch the area. When the pressure is removed, the normal nail color should return immediately. If the area does not blanch, this is also significant because it indicates local congestion and lack of good circulation.
Pulselessness	A pulse in an extremity cannot be found (when the area to be palpated is accessible).
Paralysis	Toes or fingers cannot be moved properly by the child.
Paresthesia	Patient feels numbness and tingling.
Passive stretch	Extending toes or fingers causes significant pain.

and lower or anterior and posterior shell. The inner wrappings should also be cut, since they may cause considerable pressure. The extremity may be maintained in the shell with the halves held opposite one another by elastic bandage. Such a cast is said to be *bivalved*. Occasionally, physicians intentionally plan to bivalve casts; such casts provide support but also allow some movement and exposure and facilitate the skin care of an area. Bivalved casts are often used as splints in conjunction with elastic bandages.

Even when the cast is dry and relatively old, the daily care of the patient in a body cast or a hip spica cast should continue to include observation for disturbance in circulation and possible areas of pressure, skin breakdown or infection. A peculiar, sweet, musty odor may indicate the presence of pus. The skin next to the cast edges must be carefully inspected and massaged. Alcohol or lotion may be used sparingly. The heel and heel cord and the perineum especially should be watched for signs of irritation.

TURNING THE PATIENT

The patient in a dry body cast is routinely turned at east every 2 or 3 hours in an attempt to prevent pressure sores and promote respiration and elimination. The number of people needed to turn a patient in a body cast depends on the size and general condition of the patient and the age of the cast. Remember the following when turning a patient in a large body cast:

1. If there is a choice, plan to turn the patient toward the nonoperative side.
2. Before turning the patient, pull or lift the child to the side of the bed, placing the "turning side" toward the center of the bed. Have the patient lift the hands above the head or, if this is not feasible, have them held against the sides with a towel or diaper placed between the hands and the cast just before turning to prevent injury. Do *not* use the abductor bar to turn the patient. It is held in place with only a few turns of plaster bandage. It helps support the cast, but it is not a handle.
3. If possible, place the protective pillows needed under the cast in the new position before the patient is turned.
   a. If the patient is placed *on the abdomen*, a flat pillow just below the chest area sometimes helps chest expansion and respiration. A small pillow for the head increases comfort.

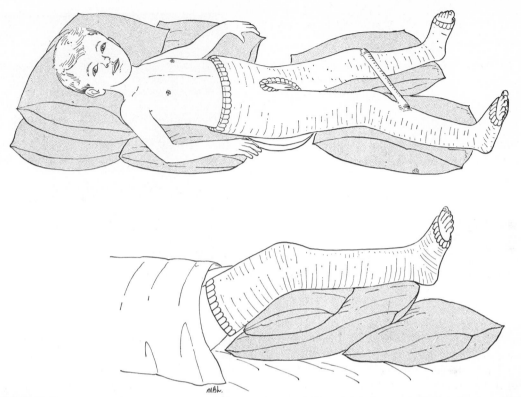

FIG. 27-13 Methods of using pillows to support a cast. The child shown at the top is on a bedpan.

Legs should be supported to prevent the toes from digging into the bedding and the problem of foot drop. Curved up-and-down contours of the cast also should be protected from strain. The abdominal position is preferred for older children at mealtime to aid in swallowing and self-help.

  b. If the patient is *supine*, place a small pillow under the head. Curved up-and-down contours of the cast should be protected from strain and the heels lifted from the mattress.

  c. Be sure that the edges of the cast do not press against the skin. The patient should be made as comfortable as possible.

  d. A young child who is incontinent and does not have a cast board may be placed on a horseshoe-shaped pillow arrangement, and a

small bedpan or large kidney-shaped basin may be positioned under the patient with a plastic strip tucked under the cast leading to the pan or basin (Fig. 27-13). Such a pillow support should elevate the child on a slight incline to prevent urine backflow into the cast.

SAFETY FACTORS

Children in casts of any type must be carefully observed and taught not to put *anything* down into the cast. Small objects, such as crayons and bobby pins, can cause pressure areas, pain, and infection. The nurse must also be vigilant regarding the use of so-called scratchers, employed to relieve itching. If scratchers are allowed at all, they must be relatively soft, such as a strip of gauze that has been strategically placed before the cast application is begun. Even pipe cleaners may cause excoriation and are not recommended for such purposes. Blowing air from a syringe—or from a hair dryer set on cool air—under the rim of the cast may be soothing. One must be sure that the child is not scratching a healing surgical incision.

GENERAL NURSING CONSIDERATIONS

Bathing. Parts of the body that might be overlooked during the daily bath are the fingers and the areas between the toes. Plaster crumbs may collect between the digits and cause pressure areas. Cotton-tipped applicators dipped in baby oil help clean these areas satisfactorily.

Diet and fluids. The child who is immobilized not only needs meticulous skin care but also special attention to the diet and fluid intake to promote healing and avoid constipation and urinary stasis. A liberal fluid intake should be maintained, and a high-protein diet is often encouraged. At times prune juice or some mild laxative may be indicated.

Support of a casted extremity. When a child with a casted extremity is allowed to be up in a chair, the cast should be elevated and not allowed to become dependent. The physician may order that a casted arm be supported in a sling. Several types of slings are available. The classic sling is formed from a triangular bandage. The fingers are exposed but the wrist is supported and the hand is higher than the elbow. The knot should not rest over the cervical spine; this is uncomfortable and may cause a pressure area. Fig. 27-14 shows a commercially prepared hammock-type sling. It is available in several sizes.

When local swelling of an extremity is present or possible, some physicians order that the arm be elevated with pillows. If such elevation is to be effective, the child's wrist must be higher than the elbow, the elbow must be higher than the shoulder, and the entire extremity must be elevated above the level of the heart.

Diversion and intellectual stimulation. A person may be clean, free from pain, on the mend physically, but not particularly happy. The nurse who is

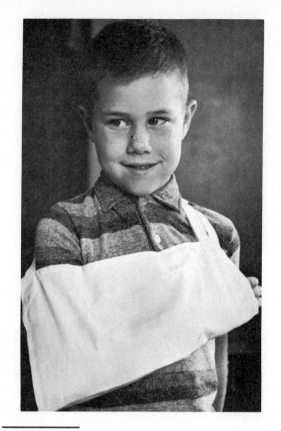

FIG. 27-14

A commercial hammock-type sling. Note that the arm enters the sling from the top, not from the side.

interested in the total patient, not just the body in the cast, should help provide proper diversion, intellectual stimulation, and interpersonal contacts for her patients. During such a time older children can develop constructive hobbies and lasting interests.

Discharge. Many casted patients do not remain in the hospital for very long. Often the cast is applied, dried, protected, and petaled, and the patient's discharge is written within 48 hours or less. The family must be instructed in detail concerning skin care, observation for circulatory problems, cast protection, and cleansing if they are not already familiar with cast care. Using proper body mechanics and seeking assistance when necessary may prevent injury to both parent and child. Appropriate transportation must be arranged. Patients in long leg casts or hip spica casts cannot be comfortably placed in all automobiles!

BRACES

A removable, external support used to maintain position or provide strength to a body part is called a brace. A brace may be made of numerous kinds of material but characteristically is constructed of metal, leather, felt, and lacings. Braces are expensive but helpful pieces of equipment. They are individually fitted and produced, and they demand the respect of both patient and nurse. Braces furnish support by exerting pressure on at least three points of the body. There are many different types of braces. The Milwaukee brace for the treatment of scoliosis is one example of a body brace (p. 628). Short, below-the-knee braces are available for ankle or foot support or full-length leg braces for both knee and ankle stabilization. Some patients (cerebral palsy victims) must have combined body and long leg braces because of extensive muscle paralysis. Many braces include movable joints that may be locked with various mechanisms to provide greater stability for weight bearing.

Maintenance of the brace

The routine care of a brace includes protecting it from rust, carefully cleaning and oiling any hinges with a fine-grade oil, and removing any excess oil to prevent staining of leather supports or clothing. It also includes the care of any leather parts by the periodic application of saddle soap, followed by polishing. Cleaning fluids may be used on felt pads. Laces should be maintained intact and free from pressure-causing knots. Shoes incorporated in any leg brace should be frequently inspected for abnormal wear. Any missing parts (such as felt kneepads

or screws) should be promptly reported because the loss may seriously jeopardize the brace's function.

Nursing responsibilities

The nurse and patient should be familiar with the purpose of each brace, the way in which it should be applied and positioned, when it should be worn, the length of time it should be worn, and its mechanism and maintenance. Patients wearing braces should be frequently inspected for bruises and pressure areas. Bony prominences can be protected beforehand by rubbing tincture of benzoin or a wet tea bag over the skin area. Trial periods should be gradually lengthened (p. 410). Those wearing leg braces should have well-fitted, "nohole" stockings. A body brace is usually worn over a cotton shirt. It should be applied with the patient lying flat in bed. Back braces are buckled or laced from the bottom up. They are then adjusted as necessary with the patient in standing position. A good orthotist (a maker and fitter of braces) and a cooperative patient and family are essential to the successful use of any brace.

CRUTCHES

Often a patient is required to use crutches, with or without braces, to be ambulatory. The physical therapist is usually responsible for teaching crutch walking and the particular gait best suited to the individual patient. However, the nurse may be asked to measure patients for crutches and assist them in developing good habits involving their use.

One method of measuring a patient in supine position for standard-type crutches is to measure the distance from the patient's axilla to a point 4 to 8 inches (10 to 20 cm) out from the patient's heel as the leg is extended and adducted. Ideally patients will be wearing the shoes that they will be using while walking. Another method involves subtracting 16 inches (41 cm) from the patient's height. Crutch length will depend also on the condition of the patient and the gait selected.

The nurse should be sure that the rubber guards on the crutch ends are not worn smooth. The patient should not lean on the "armpit rests." The weight of the body should be borne by the hands. It is easier for a patient using crutches to rise from a firm rather than an overstuffed chair. When walking with a patient who is learning to use crutches, the nurse should walk behind her patient. In case of difficulty she may grasp the patient by the belt, trousers, or waist.

• • •

Orthopedic nursing can be extremely satisfying. It may take much skill, patience, determination, and time to achieve a straightened back or a corrected foot, but they are well worth all the effort involved.

CHAPTER 28

Methods of temperature

control and therapeutic uses

of heat and cold

The regulation of body heat and the effects of localized temperature change on body parts are significant considerations in the medical and nursing care of many patients. The regulations of body temperature through the use of therapy not only may bring greater comfort to the patient but also may avoid complications that occur in the presence of high temperature or abnormal loss of body heat. Appropriate temperature maintenance may be particularly lifesaving for small infants by conserving calories and avoiding acidosis.

Occasionally extremes of body temperature have been induced for therapeutic reasons. Local hot and cold applications are commonly used for treatment. Both the regulation of general body temperature and local reactions to temperature extremes will be discussed in the following paragraphs.

BODY TEMPERATURE

Regulation (Fig. 28-1)

Although the normal oral temperature is usually cited as 98.6° F, or 37° C, the figures indicate only the average normal temperature. Oral temperatures ranging from 97.6° to 99° F (36.4° to 37.2° C) are not considered abnormal. Rectal temperatures *average* 1° F higher than oral readings, whereas axillary temperatures register 1° F lower, *on the average*. Normal body temperature in a human being represents a balance between heat production and heat loss in the body. The main source of body heat is inadvertently created in the process of carrying out normal body functions. Production of body heat is the result of the activity of all cells, made possible by the oxidation, or burning, of foodstuffs within those cells. Blood, flowing through the various parts of the body, helps distribute heat; and although measured body temperature differs depending on the method by which it is determined (oral, rectal, axillary, or skin probe), the remarkable fact is that these various measurements record temperatures so similar. Body heat is conserved by the involuntary constriction of the blood vessels of the skin, forcing more blood into the warm interior of the body and cutting it off from cooler areas near the skin's surface; it is also conserved by the automatic reduction of perspiration. Of course, the maintenance of body heat is also aided by the voluntary activity of the person. Adding a sweater or coat to provide better insulation or exercising to increase metabolism and circulation increases the tolerance of cold environmental conditions. Much heat is produced through the activity of the skeletal muscles. When additional warmth is necessary, these muscles may even contract involuntarily to produce heat, a process called

CONTROL OF BODY TEMPERATURE

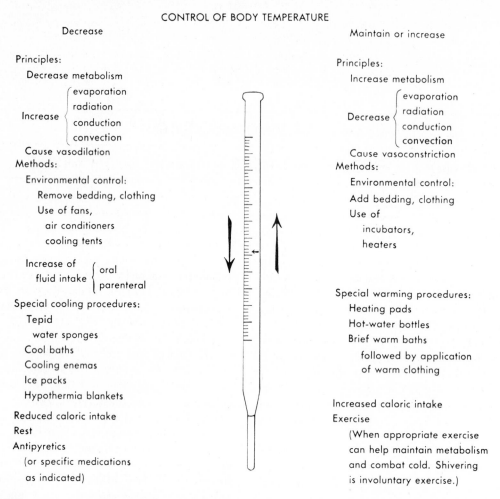

Decrease

Principles:

Decrease metabolism

Increase { evaporation / radiation / conduction / convection

Cause vasodilation

Methods:

Environmental control:

Remove bedding, clothing

Use of fans,

air conditioners

cooling tents

Increase of fluid intake { oral / parenteral

Special cooling procedures:

Tepid

water sponges

Cool baths

Cooling enemas

Ice packs

Hypothermia blankets

Reduced caloric intake

Rest

Antipyretics

(or specific medications

as indicated)

Maintain or increase

Principles:

Increase metabolism

Decrease { evaporation / radiation / conduction / convection

Cause vasoconstriction

Methods:

Environmental control:

Add bedding, clothing

Use of

incubators,

heaters

Special warming procedures:

Heating pads

Hot-water bottles

Brief warm baths

followed by application

of warm clothing

Increased caloric intake

Exercise

(When appropriate exercise

can help maintain metabolism

and combat cold. Shivering

is involuntary exercise.)

FIG. 28-1   In health, the body keeps its temperature within safe ranges. However, during unusual conditions or illness, normal temperature controls may be disturbed, and special regulating measures may be needed.

shivering. Conversely, removing insulation, increasing surface evaporation, and reducing muscular activity decrease body heat.

Body heat is lost primarily through the dilatation of the capillaries in the skin, the *evaporation* of increased perspiration on the skin's surface, and the process of warming inspired air, which is subsequently exhaled. Heat naturally moves from a warmer to a cooler area or surface. Heat transfer occurs even though objects of different tempera-

tures may not touch. This heat loss, called *radiation*, is more rapid if a significant difference in the temperatures of neighboring objects exists. Placing a body part directly in contact with a surface cooler than itself causes heat loss by *conduction*. Some surfaces remove body heat much more rapidly than others. They are termed "good conductors of heat." Cooler air flowing on the body, particularly the face, can be the source of considerable heat loss by *convection* (conduction to air). All of these mechanisms of heat transfer or loss may become operative, and the nurse trying to conserve a patient's body heat must understand them. For example, a wet, nude newborn may be in serious jeopardy if placed in a draft or in contact with rapidly flowing oxygen while lying on a cool surface near cool walls and supply tables.

The part of the body that ultimately controls the unconscious processes necessary for the regulation of heat production, heat maintenance, and heat loss is thought to be located deep in the brain. The part of the brain considered most responsible for heat regulation is the hypothalamus, often dubbed the "thermostat" of the body. It probably controls the processes of vasoconstriction and vasodilatation, the associated activity of the sweat glands, and the involuntary skeletal muscle motion. Perhaps indirectly it influences the appetite and digestive and metabolic regulation through glandular stimulation or control.

In infants and young children temperature regulation is not perfected, and rather wide swings in body temperature occur readily. During the first days of life an infant is more likely to be influenced by the temperature of the environment; hence the frequent use of incubators. Toddlers and young school-age children often react to the common infectious diseases of childhood by running temperatures of 104° F (40° C) or more. A child may initiate a temperature elevation during a hard crying spell.

Causes and effects of elevated body temperature

At times a temperature elevation may produce a beneficial effect. In fact, fever is often looked on as a protective mechanism, since it helps kill certain heat-susceptible microorganisms and warns the individual of the possible presence of a pathologic process. In the past fever was even artificially induced in the treatment of certain infectious diseases.

Fever is described as a resetting of the body's thermostat in response to the presence of toxins produced by infection. This resetting of the thermostat interrupts normal heat-dissipating mechanisms. The capillaries at the skin's surface contract, causing patients to feel cold, and they shiver, sometimes violently, to reduce the feeling of cold. The muscular activity of shivering further elevates the body temperature.

The skin of chilled patients should be kept sufficiently warm to halt shivering while other means of combating excessive internal temperatures or eliminating the initial cause are instituted. An exaggerated elevated systemic temperature—whether initiated by infectious processes, certain chemicals, or elevated environmental temperatures (heat exhaustion, sunstroke)—can cause serious injury, especially if it is prolonged. It can cause dehydration if adequate fluid intake is not maintained. On the other hand, an abnormal rise in body temperature may result from dehydration due to any cause (vomiting, diarrhea, or poor fluid intake). A frequent companion to high temperature in children is a convulsion. A common phrase in a pediatric setting is "febrile convulsions." The word "febrile" refers to the state of being feverish. A person who has no abnormal temperature elevation may be called "afebrile."

Causes and effects of depressed body temperature

A depressed body temperature may simply reflect inactivity. The early morning temperature reading may be low, only because body processes are at a naturally low ebb. However, an abnormally low systemic temperature may also indicate circulatory collapse or the tiring of basic body processes before death.

For patients undergoing cardiac and thoracic surgery it may be particularly desirable to slow down metabolism during surgery and postoperative care by cooling the body to extremely low temperatures to rest the heart and respiratory system. The narrowing of the blood vessels in the skin that results from surface cooling forces the blood into the interior of the body, increases viscosity (thickens the blood), slows the blood flow, and necessitates less oxygen intake. Uncompensated by muscle activity, the drop in temperature is of therapeutic importance. However, such a severe reduction in metabolism requires special equipment and personnel and cannot be safely maintained indefinitely.

A less drastic reduction in body temperature may increase metabolism because of the body's continuing compensatory efforts to maintain a normal temperature. Such efforts may decrease blood glucose used for fuel and consume more oxygen. This is particularly important to remember when caring for the neonate. At-risk infants subjected to this type of continued cold stress rapidly become hypoglycemic and, in addition, are unable to increase their oxygen intakes sufficiently to meet their metabolic needs. Cellular metabolism in the absence of adequate oxygen produces lactic acid, and acidosis results. Such a sequence of events is to be avoided by maintaining a neutral thermal environment in which an infant is able to maintain body temperature with the least expenditure of energy, enhancing adequate weight gain and proper acid-base balance. A neutral thermal environment for a baby is usually achieved when the abdominal skin temperature registers between 96.8° F (36° C) and 98.6° F (37° C).

Raising body temperature

At times it becomes the duty of the nurse to carry out techniques to maintain or raise body temperature. This may be done to provide comfort, regulate metabolism, or combat exposure. It may be accomplished most simply by increasing room temperatures, applying more blankets, adding clothing, and offering warm but not hot drinks. In the home situation, placing children who have been chilled in a *brief* warm bath, dressing them warmly, and tucking them in bed is a time-honored technique.

In an emergency situation in which no incubator is available, the warmest place for a newborn infant would be directly next to the mother, who could share her own body heat. However, an infant can be most easily warmed by the use of an incubator, a cozy box supplied with a built-in heating unit, or one of the open, radiant-heat infant warmers.

Infant incubator. Incubators are often used to help maintain or gradually increase the body temperature of newborn infants. They allow close observation of a nude or partially clad baby without jeopardizing body temperature. Incubators are plastic enclosures that also may provide additional humidity and oxygen for their small residents. Three basic designs are available: (1) those that have hinged lids that are lifted up to expose the infant; (2) those that, in addition to a hinged lid, provide special portholes or panels for access to the infant (Fig. 28-2); and (3) those that lift up from the side, creating an open, horizontal slitlike access to the infant (Fig. 28-3). Before opening any part of an incubator, the nurse should read the environmental temperature of the air inside and record any oxygen concentration percentage. The baby's body temperature should be recorded with that of the ambient air temperature on the baby's graphic chart. How warm an incubator will be kept to conserve the infant's energy will depend on the baby's gestational age when born, weight, and age postbirth.

In some models of incubators the temperature of the artificial environment may be automatically controlled by the baby's own skin temperature through the use of a heat-sensitive probe taped to the baby. This may be advantageous in maintaining body temperature. Abdominal skin sensor temperatures within a range of 97° to 99° F taken in such an automatically controlled incubator probably indicate a reasonable environmental temperature. However, an early abnormal rise in an infant's temperature may be masked unless the simultaneous records of the temperature of the incubator and the skin of the infant are compared, because as the infant's temperature rises, the heat source will not

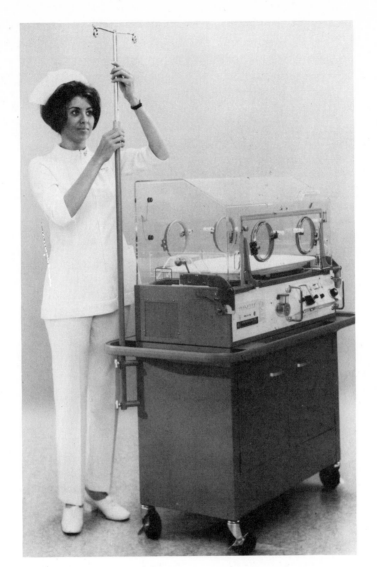

FIG. 28-2   Isolette infant incubator, Model C-86.

Courtesy Isolette—a Narco Medical Co., Warminster, Pa.

be activated and the incubator temperature will decrease. Conversely, if the probe becomes detached from the infant undetected, the unit may overheat. The temperature setting of incubators may also be adjusted manually, depending on the results of intermittent temperature readings.

The application of local heat is helpful in raising total body temperature. The use of hot-water bottles, various heating pads, and hypothermia blankets, which may be regulated to function like giant heating blankets, are discussed in detail on p. 557.

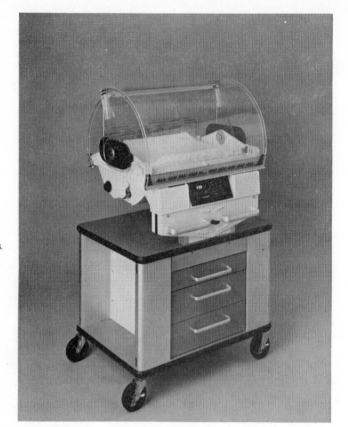

FIG. 28-3

Intensive care incubator.

Courtesy Ohio Medical Products.

Reducing body temperature

A sponge bath is only one method of reducing temperature, and it is usually not the first or only method employed. Approximately six basic ways exist by which one may try to reduce fever or lower body temperature.

Fluid intake. The first method of body temperature reduction involves encouraging fluid intake. It has already been noted that fever may result from dehydration. If oral fluids are impractical because of the state of the gastrointestinal tract or exaggerated body need, frequently fluids must be administered intravenously.

Environmental control. Body temperature may be lowered and the patient made more comfortable by attention to the immediate environment. The removal of extra blankets and heavy clothing (unless the patient is complaining of chills and shivering) is often helpful. A well-ventilated, draft-free room may also be an aid. In warm weather well-placed fans that circulate the air without blowing on the patient directly may be used.

Medication. Medication may be ordered to help reduce fever; such medications are called *antipyretics*. The most frequently prescribed medications are acetylsalicylic acid, commonly known as aspirin, and acetaminophen (Tylenol or Tempra), the nonsalicylate analgesic and antipyretic. They seem to reduce temperature chiefly by producing greater amounts of perspiration and therefore greater cooling by evaporation.

Sponge bath and tepid bath. Tepid water sponge baths are also administered to reduce fever; these are described on p. 561. Sometimes the child will be placed in a tepid tub bath, especially if the child is not sufficiently responsive to other therapy. The temperature of the water is gradually reduced by the addition of cooler water. The child should never be left alone while undergoing such treatment.

Cooling enema. Another method that has been used to reduce fever is the cooling enema. This procedure usually consists of the intermittent administration of cool tap water per rectum. The infant and toddler have little or no sphincter control, and the solution usually returns fairly quickly even before the amount to be given has been completely administered. When treating children of this age group, it is usually unrealistic to speak of clamping the tube for several minutes and then siphoning out the remainder of the fluid before repeating the process. However, even the brief introduction of cool fluid into the lower gastrointestinal tract may prove helpful if the child does not become too upset. Infants under 6 months of age usually do not tolerate more than 100 ml of fluid administered at one time. Infants 6 months and older or toddlers usually are not given more than 250 ml at one time. The efficiency of the enema should be checked by taking the child's temperature 30 minutes after termination of the treatment.

Hypothermia blankets. Patients with temperature elevations that are exaggerated or fail to respond to other methods of treatment may be placed on so-called hypothermia blankets (sort of K-pads in reverse).

Several hypothermia blankets are manufactured. Although the operating instructions on each may differ, the principles involved are similar. Cold, distilled water or alcohol and distilled water (depending on the model) are circulated through tubes embedded in a plastic mat or mats. The water is cooled and circulated by a refrigeration pump unit to which the pads are attached. With some units adjustment of the pad temperature is accomplished manually by the nurse, depending on the patient's temperature. With others a rectal probe is inserted, facilitating continuous monitoring of the patient's temperature. The temperature of the patient registered by the probe may regulate the temperature of the pads automatically, according to predetermined temperature settings. Several pads of various sizes may be used both under and over the patient according to need. A light bath blanket or sheet is always placed between the patient and the plastic pad. The pad should not be folded or creased, and no pins should be used to secure them. The temperature desired and the time it should be maintained should be ordered by the attending physician.

LOCAL APPLICATION OF HEAT OR COLD

Local application of heat

Local application of heat and cold for the treatment of disease may be ancient therapy, but it is also very contemporary. Local heat is frequently ordered to prevent chilling, relieve pain, hasten superficial abscess formation or the drainage of an infected wound, and relieve congestion in one body part by increasing the blood supply to another.

EFFECTS

The primary effect of locally applied heat is vasodilatation of the treated area (the skin becomes warm and pink). Locally applied heat also speeds up metabolism, enhances associated muscle relaxation, increases the temperature of the underlying skin, subcutaneous tissue, and muscle, and even raises the skin temperature of remote body areas. Studies have shown that immersion of an arm in a hot soak will raise the temperature of the big toe. Controversy exists regarding the degree of reflex vasodilatation achieved in *deep* tissues through the application of surface heat. When the effects of heat are desired in the deep-lying organs of the body, diathermy treatments, using high-frequency currents or ultrasound, are often ordered. These treatments are administered using special equipment and are seldom part of the nurse's responsibility. They more properly lie within the sphere of the physical therapist.

DANGERS

The surface application of heat is not without danger. The nurse should never apply heat (other than in the form of extra blankets) without a physician's order.

When an internal abscess or localized infection is suspected (such as appendicitis), local heat should never be applied because of the danger of rupture, subsequent spread of infection, and peritonitis.

Skin temperatures over 110° F (43.3° C) cause tissue damage. However, compresses or soaks that are prepared with solutions above 110° F do not necessarily raise skin temperatures to 110° F. Skin temperatures depend on the extent of the exposure to heat, considering body area, time, method employed, and temperature of the solution.

Water temperatures have been placed by several authors in the following descriptive classifications:

Neutral (warm)	93° F (33.8° C) to 98° F (36.6° C)
Hot	98° F (36.6° C) to 105° F (40.5° C)
Very hot	105° F (40.5° C) to 115° F (46.1° C)

The area receiving heat treatments should be observed frequently for signs of congestion and tissue damage. Nerve endings that detect the presence of hot and cold have the capacity to adjust when temperatures are not extreme and become less sensitive to variations. Temperatures may be increased to an injurious level unless this loss of sensitivity is recognized. Fair-skinned individuals are more likely to be burned than dark-pigmented individuals and should be observed especially closely. Special precautions should be observed when the area to be treated reveals poor circulation or sensory loss. Patients may sustain tissue damage from burning and not realize that they are being burned because of the lack of feeling in the area.

The time interval ordered for heat application should be carefully observed, because if significant warmth is applied to a local area longer than approximately an hour (some say 30 to 45 minutes), a reflex vasoconstriction may reduce the blood supply to the area, and a reverse effect may occur.

METHODS

Dry heat. Dry heat may be administered by an electric heating pad, a hot-water bottle, or a unit that circulates warm water through a plastic pad. An electric heating pad is rarely used in a hospital setting because of the danger of electrical malfunction and the problems of maintenance and disinfection. Hot-water bottles are not recommended because of the many instances of accidental burning that have resulted from their use. If hot-water bottles are employed for infants and young children, they should never contain water hotter than 115° F (46.1° C), although temperatures up to 120° F (48.8° C) are permitted for older children and adults. They should be emptied of excess air, tightly stoppered, and turned upside down to check for leaks. A dry, warm cloth cover should be placed on the bottle to provide proper insulation. Hot-water bottles should not be placed between skin surfaces or under the back.

A plastic pad is often used that contains tubing through which warm water may be circulated at a preset temperature from a bedside heating unit. A well-known appliance of this type is the K-pad (Fig. 28-4). Such an apparatus uses distilled water, which is periodically added to a reservoir at the top of the heating and circulating unit. Warm water is pushed out of the unit, flows through the continuous pattern of tubes embedded in the plastic pad, and returns to the heating unit. No pins should be used in stabilizing the position of the various sized pads available. Pads may be tied or taped in place; however, if they are bent, the warm water may not circulate properly. Ideally, a pad should be neatly wrapped in a pillowcase or towel and the tubing covered with stockinette. Detailed operating instructions accompany the unit.

A commercially available chemical mixture con-

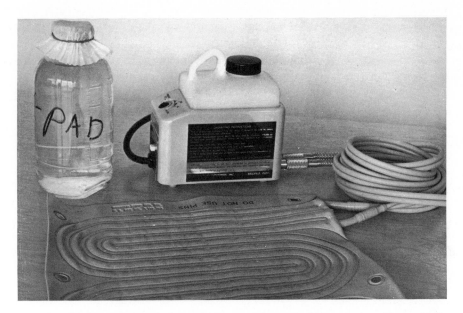

FIG. 28-4   The K-pad circulates distilled water through tubing in a plastic pad at a preset temperature.

Courtesy Grossmont Hospital, La Mesa, Calif.

tained within a waterproof envelope, activated by abruptly striking a premarked spot, represents another method of obtaining dry heat. These units are convenient, disposable, and efficient, but somewhat expensive. In miniature form they may be used as infant heel warmers to enhance capillary dilatation before blood samples are obtained.

Moist heat. Moist heat therapy is more penetrating and faster acting than dry heat therapy. Moist heat is usually applied locally in the form of hot soaks or compresses.

Hot soaks. If the condition of the young child permits such treatment, soaks of body parts when no open skin areas are involved may be carried out as part of a general bath, depending on the reason for the order. If this is not feasible, basins of water or other ordered solution may be provided at the bedside. If the area to be soaked involves an open lesion or wound that is not too extensive, a sterile container is provided for sterile water, tap water, or other solution. (Tap water from an approved

water system is generally accepted as free from disease-producing microorganisms.) However, normal saline solution (properly called physiologic saline solution or sodium chloride, 0.9%) is often preferred because it contains approximately the same salt concentration as normal tissue fluid and therefore will not cause abnormal drying or bogginess in the body tissues. Because sterile physiologic saline solution is usually readily available in the hospital setting, it is often used for soaks involving small body areas. (Physiologic saline solution may be prepared in the home by adding 2 teaspoons of salt to 1 quart of water.) The temperature of hot soaks for children, unless ordered otherwise, is 105° F (40.5° C). The duration of the soak may vary according to orders, but the treatment is usually prescribed for 20 minutes. When the soak is terminated, any open skin area is dried and dressed as ordered.

Soaks involving large body areas are usually carried out in a bathtub. The tub is disinfected before and after use, but the procedure is not really sterile, just clean. Tepid (about 98° F [36.6° C]) body soaks are often ordered for severely burned patients. The soak, in these cases, is not administered as a heat treatment but for the cleansing and debriding action that occurs when the patient's inner dressings are removed in the water and the tub solution is agitated. Frequently such soaks, followed by the application of sterile dressings, are performed in a physical therapy department using a whirlpool bath.

Hot compresses. Application of hot or warm compresses, however, is commonly part of a nurse's responsibilities. They may be applied to speed superficial abscess formation, promote wound drainage, or improve circulation. If the skin in the area to be compressed is broken, sterile gauze is used. The following are general suggestions for warm compress application (usually several alternatives are possible):

1. The procedure should be explained to patients according to their ability to understand and cooperate.

2. The area under the body part to be compressed should be protected by a clean, waterproof material overlaid by an absorbent towel or bath blanket.

3. The sterile gauze pads may be placed in a hot (110° F [43.3° C]) sterile solution as ordered (usually physiologic saline) and wrung with two sterile forceps until dripping stops. The pads may be placed on the designated area and replaced with new compresses about every 2 minutes.

4. In areas where the additional weight will not cause pain or injury, two or three warm compresses may be quickly covered by sterile, lightweight waterproof plastic, and the body part may be wrapped or covered by an insulating towel warmed by an overlying K-pad, hot-water bottle, or low-set electric pad.

Clean warm compresses are applied in much the same manner, except that sterile precautions need not be observed. Wriggly toddlers usually need to have the compresses gently tied in place and fairly constant nursing attendance to prevent the dismantling of the nurse's handiwork. Great care

should be taken not to burn the child. Children should not be left in a position in which they may come into direct contact with the hot water used for heating the compresses.

Local application of cold

EFFECTS

The local application of cold may also be therapeutic. Cold applied to the skin surface for brief periods (30 to 45 minutes) produces vasoconstriction of the area treated, which helps in the prevention (but not treatment) of swelling, the control of hemorrhage, and the retardation of any inflammatory process. Cold applied for a sufficient period will significantly cool muscles and other underlying organs, either directly or by reflex action. Cold also has an anesthetic quality that may sometimes become of primary importance. If applied to the skin for longer periods, cold may trigger a reverse reflex mechanism that results in vasodilatation.

DANGERS

The local use of cold applications, like that of heat, is not without hazard. The skin surface must be frequently observed for mottling and tissue damage. Cold applied to areas in which circulation is inadequate may produce injury (frostbite) and lead to gangrene. The anesthetic quality of cold may make the patient unaware of injury inadvertently produced by other factors.

METHODS

Like heat, cold may be used therapeutically in dry or moist form. Moist cold is more penetrating than dry cold.

Dry cold. An example of the application of dry cold would be the typical ice bag or ice collar. Some of these, like the Freez-A-Bag, are prefilled and sealed. Others must be filled. Small cubes and a small amount of cold water are used to fill two thirds of the bag; all air is pressed out (it delays the transfer of cold), and the bag is capped. The bag should be wrapped in a cover to prevent condensation from wetting the patient or bedding. For effective local reaction an ice cap or ice bag should be removed approximately every 30 to 45 minutes to observe the skin and allow it to return to normal and to enable the cold to continue its process of vasoconstriction when reapplied.

Moist cold. Moist cold may be applied in the form of cold, damp compresses, cold soaks, or sponge baths.

Cold compresses. If the body part compressed can tolerate weight, clean cold compresses are best made from washcloths or towels. If a delicate organ like an eye or an extremely tender body part is to be treated, gauze compresses may be used. The adjoining area is protected by a waterproof plastic or rubber sheet lined with an absorbent layer. A basin of water and ice, large enough to accommodate the compresses, should be at hand. The compresses should be wrung out well to avoid dripping, and once applied, they should be left exposed. Covering it would soon make it only tepid as a result of the heating capability of the body. The compresses have to be changed frequently, depending on their size and density and the temperature of the body part to which they are applied.

It is difficult to apply sterile cold compresses because ice is not sterile. However, if sterile technique is necessary, sterile cold solutions may be maintained in a refrigerator and the sterile container packed in ice at the bedside during the treatment. Sterile compresses may be handled in an aseptic manner with forceps or gloves. We do not recommend the use of forceps around the eyes and faces of young children in the usual bedside setting. Their movements are too unpredictable. Wearing gloves is much less cumbersome and is safer.

Light gauze compresses usually must be changed about every minute to maintain their temperature. If any drainage or open skin area is present, the compress should not be reused but discarded.

Cold soaks. Cold soaks, often recommended to prevent the swelling of a twisted or sprained ankle, usually consist of cold water in a basin into which an extremity is placed for about 20-minute intervals. Occasionally alternating cold and hot soaks are ordered to stimulate circulation.

Sponge baths. Tepid water sponge baths to reduce body temperature are fairly frequent procedures in a pediatric setting. A suggested procedure follows.

Tepid water sponge bath

Purposes: To reduce body temperature and relieve discomfort.

Materials:
1. Waterproof sheet
2. Absorbent bath blanket or towels, depending on the size of the child
3. Light bath blanket to place over the patient
4. Basin of tepid or cool water at approximately 70° F (21.1° C)
5. Small supply of ice to add to the sponging solution, if necessary
6. Four washcloths

Procedure:
1. Explain the procedure to the patient as much as possible.
2. Place the child on top of a waterproof sheeting and absorbent blanket (unless this is already part of the base of the bed) fairly close to the side of the bed so that the child may be easily reached. Remove any pillows.
3. Undress the child and cover with the light bath blanket.
4. Rub the skin of the anterior trunk and extremities briefly with a dry washcloth to bring the blood to the surface, decreasing the sensation of chilling and aiding in heat reduction when the cool moist washcloths are applied.
5. Place cool, moist, but not dripping, folded washcloths on the axilla and groin on the side of the child that you will sponge last.
6. Wash the patient's face and neck with the solution.
7. Expose only the area being sponged. Use firm, long strokes in sponging the upper extremity, thorax, abdomen, and lower extremity on the side farthest from you. Place the washcloths on the groin and axilla of the opposite side. Continue sponging the patient, first the upper extremity, then the thorax, abdomen, and lower extremity.

8. During the sponge bath, periodically evaluate the patient's reaction. How are the child's color, pulse, and respirations? If the child seems to be chilling or shivering excessively, protests and becomes agitated, or if other untoward reactions occur, stop the treatment, lightly cover the patient, and report to the supervising nurse.

9. Turn the patient on the side. Rub and sponge the back firmly.

10. Gently pat the skin dry at the end of the sponge bath with a towel and dress the child in a light gown. The procedure should take about 20 to 25 minutes.

11. Cover the child with a light sheet or blanket. Remove the bed protectors and encourage rest.

12. Check the patient's temperature, pulse, and respiration 30 minutes after the sponge bath and report them to the supervising nurse.

13. Record the procedure, patient's reaction, and results.

The local use of heat or cold applications can be of strategic importance in patient care. It may involve old principles, but they have proved worthy of study and application.

UNIT **8**

SUGGESTED SELECTED READINGS AND REFERENCES

GENERAL

Brunner, L.S., and Suddarth, D.S.: The Lippincott manual of nursing practice, ed. 3, Philadelphia, 1981, J.B. Lippincott Co.

Committee on Standards of Child Health Care, American Academy of Pediatrics: Standards of child health care, ed. 3, Evanston, Ill., 1977, The Academy.

Droske, S.C., Francis, S.A.: Pediatric diagnostic procedures with guidelines for preparing children for clinical tests, New York, 1981, John Wiley & Sons.

Fochsman, D., and Raffensperger, J.G.: Principles of nursing care for the pediatric surgery patient, ed. 2, Boston, 1976, Little, Brown & Co.

Hughes, W.T., and Beuscher, E.S., Pediatric procedures, ed. 2, Philadelphia, 1980, W.B. Saunders Co.

Leifer, G., Principles and techniques in pediatric nursing, Philadelphia, 1982, W.B. Saunders Co.

Pike, B.H., editor: Massachusetts General Hospital manual of pediatric nursing practice, Boston, 1981, Little, Brown & Co.

Whitson, B.J., and McFarlane, J.M.: The pediatric nursing skills manual, New York, 1980, John Wiley & Sons.

PREPARATION FOR HOSPITALIZATION

Atkins, D.M.: Evaluation of a preadmission preparation program: goals clarification as the first step, Child. Health Care 10:48-52, Fall 1981.

Crocker, E.: Preparation for elective surgery: does it make a difference? J. Assoc. Care Child Health 9:3-11, Summer 1980.

Eichelberger, K.M., et al: Self-care nursing plan: helping children to help themselves, Pediatr. Nurs. 6:9-13, May-June 1980.

Gohsman, B., and Yunek, M.: Dealing with the threats of hospitalization, Pediatr. Nurs. 5:32-35, Sept.-Oct. 1979.

Johnson, M., and Salazar, M.: Preadmission program for rehospitalized children, Am. J. Nurs. 79:1420-1422, Aug. 1979.

PREPARING CHILDREN FOR PROCEDURES

Bubb, D.: Teaching patients about brain scans, RN 44:64-65, Dec. 1981.

Campbell, J.: The BSA method of calculating pediatric drug dosages, Am. J. Mat. Child Nurs. 3:357-360, Nov.-Dec. 1978.

Evans, M.L., and Hansen, B.D.: Administering injections to different-aged children, Am. J. Mat. Child Nurs. 6:194-199, May-June 1981.

Fassler, D., and Wallace, N.: Clinical essay: children's fear of needles, Clin. Pediatr. 21:59-60, Jan. 1982.

Hansen, B.D., and Evans, M.L.: Preparing a child for procedures, Am. J. Mat. Child Nurs. 6:392-397, Nov.-Dec. 1981.

McConnell, E.: Injections with finesse, RN 45:24-34, Feb. 1982.

Mills, G.C.: Preparing children and parents for cerebral computerized tomography, Am. J. Mat. Child Nurs. 5:403-407, Nov.-Dec. 1980.

Newton, D.W., and Newton, M.: Route, site, and technique: three key decisions in giving parenteral medications, Nurs. '79 9:18-25, July 1979.

HOSPITAL PROCEDURES

Bell, E.A.: Charting: how to get out of a rut, Nurs. '81 11:43, Mar. 1981.

Bishop, B.: How to cool a feverish child, Pediatr. Nurs. 4:19-20, Jan. 1978.

Eggland, E.T.: Charting: document your care daily and fully, Nurs. '80 10:38-43, Feb, 1980.

Freeman, P., and Boyer, J.: How to get the most out of op-site, RN 45:36-39, Jan. 1982.

Hoppe, M.: The new tube feeding sets: a Nursing '80 product survey, Nurs. '80 10:79-85, Mar. 1980.

Schreiner, R.L., et al: Infant lumbar puncture: a teaching simulator, Clin. Pediatr. 20:298-299, Apr. 1981.

VITAL SIGNS

Castle, M., and Watkins, J.: Fever: understanding a sinister sign, Nurs. '79 9:26-33, Feb. 1979.

Eoff, M.J., and Joyce, B.: Temperature measurements in children, Am. J. Nurs. **81**:1010-1011, May 1981.

Fisher, R.E.: Measuring central venous pressure: how to do it accurately—and safely, Nurs. '79 **9**:74-78, Oct. 1979.

Harris, R.D., et al: The child-adolescent blood pressure study. I. Distribution of blood pressure levels in the Seventh Day Adventist (SDA) and Non-SDA children, Am. J. Public Health **71**:1342-1349, Dec. 1981.

Kinnebrem, M.N.: Add paradoxical pulse to your assessment routine, RN **44**:32-33, Nov. 1981.

Pepler, C.J.: Your fingers on the pulse: evaluating what you feel, Nurs. '80 **10**:32-39, Nov. 1980.

Stright, P.A., and Soukup, S.M.: How to hear it right: evaluating and choosing a stethoscope, Am. J. Nurs. **77**:1477, Sept. 1977.

COLLECTING LABORATORY SPECIMENS

Gurevich, I.: The new urine meters: a Nursing '80 product survey, Nurs. '80 **10**:47-52, Dec. 1980.

Hargiss, C.O., and Larson, E.: How to collect specimens and evaluate results, Am. J. Nurs. **81**:2166-2174, Dec. 1981.

Hutton, N.M., and Schreiner, R.L.: Urine collection in the neonate: effect of different methods on volume, specific gravity, and glucose, JOGN Nurs. **9**:165-169, May-June 1980.

Marchiondo, K.: The very fine art of collecting culture specimens, Nurs. '79 **9**:34-43, Apr. 1979.

McArthur, B.J.: Microbiology: a concern for nursing, Nurs. Clin. North Am. **15**:655-688, Dec. 1980.

Shetler, M.G., and Bartos, H.: Collecting synovial fluid and wound drainage cultures, RN **44**:50-53, Feb. 1981.

Shetler, M.G., and Bartos, H.: Culture specimens: how to collect, what to expect, RN **43**:65-69, Sept. 1980.

Shetler, M.G., and Bartos, H.: Eye and ear cultures, RN **44**:58-61, Mar. 1981.

Shetler, M.G., and Bartos, H.: Spinal and peritoneal taps, RN **44**:50-53, Jan. 1981.

Shetler, M.G., and Bartos, H.: Stool specimens: key to detecting intestinal invaders, RN **43**:50-53, Oct. 1980.

Tucker, J.B., et al: Throat culturing techniques in the family practice model unit, J. Fam. Pract. **12**:925-931, May 1981.

TRACTION

Mentink, D.: Especially for those in traction, J. Assoc. Care Child Health **8**:36-38, Fall 1979.

Nursing care of a patient in traction: programmed instruction, Am. J. Nurs. **79**:1771-1798, Oct. 1979.

Swanson, V.M.: The school-age traction patient: toward better behavior patterns, J. Assoc. Care Child Health **9**:12-14, Summer 1980.

BLOOD GASES

Brantigan, C.O.: Hemodynamic monitoring: interpreting values, Am. J. Nurs. **82**:86-89, Jan. 1982.

Clark, B.: Getting those blood samples right, RN **44**:36-41, Dec. 1981.

Milhorn, H.T.: Understanding arterial blood gases, Am. Fam. Physicians, **21**:112-120, Mar. 1980.

Shrake, K.: The ABCs of ABGs—or how to interpret a blood gas value, Nurs. '79 **9**:26-33, Sept. 1979.

Worthington, L.: What those blood gases can tell you, RN **42**:22-27, Oct. 1979.

INTRAVENOUS THERAPY

Aisenstein, T.: Those all-too-common IV complications, RN **44**:38-44, Mar. 1981.

Bjeletich, J., and Hickman, R.O.: The Hickman indwelling catheter, Am. J. Nurs. **80**:62-65, Jan. 1980.

Buickus, B.: Administering blood components, Am. J. Nurs. **79**:937-940, May 1979.

Cullins, L.C.: Preventing and treating transfusion reactions, Am. J. Nurs. **79**:935-936, May 1979.

Guhlow, L.J., and Kolb, J.: Pediatric IVs: special measures you must take, RN **42**:41-51, Mar. 1979.

Huxley, V.: Heparin lock: how, what, why, RN **42**:36-41, Oct. 1979.

Intravenous therapy: fundamentals of IV maintenance: a programmed unit, Am. J. Nurs. **79**:1274-1287, July 1979.

Masoorlie, S.T.: Trouble-free IV starts, RN **44**:20-27, Feb. 1981.

McGrath, B.J.: Fluids, electrolytes and replacement therapy in pediatric nursing, Am. J. Mat. Child Nurs. **5**:58-62, Jan.-Feb. 1980.

Newton, M., Gilbert, J.P., and Newton, D.W.: Parenteral antibiotics: the hazards to watch for, RN **44**:44-51, Mar. 1981.

Parfitt, D.M., and Thompson, V.D.: Pediatric home hyperalimentation: educating the family, Am. J. Mat. Child Nurs. 5:196-202, May-June 1980.

Piercy, S.: A care plan that really works for children on long-term IV therapy, Nurs. '81 11:66-69, Sept. 1981.

Schmidt, A., and Williams, D.: The amazing Hickman and its easy home care, RN 45:57-61, Feb. 1982.

Thomas, S.F.: Transfusing granulocytes, Am. J. Nurs. 79:942-944, May 1979.

Woodland, C.: How to make infusion control devices work for you, RN 44:58-63, Nov. 1981.

SUPPORTING RESPIRATION

Albanese, A., and Riley, J.: Caring for the intubated patient, RN 43:38-43, Apr. 1980.

Albanese, A., and Toplitz, A.: A hassle-free guide to suctioning a tracheostomy, RN 45:24-29, Apr. 1982.

Benchot, R.S.: Tracheostomy care in infants and young children, Ethicon/Point of View 18:8-9, 1981.

Bolton, M.E.: Hyperbaric oxygen therapy, Am. J. Nurs. 81:1199-1201, June 1981.

Erickson, R.: Chest tubes: they're really not that complicated, Nurs. '81 11:34-43, May 1981.

Erickson, R.: Solving chest tube problems, Nurs. '81 11:62-68, June 1981.

Foster, S., and Hoskins, D.: Home care of the child with a tracheostomy tube, Pediatr. Clin. North Am. 28:855-857, Nov. 1981.

Fuchs, P.L.: Getting the best of oxygen delivery systems, Nurs. '80 10:34-43, Dec. 1980.

Fuchs, P.L.: Understanding continuous mechanical ventilation, Nurs. '79 9:26-33, Dec. 1979.

Haghenbeck, K.: Quick! Your first move when a patient chokes? RN 42:55-62, Dec. 1979.

Hoops, E.J.: Cardiopulmonary resuscitation of children, Nurs. Clin. North Am. 16:623-634, Dec. 1981.

How to do postural drainage, Am. J. Nurs. 81:525-526, Mar. 1981.

How to work with chest tubes: programmed instruction, Am. J. Nurs. 80:685-712, Apr. 1980.

Kennedy, A.H., Johnson, W.G., and Sturdevant, E.W.: An educational program for families of children with tracheostomies, Am. J. Mat. Child Nurs. 7:42-49, Jan.-Feb. 1982.

Kulberg, A.: CPR in the very young, Emerg. Med. 13:154-176, Sept. 1981.

McFadden, R.: Decreasing the infant's respiratory compromise during suctioning, Am. J. Nurs. 81:2158-2161, Dec. 1981.

Monitoring with telemetry, Nurs. '80 10:61-64, Oct. 1980.

Orlowski, J.P.: Cardiopulmonary resuscitation in children, Pediatr. Clin. North Am. 27:495-512, Aug. 1980.

Preventing and correcting tube and cuff problems in artificial airways, Nurs. '80 10:65-67, Jan. 1980.

Proctor, A.: Pediatric arrest: scaling down CPR, RN 42:58-64, Sept. 1979.

Pulmonary function tests in patient care: programmed instruction, Am. J. Nurs. 80:1135-1161, June 1980.

Tecklin, J.S.: Positioning, percussing and vibrating patients for effective bronchial drainage, Nurs. '79 9:64-71, Mar. 1979.

Waldron, M.W.: Oxygen transport, Am. J. Nurs. 79:272-275, Feb. 1979.

Worthington, L.: Hypoxemia: giving oxygen isn't enough, RN 43:48-53, May 1980.

COMMON PEDIATRIC PROBLEMS AND THEIR NURSING CARE

CHAPTER **29**   Conditions involving

the integumentary system

The integumentary system consists of the skin as well as the hair, nails, sweat and oil glands, and superficial sensory nerve endings. These organs form the first line of defense against body injury. The integumentary system prevents both excessive loss of fluid from the body and the entry of certain poisons and microbes into the body. It is of special importance in the regulation of body temperature, principally through capillary dilatation and constriction and the formation of cooling perspiration. The skin can be an important avenue of fluid loss. However, it has only limited powers of absorption. It is of considerable aid in the evaluation of environmental conditions and therefore in the determination of individual safety. Embedded within the tissues of the integumentary system are nerve endings that relay to the brain sensations of pressure, touch, hot, cold, and pain.

The health of the skin is often a reflection of the health of the individual. Skin color, hydration, and the presence of detectable surface irregularities and disturbances in sensation may reveal significant information about an individual's health habits and status. The skin may also give clues to a patient's emotional reactions. Involuntarily, a person may blush with embarrassment or pale with fright.

LAYERS OF THE SKIN (FIG. 29-1)

The epidermis is paper thin and consists of several microscopic layers. The uppermost layer consists of dead cells ready to be shed from the body's surface. They are constantly being replaced by new cells, which are formed in the lower layers. The lower layers of the epidermis secure their nourishment from the dermis, or true skin, over which they lie.

The dermis, also called the *corium*, is a dense layer of connective tissue well supplied with blood vessels and nerves. It also contains sweat and oil glands and hair follicles, some of which may extend into the deeper subcutaneous tissue. Small muscle fibers may be attached to the hair follicles.

The subcutaneous layer is chiefly fatty tissue in a framework of elastic and fibrous tissue. It serves multiple functions including those of lipid storage and insulation.

The observation of the skin and the description of its condition is often the nurse's responsibility. Her patients may not be hospitalized primarily because of skin problems. Skin difficulties may be, at times, of secondary importance in the diagnostic picture. However, the condition of the skin is always of significance as the nurse views her patient's total needs.

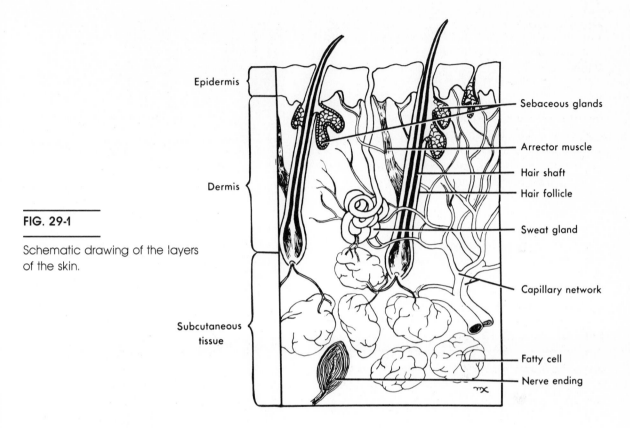

Epidermis

Dermis

Subcutaneous
tissue

Sebaceous glands

Arrector muscle

Hair shaft

Hair follicle

Sweat gland

Capillary network

Fatty cell

Nerve ending

FIG. 29-1

Schematic drawing of the layers
of the skin.

KEY VOCABULARY

Physicians commonly use certain terms to describe the condition of the skin. Some of the words the nurse may wish to use in her own recording. Others she may not employ, but she should be able to interpret their meanings. These terms are simply defined as follows:

abrasion (adj., abraded) Loss of superficial tissue by friction (chafing).

contusion (adj., contused) A bruise; a black-and-blue mark.

crust (adj., crusted) Temporary covering of a lesion formed primarily by dried blood or serum (scab).

ecchymosis (adj., ecchymotic) Black-and-blue mark.

erosion (adj., eroded) Moist, circumscribed, often depressed lesion.

erythema (adj., erythematous) Reddened areas of the skin.

excoriation (adj., excoriated) Superficial laceration; a scratch.

jaundice or *icterus* (adj., jaundiced or icteric) Yellow tinge to the skin or sclerae.

laceration (adj., lacerated) Jagged cut or tear.

lesion Any change or irregularity in tissue caused by disease or injury.

macule (adj., macular) Flat spot or stain; the typical measles rash is macular.

papule (adj., papular) Small, solid elevation on the skin; the typical early stage of a pimple is papular.

petechia (adj., petechial) Small bluish purple dot caused by capillary hemorrhage.

pruritus (adj., pruritic) Itching.

pustule (adj., pustular) Pus-filled vesicle; a superficial cutaneous abscess.

ulcer (adj., ulcerated) Raw area often depressed or forming a cavity, caused by loss of normal covering tissue.

urticaria (wheals and hives) (adj., urticarial) Large, slightly raised, reddened or blanched areas, usually accompanied by intense itching.

vesicle (adj., vesicular) Small elevation of the skin obviously containing fluid such as a blister.

A skin lesion should be described in such a way that the following information is included:

1. Size (described in metric measurements, such as 1 cm in diameter)
2. Elevation (raised, flat, depressed)
3. Quality (smooth, rough, scaly, moist)
4. Color
5. Distribution (localized, scattered, etc.)
6. Associated sensory disturbances (numbness, itching, pain, burning, etc.)
7. Type of any drainage or exudate noted

COMMON SKIN PROBLEMS

The infant and toddler

MILIARIA RUBRA (PRICKLY HEAT, OR HEAT RASH)

Miliaria rubra is a common problem caused by blockage of the sweat pores. The exits of the sweat ducts are plugged, causing sweat to seep into the dermis or epidermis. This produces a red, pinhead-sized vesicular-papular rash associated with underlying erythema, especially in areas where perspiration is common or friction is frequent. It may be accompanied by considerable itching. Occasionally the rash may include pustular lesions. Prevention is easier than treatment; avoid overdressing children. Any procedure that will reduce the need for perspiration will help improve the condition. Light dusting of the skin with a fine cornstarch or baby powder may be beneficial. Some dermatologists may recommend the use of a skin lotion containing hydrocortisone. In the event of secondary infection an antibiotic drug may be prescribed.

INTERTRIGO

Intertrigo, often simply called *chafing*, is commonly found in the folds of the skin where friction is frequent and hygiene may be lacking. Examples

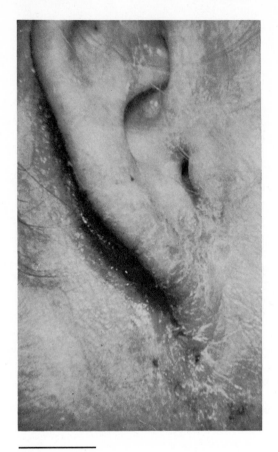

FIG. 29-2

Seborrheic dermatitis.
Courtesy W.W. Duemling, M.D., San Diego, Calif.

of problem areas include the creases in the neck and in the folds of the groin and gluteal muscles, where the skin may become inflamed. As in miliaria rubra, prevention is more simple than cure. Meticulous hygiene and keeping the area dry and lightly powdered is of great importance.

SEBORRHEIC DERMATITIS (FIG. 29-2)

Seborrheic dermatitis is a common dermatitis of infants up to 3 months of age. It is a disorder of unknown origin, usually benign and self-limited, but it can be chronic and is often confused with atopic dermatitis. Seborrheic dermatitis is characterized by a scaly eruption (scales may be dry or greasy) on an inflammatory base; it chiefly affects the scalp, eyebrows, eyelids, and pubic regions. In infants seborrheic dermatitis is seen most commonly as "milk crust" or "cradle cap," yellowish, slightly adherent large scales found principally on the top of the head. It sometimes is related to a parent's reluctance to wash the soft spot on the baby's scalp for fear of causing injury. It also develops fairly often in the groin and may become secondarily infected with yeast (*Candida* or *Monilia*) or bacteria. Frequent shampooing and the use of mild medications containing sulfur, salicylic acid, or hydrocortisone are often prescribed for seborrheic dermatitis. In adolescents it is often associated with acne. When the condition involves the scalp, the common name is dandruff.

Some children are affected by another form called intertriginous seborrhea, which is usually moist and involves areas behind the ear and the axillary and inguinal regions.

DIAPER RASH

Infants with diaper rash are believed to have an irritant dermatitis, but seborrhea dermatitis and eczema are other considerations. The rash may take multiple forms from simple erythema to blisters and ulceration, depending on the causes. As a group, children with irritation of the diaper area usually have sensitive skins—a predisposition said to be inherited. Unfavorable conditions quickly trigger an unfavorable response. Situations that often set the scene for skin problems are poorly washed and rinsed diapers, infrequent diaper changes aggravated by prolonged use of plastic diaper covers, and incomplete or infrequent washing and drying of the diaper area. Careful attention to cleanliness is necessary. However, overzealous ministrations can cause problems, too!

To reduce the formation of irritating ammonia produced by the action of bacteria on urine, every effort is made to cut down the bacterial population on the diaper area. The use of a gentle antiseptic final rinse, such as methylbenzethonium chloride (Diaparene), is often recommended. The use of antiseptic rinses by diaper laundries is standard practice.

The cautious application of dry heat to diaper rash often improves the skin condition. A gooseneck lamp with a 25-watt bulb may be positioned over the prone infant. Precautions against burning should be observed. The lamp should be out of the child's reach and away from the bed linens. The bulb should be at least 12 inches (20.3 cm) from the child's buttocks. During heat treatments the diaper area should be free of medications. If the application of heat is difficult, simply exposing the area to the air is frequently helpful. Sunshine, if present, can be used for brief periods, but an infant should be carefully watched for overexposure.

Cornstarch or a fine baby powder to decrease area moisture is usually an aid. Desitin, hydrocortisone, and certain antimicrobial agents, such as Polysporin and nystatin cream, may be ordered, depending on the needs of the particular patient. In general occlusive medications should be avoided (for example, nystatin cream is preferred to nystatin ointment).

INFANTILE ECZEMA (ATOPIC DERMATITIS) (FIG. 29-3)

Infantile eczema most often appears after the second month of life. It often subsides considerably after the second year. It is characterized by skin lesions, which first appear as localized, scaling, red areas, usually on the head, neck, wrists, flexor surfaces of the elbows, and knees, although involvement may become progressively more extensive. Fairly rapidly, small vesicles, which break and weep serum (a yellow, sticky fluid) develop in these reddened areas. The fluid dries, forming crusts on the skin. Lesions on various parts of the body may be in different stages of development—some moist, others dried and scaling. The skin may become thickened and fissured. Since itching is intense, the child invariably scratches the lesions, and thus secondary infection is usually present. For this reason different types of topical medications may be applied to the parts of the body, depending

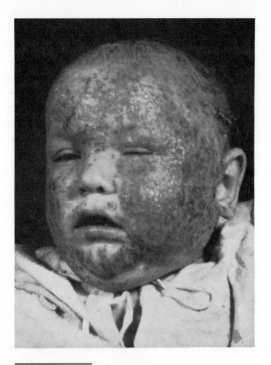

FIG. 29-3

Infant with severe eczema.

Courtesy R.B. Pappenfort, M.D., San Diego, Calif.

on the aims of the treatment. Seborrheic dermatitis and fungal infections may be associated with atopic dermatitis. Permanent scarring does not usually occur unless the lesions become secondarily infected or deeply excoriated.

Infantile eczema is considered to be essentially an allergic response. It is, more properly, a symptom of a disorder rather than the disorder itself. Infantile eczema has been called the most frequent manifestation of the allergic state in infancy. It is not always clear, however, just what agents, or *allergens*, cause the dermatitis. Exposure to allergens may occur in any of the following ways:

1. By ingestion (common foods causing difficulties in infancy are cow's milk, egg whites, wheat products, and citrus juices)
2. By inhalation (dust, pollen, and animal dander)

3. By skin contact with some medications and materials (rubber, plastic, and wool)

Many investigators believe that child-parent relationships and emotional stress play a significant role in the initiation and course of the disease. There is often a family history of allergy manifested by eczema, asthma, or hay fever. Eczema usually improves during the summer months and worsens during the winter.

Many factors must be considered in the treatment of eczema. If possible, the offending allergens should be identified and eliminated from the infant's environment. Secondary infection, if present, should be treated, and itching, scratching, and exposure to known infections should be avoided. Treatment of the lesions to clear scaling, minimize discomfort, and improve appearance is continued. Psychologically, supportive care for the child and the family is of great importance.

To identify those substances that may initiate the dermatitis, a careful history is taken by the physician. For the infant or toddler an elimination diet is often prescribed in which the foods that are allowed are listed in detail. If the baby is not breast-fed, evaporated milk, goat's milk, or soybean milk may be prescribed. The importance of rigidly following the diet must be impressed on the parents. As time goes on, more foods are added, one by one, to the diet. The child is carefully observed for changes in skin condition and general health after each addition.

The home environment of the infant must be carefully controlled also. Since many children with allergic symptoms of the respiratory tract show sensitivity to dust, their nurseries are stripped of all drapes, rugs, and fuzzy toys. The crib mattress is encased in a nonallergenic cover, and wool blankets or clothing are eliminated. Although infants do not usually have pets, the presence of a dog or cat in the household may cause significant problems, and so, sad to relate, pets must sometimes find new homes. However, fish and turtles generally do not cause allergies. The house should be frequently vacuumed with special attention to the child's sleeping quarters. Skin testing with special patches and scratch technique in an effort to determine allergens is usually reserved for older children.

The child with eczema should be protected against contact with people who have staphylococcal, streptococcal, or viral infections such as herpes simplex (the cause of the common fever blister). In many hospitals the child with eczema is placed on isolation precautions; however, routine isolation creates problems of its own—psychologic stress and financial strain!

To help reduce scratching, which increases the possibility of secondary infection, various methods are used. Efforts are made to decrease the itching by the use of a minimum of clothing, all softly textured. Diapers are changed frequently. Fingernails and toenails are trimmed short. Formerly the baby's arms were restrained in some way. Restraints are no longer recommended unless all other methods of control fail.

Different types of medications are used. Systemic antihistaminic drugs may be tried to ease itching. Sedation may be ordered to allow the infant to sleep. Erythromycin may be useful in combating secondary infection. Bacitracin and neomycin are recommended for local application for the same reason. Various topical creams containing hydrocortisone may be used to reduce inflammatory response if infection is not present.

If coal tar preparations are used, care should be taken not to expose the areas to sunshine because a chemical reaction, which in itself is irritating to the skin, may take place. Jars containing coal tar preparations should be tightly closed to prevent deterioration. Coal tar ointment should be removed in special baths or with liquid petrolatum before a new application is made.

Medications are applied with clean hands or a finger cot or glove. They are generally used on a small area on a trial basis to test skin reaction. Many of these medications are expensive and should not be wasted.

Sometimes special baths or soaks are prescribed for the infant to help remove crusts and reduce pruritus and weeping. Common ingredients added to the bath water are cornstarch, oatmeal preparations (such as Aveeno), or bicarbonate of soda solutions. The water should be tepid, about 95° F (35°

C). If possible, a small baby bathtub should be used. Sometimes the skin of the infant is so dry that the physician restricts bathing. In routine bathing a soap substitute is regularly used.

Continuous, tepid, wet, medicated compresses are sometimes employed to dry weeping crusted lesions. Therapeutic compresses must be *kept wet* to accomplish the aim of the treatment. This type of compress or gauze bandage is not covered by waterproof material but is left exposed to cool the area by evaporation.

Older children may undergo so-called desensitization procedures. Through the injection of small but gradually increasing amounts of allergen, the body is sometimes able to tolerate the substance eventually without untoward reaction.

The course of infantile eczema is usually not one of steady improvement. The child will improve, have a relapse, and improve again. The parents should be told to prepare themselves for a rather long siege of skin difficulty. However, after 2 years of age a respite can usually be expected. Unfortunately, as eczema disappears other types of allergy manifestations such as asthma or hay fever may develop. The child with eczema is infrequently hospitalized because of the increased exposure to infection (despite precautions), the emotional upset that may occur in the child as a result of the change of environment, and the need for the "maternal figure." However, parental exhaustion and tension may be considered a factor in obtaining an admission to the pediatric unit of a hospital.

The preschool-age and young school-age child

IMPETIGO (FIG. 29-4)

Impetigo is a skin infection caused by either coagulase-positive staphylococci or beta-hemolytic streptococci. It is highly contagious and serious in newborn infants and fairly contagious but less serious among children and adults. It is often associated with poor hygiene. Inflammation begins with the appearance of reddish spots on the skin, which

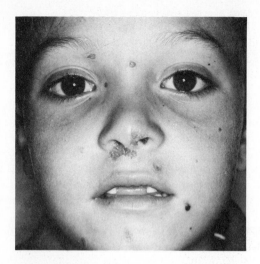

FIG. 29-4

Impetigo.

Courtesy David Allen, M.D., San Diego, Calif.

develop into small blisters. These blisters become pus filled and break, causing thick yellow-red crusts on older children but few crusts on infants. When the crusts are removed, small superficial erosions are seen. The face and hands are the areas most frequently affected, but other body areas may become involved. In the hospital, isolation is indicated.

Treatment includes careful cleansing and removal of the crusts, with compresses if necessary, and the use of neomycin-bacitracin ointment. A course of penicillin or erythromycin administered systemically is recommended because of the demonstrated association between certain strains of beta-hemolytic streptococci and nephritis. Also, a more rapid improvement of the lesions is seen when systemic therapy is used. The nurse should be especially cautious in the care of the lesions and disposal of infected material because the infection spreads easily. The child's fingernails should be clipped short. The dermatitis usually responds well to treatment.

FURUNCLES AND CARBUNCLES

Furuncles and carbuncles are deep infections of the hair follicles. They may occur singly or in groups. If the furuncles run together, forming one sore with several draining points, the resulting lesion is called a carbuncle. Carbuncles are uncommon in small children but are seen with greater frequency among adolescent boys. A furuncle begins as a single papule associated with a hair. The papule becomes a pustule, which enlarges and forms a head. At this time the physician incises and drains the "boil." Warm compresses or soaks may be ordered to prepare the lesion for lancing. If multiple furuncles are present, systemic antibiotic therapy may be prescribed.

STY, OR HORDEOLUM

A sty, an infection involving an eyelash follicle, will usually clear spontaneously or may be incised.

RINGWORM OF THE SCALP, SKIN, AND FEET (FIG. 29-5)

Ringworm of the scalp, or *tinea capitis*, used to be fairly common among school-aged children and is still seen from time to time, particularly in urban areas. It can be caused by several kinds of fungi. Some types of fungi are contracted from human beings, whereas others are contracted from animals. The fungus attacks hairs at their bases, causing them to break off close to the skin and leave circular balding areas. The scalp in the area of the hair loss may become red and scaly. Mild itching may be present. Diagnosis is usually made on the basis of the clinical history, an ultraviolet light called *Wood's lamp,* or a microscopic examination of the affected hairs. Some fungi that commonly cause ringworm of the scalp fluoresce brightly when exposed to the rays of Wood's lamp. In the past, treatment of ringworm was difficult, and the disease had a tendency to become chronic, usually healing spontaneously at puberty. Treatment included shaving the head. Boys and girls wore little stocking caps in an effort to cover the hair loss and prevent the spread of the disease. X-ray treat-

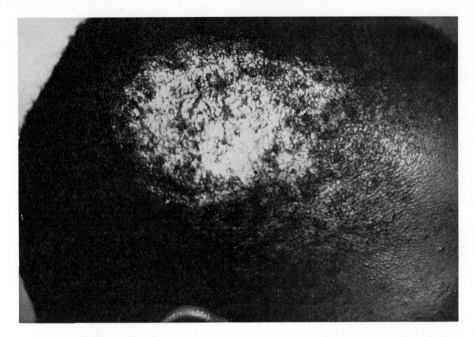

FIG. 29-5   Tinea capitis (ringworm of the scalp).

Courtesy W.W. Duemling, M.D., San Diego, Calif.

ment was sometimes prescribed. The oral administration of the antibiotic griseofulvin has been successful. The drug does not kill the fungus but prevents its spread into uninfected cells. As the infected cells are shed or removed, they are replaced by healthy cells. Clipping of the affected hair after a few weeks of treatment is also desirable. In addition, a local antifungal ointment may be ordered.

Ringworm of the skin may involve various areas, including the face, neck, arms, and hands. Although there are exceptions, the classic lesion of ringworm of the skin is rounded or circular with a gradually extending, small, raised vesicular border with central healing. The lesion may vary considerably in size, but it is usually about the size of a quarter. Treatment consists of prevention of scratching and application of one of several topical remedies such as Tinactin (tolnaftate 1%), haloprogin (Halotex), Monistat-Derm and clotrimazole (Lotrimin). Local treatment is combined with sys-

temic use of griseofulvin in some cases.

Ringworm of the feet, *tinea pedis*, or so-called athlete's foot, is essentially limited to postpubescent children. Younger children with scaling of the feet usually have some form of eczema. However, it is discussed here with the other types of ringworm. Ringworm of the feet is most often characterized by itching or burning of the feet, blisters, and painful cracks between the toes. At times it may extend to involve other areas and become serious. It is caused by several kinds of fungi. Treatment consists of the use of griseofulvin or Nizoral. Better ventilation of the feet and the reduction of sweating in the area are helpful. Frequent changing of socks is a necessity. If the infection has been intense and tends to recur, the advisability of discarding shoes worn during the infection should be considered. Antifungal preparations such as Desenex or Whitfield's ointment, in addition to those already mentioned, are often used locally but are ineffective unless combined with griseofulvin. The feet should be carefully dried. A prophylactic anti-fungal dusting powder is often advised for susceptible persons. For the protection of other people, victims should not use public showers or swimming pools.

PEDICULOSIS, OR LOUSE INFESTATIONS

Although there are three types of lice—head lice, body lice, and pubic lice—only one type is of significance to children, *pediculosis capitis*, or infestation of the hair of the head by lice. This condition is often seen in neglected children of lower socioeconomic levels. However, children who are well cared for may inadvertently become exposed and contract the infestation, much to their parents' shock!

The parasitic head louse causes itching as it travels on the scalp. Small, grayish, oval eggs called *nits* are laid and attached to the base of the hair shafts with a type of mucilage produced by the louse (Fig. 29-6). As the hair grows, the nits become more visible; they resemble tiny flakes of dandruff except that they do not brush out. New lice hatch within 1 week, and the cycle repeats. Pediculosis is often accompanied by excoriation and secondary infection caused by scratching.

Old-style treatment involved the local use of crude oil or kerosene. More acceptable and highly effective are shampoos of lindane (Kwell) or crotamiton (Eurex). Because of the potential systemic absorption of lindane and potential nervous system toxicity causing convulsions if product directions are not observed, some clinicians are prescribing crotamiton for children under 50 pounds. At the end of the treatment, the hair should be combed with a fine-tooth comb to remove the devitalized nits. Warm vinegar solution also aids in the mechanical detachment of nits. The entire family of an affected person should be treated, if possible.

SCABIES

Scabies is a superficial infestation by the itch mite (*Acarus scabiei*, or *Sarcoptes scabiei*). The female mite burrows under the skin, making a tunnel about ½ inch (1.2 cm) long, which is visible as

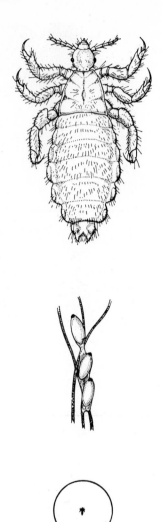

FIG. 29-6

Top, the female head louse (enlarged); center, an enlargement of nits on hair shafts; bottom, life-sized louse.

an elevated line from the skin's surface. The insect is so small that it is rarely visible to the naked eye. Scabies usually involves those body areas where the skin is moist and thin—between the fingers and toes, in the axillae, and on the groin and abdominal areas. The itch mite causes itching, as the name indicates. Various treatments are now available. Lindane (Kwell) may be applied in cream form to cool, dry skin. Instructions for application and removal should be carefully followed. The entire family of an affected person should receive therapy, if possible.

The adolescent

ACNE VULGARIS

Vulgar means "common," and acne vulgaris is a skin inflammation that is exceedingly common among teenage boys and girls. It may exist in a very mild form, or it may be extremely severe. There are probably several causes that, appearing together, produce the problem. When acne is present, it first appears, almost without exception, at the time of puberty. Hormone levels in the body are believed to play a role. Many times the parents of the affected child also experienced similar difficulty; therefore hereditary factors are not discounted.

The production of sebum, or fatty secretion of the oil glands, is stimulated by certain hormones during adolescence, and several types of skin microorganisms utilize sebum as a food source and change it into irritating fatty acids that cause acne. The pores clog, and blackheads (plugs of keratin, sebum, and microorganisms, also called *comedones*, the primary lesions of acne) form. The pores may also be clogged with dirt, but blackheads are not commonly caused by dirt particles but by oxidation of the top of the plug, a process that may occur no matter how carefully the adolescent washes. Plugging of the oil ducts may lead to papules, pustules, and, at times, cyst formation and permanent scarring.

Since acne most often occurs on the face, shoulders, and back, it is of great cosmetic and psychologic concern. The teenager should be given professional help during this distressing period so that the interval is as short and free from complications as possible. Acne fosters a sense of inferiority and social insecurity at a difficult period in life.

Treatment includes a review of general health habits. Little emphasis is now placed on avoidance of carbohydrates and fatty foods such as chocolate, nuts, and peanut butter, and a well-balanced diet is stressed. Lack of sleep, nervous tension, and menstrual problems may lead to a flare-up. Mild cases are treated with topical measures such as antibacterial detergent soaps or skin cleansers (Fostex or Acne-Aid) and lotions containing *keratolytic* compounds (salicylic acid, resorcin) or other agents (Benzoyl Peroxide, tretinoin [Retin-A]). Girls are advised to avoid oily makeup and moisturizers, but there are numerous tinted antibacterial creams or lotions available that help heal and mask the lesions—a very important psychologic consideration. Frequent shampooing is often helpful. Patients should be instructed not to press or scratch the lesions, because this may break down tissue walls and spread infection. However, despite this advice, most patients find it extremely difficult not to tamper with the lesions they see in the mirror. The physician may remove comedones in the office with a special extractor or give careful instructions to the patient's family regarding the removal of comedones. The drug treatment of choice in advanced cases includes either tetracycline or erythromycin to kill the bacteria.

Usually acne is self-limiting and subsides in 3 or 4 years. However, severe cases may persist into middle age. The partial removal of scarred tissue may be accomplished, in selected cases, by superficial abrasion, a technique called *dermabrasion*. X-ray treatment is no longer recommended by many dermatologists because of the possibility of causing skin changes later in life and the availability of other therapeutic alternatives.

HERPES SIMPLEX (TYPE 1)

Herpes simplex type 1, a viral infection, usually causes an irregular vesicular lesion on the margin of the lip (fever blister) or gums. The blister breaks, and a crust develops and eventually clears. These lesions have a tendency to recur in the same area, causing considerable annoyance, discomfort, and cosmetic concern. Occasionally herpes simplex will take on a more important aspect. It is serious when a newborn infant or very young child is involved, because the lesions have a tendency to multiply, and it is serious when the eye is involved, because an impairment of vision may result. Acyclovir, a recently developed antiviral agent, appears to have promise in the management of herpes simplex. (See also p. 165)

DERMATITIS VENENATA

Dermatitis venenata may be seen at any age; it is an inflammatory skin response resulting from external contact with some irritating substance, such as fibers, plants, synthetics, or adhesive tape. However, it is most often observed in those groups who go hiking in the midst of some poison oak or poison ivy. Signs of skin irritation usually occur several hours after exposure and consist of redness, swelling, and small blisters at the point of contact. Itching is intense. If patients know that they have been exposed, the best immediate treatment before the appearance of symptoms is washing the area well. Of course, the best course of action is proper identification of the offending plants in the first place and a prudent detour. After the blisters have developed, the urge to scratch must be resisted to prevent spreading. Calamine lotion and cortisone preparations applied locally may help relieve itching.

BURNS

Another problem, which primarily involves the skin but may finally affect many organs and processes of the body, is burns. Burns may be caused by exposure to hot liquids, strong chemicals, direct flame, radiation, sunlight, or electric current. Toddlers and young children are most often scalded by hot coffee, grease from frying pans, or hot water from unguarded bathroom faucets. Older children are frequently burned when their clothes catch fire while they are playing with matches, using kerosene, or standing too close to household heaters. In the United States approximately 5,000 children are hospitalized each day because of burns and about 3,000 die each year from burns.

Classification

Burns are classified into four categories, depending on the depth of penetration of the body's surface.

A *first-degree* burn (partial thickness) involves only the epidermis. It is very superficial; a tender, slightly swollen redness results. A common illustration of a first-degree burn is the typical summer sunburn. A *second-degree* burn (partial thickness) involves the epidermis and dermis. This category is further divided into superficial and deep dermal burns. Some epidermal appendages must be intact for these burns to heal spontaneously. Deep dermal burns may change from partial-thickness to full-thickness wounds by infection, trauma, or obliteration of the blood supply to the affected part. A second-degree burn is characterized by blister formation or a reddened, discolored region with a moist, weeping surface. A *third-degree* burn (full thickness) involves the entire dermis and portions of the subcutaneous tissue. The region affected has a brown, leathery appearance with little surface moisture. A *fourth-degree* burn (full thickness) involves subcutaneous tissue, fascia, muscle, and perhaps bone. The tissue appears blackened and contracted. Partial-thickness burns can heal without grafting. Full-thickness burns must be grafted for healing to occur. Evaluation of the depth of a burn is not always easy immediately after the injury.

It is not only the degree of burn that is significant but also the amount of body surface affected. A person can usually survive a rather extensive superficial burn but may tolerate a deep burn only if a small area is involved. In evaluating the extent of a burn on an adult, the so-called rule of nines may be applied; it gives a certain percentage value to each part of the body—a percentage that is almost always nine or a multiple of nine. This method of calculation, unless modified, is not helpful when working with children because of the relatively large size of a baby's or young child's head and the reduced length of the legs. (One example of modi-

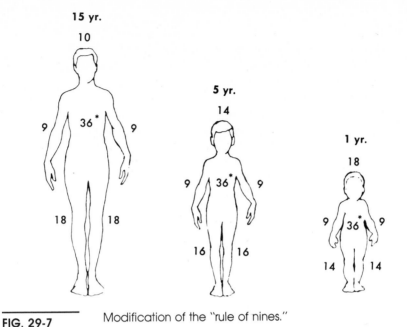

FIG. 29-7   Modification of the "rule of nines."
Courtesy Burns Institute, Galveston Unit, Shriners Hospital for Crippled Children.

fication based on size differences is illustrated in Fig. 29-7.)

The area, extent, and depth of a burn determines its severity, and treatment is planned according to severity. *Minor burns* are described as partial-thickness first- or second-degree burns covering less than 15% of the body surface and not involving strategic areas such as the face, hands, feet, or genitalia. Minor burns are treated on an outpatient basis. *Moderate burns* are described as partial-thickness second-degree burns covering over 15% but less than 30% of body surface or as full-thickness burns involving less than 10% of body surface. Moderate burns usually require hospitalization. *Major burns* are described as partial-thickness second-degree burns covering at least 30% of the body surface or as full-thickness third-degree burns involving more than 10% of the body surface. Most burns—either partial- or full-thickness—that involve a large part of the face, hands, feet, or genitalia are considered major burns. Children with major burns always require hospitalization, and

children with critical burns are transferred to a major burn center if possible.

Therapeutic management and nursing responsibility

INITIAL CONSIDERATIONS

Any person who is at the scene when someone is burned should first extinguish the fire if the victim's clothes are aflame. If an abundant source of water from a hose or bucket is readily available, it should be used; if not, handy blankets or throw rugs may be employed to smother the flames, since fire cannot continue in the absence of oxygen. If neither water nor blankets are available, the victim should be rolled on the ground or floor to help smother the flames. When the fire has been extinguished, the burned area should be rinsed with cold water. The victim should be taken immediately to a physician's office or, preferably, a hospital for evaluation and care. The victim should be transported wrapped in a clean sheet and blanket. No time should be expended on trying to remove the child's clothes unless they are smouldering. No medication of any type should be administered.

When a burned child is admitted to an emergency room or other hospital receiving area, the clothes should be removed gently, cutting along the seams of the garments if necessary. The child should be placed on and covered by sterile sheets in a room with good lighting. All those in attendance should wear face masks. Those in contact with the patient should be provided with sterile gowns and gloves. The severity of the burns will be estimated by the attending physician, and the need for hospitalization will be determined.

Minor burns. The technique of immediately immersing the area briefly in cold water or holding an ice cube on the injured surface to reduce pain and edema has become popular. Care of minor burns usually consists of cleansing the area with mild soap and water. Iodophor soaps are currently used for their antibacterial effect. The area may be covered with a fine-mesh gauze lightly lubricated with water-soluble antimicrobial cream (for example, nitrofurazone, neomycin, or bacitracin) and wrapped with a bulky protective dressing. Depending on the condition of the dressing, the condition of the patient, and the physician's preference, this dressing may be left in place for 4 or 5 days. The child's tetanus immunization should be validated and given if not documented as up to date (see p. 375). Acetaminophen (Tylenol) may be prescribed for pain, and the patient should return to be seen by the physician in 48 hours.

Moderate or major burns. The first phase of therapy when moderate or major burns are present includes maintenance of an airway and prevention of shock. The airway is not a problem in all cases, but occasionally, because of the location of the external burn, the inhalation of fumes, or internal burning of the respiratory tract, it is of great importance. Blood gas analysis is mandatory, and a complete blood count, electrolyte determination, and blood typing provide a baseline that is vital for evaluating the child's state of health on admission. An

endotracheal tube may be needed. Humidified oxygen should be administered and the airway suctioned as necessary.

A nasogastric tube (double lumen sump) may be inserted to prevent tachypnea, associated with acute gastric dilatation and vomiting. Paralytic ileus, a complication associated with circulatory problems in small children, may also be prevented by nasogastric drainage.

Intravenous fluid therapy is the most important aspect of the early care of the burn patient. Loss of plasma into the burn area and evaporation of water from the burn results in a rapid decrease in plasma volume, a concentration of red blood cells, and ultimately an increase in hematocrit. Fluid replacement must be initiated immediately and continued at a high rate for about 24 hours, after which a plasma shift occurs. Fluid that has leaked into the burn area returns to the vascular area. In young children a peripheral cutdown is performed or a central venous line is inserted. An indwelling urinary catheter is usually also necessary. The amount and type of urine formation is observed and recorded hourly to determine the rate of intravenous therapy and to provide an index of the patient's general condition. An initial specimen should be sent to the laboratory for a baseline urinalysis and specific gravity and electrolyte studies. A dwindling urinary output may serve as a warning of developing hypovolemia and possible circulatory collapse. A urinary output of 0.5 to 1.0 ml/kg/hr for a child is desirable (approximately 10 to 30 ml/hr). Signs of overhydration revealed by excessive output require a reduction in fluids given intravenously. Electrolyte, specific gravity, and BUN/creatinine levels are followed regularly and frequently. It is extremely important to report irregularities in the urinary output, loss of a urine specimen, or an error in the measurement of a urine specimen because of the danger of miscalculating the rate and amount of intravenous fluids needed. Overloading the circulatory system is a real possibility unless great care is exercised. The patient is weighed to provide a baseline for subsequent weight loss or gain. Vital signs are checked frequently, although meaningful blood pressure readings may be difficult to secure because of the age of the child and location of the burn area. Some children need central venous pressure determinations.

Hospitalized children with serious burns are sometimes treated with low doses of parenteral penicillin to prevent infection by the staphylococci and streptococci present on the skin. Although prophylactic antibiotics are controversial, they are given as indicated by the patient's clinical course and specific cultures of the wound. Pain medication is administered intravenously to help control shock. The child should be made comfortable but should not be oversedated. More pain accompanies a partial-thickness burn than a full-thickness burn, because in the partial-thickness burn, some nerve endings are still intact. The shock phase of the body's response to extensive burns is usually considered to last from 48 to 72 hours. Many hospitals routinely isolate their burn patients in an effort to prevent or reduce infection.

After 48 hours, the initial ileus that may be seen with major burns has passed, and either oral or nasogastric feedings should be initiated. Hypermetabolism is seen in all patients with extensive burns and continues until the wound is covered. Calorie and protein intake must be increased to facilitate wound epithelialization and graft acceptance. Increased nutritional requirements often necessitate tube feedings to supplement oral feedings. An antacid is given either orally or through the tube to prevent Curling's ulcer, which is a stress ulcer associated with serious burns. Frequent milk feedings, which children usually take well, provide greatly needed calories and fluid. Children usually require about 80 cal./kg of body weight and 3 g of protein per kg of body weight daily. Adequate nutrition will maintain basal weight and enhance wound healing, helping to prevent infection.

The vocational nurse should not be assigned the total bedside responsibility of a severely burned child during this critical period, although she may skillfully assist the registered nurse in important aspects of the care. The vocational nurse must understand the principles of the patient's treatment and, as the patient's condition becomes more stable, she will participate more fully in the patient's care.

Wound care

After the patient is initially stabilized the burn wound is treated. Hair adjacent to the burn wound should be shaved carefully and the burned area cleansed with water and small amounts of iodophor soap or saline solution. Cleansing is preferably done in a hydrotherapy tub. At the time of admission the loose skin and blisters of partial-thickness burns are surgically removed by the physician in a procedure called *debridement*. Gradually a thick black crust (eschar) composed of the drying wound secretions and nonviable tissue forms. An escharotomy may be necessary to relieve compression from circumferential burns. For the little girl in Fig. 29-8, an incision through the eschar was required to release pressure and to permit adequate respirations.

A modified exposure treatment is used for the immediate care of moderate and major burns. Partial-thickness burns are prepared for spontaneous healing by covering the area with fine-mesh gauze that is impregnated with antibacterial ointment or cream. The gauze is held in place by elastic netting or a Surgifix dressing. A sterile blanket may be applied to prevent chilling, and burned extremities should be elevated to minimize accumulation of edema.

The surface of the burn wound must be kept clean by vigorous daily cleansing in the form of povidone-iodine (Betadine) tub baths, whirlpool treatment, or local soaks. All dressing materials should be ready to reapply in a sterile manner after the soak. Soaking in the hydrotherapy tub facilitates removal of loose, sloughing tissue, exudate, and the topical medication.

Days later, as the eschar begins to separate, the physician will cut away portions of the dried crust, revealing new granulation tissue. When the granu-

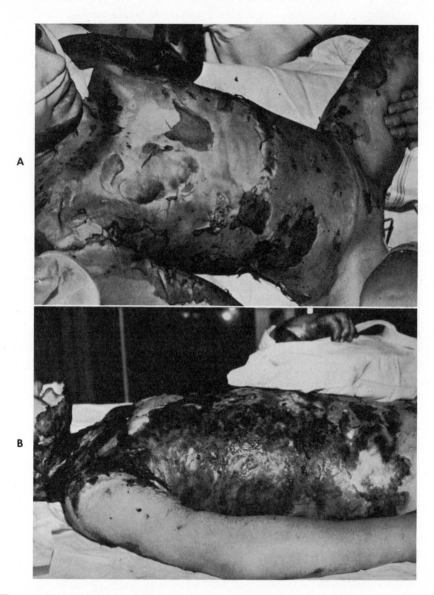

FIG. 29-8 **A,** This 6-year-old child has just been admitted to an emergency room because of second- and third-degree burns. She is receiving oxygen by nasal cannula. **B,** A heavy eschar formed over the trunk. **C,** Escharotomy incisions performed to permit deeper respirations.

Courtesy Matthew Gleason, M.D., San Diego, Calif.

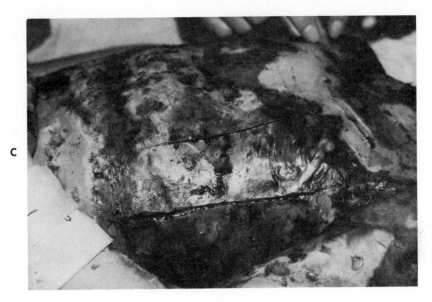

C

Fig. 29-8 cont'd   For legend see opposite page.

lation tissue is exposed (by removal of the eschar), antibiotic gauze is usually laid over the open granulation areas. Through soaks and redressings or intermittent surgical debridements, the burned areas are cleaned and the developing granulation tissue is prepared for elective grafting, which will save time and give a better end result. Granulation tissue is a deep-pink, fragile tissue that bleeds easily. When the tissue is sufficiently prepared, the child will undergo grafting. Donor sites are selected on the patient's body. The donor site is usually covered with fine gauze and a pressure dressing. Later, when bleeding has been controlled, the outer pressure dressing may be removed. Donor sites heal in about 2 weeks. The newly grafted area is kept covered. The dressing should be observed for amount and type of drainage and odor. Exposed adjacent areas are observed for edema and circulatory problems. Grafts are usually firmly attached by the twelfth day after the grafting procedure.

Full-thickness major burn wounds are now being treated soon after admission by primary (tangential) excision. In the operating room under hypo-

tensive anesthesia, which minimizes bleeding, devitalized burned tissue is cut down to the live tissue, and skin grafts are immediately applied. The primary objective of wound care is to reduce the size of the wound as rapidly as possible, thereby increasing the patient's chance for survival. When the wound is reduced to less than 20% of the body surface area, the chance for survival approaches 100%. Full-thickness major burns are, preferably, covered with the patient's own skin. These *autografts* from undamaged parts of the patient's own body provide permanent coverage (see box on p. 582). Unfortunately, often too little skin remains, and homografts, heterografts, and synthetic grafts are used as temporary surface coverings. Donations from other individuals (other than an identical twin) may "take" temporarily but are later rejected. These biologic dressings are used to cover the wound and prevent infection in preparation for skin autografts.

Immediate coverage of the burn wound with grafts or medication following debridement or primary excision is very important to the child's recov-

TYPES OF SKIN GRAFTS

Permanent

Isografts (autografts)	Undamaged tissue from the patient's own skin. (May also be from patient's identical twin if the patient is so fortunate!)

Temporary

Allografts (homografts)	Tissue taken from a different member or cadaver of the same species
Xenografts (heterografts)	Tissue taken from another species, e.g., pigskin (porcine xenograft)
Synthetic grafts (Epigard)	Man-made grafts

ery. Such treatment should forestall pain, fluid loss, and infection, and provide the best environment for wound healing.

After surgery the child is placed in protective isolation. Twenty-four-hour personalized nursing care is essential, with particular attention to respiratory therapy, nutrition, the newly grafted area, and prevention of complications. The use of biologic dressings in the treatment of deep dermal and full-thickness burns has revolutionized the treatment and rehabilitation of burn patients.

TOPICAL MEDICATIONS

Because systemic antibiotics cannot reach the damaged area due to thrombosed or burned vessels, topical medication is an essential means of therapy. A thin layer of medication may be applied directly to the injured area with a sterile glove or tongue blade, or the medication may be embedded in sterile gauze strips that are positioned as needed. A spray form may also be available. (See Table 29-1.)

Mortality caused by infection has declined as a result of the effectiveness of new and improved topical antimicrobial agents. The most desirable topical agent should be inexpensive, painless, non-allergenic, easy to apply, and effective against all microbial contaminants. It should also penetrate the wound without causing systemic effects or harm to viable tissue. Unfortunately, although several topical agents have led to excellent results, no single agent offers all the above-mentioned characteristics.

Mafenide hydrochloride (sulfamylon cream), povidone-iodine (Betadine) ointment, and silver sulfadiazine cream are useful for exposure treatment, combined with frequent hydrotherapy and reapplication of the agent.

CONTINUING CONCERNS

No matter what methods of burn therapy are selected, all treatment is done to accomplish the following aims:

1. Preserve life
2. Promote healing
3. Prevent infection
4. Prevent deformity
5. Provide emotional and physical rehabilitation

Maintaining good nutrition is essential for the survival and satisfactory healing of extensively burned children. An important aspect of the nurse's responsibility is the provision of a good nutritional intake. Initially the child with extensive burns will probably be maintained on tube feedings, but fairly soon the patient may be fed orally with or without a nasogastric tube, depending on the child's progress. It is very important for the nurse to keep an accurate record of all nourishment and fluids taken. Many physicians will request a detailed daily intake record kept to be analyzed by the dietitian for caloric and foodstuff (protein, fat, carbohydrate, and mineral) content. Protein consumption is particularly important. Usually supplemental vitamins and iron will be ordered. Vitamin C and zinc are substances believed to be particularly helpful in aiding tissue healing.

Frequent milk feedings and the prophylactic administration of antacids may prevent a Curling's

TABLE 29-1 COMPARISON OF THREE COMMON TOPICAL ANTIMICROBIALS

Agent	Cost	Advantages	Disadvantages
Mafenide cream 10% (Sulfamylon)	Least expensive	Penetrates eschar Easy application Effective against all gram positive and gram negative organisms	Tendency to cake; should be removed by tub bathing Burning pain on application May cause metabolic acidosis Requires a minimum of two applications daily Patient may develop sensitivity rash
Betadine ointment 10%; also available in foam preparation (Helafoam)	More expensive	Very wide spectrum Effective against gram positive and gram negative organisms, fungi, yeasts, protozoa and viruses Sensitivity is infrequent	Ointment becomes liquid and runs off surface, staining linen Mild burning on application Foam dries out rapidly to a thick powder Inactivated by wound exudate
Silver sulfadiazine cream 1% (Silvadene)	Most expensive	Painless Effective against gram positive and gram negative organisms and *Candida albicans* Sensitivity is infrequent No discoloration	Poor penetration Supplemental systemic therapy usually needed

ulcer, but the nurses should be alert for any signs of blood in the stool or nasogastric tube. The child's appetite should not be discouraged with servings that are too large. Feedings should be judiciously planned. The patient should not be expected to eat directly after an exhausting dressing change. A different schedule for the kitchen on some days or better planning of procedures on other days may be necessary, but patients should receive their meals when they can best *eat*. Likes and dislikes should be noted. The foods selected should be high in calories as well as protein. Sometimes permission to bring food in from home brings forth happy cooperation by both parents and patients. Children must be weighed periodically to help determine their nutritional status.

The immediate and long-term positioning of a seriously burned patient is critical in preventing extensive deformity. Although the position of flexion may be the position of greatest comfort to the patient, it will also become the cause of crippling contractures. The posture of extension may at first appear "heartless," but in the final analysis such placement of the head and extremities may save the patient weeks, if not months, of needless hospitalization and additional pain. The neck splint pictured in Fig. 29-9, *A*, is made of a type of plastic, "Orthoplast" Isoprene, which, when molded and fitted to the individual patient, has been successful in preventing deformities that had previously been difficult to avoid. (Fig. 29-9, *B*.)

Active and passive exercises of the affected body parts, if neglected when ordered, may retard convalescence significantly. It is the responsibility of the nurse (and the physical therapy staff) to see that these important movements, which the patient

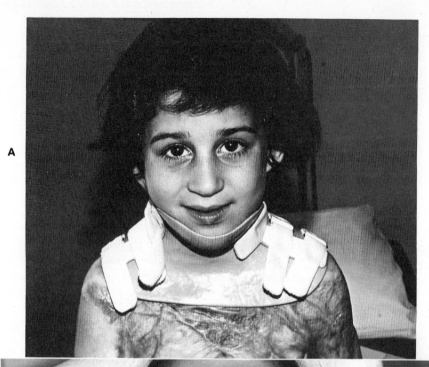

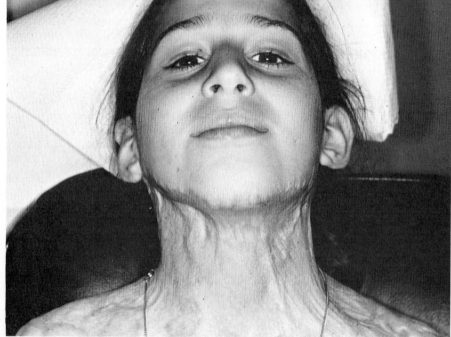

FIG. 29-9

A, Same patient as in Figure 29-8. Splint to prevent neck contractures. **B,** Same child 5 years later. Treatment included skin grafting and splinting.

Courtesy Matthew Gleason, M.D., San Diego, Calif.

often resists, are carried out. Appropriate exercises plus good positioning to avoid flexion contractures can contribute greatly to the early rehabilitation of the patient.

During the entire period of treatment and observation of the extensively burned patient, the morale of the parents and their child is of tremendous importance. Often the parents feel guilty concerning their child's accident. They may be appalled at the condition and appearance of the child. Some will be overly protective; others may hardly be able to make themselves approach the child. All will be extremely upset, whether they appear so or not. Children may have serious guilt feelings if they consider themselves responsible for the injury. Children who have extensive burns characteristically regress in their behavior. Frequent and consistent parental visits are extremely important. Some children who have had a history of emotional disturbance before their accident develop extreme hostility toward their parents and others involved in their care.

Good communication between the physician, the nursing staff, the parents, and the burned patient is essential. Parents need to be informed of the child's progress and helped in their efforts to cope with their feelings while providing support to the child. A feeling of acceptance and freedom to talk without being criticized for talking are important for both the child and his parents. Simple explanations of treatments take time at the beginning, but they save much time and anguish later on.

Play therapy, availability of toys and television, and an empathetic approach to painful procedures are all helpful. Often additional specialized assistance is needed to meet the needs of the patient and family. The social worker, psychologist, or psychiatrist should be called upon to help maintain a healthy support system whenever necessary.

REHABILITATION

The rehabilitation of a burned child may be long and exhausting, but despite the pain and fatigue, the end result is well worth the continuing effort. Fortunately, with the use of new surgical techniques, the time needed for rehabilitation promises to become much shorter. Splinting, traction, and frequent visits to the physical therapy department's pool or exercise room may be necessary. Plastic surgery may be needed in some cases to relieve contractures or remove keloid formation (exaggerated scar tissue). Special tutoring may be required to prevent educational loss, and social contacts must be maintained, particularly for older children. A positive, constructive attitude toward therapy should be encouraged.

Patients who have been seriously burned will probably be among the nurse's most challenging and difficult responsibilities. They will also be among her most rewarding.

CHAPTER 30　Isolation technique and communicable childhood diseases

The student nurse often contemplates her experience with patients suffering from contagious disease with a fascinating mixture of eager anticipation and fear. Both these emotions, when under control, work to her advantage. She has much to learn about the needs of the patients and about safe methods of meeting their needs. There are new words, new techniques, and a new awareness of the unseen. The student must be impressed with the importance of carrying out the isolation, or barrier, techniques recognized in the area where she is working. Any lapse in technique by *anyone* jeopardizes other patients, the entire staff, and, indeed, perhaps the entire hospital.

KEY VOCABULARY

The following list includes some of the new words the nurse may encounter when working in an isolation area:

antitoxin Preparation, often *horse serum* rich in specific antibodies, designed to produce passive immunization. (The antitoxins are produced by injecting a horse with a toxoid; after a period of time, antibodies are manufactured and identified in the horse's blood serum; this serum is modified for injection. Some people are allergic to the serum containing the antibodies. Extreme caution must be taken in administering antitoxin.) This animal hyperimmune serum is being replaced when possible by specific human hyperimmune globulin.

carrier Person or animal capable of transmitting a contagious disease while showing no outward sign of the disease.

contagious diseases Disorders caused by living microorganisms or their toxins, which may be communicable by contact with other persons harboring the organism, their body discharges, or objects, touched by them. Spread by contact or airborne droplet.

contaminated In isolation technique, or medical asepsis, this adjective is applied to any person or thing that has touched a patient with a contagious disease, has touched anything the patient has touched, or has undergone prolonged exposure to such a patient before proper disinfection has occurred. (The student should remember that the word "contaminated" used in a surgical setting means "touched by anything not sterile." In isolation technique it means "touched directly or indirectly by the patient or the patient's excretions or discharges.")

immunity Ability to protect oneself against development of a contagious disease. Immunity may be natural or acquired.

　Natural immunity may be hereditary—related to racial strengths and the individual capacity for protective antibody formation.

　Acquired immunity may be active or passive.

　　Active acquired immunity occurs with formation of protective antibodies by the individual as a result of having actually contracted the disease or of having been protected by the intentional introduction into the body of a vaccine or toxoid. Protection is relatively long lasting.

　　Passive acquired immunity occurs with protection gained through introduction into the individual of antibodies already manufactured by some other person or an animal. Passive immunity may also be transmitted via the placenta from a mother to her unborn child or from a breast-feeding mother to her nursing infant. Protection is relatively brief.

incubation period Time that must elapse between the infection of an individual at a time of exposure until the appearance of signs or symptoms of the disease.

infectious diseases Disorders caused by microorganisms that invade tissue and cause symptoms of illness. (Most infectious diseases are also communicable, but there are exceptions. A person with a disease caused by an organism that is present everywhere but causes disease only when introduced unnaturally into the body, such as an *Escherichia coli* urinary tract infection, would have an infectious disease, but it would not be considered contagious.)

isolation Observance of certain barrier techniques designed to stop the spread of illness by preventing unguarded contact with a person with contagious disease during its period of communicability.

portal of entry The way that infectious agents gain entrance into a person's body (for example, respiratory tract, digestive tract, skin, and mucous membranes).

quarantine Confinement of a person or group of persons who have been exposed to a contagious disease to a specific place without outside contacts for the duration of the longest usual incubation period of the disease in question.

toxoid Preparation containing a toxin or poison produced by pathogenic organisms; it is capable of producing active immunity against a disease but is too weak to produce the disease itself.

vaccine Preparation containing killed or weakened (attenuated) living microorganisms, which, when introduced into the body, cause the formation of antibodies against that type of organism.

ADMISSION TO AN ISOLATION UNIT

Parental needs and fears

Almost without exception, admission to the hospital is a stressful period for parents and child. The anxiety and feeling of helplessness often experienced by parents is increased considerably when the admission necessitates the use of certain barrier techniques or entry into a special ward or room labeled "Isolation." The sight of the medical and nursing staff wearing gowns and perhaps masks and the sound of potentially alarming terms such as

"contaminated" and "contagious" does not tend to reassure parents. Everything seems so strange. Disquieting and not always accurate deductions often disturb their peace of mind. "If Johnny has to be here, he must be terribly ill. I wonder what the other children here have. Couldn't Johnny catch something else from them?" Parents need a lot of support and instruction at such a time, and both physicians and nurses must contribute the necessary time and effort to provide it.

Unit preparation

Usually the admission of a new patient is anticipated, and an individual isolation unit is set up before the child's arrival. Patients are not usually placed in the same room unless it is confirmed that their diagnoses are the same and the attending physicians involved grant permission. However, patients assigned "wound and skin or enteric isolation" may sometimes share a room, having the same type of isolation while maintaining separate bed units. The room should be comfortably warm and well ventilated. In addition to a correctly sized bed or crib, bedside stand, and overbed table found in all standard patient units, an isolation unit should include the following items:

1. Access to a sink, running water, and a toilet
2. Antimicrobial detergent (such as Betadine) for hand and arm care of the attendants
3. Paper towels in a dispenser
4. Laundry hamper support and plastic isolation laundry bags
5. Plastic isolation bags for wrapping or collecting objects for home transport and for collecting and preparing trash for discard
6. Clothes tree or hook where gowns, if they must be reused, may be hung in a special way (paper disposable gowns are recommended)
7. Disinfectant used to wipe down the furniture after the patient's basic care
8. Clean masks, gowns, gloves, and plastic bags readily available in cart or table outside door

The following articles, usually necessary for an admission, should also be at hand:

1. Appropriately sized gown or pajamas; diapers and pins, if appropriate
2. Bath towel set
3. Washbasin and emesis basin
4. Bedpan and urinal, toilet paper or wipes
5. Coloplast bag or other means to help obtain a urine specimen from an infant or young child, if appropriate
6. Correctly sized blood pressure cuff (plastic coated if possible) and sphygmomanometer
7. Thermometer, petrolatum, and cellulose wipes (electronic thermometers are usually not used, depending on type of isolation)
8. Scales, properly draped and balanced
9. Soap, lotion or powder, toothbrush and toothpaste, and comb (To cut down on waste, dispensable supplies in small sample sizes are often used.)
10. Emergency equipment, oxygen, suction, etc., if needed

It is important that all equipment be in readiness, because much time is lost if the nurse must leave the patient to obtain equipment. However, unnecessary equipment should not be brought into the unit, since it would be needlessly exposed to contamination. The safety of an individual patient's unit also depends on adequate, well-planned utility and laundry rooms.

Admission modifications in isolation

In-room visitation by family members of isolated patients is now much more liberal than in the past. Just who would be allowed to enter would depend on the type of isolation technique ordered and the visitor and patient being considered.

The child's clothes are usually placed in a clean bag and returned to the parents. Parents often ask, "What do we do with Johnny's clothes when we get them home?" and "What about all the things that Johnny used at home while he was sick?" Usually it is sufficient to tell the parents to wash the child's clothes separately, using a hot water setting on an automatic washer, regular laundry detergent, and 1 cup of household bleach if the clothes are colorfast.

The former sickroom or sickrooms should be carefully cleaned (preferably vacuumed), damp dusted with disinfectant, and well aired. Objects that the child had handled should, whenever possible, be washed.

Parents should be shown where they may store their coats and purses outside the patient's room when visiting, where the supply of clean gowns are kept, and how to put them on. They should be taught simply to take the gowns off, place them in the laundry hamper, wash their hands just before leaving, and open the door with a paper towel. They should be told always to check at the nurses' desk before taking anything in to the child, since all objects cannot be adequately disinfected, and if an article is brought to a child with a serious disease, it may have to be destroyed when the child goes home. This might cause unnecessary distress! Expendable toys are therefore encouraged. (Television sets are also usually appreciated by the patient.)

When weighing an isolated patient, the nurse must drape and balance the scale before bringing it into the patient's room. The child is weighed and the drape discarded in the laundry hamper. The scale is then cleaned and sprayed with disinfectant.

Urine and stool specimens are collected in the usual way, but the outside of the container used to send them to the laboratory should be clean. The specimen container may be held by a "clean nurse" while the "contaminated nurse" places the specimen in the container. The clean nurse is then responsible for capping and labeling the specimen. If only one nurse is available, the open specimen container may be set on a clean technique paper (a clean paper towel). The specimen is then transferred to the container, and the nurse ungowns, washes her hands, covers the specimen, and labels it outside the patient's room.

ISOLATION TECHNIQUE

Types of isolation

Isolation techniques are designed to accomplish two main objectives: to prevent the spread of any communicable disease that the isolated patient may have and to protect the isolated patient from any outside source of infection.

The first objective is accomplished by erecting barriers between the patients, their environment, and their body excretions or discharges and the rest of the hospital and hospital staff. Special protective coverings may be worn by the nursing staff, and special hand-washing instructions are observed. Articles *coming out* of the unit—that is, articles that have been exposed to the patients for a prolonged period or have directly contacted their persons or units—must generally undergo some type of disinfection. This technique also helps to reduce the introduction of secondary infection from outside the unit, because the attendants usually wear gowns that are worn nowhere else in the hospital over their uniforms while directly caring for patients.

When the second objective is paramount, as in the care of a patient without normal defenses against disease, a type of reverse or protective isolation is practiced. Good hand washing before and after patient care is stressed and clean gowns and possibly masks are used. No special precautions are taken to remove objects and materials from the room, but there are restrictions regarding the kind of things *going into* the room for use. A similar type of protective technique may be employed with certain burn cases, but sterile linens and gloves may be required. In fact, burn cases may require the observance of both protective and strict isolation techniques concurrently. (This makes nursing doubly interesting and the laundry problem tremendous!) Reverse isolation may also be employed with leukemic children who are receiving immunosuppressive therapy in the hospital.

In 1975 staff members of the Center for Disease Control of the Department of Health, Education, and Welfare in Atlanta, Georgia, prepared for government publication the second edition of a booklet entitled *Isolation Techniques for Use in Hospitals*. This publication describes five different types of isolation, or precautionary techniques, based on the characteristics of the disease and the patient being treated. These different types of isolation may be modified as necessary to fit the individual needs of patients and different patient care areas. *All techniques involve good hand washing* on entering and leaving the room, as well as limitation of visitors. In modified summary they are as follows:

1. *Strict isolation* includes a private room with the door kept closed; gowns, masks, and gloves on entering room; and special discard or disinfection of articles. Examples of diseases requiring strict isolation are staphylococcal and streptococcal pneumonias and congenital rubella syndrome.

2. *Enteric precautions* include a private room for children, gowns and gloves for persons in direct contact with either the patient or articles contaminated with fecal material, and special discard or disinfection of eating utensils, dishes, or any articles contaminated with urine or feces. Examples of diseases requiring enteric precautions are salmonellosis (including typhoid fever) and shigellosis.

3. *Wound and skin precautions* include gowns for all persons having direct patient contact, gloves if contact with infected area or its drainage is anticipated, masks only during dressing changes, and special discard (or disinfection) procedures used during dressing changes and bed making. The mattress and pillows should be covered with clean, impervious plastic. Examples of conditions requiring wound and skin precautions are staphylococcal and streptococcal skin infections not associated with extensive burns.

4. *Respiratory isolation* includes a private room with the door kept closed, masks for those who must enter the room and who are susceptible to the disease, and special discard or disinfection of articles contaminated with secretions. Gowns and gloves are not considered necessary. Examples of

diseases requiring respiratory isolation are pertussis and pulmonary tuberculosis.

Note: Pediatric nurses routinely wear overgowns with young children on respiratory isolation because of their developmental level. Barrier gowns are used when caring for all infants and toddlers, whether isolated or not. To help prevent spread of the airborne organisms, patients needing respiratory isolation are best placed in a specially ventilated, double-doored room that exerts a slight negative pressure when entered, thereby retaining contaminated air.

5. *Protective isolation* includes a private room with the door kept closed. As described by the Center for Disease Control, protective isolation includes gowns, masks, and gloves. However, many times it may be modified to omit masks and gloves, depending on the condition of the patient. Articles brought into the room should be clean. In some hospitals and situations, all linen in direct contact with the patient is sterilized prior to use. Mattresses and pillows should be covered with impervious, clean plastic. Use of only fresh cleaning equipment is necessary for such units. Persons requiring protective isolation include certain patients receiving immunosuppressive therapy and those with extensive skin lesions vulnerable to infection.

Note: Details of care using these classifications may be obtained from CDC government publications. In addition to the five categories of isolation, precautions in dealing with secretion, excretion, and blood (body discharges) of patients with specific diseases and safe barriers against possible spread of infectious material, are discussed in the 1975 booklet. A third edition is now being prepared.

Personal precautions

The nurse working with patients in isolation must take certain personal precautions for her own safety and for the safety of her co-workers and other patients. Some of these are essential for every nurse to follow, regardless of the area in which she finds herself; others are particularly important when dealing with known infectious conditions. The following precautions should be noted:

1. Fingernails should be short and clean.
2. The nurse should be free from symptoms of contagious illness (upper respiratory tract infections, skin infections, diarrhea).
3. Any open lesion on the hands or face should be reported and evaluated before going on duty. Perhaps a change of assignment would be prudent to protect the nurse.
4. No rings should be worn. A watch, although used, should not be kept on the wrist.
5. Eyeglasses, if worn, should be periodically disinfected.
6. Shoes should be kept off chairs and other clean areas. Think where they have been!
7. The nurse's hands should not touch her face.

Certain areas in a hospital are always considered contaminated. All floors are contaminated regardless of the location. In most hospitals the entire room of a patient with a communicable disease is considered contaminated *with the exception* of the supply of paper towels inside a dispenser near the sink. This supply is located as far from the patient as possible. At times there is an adjoining anteroom where such supplies are kept, and washing, laundry, and discard facilities are available.

The isolation gown

OCCASIONS FOR USE

An isolation gown should be worn in a unit whenever a possibility exists of contact with the patient or any contaminated equipment in the room. When strict isolation is ordered, anyone going into the room, whether or not she will be touching anything, should wear a gown, mask, and perhaps gloves (depending on what will be done). However, in other types of isolation, the attendant may enter several times to bring in supplies and equipment without touching anything already in the room and not be required to gown or wash her hands—if she is *careful*. If the nurse touches something contaminated with her hands, she should, of course, follow the hand-washing technique before leaving the room. A gown should not be worn outside a patient's room once it has been worn inside the room, with the following exceptions only:

1. When transporting a patient for an ordered procedure in another room.
2. When transporting a patient to some other department for x-ray examinations, therapy, or a change in room or unit.

When a contaminated gown must be used outside the patient's room, the nurse should be very discreet about what she touches and where she goes. When it is necessary to transport a child with a communicable disease through the hospital corridors, the wheelchair or gurney should be draped with clean linen. The child should wear a mask if the disease is spread through droplet contamination. The child should be properly restrained to prevent falling and covered to prevent chilling. If the trip will be long or the wait protracted, an appropriate fluid, if allowed, may be taken along for an infant. The child's chart should be placed in a bag for protection. The chart itself should be handled only by people with clean hands.

GOWN TECHNIQUES

Gowning. When a clean gown is required, the nurse should put it on before entering the patient's unit or room. Since the gown and the nurse are "clean," any part of the gown may be touched by the nurse as she puts it on. It should be tied at the back of the neck and then the back of the gown

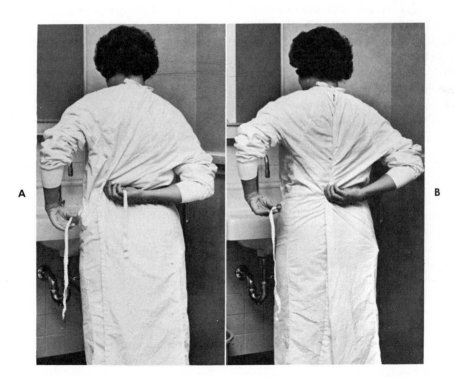

FIG. 30-1   Two methods of gowning. **A,** Right side over left. **B,** Back inside edges together; then roll until snug.

Courtesy Children's Hospital and Health Center, San Diego, Calif.

adjusted in such a way that no part of the nurse's uniform is exposed. Following are two ways by which a gown may be closed:

1. Pull the left-hand side of the back of the gown as far to the right as possible and lap the right-hand side over the left. Pull the belt around, cross it at the back, and tie it in the front. Push the sleeves up above the wrists (Fig. 30-1, *A*).
2. Hold the right and left inner edges of the back of the gown together and fold over until snugly closed against the wearer's back (Fig. 30-1, *B*). Continue as in Step 1.

Note: Reuse of isolation gowns is not recommended if it can be avoided. Many hospitals are now using paper gowns, which are discarded in the trash.

Removing a gown. The steps for removing an isolation gown are basically the same whether the gown is to be discarded or saved for further use. The procedure is as follows:

1. Untie the belt, letting the ends drop to the side.
2. Turn on the running water.
   a. If faucets are used, they are opened with unwashed hands and closed with clean hands protected by a paper towel.
   b. If a knee lever is used, it is turned on and off with a knee covered by the isolation gown.
   c. If foot pedals (the preferable device) are used to control the water flow, one does not need to consider the possibility of contaminating clean hands. Shoes are always considered contaminated.
3. Carefully wash the hands and exposed portion of the arms for 1 minute with an antimicrobial detergent, using considerable friction. The use of a brush is overly irritating and unnecessary. The areas are rinsed and patted dry with paper towels. The hands should be kept lower than the elbow when washing, as part of isolation technique, to avoid increasing the area of possible contamination.
4. Untie the neckband with newly washed hands.

5. After discarding the gown, rewash your hands and arms using the same technique described previously, *except*, if a knee lever is used to control the water flow, open it with a hand before washing. If the lever is opened with knee action at this point, the nurse's uniform becomes contaminated. After the hands are washed, close the faucet or knee control with a hand protected by a paper towel.

Leaving the patient's room

The following precautions are taken when leaving the room of an isolation patient:

1. Open the door with the paper towel used to turn off the water. Walk through.
2. Turn around before letting the door close and discard the paper in the wastebasket.
3. All doors to isolation rooms should routinely be kept closed.

Use of masks

Masks may help filter out bacteria, thus protecting the wearer or the patient. Newer models are said to be effective approximately 6 hours unless they become very damp. Masks also keep the attendant's hands away from her face!

The following techniques are important in the use of masks:

1. Store masks conveniently outside the patient's unit. Many times they are placed in a paper bag taped on the outside of the patient's room where they are required to be worn.
2. Position the mask in place before entering the room.
3. Remove a mask after your hands are washed by touching only the supporting ties or band and dropping it directly into the trash.
4. Never leave a patient's room with a mask dangling around your neck!

Use of technique papers

A technique paper enables a nurse to carry out a procedure with greater skill and observance of asepsis by providing a temporary barrier between contaminated and clean objects. A clean paper towel usually serves as a technique paper. Taken directly from the dispenser, it is folded to form at least two layers of paper. It may be placed on a dry contaminated surface with clean hands, serving as a temporary island of cleanliness on which to place articles such as watches, pencils, and perhaps specimen bottles. (The underside of the paper touching the bedside table is contaminated; the upper side is not considered contaminated.)

A watch should not be worn in an isolation situation because hands and arms cannot be properly washed with a watch in place, and a contaminated watch may come into contact with a patient during care. A watch cannot be sprayed or soaked with disinfectants—both procedures seem to do something to its insides! However, since a watch is necessary to the nurse, it may be enclosed in a clear, small, waterproof plastic bag or box or placed on a technique paper for a brief period in such a position that the dial may be easily seen.

Neither the chart nor the nursing assignment sheet should be taken into the isolated patient's room.

Service of meals

1. All food prepared for isolation patients in the hospital should be served with disposable dishes and utensils, or, if facilities are available, ceramic dishes and serving tray may be placed in a special clean sack that dissolves during a subsequent sterilization process.
2. If paper dishes are used and no appropriate sterilization procedure is available for the tray, the tray should not be brought into the room.
3. The food should be served as soon as possible.

No one enjoys cold meals. The setting can be prepared for the children who can feed themselves and, then others who need assistance can be helped.

4. Uneaten solid food should be scraped into a paper dish or cup and placed in a refuse sack in the wastebasket. Unfinished liquids may be poured into the toilet.
5. If intake-output records must be kept, the record is posted outside the isolation room, usually on the outside of the patient's door.

Care of linen, trash, and diapers

1. Soiled linen, usually with the exception of cloth diapers, should be placed in a laundry hamper in the patient's unit. Disposable diapers are usually recommended. Handle soiled linen carefully. Do not "wave it in the breeze." Remember, careless handling of linen increases the organism count in the air. (See Fig. 30-2.)
2. At the end of each tour of duty or when the hamper in the room is two-thirds full, close the top of the bag and place it upside down in a clean hamper or a clean bag held by another nurse just outside the door. If the inner bag is made of water-soluble plastic, handling of these contaminated linens is reduced. The outer plastic bag ideally should be red or distinctly marked to alert the housekeeping department of potentially infective material.

Note: A "contaminated nurse" may touch only that part of the outer laundry bag that will be on the inside of the bag when it is closed.

3. Contaminated trash is collected in a plastic bag, which lines the wastebasket. At the end of a tour of duty or when appropriate, the bag is carefully closed and placed in a clean outer bag just outside the door for disposal.
4. Double-bagged linen or bags of trash should be completely closed as soon as the nurse is able to remove her gown and wash her hands so that contaminated material does not

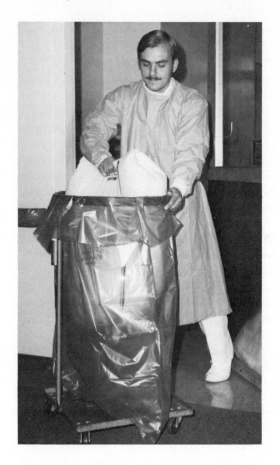

FIG. 30-2

He's glad he didn't forget to properly clear his isolation room of dirty linen.

Courtesy Children's Hospital and Health Center, San Diego, Calif.

remain unattended in the corridors. Sometimes it is possible for two or more nurses to work together to facilitate the removal of contaminated linen and trash. One will work in the patient's room, and the other(s) will close all the clean outer bags and place them in the approved areas for removal.

5. The handling of contaminated diapers depends on the facilities and services available. Some hospitals use professional diaper services. The instructions of these companies regarding the pretreatment of diapers (if necessary) and collection should be followed. Any diaper pails used for collections should be closed, ideally with lids that are operated by a foot pedal.

Disposal of urine, feces, emesis, and other body discharges

1. Bedpans and emesis basins are usually emptied directly into the toilet in areas where urban sewage facilities are available. The hospital staff should know the sewage precautions needed in its own community. It is strongly recommended that each isolation unit have its own toilet facilities. In certain situations special precautions may have to be taken in the event of the occurrence of typhoid-related illnesses.
2. Any patient with nasal discharge should have a small paper sack attached to the bedside in

which to put used cellulose wipes. When this bag is almost full, it should be closed and added to the trash in a large plastic bag in the wastebasket.

Disinfection of equipment

1. Disposable equipment is used in an isolation unit as much as possible.
2. Only essential equipment should be taken into an isolation room.
3. Nondisposable, washable items (such as basins, bedpans, spoons, and hemostats) may be washed in the patient's room, sprayed with a disinfectant, and preferably transported directly to a dishwasher that disinfects the utensils. If this method is impossible, they may be boiled in water or soaked in disinfectant.
4. Stethoscopes, percussion hammers, and flashlights are usually sprayed with disinfectant. Sphygmomanometers are wiped off with disinfectant. Blood pressure cuffs should have plasticized washable surfaces.
5. If at all possible, disposable needles and syringes should be used. These should be destroyed after use to prevent reuse. The needles should be covered with their protective hoods, placed in a rigid pierce-proof container, and double bagged.

SUGGESTIONS FOR NURSING ORGANIZATION

Suggestions for organizing and completing your daily work in isolation are as follows:
1. Try to have *everything* you need in the room or just outside the room before gowning, including the following:
   a. Linen for the bed
   b. Clean clothes for the patient
   c. Hygienic supplies
   d. Supplies for early morning treatments
   e. Liquids to encourage fluid intake, if appropriate.
   f. Plastic sacks, to replace those you will remove when emptying trash or removing diapers or laundry
2. Before ungowning, always ask your patients (if they talk!) if there is anything more they wish.
3. Use the intercom for assistance, if one is available.
4. Remember, charting and clearing your unit of contaminated linen and waste takes time. Plan your working schedule with this in mind. Be sure you have taken any unnecessary equipment, such as bottles, from the room before you report off duty. At the completion of your morning care, the table tops, bed, and counters in the isolation room should be wiped down with a paper towel moistened with disinfectant.

TERMINATION OF ISOLATION

If isolation precautions are discontinued before a previously contagious patient is discharged from the hospital, a "termination of isolation" bath may be given. If the child's condition is satisfactory and the physician is agreeable, a shampoo followed by a tub bath is ideal. After the tub bath the child is dressed in clean clothes and returned to a new bed and unit or is kept on a clean gurney in another room until the old room can be wiped down and aired or otherwise disinfected.

Everything transferred from the patient's old isolation unit to the new uncontaminated unit must undergo some type of disinfection. The former isolation room is stripped of everything easily moveable that can be best disinfected in the utility room (including any wall oxygen and suction equipment). The linen is double bagged. All paper goods are discarded in the trash. The stripped room is then either wiped down with a disinfectant (or exposed to ultraviolet light if the organism involved was the tuberculosis bacillus), and the room is completely cleaned.

Text continued on p. 611.

TABLE 30-1 COMMUNICABLE CHILDHOOD DISEASES

Disease	Infectious agent and general description	Importance	Mode of transmission	Communicable period
Bacillary dysentery (shigellosis)	*Shigella dysenteriae* and *Shigella paradysenteriae* Acute inflammation of colon	Extremely widespread in areas with poor sanitary facilities and hygiene practices Disease often severe in infancy but mild after 3 yr of age	Direct or indirect contact with feces of infected patients or carriers Contaminated food, water, and flies play important role (Enteric precautions needed)*	As long as patients or carriers harbor organisms (as determined by stool or rectal swab cultures) Healthy carriers common; they should not become food handlers In areas where sanitary treatment of sewage is not routine, stools should be disinfected
Chicken pox; see varicella				
Diphtheria	*Corynebacterium diphtheriae* (Klebs-Löffler bacillus) Severe, acute infectious disease of upper respiratory tract and perhaps skin Toxins produced may affect nervous system and heart	Rarely seen because of routine childhood immunization, more comprehensive public health regulations, and enforcement of milk standards and carrier control 5% to 10% mortality Serious complications include neuritis, paralysis, and myocarditis	Direct or indirect contact with secretions from respiratory tract or skin lesions of patient or carrier (Strict isolation)*	Variable: 2 to 4 wk in untreated persons, or 1 to 2 days after antibiotic therapy initiated Isolation until satisfactory nose and throat cultures obtained; contacts may be isolated
German measles (rubella, 3-day measles)	Rubella virus Acute infectious disease characterized chiefly by rose-colored macular rash and lymph node enlargement	Very common, frequently occurring in epidemic form Complications rare for victim but may cause deformities of fetus if contracted by pregnant woman during first trimester	Usually direct contact with secretions from mouth and nose May be acquired in utero (Strict isolation for congenital rubella; respiratory isolation for postnatal rubella)	From 1 wk before rash appears until approximately 5 days after its onset For discussion of congenital rubella syndrome see pp. 293-294; affected infants may be infectious up to 1 yr of age
Gonorrhea (pp. 164 and 610)				

*Report of the Committee on Infectious Diseases, Evanston, Ill., 1982, American Academy of Pediatrics (Red Book).

Incubation period	Symptoms	Treatment and nursing care	Prevention
1 to 7 days (usually 3 to 4 days)	Mild to severe diarrhea; in severe cases blood, mucus, and pus may be seen in stool. Abdominal pain, fever, and prostration may be present	Treatment depends on severity of infection. Ampicillin or Septra drug of choice; trimethoprim-sulfamethoxazole (Septra) best drug for the treatment of the dysenteric form of shigellosis, which is resistant to multiple antibiotics. Keep patient warm; oral fluids may be restricted; intravenous therapy may be necessary to prevent dehydration	Attack appears to confer limited immunity. No preventive known other than improved individual and community hygiene
2 to 6 days (occasionally longer)	Depend on type and part of upper respiratory area inflamed. Formation of fibrinous false membrane, which may or may not be visible in throat or nose. Nausea, possible muscle paralysis, and heart complications	Administration of antitoxin, analgesics, erythromycin, or penicillin. Prednisone lessens incidence of myocarditis in severe disease. Absolute bed rest; gentle throat irrigations; bland, soft diet; humidification. Possible need for tracheostomy. Watch for muscle weakness	Immunity after one attack, but person may be immune without history of disease. Immunity determined by Shick test. Routine primary schedule—Td booster injection recommended at 10-year intervals
14 to 21 days (usually 18 days)	Rose-colored macular rash occurring first on face, then on all body parts; enlargement and tenderness of lymph nodes; mild fever	Supportive nursing care with good personal hygiene	Rubella vaccine. Immune after one attack

Continued.

TABLE 30-1   COMMUNICABLE CHILDHOOD DISEASES—cont'd

Disease	Infectious agent and general description	Importance	Mode of transmission	Communicable period
Hepatitis, viral; 3 types identified: Type A (infectious); Type B (serum); Non-A, Non-B	All types manifest similarities and differences; may vary with age and general condition of person infected	Hepatitis of all types represented fourth most commonly reported communicable disease in 1981		
Type A, (infectious) (HAV)	Hepatitis A virus (HAV): usually abrupt onset	HAV: Highest incidence in civilian populations in persons under 15 years, typically mild in children (very common in mentally retarded children)	Person-to-person; generally thru fecal contamination; transmission is facilitated by poor sanitation and close contact; ingestion of fecally contaminated food and water (e.g., shellfish, milk) (Excretion precautions only)*	Uncertain; probably infectious 2 weeks before onset of jaundice; minimal risk 1 week after onset of jaundice
Type B, (serum) (HBV)	Hepatitis B virus (HBV): characterized by usually insidious onset	HBV more common in adults; more often complicated by relapse and prolonged liver dysfunction; typically more severe in infants and debilitated patients	HBV reported more frequently; transmitted through inoculation of contaminated blood products, needles and syringes; close and intimate contact including sexual contact (person to person); meticulous hand-washing technique needed (Blood precautions only)*	Potentially infectious for indeterminant period before and after active symptoms; carrier state possible. Neonates acquire illness from infected mother and have high risk of developing chronic active hepatitis
Non-A, Non-B viral hepatitis (NANB)	Causative agent or agents have not been identified. Clinical features resemble HBV, insidious onset	Acute hepatitis, neither HAV or HBV, affects all age groups; common among low socioeconomic status such as commercial blood donors; most common type of hepatitis associated with blood transfusion (70-80%)	Most common cause of post-transfusion hepatitis. Parenteral exposure to blood or illicit drugs (Excretion and blood precautions)*	Potentially infectious for indeterminate period before and after active symptoms; carrier state possible

Incubation period	Symptoms	Treatment and nursing care	Prevention
	Jaundice for 3 types may be inapparent, fleeting or persistent with or without itching	No specific therapy available; supportive care, rest and high-calorie diet	
15 to 50 days; average 28 to 30 days	Fever, malaise, anorexia, nausea, enlarged liver, abdominal discomfort, dark urine, weight loss Children usually have less severe clinical manifestations and illness may not be accompanied by jaundice	In fulminating hepatitis—to combat liver failure, protein withdrawn from diet; neomycin given to suppress bacterial flora in GI tract; possible use of corticosteroids; exchange transfusion for patient in coma	HAV attack confers immunity for HAV IG* recommended for HAV contact; IG is protective if given before exposure or during incubation period. Best if given within 72 hours after exposure *IG immune globulin (formerly called "immune serum globulin," ISG, or "gamma globulin")
45 to 160 days; average 60 to 90 days	Urticaria and arthralgia more characteristic of HBV Various combinations of anorexia, malaise, nausea, vomiting, abdominal pain and jaundice Occasionally a rapid, severe (fulminating) type seen characterized by mental confusion, emotional instability, restlessness, coma, and internal bleeding; usually progresses to a fatal outcome within 10 days	Bedrest for symptomatic patients; well-balanced diet as desired; supplements of all vitamins, especially B complex	HBV attack confers immunity for HBV; hepatitis B—immune globulin reserved primarily for those exposed to HBV known blood products (HBIG); optimal effect if given within 48 hours after exposure; results of IG given to HBV contacts have been inconsistent, but also efficacious, at least to attenuate the disease Effective screening of blood donors; absolute sterilization of equipment used for drawing blood, or use of disposable equipment
Mean range 15 to 180 days; average 60 days	Same as HBV; symptoms may not be as severe	Same as HBV	Unknown IG not known to be beneficial, but may offer some protection

Continued.

TABLE 30-1   COMMUNICABLE CHILDHOOD DISEASES—cont'd

Disease	Infectious agent and general description	Importance	Mode of transmission	Communicable period
Measles (rubeola, or 2-week, or red, measles)	Measles virus Acute infection characterized by moderately high temperature, inflammation of mucous membranes of respiratory tract, and macular rash	Very common, highly infectious disease frequently occurring in epidemic form Possible serious complications include pneumonia, otitis media, conjunctivitis, and encephalitis	Direct or indirect contact with secretions from nose and throat, perhaps airborne May be acquired in utero (Respiratory isolation)*	From time of "cold symptoms" until about 3 days after rash appears
Meningococcal meningitis (cerebrospinal fever)	*Neisseria meningitidis (N. intracellularis)* Meningococcus Serious, acute disease caused by bacteria that invade bloodstream and eventually meninges, causing fever and central nervous system inflammation	Occurs fairly often where concentrations of people are found (army bases, schools) because of healthy carriers Very severe or relatively mild Mortality depends on early diagnosis and treatment Complications include hydrocephalus, arthritis, blindness, deafness, impairment of intellect, and cerebral palsy	Direct contact with patient or carrier by droplet spread Organism may be found in urine (Strict isolation)*	As long as meningococci are found in nose and mouth Usually not infectious after 24 hr of antibiotic therapy
Mononucleosis, infectious (glandular fever)	Epstein-Barr (EB) virus Mildly contagious disease characterized by increase in monocyte-type white cell in blood, splenomegly, lymph node enlargement, fever, and fatigue Heterophil agglutinin studies positive fairly late in course of disease	Typically, disease of teenagers or young adults Trauma may rarely cause ruptured spleen; hepatitis in 8% to 10% of cases May involve prolonged convalescence	Probably droplets from nose and throat, saliva, or intimate contact (Respiratory isolation)*	Not known Probably only during acute stage

Incubation period	Symptoms	Treatment and nursing care	Prevention
About 10 days	Catarrhal symptoms, like a common cold; conjunctivitis; photophobia Fever followed by macular, blotchy rash involving entire body Koplik's spots (eruption on mucous membrane of mouth) diagnostic	Antibiotics (for treatment of secondary bacterial infections) Aspirin and tepid sponge baths for severe cases; various soothing lotions Boric acid eye irrigations; protection from bright lights—eyeshade Observation for onset of pneumonia or ear infection	Live measles vaccine; immune globulin (IG) may lessen disease Usually immune after first attack
1 to 7 days (usually 4 days)	Sudden onset of fever, chills, headache, and vomiting (convulsions fairly common in children) Cutaneous petechial hemorrhages; stiffness of neck; opisthotonus; joint pain; possibly delirium; convulsions	Spinal tap and culture needed to confirm diagnosis Temperature control; penicillin G, or ampicillin, analgesics, and sedatives Watch for clinical signs of increasing intracranial pressure or meningeal irritation and eye and ear involvement Maintain dim, quiet atmosphere; turn gently; watch for constipation and urinary retention; attention to fluid balance	Meningococcal polysaccharide vaccines for group A and C meningococcal infections Extent of immunity after attack unknown Sulfonamides have been used prophylactically during epidemics Rifampin and minocycline Rifampin prophylaxis for sulfonamide-resistant organisms
Unknown (probably 2 to 8 wk)	Sore throat, malaise, depression, enlarged spleen, liver, and lymph nodes Possible jaundice with liver damage	Symptomatic, no specific therapy known Bed rest, high carbohydrate, protein intake Possible use of corticosteroids with severe throat involvement and airway obstruction	No immunization available

Continued.

TABLE 30-1 COMMUNICABLE CHILDHOOD DISEASES—cont'd

Disease	Infectious agent and general description	Importance	Mode of transmission	Communicable period
Mumps (infectious parotitis)	Virus Acute infectious disease causing inflammation of salivary glands and, at times, testes and ovaries	Possible serious consequences for male after puberty, when an attack is more severe; sterility can be complication Meningitis or encephalitis occur infrequently Mild pancreatitis may be encountered	Direct or indirect contact with patient by droplet spread (Respiratory isolation)*	From several days before apparent infection until swelling disappears
Rabies (hydrophobia)	Virus Only two nonfatal cases reported, acute infectious encephalitis, causing convulsions and muscle paralysis	Exceedingly dangerous Household pets may acquire rabies through bite of rabid wild animals All dogs should be immunized periodically; cats may also be carriers, but impractical to insist on immunization	Bite of rabid animals or entry of infected saliva through previous break in skin or mucous membrane (Strict isolation)*	During clinical course of disease plus 3 to 5 days before appearance of symptoms (as demonstrated in dogs and cats)
Staphylococcal infections	Coagulase-positive staphylococci *(Micrococcus pyogenes,* var. *aureus)* pus-producing coccus Descriptions variable	Found almost everywhere; causes many hospital infections; does not respond well to usual antibiotic therapy; extremely difficult to control; anyone may be carrier at intervals Complications include skin lesions, pneumonia, wound infections, arthritis, osteomyelitis, meningitis, and food poisoning	Depends on body area infected Via hands of hospital personnel Asymptomatic nasal carriers common Open suppurative lesions May be airborne Direct or indirect contact with infected secretions (Type of isolation depends on area infected)	As long as lesions drain or carrier state persists

Incubation period	Symptoms	Treatment and nursing care	Prevention
14 to 21 days (usually 18 days)	Tender swelling chiefly of parotid glands in front of and below ear Headache; moderate fever; pain on swallowing	Bed rest; bland, soft diet; analgesics; warm or cold applications to swollen glands Watch for tenderness of testes—scrotal support may be necessary	Mumps vaccine Usually immune after first attack
Usually 2 to 6 wk	Mental depression, headaches, restlessness, and fever Progresses to painful spasms of throat muscles, especially when attempting to drink Delirium, convulsions, and coma	No effective treatment known Supportive nursing care to help prevent convulsions; analgesics Death usually occurs in about 7 days	Vaccination of dogs; 10-day confinement of any dog who has bitten human Laboratory investigation of brain of dog that dies during this period; if rabies is diagnosed, person bitten must receive rabies vaccine; consult Red Book for specific treatments
Variable; 1 to 10 days to several weeks	Depend on area infected Fever and characteristic signs of inflammation typical	Antibiotics according to drug sensitivity pattern of organism; methicillin, oxacillin, cephalosporins Topical antibiotics: bacitracin, neomycin, polymyxin	Good hygiene and aseptic technique best preventive

Continued.

TABLE 30-1   COMMUNICABLE CHILDHOOD DISEASES—cont'd

Disease	Infectious agent and general description	Importance	Mode of transmission	Communicable period
Streptococcal infections	Strains of beta-hemolytic streptococci, usually group A Diseases include septic sore throat, scarlet fever (scarlatina), erysipelas, impetigo, puerperal fever	Interrelated group of infections; septic sore throat probably most common Early complications include otitis media May cause serious complications not contagious in themselves—nephritis and rheumatic fever, with possible arthritis and carditis	In septic sore throat and scarlet fever, direct or indirect contact with nasopharyngeal secretions from infected patient; probably airborne In erysipelas, impetigo, and puerperal fever, direct or indirect contact with discharges from skin or reproductive tract (Type of isolation depends on area infected)	Variable
Syphilis (see pp. 162 and 610)				
Tetanus (lockjaw)	Bacillus *Clostridium tetani* Acute infectious disease attacking chiefly nervous system Wounds deprived of good oxygen supply especially vulnerable	Always considered in event of burns, automobile accidents, or puncture wounds Mortality of about 35%	Entrance of spores into wounds through contaminated soil Direct or indirect contamination of wounds (No isolation recommended except possibly gloves for wound care)*	None

Incubation period	Symptoms	Treatment and nursing care	Prevention
2 to 5 days	Depends on manifestations Septic sore throat, severe pharyngitis and fever Scarlet fever, pharyngitis, fever, and fine reddish rash and strawberry tongue Erysipelas, tender, red skin lesions, and fever often recurrent Impetigo, refer to p. 571 Puerperal fever, refer to pp. 5 and 204	Depends on manifestation Penicillin for at least 10 days	No artificial immunization available Penicillin prophylaxis may be used with special groups Good asepsis important
3 to 21 days (usually 8 days)	Irritability, rigidity, painful muscle spasms, and inability to open mouth Exhaustion and respiratory difficulty	Specific—tetanus immune globulin (human); TIG preferred over tetanus antitoxin Sedation plus muscle relaxant Quiet, dim room Possible suction and tracheotomy Observation of fluid balance; watch for constipation and respiratory distress; protect from self-injury during convulsions	Routine primary immunization; booster at school age and Td every 10 yr (see p. 376)

Continued.

TABLE 30-1   COMMUNICABLE CHILDHOOD DISEASES—cont'd

Disease	Infectious agent and general description	Importance	Mode of transmission	Communicable period
Tuberculosis	*Mycobacterium tuberculosis* (tubercle bacillus) Typically chronic infection that may affect many body organs Human type most often causes pulmonary infection Bovine type causes much of tuberculosis affecting areas outside lungs	Serious world health problem, particularly in economically deprived areas Infants and young children highly susceptible Pulmonary complications, hemoptysis, spontaneous pneumothorax, or spread to other organs with varied symptoms; possible orthopedic problems	Direct or indirect contact with infected patients; body excretions or droplet spread (depending on type) Respiratory tuberculosis often airborne; bovine type may result from drinking milk from infected cows (now rare in U.S.) (Respiratory isolation for pulmonary tuberculosis; secretion precautions for draining lesions)*	Children with uncomplicated primary TB are usually noninfectious because of minimal pulmonary lesions; in chronic TB as long as organism is discharged in sputum or other body excretions Communicability may be reduced by medication, therapy, and teaching cough control and asepsis to patients Body often walls off a primary infection, controling spread and preventing active disease
Typhoid fever (enteric fever)	*Salmonella typhosa,* a bacillus (many types have been identified) Relatively severe febrile systemic infection (sepsis) with symptoms involving lymphoid tissues, intestine, and spleen, which may be accompanied by complete prostration and delirium Condition has prolonged course and convalescence	Always of potential public health importance when community hygiene breaks down Carrier states may persist Complications include intestinal hemorrhage and perforation, thrombosis, cardiac failure, and cholecystitis	Direct or indirect contact with urine and feces of infected patients and carriers Food and water supplies may be infected by contaminated *flies* or unsuspected *carriers;* community sewage facilities should be evaluated; excreta may have to be disinfected before being added to local system (Enteric precautions)*	As long as typhoid organism appears in feces or urine 2% to 5% of those affected become permanent carriers

Incubation period	Symptoms	Treatment and nursing care	Prevention
From infection to primary lesion, 2 to 10 wk Time of appearance of active symptoms variable	Active pulmonary tuberculosis: anorexia, weight loss, night sweats, afternoon fever, cough and dyspnea, fatigue, and hemoptysis; in children dyspnea and cough often absent Diagnosis based on symptoms and microscopic studies of sputum, gastric washings, and chest x-ray examination	Specific—isoniazid (INH), plus ethambutol or rifampin Nursing care includes provision for mental and physical rest; nutritious diet; observation for toxic drug reactions and increasing respiratory distress; provision for and instructions in personal hygiene; moral support	BCG vaccine to build up immunity in high-risk populations advised by some Early detection and control of known cases through periodic x-ray examination, possible skin tests, and close medical supervision
1 to 3 wk (usually 2 wk)	In children symptoms may be atypical, may at first resemble upper respiratory tract infection; intestinal tract becomes inflamed and even ulcerated; spleen enlarges; fever mounts; pulse relatively slow; rash, "rose spots" may be present	Ampicillin or chloramphenicol for typhoid fever Supportive nursing care; liquid to bland, soft diet as tolerated; bed rest Watch for abdominal distention and hemorrhage; small enemas may be ordered; observation of fluid balance	Immunity usually acquired after one attack Vaccine available

Continued.

TABLE 30-1   COMMUNICABLE CHILDHOOD DISEASES—cont'd

Disease	Infectious agent and general description	Importance	Mode of transmission	Communicable period
Varicella-zoster infections	Virus capable of causing varicella (chicken pox), or zoster (shingles)		Direct or indirect contact with secretions from mouth or moist skin lesions of varicella or zoster (Strict isolation)*	Approximately 1 to 2 days before rash appears until 6 days after its onset; dried crusts not contagious.
Varicella (chicken pox)	Varicella—response to primary infection Mild, chiefly cutaneous infectious disease	Very common, highly contagious, usually mild disease Complications other than secondary infection from scratching rare; however, encephalitis possible		
Zoster (shingles)	Zoster—reactivation in debilitated persons or in persons receiving immunosuppressive therapy	Overwhelming severe infection seen in children receiving immunosuppressive therapy CAUTION: Contact!	Zoster less contagious, but susceptible children exposed to zoster lesions may develop chicken pox	
Whooping cough (pertussis)	*Bordetella pertussis* (pertussis bacillus) Acute infection of respiratory tract, characterized by paroxysmal cough ending in "whoop," often accompanied by vomiting	Severe disease in infants, may terminate fatally Complications include bronchopneumonia and convulsions, widespread hemorrhages, hernia, and possible activation of pulmonary tuberculosis	Direct or indirect contact with nasopharyngeal secretions of infected patients (droplet infection) (Respiratory isolation)*	From 7 days after exposure to 4 wk after onset of typical cough Greatest in catarrhal stage before onset of paroxysms

Incubation period	Symptoms	Treatment and nursing care	Prevention
10 to 21 days (usually 14 days)		Keep fingernails short and clean to minimize secondary infections caused by scratching Calamine lotion, oral antihistaminics reduce pruritus	None; immune after one attack Passive immunization of susceptible immunodeficient patients exposed to varicella-zoster virus may be obtained with varicella-zoster immune globulin (VZIG) given within 96 hours of exposure Distributed by the American Red Cross Blood Services Regional Centers
	Slight fever; malaise; rapidly progressing papulovesiculopustular skin eruption in all stages of development, first appearing on trunk and scalp	Children with varicella should not be given salicylates because of potential development of Reye's syndrome	
	Zoster lesions confined to skin over sensory nerves preceded by local pain, itching and burning		
5 to 21 days (usually within 10 days)	Early symptoms resemble typical common cold Cough worsens and may become violent and paroxysmal Vomiting may be caused by coughing or nervous system irritation; cough may linger after convalescence	Diagnosis confirmed with bacterial studies of mucus from the nasopharynx; immunofluorescent antibody technique will identify organism after it has been isolated Immune pertussis globulin (human); erythromycin antibiotic of choice; provision for rest and quiet; sedatives Light nutritious diet; judicious fluid intake to prevent dehydration; weight determinations Observed for onset of respiratory distress or other complications	Immunity usually produced after one attack Routine primary schedule plus boosters

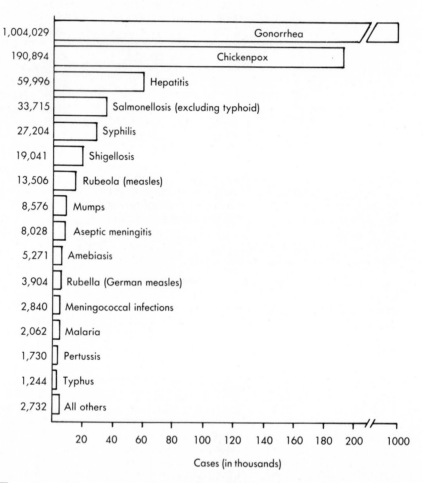

FIG. 30-3 Cases of communicable diseases (in thousands) in the United States for 1980. Total number of reported cases of specified notifiable diseases.

Statistical data from Morbidity and mortality weekly report, annual summary, 1980, **29**:3 HHS Publication No. (CDC) 81-8241, Sept. 1981.

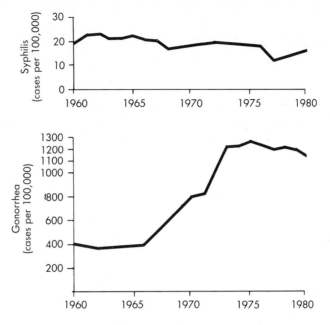

FIG. 30-4   Reported incidence of primary and secondary syphilis and gonorrhea in the United States for ages 15 to 19 years from 1960 to 1980.

Statistical data from Morbidity and mortality weekly report, annual summary, 1979 **28**:36, 83, HHS Publication No. (CDC) 80-8241, Sept. 1979, and Morbidity and mortality weekly report, annual summary, 1980, **29**:38, 82, HHS Publication No. (CDC) 80-8241, Sept. 1979, and Morbidity and mortality weekly report, annual summary, 1980, **29**:38, 82, HHS Publication No. (CDC) 81-8241, Sept. 1981.

SIGNIFICANT COMMUNICABLE DISEASES OF CHILDHOOD AND THEIR NURSING CARE

Descriptions of some of the communicable diseases seen or mentioned most often in pediatrics are included in Table 30-1. Also summarized are nursing points to remember in each case. Fortunately, not all the diseases described will be encountered by nurses today. However, all those described, and some not included, pose a potential threat to communities (Figs. 30-3 and 30-4). Diseases such as diphtheria, typhoid, and polio, for which proved preventives exist, could again ravage the population if public health standards decline and public education and support for immunization programs are not constantly maintained.

CHAPTER 31   Conditions involving the
neuromuscular and skeletal systems

All the systems of the body are intimately related. If a difficulty in one part of the body is severe enough or sufficiently prolonged, many body systems—in fact, the entire person—will react. The interdependence of the neuromuscular and skeletal systems is especially noteworthy.

Traumatic, infectious, or toxic injury to the nerve centers or nerve fibers that control the skeletal muscles often leads to wasting of those muscles and an inability to control or perhaps even initiate motion in related parts of the body. Poorly developed, abnormal, or damaged muscles may cause orthopedic deformities. Broken bones frequently cause muscle spasm and pain.

This chapter will present or review some of the more common neuromuscular and skeletal problems found in children, the methods of treatment, and, of course, the nursing care involved. Because of the amount of material, the presentation has been divided into three parts. Part 1 discusses fractures, joint and extremity problems, and other conditions involving the bones and muscles; Part 2 considers nervous system diseases that affect the bones and muscles; and Part 3 includes an assessment of vision and hearing and related pediatric disorders.

A number of the problems affecting these interrelated systems are present at birth or are congenital in nature. The more common of these congenital defects were discussed in the chapter treating abnormalities of the newborn infant. For a brief description of hydrocephalus, cranial stenosis (craniosynostosis), microcephaly, spina bifida, clubfoot, congenital dislocated hip, syndactyly, and polydactylism, refer to Chapter 14.

Part 1: Fractures, and joint and extremity problems
FRACTURES

A very common problem in childhood is a broken bone, or fracture. Roller skates, skate boards, bicycles, and the rather rough-and-tumble life of youngsters (especially boys) contribute to the high incidence of fractures. Probably even more broken bones would occur in childhood if it were not for the relatively plastic condition of the child's skeletal system. Children's bones tend to bend rather than break. Frequently, if a bone does break, it is not completely severed; a portion of the bone remains intact. This type of fracture is called an incomplete, or a *greenstick*, fracture (Fig. 31-1).

Classifications

Other common types of fractures described according to the course of the break sustained include *transverse*, *spiral*, and *oblique*. A *commi-

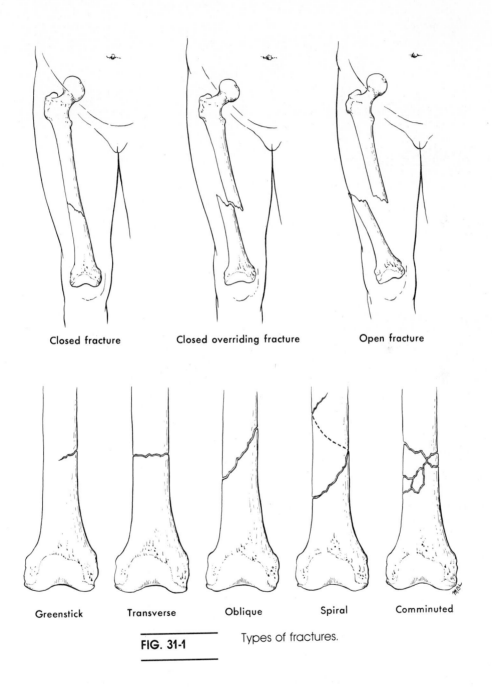

Closed fracture   Closed overriding fracture   Open fracture

Greenstick   Transverse   Oblique   Spiral   Comminuted

FIG. 31-1   Types of fractures.

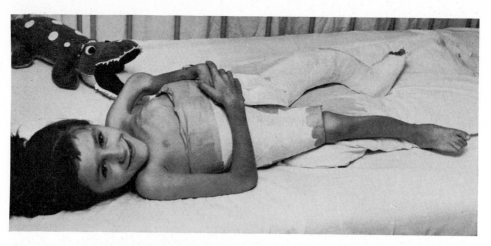

FIG. 31-2   This alert young lady is a victim of osteogenesis imperfecta congenita. She was hospitalized for corrective surgery involving previous fractures.

Courtesy Children's Hospital and Health Center, San Diego, Calif.

nuted fracture is especially difficult to repair because the bone is typically broken into several pieces. A *depressed* fraction is particularly important when the fractured bony area is the skull and abnormal pressure is exerted on sensitive brain tissue.

Fractures may result from excessive or sudden direct pressure, exaggerated muscular contractions, or a basically unsound bony structure. If an unsound bony structure is the case, the fracture is termed "pathologic." Some of the causes of pathologic fractures are osteomyelitis (infection of the bone marrow and surrounding bone cells), primary bone tumors or metastases, and osteogenesis imperfecta congenita (congenital brittle bones, a disease of unknown origin in which bones may fracture even before birth, causing characteristic skeletal malformations occasionally accompanied by deafness). If a patient has an underlying bone disease, great care and gentleness must be practiced in turning and positioning the child (Fig. 31-2).

A careful note must be made of the general condition of a child who enters the hospital with a fracture of unknown origin, multiple fractures, or a repeated fracture. Sometimes these little patients are the victims of abuse from their own parents, who are unable to meet the daily frustrations of

parenthood in a mature manner or who have deep-seated psychologic problems. Such children usually exhibit bruises and suffer from malnutrition (battered child syndrome). (See Fig. 31-3 and p. 390.)

Every fracture, irrespective of the course or extent of the break or its basic cause, may be placed in one of two main categories. If a bone is broken, but the skin overlying the fracture has not been pierced by the end of the broken bone and no opening in the skin has occurred through which organisms could be introduced from the exterior to the bone, the result is called a *simple*, or *closed*, fracture. If, however, the skin has been broken, exposing the bone to infection, the resulting trauma is called a *compound*, or *open*, fracture. Open fractures are surgical emergencies because of the increased danger of infection and extensive soft tissue damage usually involved.

First-aid considerations

A nurse encountering an accident victim with unknown injuries should take the following action:

1. Evaluate the safety of the immediate environ-

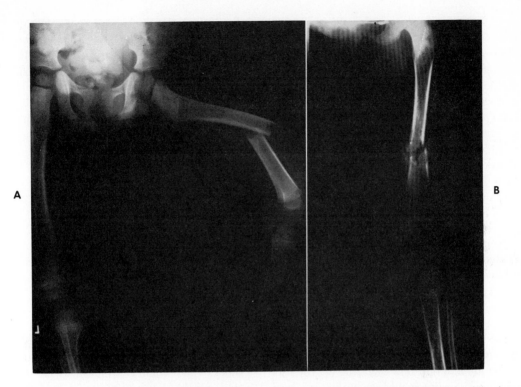

FIG. 31-3   **A,** X-ray film of the left femur of a 19-pound, 2½-year-old child who entered the hospital with multiple body bruises. Provisional diagnosis was "nonaccidental injury." **B,** X-ray film showing the same leg after reduction of the fractured femur. The shadowy outline around the break is callus.

Courtesy Naval Regional Medical Center, San Diego, Calif.

ment. (Turn off ignition of car, set out warning flares if on the highway, etc.) Send someone for help, if possible.

2. Establish an airway, if respirations are not present.
3. Control hemorrhage, if present.
4. Restore and maintain breathing, if necessary.
5. Evaluate for spinal injury and fracture. Do not move victim until proper help is available.
6. Keep the patient warm and quiet to prevent and treat shock.

If a victim with spinal injury is moved improperly, the injury may be increased and permanent paralysis or even death may occur. If the victim is conscious but cannot move any extremity, the nurse must consider the possibility of a cervical fracture or a fracture of the thoracic spine. A patient with a possible broken neck should be moved by a team so that no twisting or injurious movement of the spine will take place. The individual should be securely positioned with sand bags and other restraints and carefully transported on a rigid support while supine, chin up. Persons with suspected spinal injuries should be moved as little as possible. They should be frequently observed to detect the onset of respiratory difficulty and abdominal distention. The higher the injury on the spinal cord, the more body functions will be affected. Nonspinal fractures are less serious but still necessitate careful attention and first aid.

Indications of fracture. Fracture of an extremity may reveal itself early through the presence of the following:

1. Deformity in alignment and swelling
2. Pain or tenderness at the fracture site
3. Loss of function or abnormal mobility of the part
4. A "grating sensation" heard or felt at the suspected point of fracture (crepitus)
5. Black-and-blue areas caused by subcutaneous hemorrhage (ecchymosis)

However, the real proof of the presence of fracture must be detected by x-ray examination. Sometimes clinical symptoms are virtually lacking or very inconclusive, but the x-ray film reveals a break. Every suspected skeletal injury should be treated as a fracture until proved otherwise.

Use of splints. First-aid treatment of a possible fracture includes limitation of the movement of the injured part by stabilizing the part and the joint above and below the break to relieve muscle spasm and pain and prevent further injury. A rolled newspaper, a cardboard box, or a magazine may be used for a splint. The splint should be applied in a position comfortable for the patient. The arm or leg should be splinted without an attempt to correct any deformity. No attempt should be made to straighten it, because this may cause still further damage. No attempt should be made to push back a broken bone protruding from the skin in the case of a compound, or open, fracture. The area should simply be covered. If bleeding is present, direct manual pressure to obtain control should be used. A tourniquet is a potential hazard, because prolonged application can cause gangrene and loss of a limb. It should be used only as a last resort. If a tourniquet is used, it should be applied for 15 to 20 minutes and then removed. Rings and bracelets on a fractured upper extremity should be removed to avoid difficulty in the event of swelling. The application of ice bags may decrease the possibility of swelling. Heat should not be applied. For bleeding from an arm or leg, the part should be elevated if possible.

When a fracture involving the bones of an extremity occurs, usually the muscles attached to the broken bone, which have been under a certain amount of tension, contract as a result of loss of proper skeletal support. The pain associated with the fracture causes the muscles to go into spasm in an effort to splint the injured part. If this spasm is exaggerated, the severed ends of the broken bone may be pulled further out of alignment or may override, causing abnormal shortening of the limb.

Hospital care

Observation. When patients with possible bone fractures are first admitted to the hospital, their general condition is evaluated in detail. Vital signs (temperature, pulse, respiration, and blood pressure recordings) are obtained. Elevated blood pressure is important to report because of the possibility of skull fracture. Low blood pressure is equally important because of the possibility of shock. The level of consciousness should be evaluated and the pupils of the eyes checked for abnormal pupil dilatation or inequality of pupil size (other signs of possible skull fracture and brain injury). Depending on the patient's condition, intravenous solutions or blood may be given, but no food or fluid should be given by mouth because corrective surgery may be indicated. An x-ray examination of possible fracture sites should be made.

Reduction and casting. If overriding or angulation of a fractured bone has occurred, the displaced bone will be pulled into alignment through some form of traction until the broken fragments are in proper position. The process of bringing the fragments into proper relationship is termed "reducing," or "setting," the fracture. If the fractured bone can be set without performing a surgical operation that actually exposes the involved bone, the procedure is called a *closed* reduction. If it is necessary to expose the site of the fracture to direct view to secure proper alignment and optimum healing or use some method of internal immobilization such as the installation of a nail, pin, or screws, the procedure is called an *open* reduction. Most children's fractures may be treated by closed reduction.

At times alignment may not be disturbed. The x-ray examination reveals a break, but the bony segments are still in proper relationship. If this is happily the case, no mechanical traction apparatus is needed. A plaster cast or protective splint is applied to maintain correct positioning to assure proper healing. Occasionally only a relatively minor disturbance in alignment has occurred and can be reduced easily at the time the patient is first seen or may not even require reduction. In children a fracture often stimulates the formation of bone, and, curiously enough, at times the physician may desire a certain amount of overriding to avoid excessive growth of the fractured extremity.

If satisfactory alignment is difficult or impossible to achieve and maintain, some form of constant pull, or traction, must be exerted to reduce the fracture and bring the ends of the broken bone into proper apposition. The position of the bone and the progress of healing are intermittently checked by x-ray studies. When a sufficient amount of new bone (callus) is formed at the fracture site to help hold the broken segment in position, traction is discontinued and a protective cast is applied, allowing the patient more mobility. For a discussion of the basic nursing care involved in the care of a patient in traction or a cast, refer to Chapter 27.

Fractures involving the legs of infants and young children are often treated by suspending both legs, wrapped in bandages from a frame hanging directly above the bed. The infant's trunk almost entirely rests on the crib mattress, and only the pelvis is raised slightly from the surface of the bed. The legs are suspended at right angles to the mattress. Such an arrangement is called *Bryant's*, or *vertical*, traction (see Fig. 27-3). It is useful in treating lower extremity fractures of children weighing under 30 pounds (13.63 kg) in the infant or toddler age groups. Even though only one leg may be fractured, both are customarily placed in traction to help stabilize the position and prevent undue twist-

ing on the part of the child. When necessary, this traction device should be changed by the physician. This type of traction is potentially dangerous to circulation. The child should not be fussy in traction and toes should not be swollen; the physician should be notified if the child appears in distress. Older children will usually be placed in types of traction similar to but smaller than those used for adults.

The healing of a broken bone, or *union* of a fracture, is accomplished through the deposit of new bone cells. In children union is usually achieved in a relatively short time. Union is seldom delayed, and it is rare indeed to see a case in which union never takes place.

Rehabilitation. After the bone has united, the weakened muscles attached to the bone may have to be gradually strengthened through a program of exercise as prescribed by the physician. This part of therapy is less necessary with young children, however, since they start using the part immediately and often do not need the encouragement required by many adults. The resources of the physical therapy department may be used on an inpatient or outpatient basis. The aims of treatment are a return of function, freedom from pain, and a normal appearance.

JOINT AND EXTREMITY PROBLEMS

The skeletal system may become distorted for reasons other than fracture. Some congenital deformities and intervening paralytic or inflammatory diseases of the skeletal system may cause muscular weakness or bone destruction, producing joint instability, which prevents normal weight bearing. Some disorders reduce joint mobility so that the usefulness of a body part is greatly reduced. Other conditions may affect the growth patterns of individual extremities. Various surgical procedures have been devised to increase the effectiveness of various body joints either by increasing their ability to bear weight (increasing joint stability) or by permitting greater motion. If a choice between motion and stability must be made, in the lower extremity the decision is made in favor of stability.

The following are a few of the basic procedures used in some cases to promote healing of or gain greater usefulness for a body part or increase its contribution to the individual's total welfare.

1. *Arthrodesis* is the fusion of a joint to gain stability for weight bearing. It may be accomplished by removing the cartilage from the opposing ends of the bones that form a joint or by grafting bone into the area and then immobilizing it in a cast for a prolonged period to promote fusion. A *triple arthrodesis* is occasionally performed on a foot; as the name implies, it involves fusion of three joints. It prohibits some lateral movements of the foot itself but preserves ankle motion. Considerable bleeding may be expected after this type of surgery, and considerable pain may be involved. Weight bearing by the newly fused part is delayed until fusion is secure, in approximately 2 to 3 months.

2. *Arthroplasty* is the reconstruction of a joint to provide greater movement. The joints usually involved in the procedure are the hip and knee. Other procedures that involve the total replacement of those joints now have largely supplanted arthroplasty.

3. *Osteotomy* is an opening into or a controlled fracture of a bone to correct a congenital or acquired skeletal deformity. In a *rotational osteotomy* the distal fragment of the bone is rotated to secure the desired correction.

4. *Bone block* is an operative procedure that incorporates a piece of bone into a joint to limit motion and help produce increased joint stability. It may precede an arthrodesis.

5. *Tendon transplant* is a procedure in which a tendon from one part of the body is transplanted to another. It may be performed for various reasons— to substitute the action of neighboring strong muscles for paralyzed or weak muscles, to replace badly damaged tendons, or to decrease a deformity caused by exaggerated muscle pull.

6. *Epiphyseal arrest* may be performed to slow the growth of one extremity that is unequal in length. Properly handled, it may also aid in the correction of deformities such as knock-knees or bowlegs. It may be accomplished by a bone block or by the placement of stainless steel staples into the epiphyseal area where bone growth takes place. This procedure stops normal growth. The staples are removed when the desired results are obtained.

CONDITIONS INVOLVING THE BONES AND MUSCLES

Because many pediatric nursing courses are organized according to developmental sequence, the following conditions are presented according to the age group primarily affected. It will readily be seen that such an approach is not without inconsistencies. Some conditions extend to children of all ages; moreover, many problems present in infancy are not diagnosed until later in childhood. In spite of these difficulties, we hope our arrangement meets the needs of nursing teachers and students.

The infant

TORTICOLLIS (FIG. 31-4)

Torticollis, or wryneck, is a congenital muscular abnormality possibly associated with birth trauma. Although the defect is minimal at birth, within 2 weeks a palpable fibrous tumor appears in the sternocleidomastoid muscle. The cause of the tumor is unknown. Within a few months the fibrous tumor gradually disappears, leaving behind a contracture (shortening) of the muscle. The head of the infant is tilted toward the side of the affected muscle, and the chin is rotated to the opposite side. When the condition is recognized early, treatment consists of passive stretching of the involved muscle. Parents are instructed in the exact maneuvers to be done four or five times daily. The reward for faithful treatment is complete and permanent correction in at least 90% of the cases. When torticollis does not

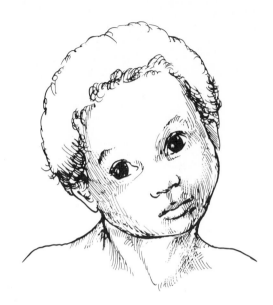

FIG. 31-4

Torticollis or wryneck; in this case, a shortening of the right sternocleidomastoid muscle.

respond to conservative measures or when treatment is not consistent, surgery is indicated. The affected muscle is divided or partially excised. The head is immobilized in the correct position for a period of time. If surgery is delayed until the child is older, postoperative exercises are necessary to prevent a recurrence.

CHILDHOOD RICKETS

One disease resulting from nutritional disturbance is common childhood rickets. The name is misleading, however, because nowadays a classic example of this disease is sometimes difficult to find in the United States. Rickets is always a potential health hazard in communities where there is little sunshine or little exposure of the children to outdoors and a diet deficient in vitamin D, calcium, or phosphorus. Vitamin D is crucial because it regulates the absorption and deposit of calcium and phosphorus. Most formulas are now specially irradiated or fortified to provide adequate levels of vitamin D to infants and children. Other rich sources are the fish-liver oils. Sunshine, if it is not screened by window glass and clothing or rendered unavailable by air pollution, is the most inexpensive source of vitamin D. Of course, vitamin preparations can be purchased. Cases of rickets may be mild and pass undetected or may be very severe and remarkable. Classic manifestations are knock-knees or bowlegs, kyphosis (humpback) or scoliosis (an abnormal lateral spinal curvature), delayed closure of fontanels and protruding forehead (bossing), thickened wrists and ankles, and enlargement of the cartilaginous area of attachment of the ribs to the sternum, forming the famous *rachitic rosary*, pigeon breast, and contracture of the pelvis. Treatment consists of greater intake of vitamin D, calcium, and phosphorus. It is possible, but not probable, to have an excessive vitamin D intake, so discretion should be used in the selection and dosage of therapeutic vitamins.

The toddler

DUCHENNE'S MUSCULAR DYSTROPHY

A number of conditions are characterized by a progressive weakening of the musculoskeletal system and eventual wasting of muscle tissue. They differ in the main muscles affected, the course of the disability, and the usual age of onset. Duchenne's, or pseudohypertrophic, muscular dystrophy is the commonest form of the progressive types of muscle weakness. The onset of this disease usually occurs within the first 3 years of life. Occasionally the onset commences between the third and sixth years. It is a hereditary, sex-linked recessive condition that is said to affect males almost exclusively. In this type of dystrophy, a fatty infiltration of the muscle cells may produce a deceptively large muscle lacking strength, hence its title "pseudohypertrophic" muscular dystrophy. This condition is seen especially in the calf muscles. Intramuscular enzymes, creatine phosphokinase (CPK) and serum aldolase, leak into the blood

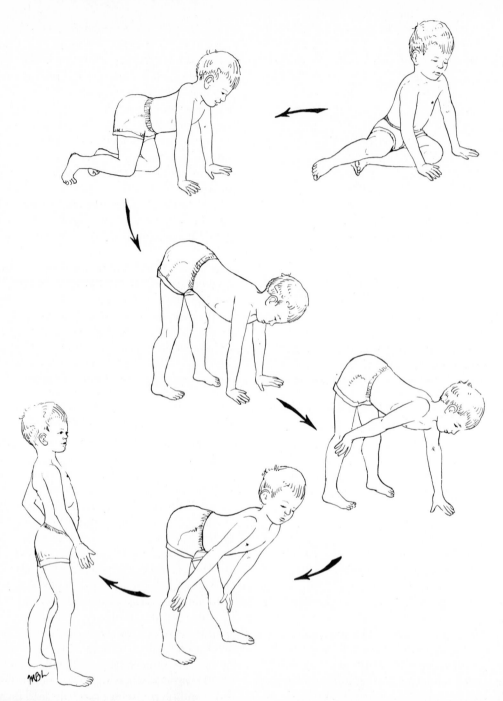

FIG. 31-5   Gower's sign, the "self-climbing procedure," characteristic of pseudohypertrophic muscular dystrophy.

serum as muscle tissue breaks down. Serum values of these enzymes are very high in the early stages of the disease but decline as the disease progresses, and in the final stages they are only slightly above normal (apparently because so little muscle tissue is left). The affected young child has difficulty in walking and falls easily as the muscular weakness attacks, in sequence, the muscles of the legs, pelvis, and abdomen. A pronounced lordosis develops as the youngster struggles to remain upright. These children display a characteristic method of supporting themselves when attempting to rise to their feet from a seated posture on the floor. They rise to their knees, extend legs and arms, grasp the lower part of their legs with their hands, and gradually push themselves upward in a self-climbing procedure. This is one of the most characteristic signs of muscular dystrophy (Fig. 31-5). The genetic background of the family, the history and examination of the child revealing the progressive nature of the problem, serum enzyme tests, electromyogram, and muscle biopsy confirm the diagnosis. Muscle biopsy is especially valuable in determining the exact type of muscular problem. Preclinical cases can now be diagnosed by determining serum enzyme levels. The CPK test is a valuable aid in identifying muscular dystrophy carriers. Counseling of affected families and carriers is an important preventive measure.

Duchenne's muscular dystrophy is a tragic model of neuromuscular disease. The term alone produces anxiety and fear in parents, so it must be emphasized that nonprogressive and indeed treatable muscle disorders may mimic Duchenne's. Only with confirmation by available techniques should parents be informed of this diagnosis.

A diagnosis of muscular dystrophy (no matter what type) is difficult for parents to accept. For the Duchenne type, life expectancy is usually limited to the teenage period. Death often results from respiratory weakness and intervening infection. The course of the disease is downhill, and it is particularly disheartening for parents who first see their children confined to wheelchairs, and then to eventually see them bedridden to the extent that they need help to turn over. Many times much can be gained if the parents of such children can meet together to share their common burdens and learn from one another how certain problems can be met. The local muscular dystrophy associations often sponsor such groups.

The nurse sees the child with muscular dystrophy in the hospital setting chiefly at the time of diagnosis, when orthopedic appliances such as braces and splints are being evaluated, or when the presence of other health problems makes it especially difficult to nurse the child at home.

JUVENILE RHEUMATOID ARTHRITIS (STILL'S DISEASE)

The most common form of arthritis encountered in pediatrics is juvenile rheumatoid arthritis (or Still's disease).

This disease affects the entire body's health. In studies it is often grouped with the collagen diseases, which affect all the connective tissues of the body. It does not confine itself to symptoms of joint pain, although this is a remarkable manifestation of the disease. The joints swell and become stiff, slightly warm, and painful with movement. Almost all the joints may eventually become involved, but the knees, ankles, and fingers are most frequently affected. The fingers often assume a spindle shape as a result of the swelling of their middle joints (Fig. 31-6).

Fever is a significant manifestation of the disease. The temperature may swing daily as high as 105° F (40.5° C) in the evening and return to normal by morning. The pattern on the temperature chart is usually characteristic and of great value in the differential diagnosis of a patient with acute juvenile rheumatoid arthritis.

Other signs and symptoms of juvenile rheumatoid arthritis include enlargement of the liver, spleen, and lymph nodes, anemia, anorexia, pallor, and possibly a salmon-colored, blotchy rash. Pericarditis, myocarditis, and uveitis are seen occasionally. Rheumatoid arthritis is aggravated by emotional stress and fatigue.

Kind and understanding parental support, pro-

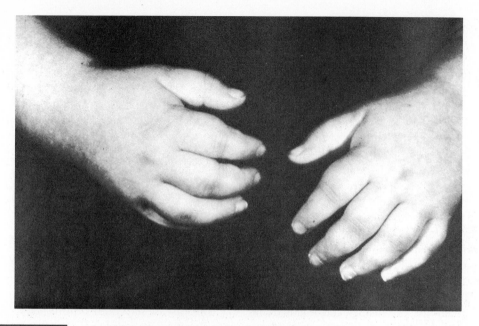

FIG. 31-6   Juvenile rheumatoid arthritis. Spindle-shaped fingers in a 2½-year-old boy.
Courtesy Naval Regional Medical Center, San Diego, Calif.

motion of general health, and physical therapy will achieve most of the therapeutic goals. No specific treatment is known. Although many medications have been tried, aspirin is the drug of choice to relieve pain, reduce swelling, and increase range of motion. It is prescribed four times daily, and the dosage is often increased to toxic levels and then reduced for best results. The children are carefully observed in the clinic and the parents cautioned about early signs of toxicity (p. 388).

A second drug for joint disease is gold salts. This medication, given with acetylsalicylic acid (aspirin) will often relieve joint symptoms in the difficult case. It is given weekly by injection. Before a patient's receiving gold therapy, a complete blood cell count and urinalysis are done, and only if they are normal is gold treatment initiated. These tests are performed weekly, since renal and hematologic complications have been reported.

In rare instances prednisone or corticosteroids may also be used for treatment of myocarditis, uve-itis, and very severe systemic disease. Steroids tend to alleviate symptoms of joint disease without affecting the basic disease process. However, the usefulness of steroids is limited by their toxicity. Toxic manifestations of such hormone therapy may include decalcification of the skeleton, altered tissue response to infections and other injuries, personality changes, moon face, abnormal growth of the clitoris in girls, and the appearance of excessive body hair (Fig. 31-7).

Unless joint activity is maintained, a joint will become permanently stiffened or immovable, a condition known as *ankylosis* of the joint. For this reason it is important to maintain reasonable joint activity by reducing pain and providing specific tasks or play goals designed to exercise the involved joints.

The rheumatoid patient, unless extremely careful, is likely to assume positions of comfort, which, if maintained for prolonged periods, will cause deformities that will interfere with motions neces-

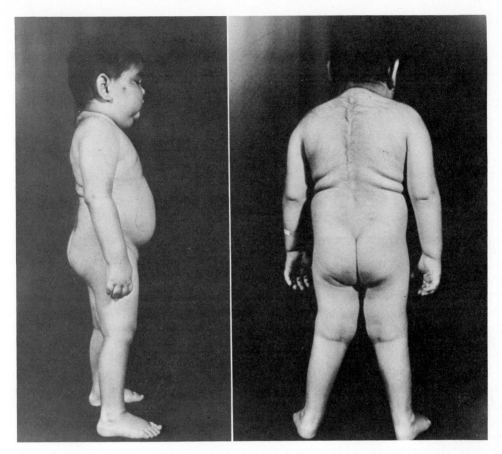

FIG. 31-7   Hypercortisolism in a 2½-year-old boy as a result of intensive steroid therapy. Note moon facies, excessive growth of hair (hirsutism), prominent fat pads, buffalo hump, and marked weight gain.

Courtesy Naval Regional Medical Center, San Diego, Calif.

sary to meet the needs of daily living. Mobility should be encouraged—as much as can be tolerated—even during periods of active disease and inflammation. When pain and inflammation are suppressed by salicylates, most children are encouraged to ambulate. The most effective, continuous therapeutic exercise program is provided through the child's own play activities. Play activities should be directed to provide the maximum exercise for the joints most involved. Play activity

and formal exercises will help prevent the stiffness and deformity that result from inactivity. The physical therapist will teach children and their parents exercises designed to give complete range of motion in each joint.

Although juvenile rhematoid arthritis may improve and then worsen over a period of years, usually it gradually subsides as puberty approaches. However, in some cases it may persist actively into adulthood and may leave difficult deformities.

ORTHOPEDIC COMPLICATIONS OF HEMOPHILIA

The problem of damaged joints should not be completely closed without at least mentioning another interesting cause of joint difficulty. The child with hemophilia, the classic bleeder, may sustain considerable joint destruction because of "insignificant initiating injuries" followed by hemorrhages into the joints of the knees and elbows. These patients must be placed in traction and protective casts fairly frequently.

The preschool child

LEGG-CALVÉ-PERTHES DISEASE (COXA PLANA)

Legg-Calvé-Perthes disease is a self-limited disease of the hip produced by lack of circulation to the femoral head. The initial degeneration of the femoral head is followed by absorption and regeneration of bone. The entire process takes an average of 4 years.

This development disease of the hip is commonly seen in children between 4 and 8 years of age and has a much higher incidence in boys. The initial complaint is usually a limp of several months' duration. Some children have a limp with pain (referred to the knee) that is aggravated by activity and relieved by rest. The primary cause of Legg-Calvé-Perthes disease is unknown. Trauma and synovitis of the hip have preceded some cases. A great variety of treatment has been used, including 4 years of bed rest. Modern successful treatment of the disease centers around two basic principles: (1) maintaining a full range of motion and (2) keeping the femoral head deep in the socket during its period of healing. In this way the physician seeks to obtain a femoral head that fits well and prevents the development of degenerative arthritis in the later years.

Treatment consists of traction until symptoms are resolved, followed by hip bracing in an abducted and slightly internally rotated position to properly maintain the femoral head in the acetabulum. Such bracing removes pressure from the avascular head of the femur. It helps to keep the child ambulatory with the least discomfort and limitation of activity during the years of necessary management. Surgery on the pelvis or femur may be indicated where conservative treatment has failed.

OSTEOMYELITIS

Inflammatory bone conditions caused by disease-producing organisms were more common in the past. With increased availability of different types of antibiotics and other helpful medications, osteomyelitis, or inflammation of the bone resulting from infectious agents, has decreased remarkably. If the term "osteomyelitis" is used without a qualifying phrase, it is assumed to mean infection of the bone by either pathogenic staphylococcal or streptococcal organisms. However, broadly speaking, osteomyelitis may also be caused by the tuberculosis bacillus, the gonococcus, or a wide variety of lesser known bacteria. The form of osteomyelitis caused by staphylococci or streptococci may be preceded by some type of local injury to the bone that either introduces the organism directly or weakens the bone so that it is more susceptible to any offending organisms brought to the area by the bloodstream from some distant source of infection.

Blood-borne infections are most common. Boys are more frequently affected than girls. Pain near the end of a long bone and fever are clinically associated with osteomyelitis. The characteristic pain is initially very severe and unremitting because pressure is building up in a closed space. When pus begins to track out under the periosteum, the area is extremely tender, more so than a fracture. Treatment is started on the basis of the clinical examination alone. The child is placed on a regimen of bed rest, and the affected limb is immobilized. Analgesics are given to lessen the pain. Although blood cultures are positive in only 50% of patients with osteomyelitis, they are taken immediately and during the first few days after examination in the hope of identifying the causative organism. Initially large doses of broad-spectrum antibiotics are given. X-ray evidence of osteomyelitis is not seen for 10 days following the onset of symptoms. Surgery is considered necessary if improvement is not seen within 36 to 48 hours after antibiotic therapy is instituted. The area of maximum tenderness is drilled to decompress the bone and to allow the pus to drain. The organism responsible for the infection is identified, and a cast is applied to the affected limb. An opening in the cast is made at the surgical site, and the wound is infused with physiologic saline or antibiotics for a period of several days before being surgically closed. Intravenous antibiotic therapy is continued for another 3 weeks. During this time the child is kept on a regimen of bed rest, and the progress of the infection may be monitored by daily sedimentation rates. When the results of this test are nearly normal, antibiotics can be stopped and, hopefully, the risk of chronic osteomyelitis and extensive bone damage has been minimized.

The school-age child

BONE TUMORS

Some of the symptoms of infectious osteomyelitis are duplicated when the cause is not pathogenic organisms but the development of abnormal cells producing a tumor within the bone. Some of these masses of abnormal tissue are *benign* and of purely local importance. They may cause pain, at times accompanied by fever, and deformity. The tumors may weaken the structure of the bone, but they do not spread (or metastasize) to distant parts of the body. Other types of bone tumors grow rapidly and metastasize early through the bloodstream. These tumors are *malignant*. An osteosarcoma originates in connective tissue (of which bone is one example) and is the most common primarily malignant tumor of bone. School-age boys are affected almost twice as often as girls. The commonest sites are those characterized by active epiphyseal growth (for example, the distal end of the femur and the proximal ends of the tibia and humerus). Initially the child complains of mild pain in the affected part, but in a matter of days to weeks, the pain is constant and severe. As the condition progresses, the tumor mass becomes obvious. Limitation of adjacent joint motion is common. Early diagnosis and immediate treatment are crucial.

X-ray studies are characteristic, but the diagnosis is made only after biopsy and pathologic studies of the tissue. Occasionally tumors of the bone in children may be secondary to tumors located elsewhere. When a tissue of bony origin is malignant, aggressive anticancer chemotherapy and radical methods of treatment, including amputation, must be endorsed in an effort to save the patient. The prognosis has been vastly improved with recent advances in surgical treatment coupled with multiple drug chemotherapy.

SPINAL CURVATURE

Spinal deformities such as scoliosis (S-shaped lateral curvature), kyphosis (humpback), and lordosis (exaggerated lumbar curvature) may be the products of many different conditions, including the following:

1. Nutritional deficiencies, such as common childhood rickets
2. Inflammation of the bony spine (osteomyelitis, tuberculosis, arthritis, or dislocation of the hips)
3. Nerve injury resulting in paralytic conditions and unequal muscle pull (myelomeningocele, poliomyelitis)
4. Primary muscle weakness or dystrophy

Scoliosis. Of the three kinds of abnormal spinal curvatures, scoliosis (or the lateral curvature), is probably the most common spinal deformity encountered in childhood. Lateral curvature of the spine can be divided into two major groups: nonstructural (functional) and structural. The patient can voluntarily correct a nonstructural curve by altering position. In functional scoliosis, a condition outside the spine (such as poor posture, pain or muscle spasm, or short leg) has caused a temporary misalignment of the vertebrae. A structural scoliosis is an irreversible lateral curvature that leads to permanent anatomic changes unless early preventive measures are taken.

Three basic types of structural scoliosis are seen:

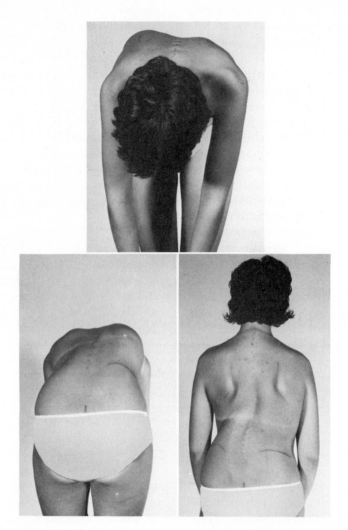

FIG. 31-8

Idiopathic scoliosis in 14-year-old girl. First visit to orthopedist. Screening positions; standing and forward bend. Observe for (1) general posture and alignment of the spine: (a) lateral angulation and (b) balance of head, neck, and shoulders over pelvis; and (2) asymmetry: (a) exaggerated flank crease—more prominent on opposite side, (b) high shoulder, (c) position of scapulae, (d) convexity on side of major curve (caused by protruding ribs), (e) prominent hip, and (f) one arm longer than the other when hanging free in the forward bend position.

Courtesy Naval Regional Medical Center, San Diego, Calif.

congenital, paralytic, and idiopathic. Congenital scoliosis results when one side of the vertebral column grows faster than the other. Surgical correction at 1 or 2 years of age may be indicated to prevent greater asymmetric growth. Paralytic scoliosis may result from poliomyelitis or other neuromuscular disorders. To prevent respiratory complications, some type of stabilization of the spine must be considered, either using an external support or surgery. Idiopathic scoliosis is the most common type, accounting for 80% of the cases classified as structural. It is called idiopathic because the cause is unknown. However, there seems to be a definite familial tendency that suggests a dominant inheritance pattern. The condition is more common in girls and is most apparent during adolescence, although it usually begins much earlier. The level of the curve may be cervical, thoracic, lumbar, or a combination of these. The most important aspect of the deformity is its progression with skeletal growth. As the lateral curvature and rotation of the spine increases, secondary permanent changes develop in the vertebrae and ribs. Misalignment of the spinal joints worsens and eventually leads to painful degenerative spinal joint disease in adult life. In addition to the "crooked back" with a high shoulder, prominent hip, and uneven legs, the deformity of the spine may compromise cardiopulmonary function and shorten the patient's life expectancy. The progression of the curvature is slow and steady, seldom arousing the concern of the parent or child. Poor posture, an uneven hemline, and inability to be fitted for a dress are common complaints that cause the parents to bring the child in for evaluation. Because pain is not associated with the progressive curve, the deformity often reaches 30 degrees before it is detected. The deformity can be clinically evaluated in three positions (Fig. 31-8). Radiologic studies confirm the extent of the deformity. The primary (major) curve is greatest in angulation and is the least flexible. It is always more marked than would be expected from the physical appearance (Fig. 31-9).

Screening. The only sure way of preventing the severe curvatures of idiopathic scoliosis, which

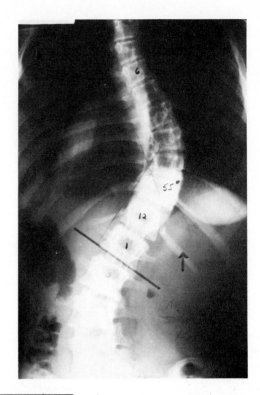

FIG. 31-9

Radiograph of 14-year-old girl (same as in Fig. 31-8) shows a 55-degree right thoracic curve of the spine.

Courtesy Naval Regional Medical Center, San Diego, Calif.

usually involve major surgical procedures and their inherent risk, is by early recognition. The presence of a mild deformity allows the use of reliable, safe, effective nonsurgical treatment. Most children who demonstrate a curve at 11 or 12 years of age have almost always had it for a number of years. Therefore screening programs for lateral curvatures should begin before 10 years of age and should include boys as well as preadolescent girls. Routine inspection of the spine by school nurses can be most rewarding.

Treatment. An orthopedist should determine the need for correction and examine the child with sco-

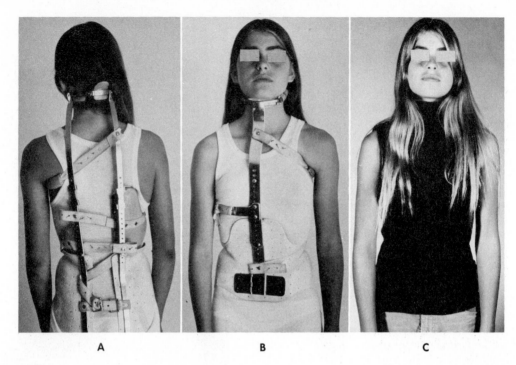

A   B   C

FIG. 31-10   **A,** Thirteen-year-old girl wearing a Milwaukee brace with right thoracic pad, left axillary sling, and left lumbar pad. Overall alignment is good. **B,** Same child front view. Brace is contoured closely to the body. **C,** It can be worn under clothing without being noticed.

liosis at regular intervals to detect any progression of the curve. Curves up to 20 degrees can probably be left alone and watched. Curves that are between 20 to 45 degrees and progressing are stabilized with a brace. The Milwaukee brace (Fig. 31-10) is the standard device used in the nonoperative treatment of mild spinal curvatures. It is designed to provide dynamic correction that incorporates a vertical pushing force between the head and pelvis through adjustable, rigid uprights as well as a lateral corrective force directed toward the convex side of the major curve. The brace is well contoured and cosmetically acceptable. To prevent worsening of the scoliosis, it is necessary to wear the brace full time (for several years), except for brief periods needed for personal hygiene, until complete maturation of the spine has occurred. Prevention of progression of the curve is likely

when treatment is begun at an early age. Normal activities (such as bike riding and skating) are encouraged while wearing the brace. In fact, an active exercise program is required to maintain good muscle tone. Most children learn to accept the brace, live with it, and have good results.

Surgical correction is usually considered for curves that are over 50 degrees. Surgery offers the best outcome for (1) curves that are cosmetically objectionable (over 60 degrees) in the preadolescent or postadolescent patient, and (2) a growing child in whom conservative measures have failed. The operation consists of a spinal fusion that is supplemented by the insertion and spinal attachment of an internal apparatus. The Harrington rod serves to obtain correction and to provide an internal type of immobilization (Fig. 31-11). After spinal fusion the patient may be placed in a body cast 10 days

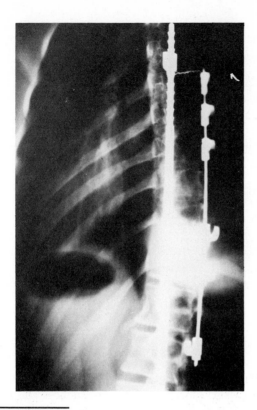

FIG. 31-11

Radiograph of back of same patient as in Fig. 31-8, 6 months after spinal fusion and Harrington instrumentation.

Courtesy Naval Regional Medical Center, San Diego, Calif.

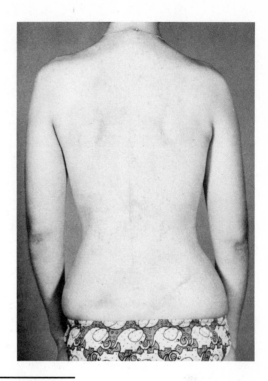

FIG. 31-12

Postoperative standing position shows girl's spine reasonably well compensated.

Courtesy Naval Regional Medical Center, San Diego, Calif.

postoperatively; then progressive ambulation in the cast is encouraged. (See Fig. 31-12.) The localizer frame devised by Dr. Risser in the early 1950s is commonly used in the application of the jacket cast (Fig. 31-13). Complete union and maturation at the fusion site takes about 1 year.

Halo traction. The halo traction is used in the treatment of a rigid spinal curvature associated with weakness or paralysis of the neck and trunk muscles. It also may be employed in the care of cervical fractures and fusions. The halo consists of a metal ring that is attached to the skull by two posterior pins in the occipital bone and two anterior

pins inserted into the temporal or frontal bones. It is attached to a weight while countertraction is exerted by weights connected to two Steinmann pins inserted into the distal ends of both femurs. The weights are increased daily as tolerated by the child until maximum correction is obtained.

When maximum correction of the curve is evidenced by x-ray examination, a spinal fusion is usually done. Weighted halo traction may be continued to prevent loss of the correction, or a body cast or jacket is applied, incorporating the halo by means of an extended frame, to maintain the gains accomplished by the original traction and fusion.

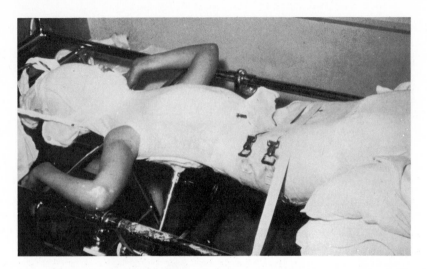

FIG. 31-13   Application of Risser cast. The cast may be applied before surgery and then bivalved for use as a postoperative holding jacket. This photograph shows neck halter, pelvic band, and a positioned localizer helping to maintain the patient's posture on the frame.

Courtesy Paul E. Woodward, M.D., San Diego, Calif.

NURSING CARE. The procedure should be explained step by step to children in words that they can understand. Their questions should be answered carefully. They may complain that the pins hurt. This usually indicates that the pins are loose, and it may be necessary for the physician to change one or more of the pins to a different site. The pins are cleaned daily with hydrogen peroxide, and the skin around each pin is painted with antiseptic.

Proper alignment of all equipment, especially the ropes, is necessary for effective traction. The little patient may prefer to remain in the supine position but should be turned at least every 2 hours, from back to side and side to back. Patients are encouraged to breathe deeply for a few minutes each time they are turned. Adequate ventilation of the lungs is extremely important, because a respiratory deficit often accompanies advanced scoliosis. Treatment includes promotion of pulmonary function, which is accomplished by specific breathing exercises.

Active and passive range of motion helps main-tain muscular strength. Careful attention is given to the skin, especially bony prominences and the heels. Neurologic and cardiac complications are not uncommon. Appropriate notice should be given to these important considerations without frightening the child. Bowel and bladder difficulties are frequent. They may be lessened by adequate intake of fluids, foods rich in bulk, and occasional laxatives. Remember that immobilization decreases appetite. Children should be given every opportunity to help select their diets when a choice is possible. Their psychologic growth is just as important as their physical well-being.

Spinal fusion. Casts, which may be worn for an extended period after a spinal fusion, make turning the patient much simpler and safer. However, if a cast is not applied after a spinal fusion, care must be exercised so that the spinal column is not twisted during changes in position. The patient's bed should be kept flat unless specific permission has been granted to allow the patient to be on a slight incline while in *supine* position (on the back). A noncasted patient who is allowed to be turned should be gently logrolled from back to side with the use of a turning sheet and at least two nurses (more if the size of the patient indicates that more hands are needed). Such a patient, casted or not, who is turned from the back to a side-lying position should have a pillow between the thighs to prevent the adduction of the top leg and pull on the small of the back. Just how much motion will be allowed a patient will depend on the physician's wishes.

Patients who have had a spinal fusion need the same basic preoperative and postoperative care required for all surgical patients. In addition, they may need the special attention necessary for all casted patients (Chapter 27). Constipation may be a particular problem; therefore the type of diet, fluid intake, and habit-times need special attention.

Therapy for severe scoliosis is usually long. It characteristically will involve innumerable visits to the physician for evaluation, hospitalization at intervals for cast changes, brace adjustments, or surgical interventions, and physical therapy. The parents and child (young woman or man) need to be constantly encouraged to continue treatment faithfully until optimum, lasting results are achieved.

Part 2: Nervous system diseases affecting bones and muscles

THE INFANT

Seizure disorders

The term "convulsive seizure" denotes an excessive and disorderly discharge from nervous tissue resulting in involuntary muscular activity or lapses in consciousness. It is really not a diagnosis but simply a description of a transient disturbance of the central nervous system (Fig. 31-14). As noted, seizures may be caused by a number of conditions. Significant fever may be the precipitating cause, especially in the age group 6 to 36 months. Seizures may also originate from congenital brain deformities, or increased intracranial pressure caused by tumors, abscess formation, or edema of the brain. Cerebral irritation resulting from toxic or infectious agents may be implicated. A chronic or recurrent convulsive disorder may also be called *epilepsy*. Some writers reserve the term "epilepsy" for recurrent convulsions of the idiopathic variety (cases of unknown cause). Opinions differ regarding the role of heredity in idiopathic seizures. Some authorities believe that heredity may be a significant cause. Because some states and communities may have laws limiting the activities of those persons who have been diagnosed as epileptic and because the public does not always understand what the word means in a specific case, many physicians hesitate to use this particular term when describing the patient's problem. The nurse would also do well to use the word very discreetly. It has been estimated that approximately 1% of the population has some type of epileptic disorder. An additional 2% have had febrile seizures.

Many types of seizures exist; the grand mal type represents one half of all seizure disorders, and the petit mal type, also known as "absence seizures," represents about 10% of all seizure disorders. Twenty percent of epileptics have mixed seizure disorders, which manifest characteristics of more than one type. Grand mal seizures affect the large muscle groups of the body. Usually the entire body becomes involved in dramatic, involuntary muscular contractions of considerable force. Petit mal seizures, on the other hand, are characterized by minor tremors or brief losses of consciousness revealed perhaps only by a prolonged blank stare or the dropping of an object held in the hand. The frequency of either type of seizure may be extremely variable. A child may experience a seizure rarely, or many times during a 24-hour period. Diagnosis is aided by a study of the child's brain waves, or an electroencephalogram (EEG).

Children who have grand mal seizures may experience a subjective warning of an impending episode. Such a warning is called an aura. It usually occurs a few minutes before the attack. It may

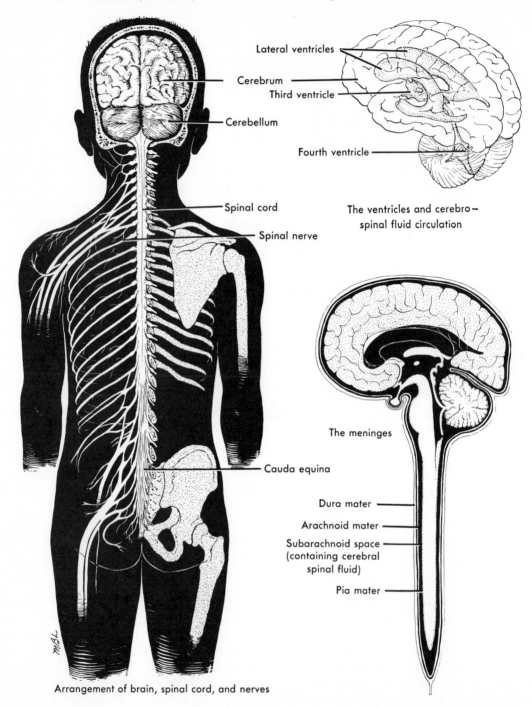

Lateral ventricles

Cerebrum

Third ventricle

Cerebellum

Fourth ventricle

Spinal cord

Spinal nerve

The ventricles and cerebro—
spinal fluid circulation

The meninges

Cauda equina

Dura mater

Arachnoid mater

Subarachnoid space
(containing cerebral
spinal fluid)

Pia mater

Arrangement of brain, spinal cord, and nerves

FIG. 31-14   Simplified central nervous system anatomy and peripheral nerve relationships.

come in the form of a vague feeling of uneasiness or as some type of sensory cue. For example, the patient may hear, see, or smell things in a particular manner. Such auras are useful to patients because they can seek out places of safety and privacy if they are forewarned of an attack. In small children the presence of an aura may only be detected through the awareness of a child's repetitive actions, such as climbing into mother's lap, preceding a seizure.

The grand mal seizure usually begins with a period of rigidity and temporary respiratory arrest. The first sign of an attack may be involuntary movements of the eyeball (the eyes rolling upward or to the side) and a stiffening of body parts. The patient temporarily suspends respirations and may become cyanotic. Saliva is not swallowed, and the patient may drool. The patient may utter a high-pitched cry. This first period, called the *tonic* phase, is usually followed by intermittent contractions of the muscles. This secondary period is the so-called *clonic* phase. During this time the tongue and lips may be bitten, and saliva, as a result, may be blood tinged.

The nursing care of a patient having a convulsion emphasizes the need to protect the patient from accidental injury and the importance of close observation and report. If possible, a patient should be placed on the side or lie with the face turned to one side to avoid aspiration. The patient should be placed in an area where the possibility of personal injury as a result of uncontrolled muscular contractions would be minimal: on the floor on a rug, if possible, or in bed. The beds or cribs of patients who experience fairly frequent convulsions of the grand mal type should be equipped with side rails padded with folded blankets or pillows. In the hospital setting nurses are taught to have a well-padded tongue blade readily accessible at the bedside for insertion into the mouth between the back teeth before the onset of the clonic phase of the seizure to prevent mouth injury. If a padded tongue blade is not available, a rolled washcloth may be helpful. In most instances the use of a blade is not required; sometimes it may cause more prob-

lems than failure to use anything at all, since loss of teeth or mouth lacerations have resulted. Nurses should not pry open a patient's mouth to insert a tongue blade. Such a maneuver may cause considerable injury and serves no practical purpose, because the damage to the mouth in most cases has already occurred. Most hospitals have discontinued the routine use of a tongue blade unless ordered by a physician. The Epilepsy Society does not advise the general public to place anything into the person's mouth. There have been too many incidents of mouth injury or aspiration caused, not by the convulsion, but by the insertion of an improper tongue protector.

After first securing a safe position for the convulsing patient, the nurse should focus her powers of observation to be able to describe the circumstances and sequence of the attack. She should note the following information:

1. When the seizure began and what type of activity immediately preceded its occurrence
2. What signs of difficulty were first noted, what part of the body was first affected, the position of the eyes, and how the convulsion progressed
3. How long the attack lasted and whether fever preceded or followed the attack
4. Whether the patient was incontinent
5. Whether prolonged cyanosis or profuse saliva appeared (may signal the need for the use of oxygen or possible suctioning)

In the great majority of cases the seizure (ictus) subsides and the child falls into a deep sleep called the postictal state. When finally awake again, the child may not remember the seizure but feel tired and sore. Children should be reassured regarding the episode and be gently questioned to determine if they had any warning, or aura, of the attack.

Almost all patients who suffer from idiopathic epilepsy and many with organically initiated seizures are receiving some type of anticonvulsant therapy. A number of medications are available, prescribed according to the individual needs of the patient. Some commonly used drugs to stop or control seizures are diazepam (Valium), diphenylhydantoin sodium (Dilantin), and phenobarbital. The time schedule established for taking anticonvulsants should be faithfully followed to avoid any interruption in treatment and the possible appearance of a seizure. Other methods to help prevent seizures limit fluids and stress a high-fat–low-carbohydrate (ketogenic) diet. Complete or almost complete control can be obtained in approximately one half of the cases. The condition of many patients can be well regulated with medical therapy, and they are able to live normal lives. A few types of epilepsy (for example, petit mal) may disappear after puberty; some change their form; others, unfortunately, persist throughout life. The nurse should realize that fatigue, illness, excitement, hyperventilation, blinking lights, and especially failure to take anticonvulsants or a change in anticonvulsant therapy may help bring on certain seizures.

The patient and family need continuous, good medical supervision and counsel. The patient should be encouraged to live life to the fullest within the limits of the disease as imposed by the community and the child's own sense of responsibility. The intelligence levels of people with epilepsy are similar to those found in the population as a whole.

The Epilepsy Societies have done considerable public education regarding the disorder, attempting to remove false ideas and any legislation that unjustly limits the activities of affected persons.

Meningitis

Meningitis, simply stated, is inflammation of the meninges. Not all types of meningitis are infectious, but the infectious types are far more common. The hemophilus influenza bacillus, meningococcus, and pneumococcus are common etiologic agents responsible for acute bacterial meningitis in children past 1 month of age. Meningitis usually affects children under 2 years of age. and *Haemophilus influenzae* is by far the most common caus-

ative agent. Whatever the cause or age of onset, the treatment of meningitis is always considered a medical emergency. Early recognition and prompt treatment are essential for a favorable recovery. A long and severe infection may result in death or lingering neurologic damage. (See Fig. 31-15.)

Typically the child is irritable and restless or drowsy. Previous upper respiratory tract infections and ear infections are frequently associated with *Haemophilus influenzae* meningitis. For this reason the nurse should impress on parents the importance of continuing medications (for otitis media or other inflammations) and all antibiotics prescribed for as long as ordered. Fever, vomiting, chills, headache, rigidity of the neck and back, and convulsions are common. In more severe cases the child may be in shock or exhibit an involuntary arching of the back known as opisthotonos (Fig. 31-16). A high-pitched cry is characteristic. Meningococcal meningitis is usually accompanied by petechiae, a hemorrhagic skin rash caused by meningococcal invasion of the bloodstream. However, meningococcemia may occur without central nervous system involvement.

A lumbar puncture is done at the slightest suspicion of meningitis. Parents and children fear a lumbar puncture. Parents should be reassured of the importance, relative safety, and necessity of this procedure. Children, if conscious and old enough to understand, should be mentally prepared just before the procedure. They should be told what is going to happen and that they are likely to feel discomfort. Reminding them that it is important to lie still during the procedure may provide a sense of control and thereby reduce feelings of helplessness. During the procedure, the child may be told that it is okay to cry but that lying still will be the best help. The assisting nurse must understand the importance of maintaining the position of the child. Several holds are possible, depending on the size of the child; however, positioning the child on the side (lateral decubitus) is usually preferred. The back of the patient is arched "like a kitten's" to provide greater room for the insertion of the needle between the vertebrae at the level of the iliac crest.

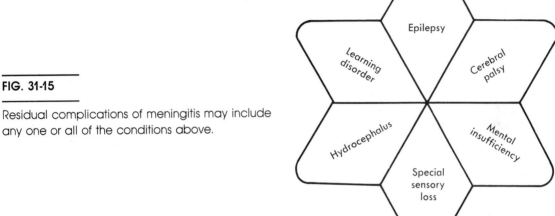

FIG. 31-15

Residual complications of meningitis may include any one or all of the conditions above.

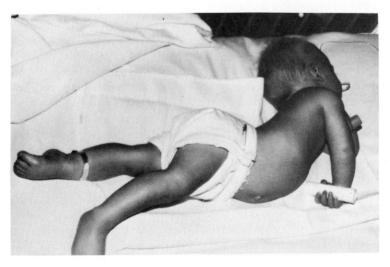

FIG. 31-16   A victim of near-drowning showing marked opisthotonos. This posture may be assumed by anyone suffering from severe meningeal irritation.

Courtesy Alan Shumacher, M.D., San Diego, Calif.

The skin is prepared with an antiseptic by the gloved physician. At the time of the lumbar puncture the pressure of the fluid within the meninges may be measured by attaching a measuring tube or manometer to the spinal needle. Three specimens of spinal fluid are usually collected consecutively in specially numbered sterile specimen containers. All three containers are sent to the laboratory, where they should be immediately examined for cellular and chemical content. From the contents of the first tube, a Gram stain and culture are done to identify any organisms that may be present. A Gram stain can often identify an organism at once, before the return of the culture report. The second tube is examined for chemical content, usually glucose and protein. The third tube is examined for blood cell content. The selection of the third tube for this procedure reduces the possibility that minor bleeding from insertion of the needle will alter the cell count. At the conclusion of the puncture procedure, care should be taken to remove iodine-containing preparations that may be used to prepare the skin. This avoids the occurrence of serious contact rashes. A Band-Aid is placed over the site of the needle insertion.

The child is isolated for 24 hours after the start of antibiotic therapy. The meaning of this isolation and why the nurse wears a gown should be explained to parents. If they are not allowed to enter the room, the crib should be turned so they might at least see the child's face.

An intravenous infusion is started as soon as the lumbar puncture is completed. Large doses of ampicillin are given intravenously with fluid and electrolyte replacement. Ampicillin is currently the drug of choice in meningitis of unknown types. Ampicillin is often given in combination with chloramphenicol (Chloromycetin.) Good supportive care requires that dehydration be corrected promptly, but the alert nurse will guard against overhydration. Symptoms of water intoxication are headache, confusion, sudden weight gain, edema, convulsions, and coma.

Effective restraints must be used to safeguard the infusion. The nurse should carefully position the restrained child on the side during intravenous therapy lest the patient convulse or aspirate vomitus. Constant nursing care and frequent observation of the child are necessary during the acute phase. Monitoring the vital signs is especially important when increased intracranial pressure is suspected. Slowed pulse, irregular respirations, and elevated blood pressure are signs of increased intracranial pressure and should be called to the physician's attention at once. Cerebral pressure may be lessened by overventilating with mask and bag, which decreases PCO_2, by infusion of drugs such as mannitol, or by surgical intervention. Such methods are often lifesaving.

The infant may be placed in an oxygen-enriched environment in an incubator. The older child may be placed in an oxygen tent. Other nursing responsibilities include control of temperature by sponging and a cool environment. Routine antipyretics are usually not recommended, because they interfere with monitoring the temperature response, which determines the length of ampicillin therapy. Accurately recording the intravenous intake and the urinary output is important (urinary retention and fecal impactions are real possibilities).

As the child progresses favorably, the nurse may safely encourage the parents to hold their infant or toddler during intravenous therapy, allowing for body contact and love, as well as position change. Granting as much freedom from restraint and provision for psychologic comforts (such as thumb-sucking) as is consistent with therapy and safety is very important.

The convalescent period should be long enough to permit the child to regain the previous physical status. The young child should be carefully reevaluated at intervals during the convalescence. Residual complications may include epilepsy, hydrocephalus, cerebral palsy (incoordination or weakness), mental insufficiency, special sensory loss, such as hearing and vision, and behavior or learning disorders (Fig. 31-15).

Aseptic meningitis syndrome. This term includes a number of viral disorders that have an acute onset and usually a self-limited course with varying meningeal manifestations. Meningismus, meningeal irritation resulting in complications such as nuchal (neck) or spinal rigidity, is present. Lumbar puncture reveals abnormal numbers of blood cells and a sterile bacterial culture. To rule out other diseases, hospitalization is necessary for at least 48 hours for observation. Treatment is supportive and symptomatic. Like bacterial meningitis, follow-up should be provided, since residual complications can occur. (See Fig. 31-15.)

Neonatal meningitis. Newborns are frequent victims of meningitis. Most often the organisms attacking these babies are *Escherichia coli* and staphylococci. About one in every 1,000 to 2,000 newborns is affected. These infections are often associated with low birth weight. Maternal infection, premature rupture of membranes, and complicated deliveries are often part of the obstetric history. Signs of meningeal irritation are minimal. The infant characteristically is lethargic and irritable and refuses to suck. Vomiting, respiratory distress, convulsions, and temperature instability, including hyperthermia and hypothermia, are not uncommon symptoms. Ampicillin, gentamicin, and other medications are given intravenously, usually be scalp vein. Abundant hair should always be shaved in advance. Intensive supportive nursing care is essential. Because of the difficulty in recognizing the disease early and the inability of the debilitated small infant to respond to treatment, survival may be as low as 60%, and children who do survive have a high incidence of residual complications.

Cerebral palsy (Fig. 31-17)

Cerebral palsy may be defined as a nonprogressive disorder of motion and posture resulting from brain injury or insult during a period of early brain growth. It is not in itself a disease but a condition that may result from numerous diseases that damage those parts of the brain that are responsible for voluntary muscular coordination. Such causes may include pressure on the brain or oxygen depriva-

tion to the brain before or during birth (cerebral anoxia), direct injury, embolus or hemorrhage, arrested hydrocephalus, and infection or toxicity occurring any time after birth. Cerebral palsy is usually diagnosed in infancy, since it is commonly caused by events associated with the prenatal or perinatal period. Treatment is directed toward limiting a disability and may continue throughout the affected person's life. It may be limited and mild or severe and far-reaching, involving many body functions. It is said that there are approximately 1.3 cases of cerebral palsy per 1,000 persons in the general population.

The child with the disorder of movement called cerebral palsy may have injuries to the brain involving other functions. Some patients with cerebral palsy may have associated seizures, mental insufficiency, behavior problems, special sensory difficulties, especially related to vision or hearing, and learning disturbances. The muscles of the mouth, tongue, and throat may be affected influencing the ability to receive, chew, and swallow food as well as to speak.

Therapists usually refer to the following main types of cerebral palsy:

1. The spastic type, the most common form affecting 65% of the patients, is characterized by increased muscle stiffness or tone, exaggerated contraction of affected muscle groups when stimulated (stretch reflex), jerky motions, and a tendency to have contractures. The lower extremities are most often involved. A scissors gait is common. The following body patterns of spastic cerebral palsy have been described:
   a. *Hemiplegia,* involving two limbs (an arm plus a leg) on the same side.
   b. *Double hemiplegia,* involving four limbs, with the arms slightly more affected.
   c. *Quadriplegia,* involving all four limbs, with the legs slightly more affected.
   d. *Diplegia,* involving all four limbs, with the legs affected to a significantly greater degree.
2. Extrapyramidal (nonspastic) cerebral palsies, comprising about 15% of cases, are character-

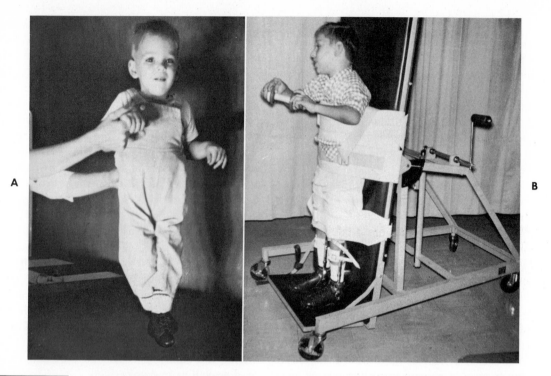

FIG. 31-17   This little fellow cannot walk at all without support. **A,** With support a scissors gait is present (one foot crossing the other caused by adductor spasticity). **B,** Many hours on the tilt-table and the consistent work and concern of therapists and parents have greatly strengthened this young child's legs.

Courtesy Crippled Children Services, Department of Public Health, San Diego, Calif.

ized by a great variability with regard to emotion, posture, and sleep states. This type includes the following:

a. *Athetoid,* characterized by involuntary, uncoordinated, purposeless movements involving joint motion rather than single muscle action. The upper extremities are more often involved.

b. *Ataxic,* characterized by loss of a sense of balance and problems in evaluating spatial relationships and the relative positions of body parts.

3. Mixed cerebral palsy combines features of types 1 and 2 and represents about 20% of affected patients.

It can be readily appreciated that the care of a cerebral-palsied child and the family cannot be the responsibility of just one practitioner. Their problems are usually too extensive. A team approach is necessary, including the pediatrician, orthopedist, physical therapist, occupational therapist, speech therapist, psychologist, medical-social worker, public health workers, office and hospital nurses, and schoolteachers.

These children and their families often have considerable emotional problems, which may be expressed in the way the parents treat the child and their aspirations for the child's future. Parents may be overprotective and do too much for their children, making it difficult for them to master the skills of which they are capable. On the other hand, they may expect too much of their children and

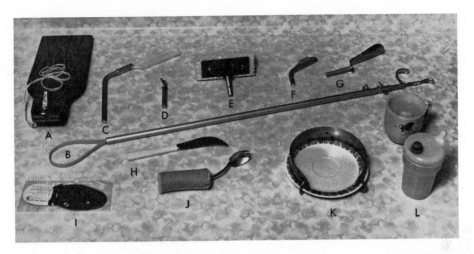

FIG. 31-18   Various aids for everyday activities for the handicapped. **A,** Nail clippers on wooden base, operated by string and foot action; **B,** gadget stick with hook attachment; **C,** comb attachment; **D,** clip attachment; **E,** mop or sponge attachment; **F,** magnet attachment; **G,** shoehorn attachment; **H,** rocker knife; **I,** elastic shoelaces; **J,** built-up handle on swivel fork (Spork); **K,** plate and plate guard; **L,** two types of weighted "trainer cups."

Courtesy Children's Hospital and Health Center, San Diego, Calif.

cause painful frustrations. They may need help in establishing realistic goals and in providing an environment conducive to good mental health as well as good physical health. The fact that the problem is not inherited should be clarified early to decrease parental feelings of guilt.

Association with other parents with similar problems and psychiatric assistance are often very rewarding. A hopeful aspect of cerebral palsy is that the initiating cause is not progressive in character, so the neuromuscular involvement, with treatment, will not worsen. Cerebral palsy is not a degenerative disease as are, for example, the muscular dystrophies, and considerable improvement can usually be gained. Through physical and occupational therapy, surgical techniques, and medication, youngsters with cerebral palsy are able to meet their daily personal needs and, in some cases, to prepare for self-supporting occupations. Special public school programs may be available in the community that are especially geared to meet the needs of such handicapped children. They may

attend some regular public school classes as well as special sessions designed to meet their individual needs during the school day.

When children with cerebral palsy are hospitalized, it is very important that the hospital staff know their capabilities as individuals. Information regarding successful feeding and dressing techniques, toileting practices, communication aids, and special problems may save hours of frustration and distress. The care of some patients will require little modification, since their total neuromuscular involvement is slight. The care of others will require considerable study and adjustment. Children who have a history of seizures or upper extremity or head involvement should not have their temperatures taken orally until the safety of the procedure is evaluated.

Each child's diet must be evaluated to make sure that it is appropriate for age, nutritional needs, and the ability to handle and swallow. Although self-feeding may take considerably more time and cause more disorder, these children should feed themselves as much as possible, using techniques they have been taught. Aids such as swivel spoons, plate guards, training cups, and rocker knives may be invaluable (Fig. 31-18). Occasionally, special weights may be attached to the child's arms to help control involuntary motion. Children who because of their condition must be fed should be assisted with patience. Since severely involved children may require the occasional use of suction, an apparatus should be available. During feedings, the nurse should hold the child in such a way that the child's arm closest to her extends behind her. This often causes the child's head to rotate comfortably to the same side (tonic neck reflex). Gentle support of the chin or stroking of the cheeks may help lip closure and swallowing. Some children who have difficulty swallowing may find carbonated drinks a problem. Waiting until the carbonation is minimal or serving other types of liquids is helpful.

Children with this condition should receive gentle, deliberate care. Excessive stimulation, sudden jarring movements, and the pressure of "having to hurry" induces greater tenseness and makes performance of relatively simple tasks extremely arduous. These children find it very difficult to relax, and they become fatigued easily. The simplest kind of controlled movement may require a tremendous amount of concentration and energy.

Whenever possible the cerebral-palsied child should have contact with other boys and girls and should not be socially deprived. Contact with other youngsters has frequently been limited. Even those who have moderately severe muscular involvement often enjoy working with Play-Doh or modeling clay, finger paints, large blocks, and hand puppets. Many can enjoy music, television, and reading. The occupational therapist may work with the children to improve skills needed to meet everyday needs. These are presented to the young child in the form of games or special projects. Progress, although at times seemingly small, should be recognized and praised. The child responds to this recognition and continues efforts to improve.

Although it may seem to some critics that a tremendous amount of time, effort, and financial out-lay is expended in community programs to help cerebral-palsied youngsters, such programs are rewarding from many points of view. In the long run it is less expensive to educate individuals to achieve their potentials than to provide the type of state-supported custodial care offered in the past. It often brings a measure of independence and a feeling of self-respect and personal worth to the individual patient. It brings hope and aid to concerned and burdened parents and inspiration to those who observe and help when they can.

THE TODDLER

Encephalitis

Encephalitis is an inflammation of the brain (encephalon). When the inflammation involves both the meninges and brain tissue, the condition is referred to as encephalomyelitis.

Encephalitis is characterized by personality change, headache, drowsiness, fever, and often convulsions. Cranial nerves may become paralyzed, affecting speech, swallowing mechanism, and protective airway reflexes. Double vision may also be reported. Encephalitis may produce the same complications as does meningitis. (See Fig. 31-16.)

Encephalitis is caused by infectious agents, most often viral. Some types of encephalitis are caused by viruses spread by vectors such as mosquitoes, ticks, or mites. Encephalitis following rubeola (2-week measles) was relatively common before immunization programs were available, occurring once in every 600 to 1,000 cases of "hard" measles.

Symptoms of encephalitis caused by toxins contacted by ingestion or inhalation are more properly referred to as encephalopathy. Lead poisoning in children, although not as common as formerly, is still reported every year. All furniture and toys used by a young child (who considers tasting at least as important as feeling or smelling) should be protected by nontoxic, lead-free paint.

The nursing care of a child with encephalitis is

very much like that of a child with meningitis. Lumbar punctures may be performed to relieve intracranial pressure, and, recently, intracranial monitoring of pressure has been frequently used. The difference between encephalitis and meningitis may not always be clinically demonstrated by symptoms. Differentiation is then made on the basis of the results from laboratory examinations.

THE PRESCHOOL CHILD

Brain tumors (Fig. 31-19)

Although brain tumors are not found as frequently in children as in adults, nervous system tumors are the second most common malignancy in childhood. Pediatric brain tumors are situated rather deeply within the brain structure, making it difficult to assure complete removal of the abnormal cells. About three fourths of the brain tumors occurring in childhood involve the supportive connective tissue of the brain, called *glial* cells. The two most common gliomas are astrocytomas and medulloblastomas. Total resection of an infiltrating cerebral astrocytoma is seldom possible, but a cystic cerebellar astrocytoma is relatively slow growing, usually encapsulated, and easier to remove. Symptoms of developing brain tumor may appear gradually in the case of a slowly progressing lesion. However, some tumors (for example, medulloblastomas) grow rapidly and cause remarkable signs and symptoms rather soon. The signs and symptoms are those caused by the increased intracranial pressure. They may include headache, dizziness, lethargy, indifference, or irritability. Emesis often occurs (many times unassociated with nausea and not always projectile in character, although projectile vomiting is significant). Double or blurring vision and speech problems are reported fairly often. The pupils may be abnormally or unequally dilated or slow to react to changes in light intensity. Balance and gait may be affected, because 60% of childhood brain tumors are subtentorial and often involve the cerebellum, a part of the brain that plays a significant role in the maintenance of equi-

librium. (See Fig. 31-19, *B*.) Rigidity, tremors, or convulsions occasionally occur. Local muscle weakness may be present. (Periodic testing of the hand-grip is sometimes ordered.) If the child is under 4 years of age, considerable enlargement of the head and fontanel may still take place, because the suture lines are not completely knitted, and interference in the ventricular drainage of the cerebrospinal fluid may be present, as well as direct pressure from the enlarging tumor itself. The blood pressure may be elevated and the pulse may be slowed when compared with the normal values for the age group represented by the patient. Respirations may be of the Cheyne-Stokes variety. Fever or wide swings in temperature occasionally occur. Diagnosis may be confirmed through various procedures: skull radiographs (x-ray films), brain scans, electroencephalograms, ventriculograms, and arteriograms, as well as clinical observation. Some of these procedures, although often necessary, are uncomfortable. The newer procedure, computerized transaxial tomography (CTT scan), may provide diagnostic confirmation of tumor with much less discomfort to the patient (p. 650).

If a nurse is responsible for the care of a patient with a possible brain tumor, she must carefully assess the child's capabilities before attempting to ambulate the chid and be sure she has sufficient help to avoid falls. Some of these patients have very poor balance. The patient should be observed for any of the signs and symptoms previously described. Observation of vital signs, including blood pressure and eye reactions, should always be part of the nursing care.

Surgery, x-ray, or cobalt radiation and chemotherapy are the treatments currently available. Surgery, of course, is preferred. The complete removal of a well-confined tumor almost always produces a more optimistic prognosis. When only incomplete removal is possible, radiation and chemotherapy are often employed to retard tumor progression.

Nursing care in the days immediately after a craniotomy, or surgical opening of the skull, is usually a complex affair. The vocational nurse may assist the registered nurse, but she should not have the

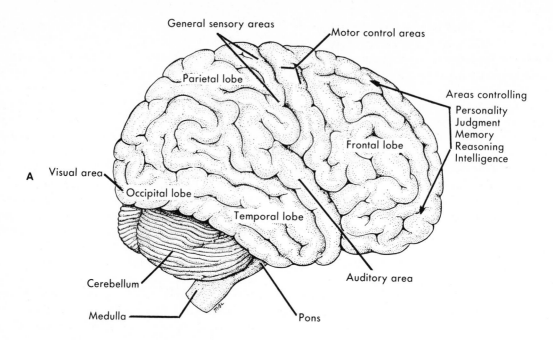

General sensory areas

Motor control areas

Parietal lobe

Areas controlling
Personality
Judgment
Memory
Reasoning
Intelligence

Frontal lobe

A   Visual area

Occipital lobe

Temporal lobe

Auditory area

Cerebellum

Medulla

Pons

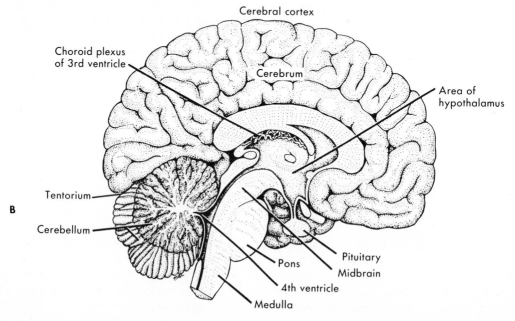

Cerebral cortex

Choroid plexus
of 3rd ventricle

Cerebrum

Area of
hypothalamus

Tentorium

B

Cerebellum

Pons

Pituitary

Midbrain

4th ventricle

Medulla

FIG. 31-19   **A,** Surfaces of the brain showing the cerebrum, cerebellum, pons, and medulla with identification of specialized areas of cerebral function. **B,** Simplified sagittal section of the brain showing internal relationships. Brain tumors in children often involve the cerebellum.

responsibility of the child's complete bedside care. The child's condition is too unstable. The patient must be turned slowly and gently to prevent dizziness, nausea, vomiting, and a rise in blood pressure. Since crying elevates the blood pressure, all measures designed to prevent fear or distress are especially important. The head dressings may become damp from cerebrospinal fluid drainage and require reinforcing until they can be changed by the physician. The face, especially the eyes, may be bruised and swollen. Special eye irrigations may be necessary to avoid infection or ulceration resulting from disturbances in tear formation and drainage because of trauma. Frequent suctioning may be necessary. The child may appear unconscious but be able to hear well. Conversations at the bedside should be prudent.

As improvement occurs, efforts to rehabilitate these patients should be made. Although the patients may eventually die, they may be able to live relatively satisfying lives for many months. Both patients and parents need much physical and emotional support to make the most of this indeterminate and occasionally prolonged period.

Neuroblastoma

A neuroblastoma is an undifferentiated malignant tumor arising during embryonic development from the adrenal medulla or from any of the nervous system's sympathetic ganglia located in the head, neck, chest, abdomen, or pelvis. It is the most common of all solid cancers of children. Both sexes are equally affected, and although the tumor may be recognized at various ages, a preponderance is diagnosed during the first 4 to 5 years of life.

Four common clinical manifestations of the neuroblastoma are (1) a mass usually involving the abdomen or lymph nodes; (2) neurologic signs such as weakness in an extremity or paraplegia; (3) pain usually in the bone or joints; and (4) orbital signs, such as local ecchymosis or proptosis (protruding eye). In addition, children with neuroblastoma

often come to the hospital with varied constitutional symptoms, including weight loss, fever, anorexia, and anemia.

When a neuroblastoma is suspected, a number of diagnostic studies must be performed at once because the neuroblastoma is a highly malignant tumor with tendencies to produce widespread metastases. The sequence of studies includes a complete blood cell count; electrolyte, glucose, and other blood chemistry determinations; a urinary assay for catecholamines; intravenous pyelogram; radioactive bone scan; chest x-ray examination; and bone marrow aspiration. In seven out of ten cases the tumor secretes excess quantities of catecholamines or metabolites or both into the blood. Urine measurements of their metabolic end products, vanillylmandelic acid (VMA) and homovanillic acid (HVA) make the 24-hour VMA and HVA urine determinations a valuable diagnostic test (p. 482). A good prognosis has generally been associated with diagnosis in children under 2 years of age who have a localized tumor. Staging of this tumor is important for planning treatment and estimating prognosis.

Stage I. Localized tumor, well encapsulated
Stage II. Tumor has extended to regional lymph nodes
Stage III. Extensive tumor spread across the midline
Stage IV. Tumor has distant metastases with bone involvement

The cure rate decreases as the extent of disease increases. Unfortunately, more than 50% of cases have metastasized at the time of initial diagnosis. However, an aggressive therapeutic approach, combining surgical excision, irradiation, and chemotherapy is used in an attempt to save a significant proportion of these children. Surgery alone is probably acceptable in Stage I. The fact that neuroblastoma is radiosensitive makes x-ray therapy to the tumor site and to any areas of local extension an indicated addition in all other cases. Palliative x-ray therapy is used for metastatic lesions in bones, lungs, liver, or brain. Chemotherapy has improved survival and is useful in shrinking previously unresectable tumors. It is especially indicated when there are tumor cells in the bone marrow, when complete removal of the tumor has not been possible, when there is evidence of distant metastases, when the urinary catecholamines remain elevated after all identifiable tumor has been removed, or when recurrence or late metastases are detected. At present three-drug chemotherapy is employed, using vincristine (Oncovin), cyclophosphamide (Cytoxan), and doxorubicin hydrochloride (Adriamycin), in addition to surgery and radiation therapy. No single chemotherapeutic agent or combination of drugs has been uniformly effective. When chemotherapy is given, control of anemia, specific antibiotic therapy for infections, and prevention of high blood levels of uric acid are necessary. Liberal fluids and allopurinol (Zyloprim) should be given to prevent kidney stone formation.

After surgery, children with neuroblastoma should be reevaluated often, since, in spite of chemotherapy and radiotherapy, results to date have been poor. Although an increasing number of long-term survivors are receiving chemotherapy, this tumor often has a rapid downhill course despite all therapy that is currently available.

THE SCHOOL-AGE CHILD

Head injuries

About 200,000 children are hospitalized annually with head injuries. Although most of these children have simple, closed head injuries, about 17% will have skull fractures. One out of ten will have active intracranial bleeding, and two out of ten will have other body injuries associated with head injury. Identifying the active intracranial bleeding and those with other injuries is a significant role of the nurse. The patients are typically boys between the ages of 4 and 9 years.

CONCUSSION

The term "concussion" implies a loss of consciousness with a temporary neuronal dysfunction due to jarring but no pathologic evidence of damage to the underlying brain. The period of unconsciousness is usually brief and is measured in terms of minutes to hours. The period of memory loss that surrounds a concussion is termed "post-traumatic amnesia" (PTA). It is important to be aware of the PTA phenomenon, because it explains why the patient often cannot provide information about the injury. Usually the longer the PTA period the greater the likelihood of brain injury rather than simple concussion. PTA is divided into retrograde amnesia, loss of memory for the period of time preceding the actual injury, and anterograde amnesia, the loss of memory for the period of time following the injury. Most patients will display some persistent residual loss of memory surrounding the period of injury. A long retrograde amnesia is particularly significant in evaluating the extent of a head injury. Any head-injured child who has loss of consciousness or shows any neurologic deficit should be admitted to the hospital for observation.

CONTUSION AND LACERATION

A contusion is actual bruising of the brain. A laceration involves tearing of cerebral tissue. This bruising or tearing of cerebral tissue is frequently accompanied by hemorrhages or bleeding into the brain substance. Contusions and lacerations, in contrast to concussion, are characterized by specific (focal) findings. Changes in motor function, speech, and vision are important clues that help determine the area of damage; for example, the left side of the brain controls the arms and legs on the right side of the body, speech is most often generated by the left side of the brain, and a visual center is located at the back of the brain. When disruption of brain tissue is associated with bleeding, intracranial pressure may begin to rise. Since the cranium containing the brain, cerebral blood vessels, and cerebrospinal fluid is rigid, any enlargement of one of these three components results in compression of the others. The brain substance is more vulnerable to compression than blood and cerebrospinal fluid, and when no further compensation is possible, intracranial pressure begins to rise. Like other tissues when the brain is subjected to injury, it becomes edematous. This swelling also causes intracranial pressure. Increasing intracranial pressure (ICP) is manifested by a deterioration in the state of consciousness, rising systemic blood pressure associated with slowing of the pulse rate, and irregularity of breathing. These are the classic neurologic signs indicating that the head-injured child is in trouble. A basic cranial check (below) is used for observing a child who is beginning to manifest subtle signs of increasing intracranial pressure or who is admitted to the hospital for observation after a head injury. Consciousness is a bihemispheric and a brain stem function. Nerve centers in the brain stem also control vital functions such as respiration, heart rate, and blood pressure. The brain stem may be directly injured, or it may be compromised by potentially reversible lesions that cause compression, such as intracranial pressure and brain shifts or lesions that cause cerebral oxygen deprivation (ischemia).

THE CRANIAL CHECK

Assessment	Technique or observation used
I. Level of consciousness	
A. Alert, oriented, responsive to:	Ask the following questions:
1. Person	1. "What is your name?"
2. Time	2. "What is your favorite TV show? What day is today?"
3. Place	3. "Where are you? Where do you go to school?"
B. Lethargic—drowsy	Patient responses are delayed.
C. Disoriented—confused	Patient gives inappropriate responses.
D. Responsive to verbal stimuli	Patient answers simple commands, e.g., "Open your eyes."
E. Responsive only to painful stimuli	Pinch patient's upper arm.
1. Purposeful	Patient withdraws from stimulus—pushes it away.
2. Nonpurposeful	Patient may only grimace.
a. Flexor response	
b. Extensor response	
F. Coma	Patient gives no response of any kind.
II. Pupil response	
A. Appearance	Observe both pupils simultaneously; pupils should be round (constricted in bright room and dilated in dark room) and equal in size.
1. Shape	
2. Size	
3. Equality	
B. Reaction to light	
1. Direct light reflex	Shine light directly into one eye; pupils should constrict briskly.
2. Consensual light reflex	Shine light into one eye to note alternate pupil constriction.
C. Extraocular movements	Ask patient to follow your finger from side to side and up and down with eyes to detect limitation in movement.

It is important to note the degree of alertness when the child is admitted to the emergency department or pediatric unit and to note the vital signs exactly. Changes in these important parameters as indicated above are classic signs that the patient is in need of prompt medical assistance. The physician should be notified at once.

Continued.

THE CRANIAL CHECK—cont'd

Assessment	Technique or observation used
III. Motor function	
A. Facial symmetry	Ask patient to show teeth—to make a "funny face."
B. Movement	
1. Upper extremities	Ask patient to raise arms and to extend both arms forward.
2. Lower extremities	Ask patient to move each leg individually upward and laterally.
C. Strength	
1. Upper extremities	Ask patient to squeeze examiner's hand or two fin-
2. Lower extremities	gers and to pull against resistance of examiner.
D. Babinski reflex	Stroke outside sole of each foot with tongue blade. Normally toes, especially big toe, turn down. Reflex is present when big toe rises (dorsiflexion) and other toes fan out. Reflex is normally present up to about 18 months of age.
IV. Vital signs	
A. Temperature	Elevation is usually associated with infection else-
B. Pulse	where unless hypothalamus (temperature-regulat- ing center) has been damaged.
C. Respiration	Slowed pulse and irregular respirations associated with rising systolic pressure indicate intracranial
D. Blood pressure	pressure.

The brain stem centers that help control vital functions are anatomically close to those which regulate pupil responses. Observations of changes in pupil size are therefore helpful in detecting damage to the brain stem.

INTRACRANIAL HEMATOMAS

Intracranial hematomas are space-occupying lesions that produce signs of intracranial pressure. They should be suspected in every case of head injury with coma or one-sided weakness. Short-term intracranial pressure may occur because of an expanding hematoma, or long-term pressure may occur because of cerebral edema caused by the injury. Unless the intracranial pressure is reduced, neurologic deterioration follows that may prove to be fatal.

EPIDURAL HEMATOMA

About 75% of epidural hematomas are associated with a skull fracture (Fig. 31-20). This lesion, located between the skull and the outer covering of the brain (dura), results from a torn high-pressure arterial system. It characteristically demonstrates a relatively rapid downhill course unless identified and treated. Since the expanding hemorrhage cannot get through the bone, the hematoma presses down on the substance of the brain. Usually a brief period of unconsciousness is followed by a lucid interval of variable duration, after which the child is progressively confused, lethargic, difficult to arouse, and finally, comatose.

Pulse and respirations become slow, and blood pressure rises. A dilated pupil and hemiparesis of the opposite side of the body, accompanied by a

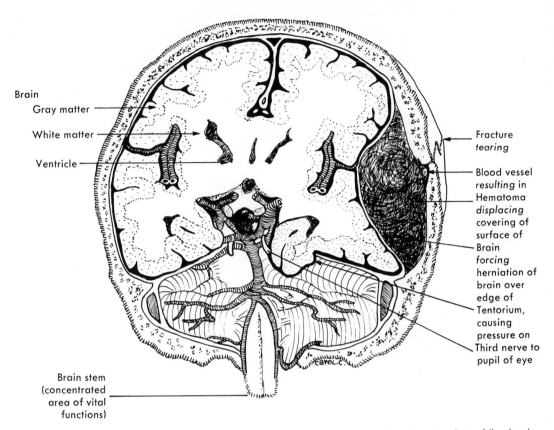

Brain
  Gray matter
  White matter
  Ventricle

Fracture
tearing

Blood vessel
resulting in
Hematoma
displacing
covering of
surface of
Brain
forcing
herniation of
brain over
edge of
Tentorium,
causing
pressure on
Third nerve to
pupil of eye

Brain stem
(concentrated
area of vital
functions)

FIG. 31-20   Epidural hematoma located between the skull and outer covering of the brain.

deterioration in state of consciousness and vital signs, indicates a prompt need for surgical intervention. The high mortality from this kind of injury usually results from failure in recognition and delay in operation.

SUBDURAL HEMATOMAS

Subdural hematomas are usually caused by rupture of low-pressure bridging veins in the space under the dura and may be associated with severe brain injury. Subdural hematomas are divided into three categories, depending on the time interval from onset of the injury to the course of symptoms. *Acute subdural hematomas* usually cause immediate unconsciousness with a rapid, downhill, pro-

gressive deterioration resulting from massive bleeding and fatal brain compression. *Subacute subdural hematomas* develop slowly because bleeding is less profuse. Clinical manifestations usually appear between 2 and 14 days after the injury. *Chronic subdural hematomas* manifest themselves weeks or months after the injury (Fig. 31-21). This condition occurs most frequently in infancy, since the subdural space, which is only present in infants, favors clot formation. A vascular membrane forms around the blood as the mass slowly enlarges as a result of leakage of plasma protein from the capillaries. Intracranial pressure mounts over a period of weeks to months and is manifested by vomiting (especially projectile type),

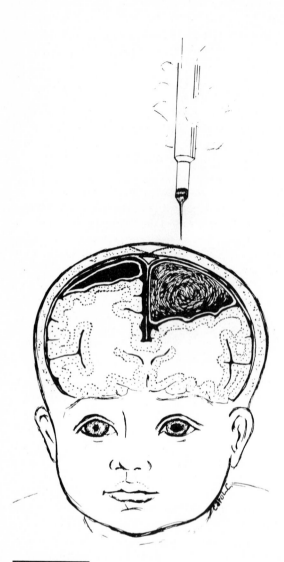

FIG. 31-21

Bilateral, chronic, subdural hematomas. Subdural taps are performed on infants by insertion of a special subdural needle through the lateral suture line.

a tense fontanel, and separation of the cranial sutures. Because chronic subdural hematomas are usually bilateral, the skull may become deformed and broad with a high forehead. The infant becomes irritable and is often underweight and anemic. Bilateral subdural taps confirm the diagnosis, and the fluid is removed. If the fluid is removed in time, repeated subdural taps may provide a complete cure; otherwise, a shunting procedure is necessary for the more persistent hematomas.

SKULL FRACTURE

Separate from but nevertheless associated with many injuries of the brain is skull fracture. A *linear* (lengthwise) fracture of the skull may often cause an underlying hematoma. This is particularly true if the fracture line crosses the normal distribution of blood vessels. In children 50% of skull fractures are in the parietal bone, and these usually will be evident on x-ray examination. *Depressed* skull fractures occur when the bone is displaced or is pressing on the brain tissue. Debridement and surgical restoration of normal contour are required. Basal skull fractures may not always be seen on x-ray examination. However, the nurse may suspect the presence of a basilar skull fracture by a variety of special findings not always present when the child is admitted. On the second day the nurse may notice black and blue marks around the eyes (raccoon sign) or ear (battle sign). A third finding is watery fluid that runs out of the ear (cerebrospinal fluid otorrhea) or a very watery discharge from the nose (cerebrospinal fluid rhinorrhea). Cerebrospinal fluid leaking from the ear or nose causes increased concern because of the danger of infection and meningitis.

Continued assessment and nursing care. Cerebral anoxia is the most frequent cause of death. Therefore the establishment and maintenance of an adequate airway accompanied by proper ventilation and circulation is critical. Obstruction of the airway not only causes atelectasis and infection but also will produce a serious abnormality in the gaseous exchange that can increase cerebral blood flow and increase cerebral edema, thus increasing intracranial pressure. When possible, blood gases should be periodically checked to validate the adequacy of ventilation. Tracheal suction may be essential to clear secretions, and tracheostomy may be necessary to maintain a patent airway. Because vomiting frequently accompanies intracranial pressure, insertion of a nasogastric tube and removal of stomach contents may prevent aspiration pneumonitis. These patients should be kept in a lateral, slightly elevated position, unless contraindicated, because of the potential for aspiration. They should be turned and suctioned hourly.

Hypotensive shock is seldom caused by head injury unless hemorrhage from a severe scalp wound occurs or the brain injury itself is so severe that the vital centers are failing and death is imminent. The presence of clinical shock should alert the nurse to notify the physician and to search elsewhere in the body for hemorrhage. Scrupulous examination of the abdomen and extremities is necessary to detect the possibility of a ruptured spleen or fractured long bone. Blood should be obtained for grouping and crossmatching because replacement of lost fluid volume by intravenous route may be life saving. The presence of shock usually means injuries involving other organs. With the exception of extradural hematoma, neurosurgical management should be postponed until other injuries are investigated and treated if necessary.

DISTURBANCES IN CEREBRAL FUNCTION

A detailed neurologic examination is included with the initial medical examination of the head-injured child. This not only allows for a more accurate diagnosis of the extent of the injury, but observations made during the examination form the baseline from which subsequent progress may be judged. The general state of the patient, the level of consciousness, heart rate, blood pressure, and breathing should be evaluated immediately with primary attention to vital circulatory and ventilatory functions on which life depends. Headache, vertigo, vomiting, increasing irritability, and restlessness often characterize the response of young children to head injury. These factors may or may not

be evidences of intracranial pressure. Restlessness may be caused by cerebral hypoxia, or it may be caused by an overdistended bladder. An indwelling catheter should be inserted to relieve an overdistention of the bladder. Other causes of restlessness include extensive soft tissue injuries, fracture, or improperly applied cast or dressing. Seizures also frequently accompany head injuries in small children. Careful systematic serial observations and recordings of changing factors and physical signs are constantly compared with the baseline. In addition to the nurse's responsibility for the care of the child, the nurse must report at once any significant change in the patient's condition. Problems associated with raised intracranial pressure demand solution before irreparable brain damage is inflicted. A *cranial check*, which includes level of consciousness, pupillary signs and extremity movement, strength and sensation, as well as vital signs, should be done every 15 to 30 minutes as necessary. Careful observation of the child, especially the level of consciousness, yields by far the most important information for further management. (See box on pp. 645-646.)

A child who is alert or is improving will not require any therapeutic measures. When serial examinations suggest that intracranial pressure is increasing significantly, various measures are employed to minimize this complication. Administration of dehydrating agents such as urea or mannitol can be given over a 4- to 6-hour period every 12 hours to control cerebral edema. Dexamethasone (Decadron) and methylprednisolone sodium succinate (Solu-Medrol) are two glucocorticoids that are commonly used to prevent cellular decompensation and increasing cerebral edema. Anticonvulsant drugs may be necessary to control seizures. Fluids should be restricted to approximately 75% of the normal daily maintenance and should be given at a uniform rate over a 24-hour period. An accurate record of fluid intake and output is essential and should be followed closely because lethargy, confusion, and convulsion may result from electrolyte imbalance and not an intracranial hematoma. Hematomas can be differentiated from cerebral edema by computerized transaxial tomography (CTT scan). This technique permits identification of hemorrhage and cerebral edema and clearly outlines ventricular cavities. The CTT scan is the safest, fastest, and best initial study for the child who exhibits further neurologic deterioration or who is comatose. If scanning is not available, cerebral angiography is used to diagnose intracranial hematomas that may need to be evacuated by craniotomy.

In summary, the nurse must remember that intracranial monitoring remains the single most important aid in determining when the previously mentioned therapeutic measures should be initiated. Although children have a remarkable capacity to survive even the most severe type of head trauma, the management of each child will remain a challenge.

Part 3: Vision, hearing, and related disorders

VISION

Fortunately only a small percentage of children are totally blind—that is, visually unable to distinguish light from darkness. The vast majority of "blind" children do have significant visual impairment, but retain some measurable or functional vision. Common causes of visual impairment in infancy and childhood include: (1) trauma, (2) strabismus (malalignment of the eyes), and (3) refractive error (image not clearly focused on the retina). In fairly recent years, four factors have contributed to the reduction of visual disability:
1. Recognition of the pathogenesis of retrolental fibroplasia
2. Prevention and control of rubella
3. Early diagnosis and treatment of developmental eye problems
4. Technological advances in eye examination and surgery

Pediatric eye examination

The gift of sight is indeed precious. Proper care of the eyes should be taught to the growing child and to the parents. Prevention of eye disease is the ideal, but early recognition of eye disorders with proper definitive treatment is the ultimate goal. Children should be observed for signs and symptoms of the following possible visual difficulties:
1. Poor vision: demonstrated by infants and preschoolers by inability to visually follow objects or visual inattentiveness to the environment; by school-aged children by difficulty with near or distant reading
2. Strabismus: intermittent or persistent crossing of the eyes; squinting, blinking, or closing one eye in bright light or with visual tasks; head turning or tilting
3. Uncorrected refractive error: irritability with near or distant visual taks or avoidance of these tasks; tearing, rubbing, or squinting the eyes; recurrent eyelid inflammations

To identify and treat visual problems as early as possible, a professional eye examination should be performed for every child immediately after birth, at 6 months, and once in the preschool years between ages 3 and 5. Annual follow-up visual screening in the schools is recommended. These examinations should include measurement of visual acuity, estimation of ocular alignment by corneal light reflexes or alternate cover testing, and examination of ocular structures for pathologic findings (Fig 31-22).

Children with the following findings should be referred to an opthalmologist:
1. Possible strabismus
2. Poor visual fixation preference (demonstrated by infants) *or* a visual acuity difference between eyes of two lines or more on the eye chart or vision in either eye of 20/40 or less (in preschool or school-age youngsters)
3. Evidence of ocular structural disease
4. Family history of retinoblastoma, congenital cataracts, or genetic or metabolic eye diseases

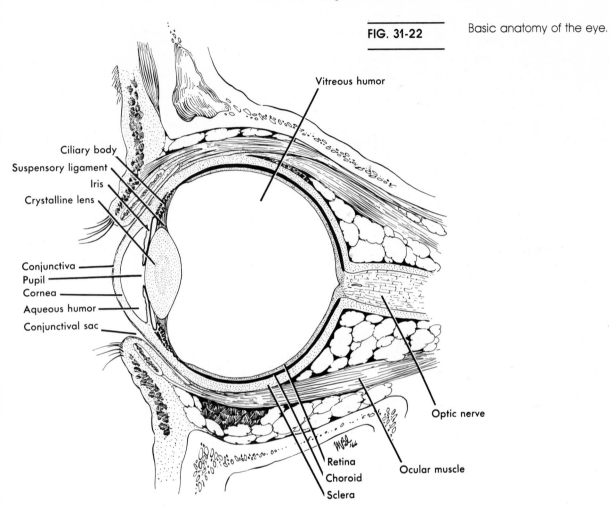

FIG. 31-22   Basic anatomy of the eye.

Vitreous humor

Ciliary body
Suspensory ligament
Iris
Crystalline lens

Conjunctiva
Pupil
Cornea
Aqueous humor
Conjunctival sac

Optic nerve

Ocular muscle

Retina
Choroid
Sclera

Retrolental fibroplasia (RLF) (retinopathy of prematurity)

Administration of oxygen, which saves the lives of numerous premature low-birth-weight infants, may also cause development of abnormal retinal vascularizations. Ultimately a contraction of this retinal scar tissue may result in a detachment of the retina and the appearance of a white fibrous sheath on the posterior surface of the lens. The incidence of RLF has decreased, but it is reemerging as the use of needed oxygen therapy rises in the salvage of high-risk infants.

Specific language disability (developmental dyslexia)

Vision is important in gathering the large amount of data demanded by our learning processes; however, provision of proper eye care for children cannot be expected to eliminate all learning problems. Developmental dyslexia may occur in children regardless of the presence or absence of visual deficit, even in children of normal intelligence. Therefore, those best qualified to deal with learning disorders are the educators and not vision specialists.

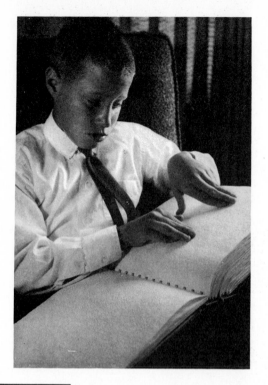

FIG. 31-23

This industrious boy, reading from his Braille Bible, is blind as a result of retrolental fibroplasia.

Amblyopia and strabismus

Strabismus (malalignment of the eyes) affects about 4% of the population. This imbalance of the extraocular muscles may lead to amblyopia (decreased vision in one eye resulting from disuse), poor binocular vision (depth perception), and an unacceptable appearance ("cross-eyed," "wall-eyed"). Although strabismus is the most frequent cause of amblyopia, the next leading cause is a notable difference in refractive error (the eye most out of focus "turns off"). Specific treatment of amblyopia may include glasses or occlusive (patching) therapy. Patching the nonamblyopic eye stimulates the increased visual maturation of the amblyopic eye. Specific treatment of strabismus depends upon the cause and may include glasses, occlusive therapy, orthoptics (visual exercises), or surgery (see Fig. 31-24). Surgical treatment of a congenital strabismus in the first year of life significantly improves chances for binocular vision and an acceptable appearance.

Strabismus surgery involves either shortening or repositioning the extraocular muscles controlling the position of the eyeball. Postoperative care is usually dictated by physician preference and the patient's needs. Although restraints have been used frequently in the past, there is no substitute for an attentive parent or nurse. Parents have usually been instructed by the surgeon to expect that the child will have red eyes. The child may become needlessly frightened by occlusive eye dressings or the inability to open the eyes because of crusted secretions on opposing lid margins. Proper postoperative care may prevent both these situations.

Refractive errors

Poor visual acuity in one or both eyes may be the result of myopia (nearsightedness), hyperopia (farsightedness), or astigmatism (see Table 31-1). Astigmatism is an irregularity in the curvature of the cornea or lens that blurs focal points; it may be associated with either myopia or hyperopia. When there is a significant difference in the ability of the eyes to focus—that is, their refractive powers—the condition is known as anisometropia. Refractive errors usually do not cause difficulties until the child reaches school age. Vision usually may be corrected to a normal level in both eyes with proper glasses. Only if amblyopia is present will uncorrected or poorly corrected refractive errors cause permanent loss of vision.

Children who wear glasses must be carefully taught to keep their glasses in a case when they are not being worn. Proper methods of handling and cleaning the lenses should also be demonstrated. When a young patient wearing glasses or contact lenses is admitted to the hospital, a note concerning them should be included in the child's admission record.

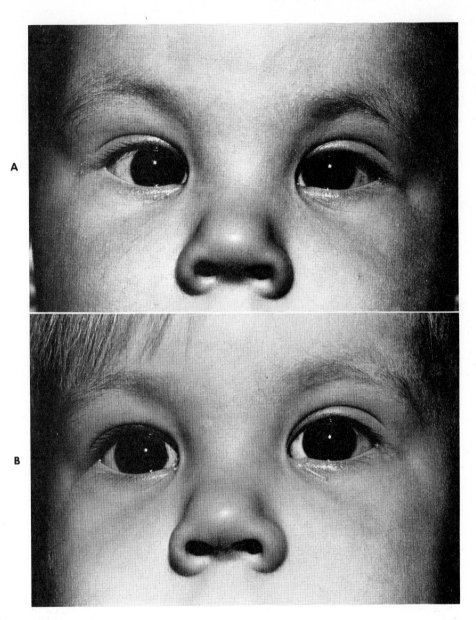

FIG. 31-24 Infantile esotropia. **A,** Age 7 months—preoperative; **B,** age 12 months—postoperative (strabismus surgery at age 11 months). Note that although postoperative alignment is straight (i.e., true strabismus has been eliminated), there are still typical facial characteristics for pseudostrabismus (flat nasal bridge, wide epicanthal skin folds, narrow interpupillary distance, and greater nasal than temporal scleral visibility).

Courtesy David G. Martin, M.D., San Diego, Calif.

TABLE 31-1 REFRACTION: THREE COMMON DEFECTS IN CHILDREN

Normal refraction	Normal eye
Emmetropia (no refractive error) Light is focused on retina	Emmetropic eye

Abnormal refraction	Cause	Optical defect	Corrected with lens
Myopia (nearsightedness) Sees near objects more clearly than at a distance	Elongated eyeball Parallel rays are focused anterior to the retina	Myopic eye	Corrected with concave lens

Cataracts

Congenital and early developmental cataracts constitute one of the most important causes of visual impairment in children. The student should note that a cataract is an abnormal opacity of the crystalline lens, located just in back of the pupil. By obstructing the pathway of light to the retina, cat-aracts can cause partial or total blindness. Cataracts may be congenital, such as those caused by maternal rubella. Some cataracts are hereditary—the most common mode of inheritance being autosomal dominant. Nonhereditary cataracts may develop as a result of trauma, infection, retrolental fibroplasia, retinitis pigmentosa, or prolonged administration of corticosteroids. Surgical removal of the

TABLE 31-1　REFRACTION: THREE COMMON DEFECTS IN CHILDREN—cont'd

Abnormal refraction	Cause	Optical defect	Corrected with lens
Hyperopia (farsightedness) Sees objects more clearly at a distance	Shortened eyeball Parallel rays are focused posterior to the retina	Hyperopic eye	Corrected with convex lens
Astigmatism (may be associated with myopia or hyperopia) Sees distorted image	Irregular corneal curvature; rays entering an eye are not refracted uniformly in all meridians	Myopic astigmatism	Corrected with myopic cylinder Axis 90'

cataract lens is the only effective method of treatment available for all but a few infants and children. The postoperative period is usually short after removal of cataracts. It usually requires a sterile eye pad and protective shield, and occasionally involves some limitation of activity. Every effort should be made to reduce crying and prevent vomiting, since they increase intraocular pressure, strain on the sutures, and possible bleeding. Occasionally the child's eyes will be bandaged. Before touching a child who cannot see, the nurse should speak so that he is not startled. A radio is a comfort when vision is limited by bandages and movement is restricted. Again, orientation to the hospital setting, preparation for the postoperative period, and parental support are extremely important.

Retinoblastoma

Retinoblastoma is a malignant tumor arising from retinal tissue. The tumor may be familial or sporadic, and may be identified by thorough eye examination at birth. Frequently the diagnosis is made because of the presence of a white reflex from the pupil (leukokoria), strabismus, or ocular inflammation. Retinoblastoma is the most frequent ocular malignancy of childhood. Early recognition and immediate treatment are essential to prevent the rapid metastasis of this foreboding tumor.

Trauma

Serious injury may be associated with a decrease in vision. Nearly one third of monocular blindness follows trauma in childhood years. Arrows and other pointed objects are the chief instruments of blinding injuries in children under 15 years of age.

Of all possible injuries to the eye, traumatic hyphema (hemorrhage within the anterior chamber of the eye) is probably the most common ocular injury necessitating hospitalization. Bleeding usually arises from a tear or laceration in the anterior ciliary body rather than in the iris itself.

Prognosis for normal vision decreases as the amount of bleeding in the anterior chamber increases. This is the primary reason for the classic preventive regimen of bed rest, bilateral eye patches, and sedation. Patients should *not* be placed on the affected side. Long-term evaluation should include careful examination of the peripheral retina for tears and periodic evaluation for development of glaucoma. Glaucoma, a condition that results from high intraocular pressure, ultimately may lead to loss of optic nerve function and blindness.

Children with a visual loss are confronted with complex, interelated problems throughout their childhood years. These problems are by no means exclusively personal. The burden is far reaching,

presenting major challenges to parents, teachers, physicians, and especially to nurses caring for such children in the hospital setting. Those who share this responsibility should be committed to assisting these children to achieve both physical and psychosocial well being so that they may develop the skills necessary to live safely and happily in our society.

HEARING

The auditory system is the primary channel through which children learn speech and language, develop educationally, and dynamically adjust to the challenges of their environment. The importance of the integrity of the auditory system is both that simple and that complex. The degree of auditory dysfunction (hearing impairment), the developmental time at which hearing impairment occurs, and the duration of the impairment all determine to what extent the child will develop normal speech, language, and education and psychosocial skills. Because hearing impairment itself is generally physically invisible and manifests itself in problems of communication, learning, and psychologic and social behavior, it has sometimes been misdiagnosed and subsequently managed as childhood autism, emotional disturbance, and mental retardation. As a result of such errors in diagnosis and treatment, many hearing impaired children have been denied the opportunity to realize their potential and to take their places as contributing members of society.

Types of loss

It is important to remember that the auditory system is divided primarily into two parts: the peripheral auditory system and the central auditory system.

The peripheral auditory system is composed of the outer, middle, and inner ears. The central auditory system is composed of afferent and efferent neurons connecting the sensory end organs of the inner ear to the brainstem and cortical structures.

The three main categories of hearing disorders are as follows: (1) *peripheral impairments*, resulting from lesions to the outer, middle, or inner ears; (2) *central impairments*, resulting from lesions to the brainstem or temporal lobe; and (3) *functional* or nonorganic impairments, which are psychologic with no physiologic basis. There may, of course, be combinations of any or all of these in a given individual.

Disorders of both the peripheral and central auditory systems can either be congenital or acquired after birth. Congenital and acquired losses can be *conductive* (caused by medically treatable pathologic conditions of the outer or middle ears); sensorineural (caused by permanent damge to the cochlea or eighth nerve); *mixed* (a combination of conductive and sensorineural); or *central* (caused by neural pathology in the central auditory nervous system).

Incidence of hearing loss

Total deafness is relatively rare, but partial hearing impairment is not uncommon. The incidence of significant hearing impairment is 1:50 in neonates discharged from intensive care nurseries, and about 1:1000 in well neonates. Most of these losses occur within the cochlea—that is, they are sensorineural hearing losses.

Common causes of hearing impairment and deafness

Hearing loss can occur during prenatal, perinatal, and postnatal stages of a child's development. The most common prenatal factors associated with hearing loss are of genetic origin or occur as a result of maternal rubella in the first trimester.

The most common perinatal factors include prematurity, low birth weight (less than 1500 g),

hyperbilirubinemia (indirect bilirubin of 15 mg or greater), anoxia, and infection (for example, TORCHES disorders). (See p.293.)

The most frequent postnatal factors are otitis media, meningitis, and other types of bacteriological and viral infections (for example, scarlet fever, measles, mumps, and encephalitis), and head injury.

An increasingly common cause of sensorineural hearing loss in the adolescent is exposure to excessively loud noise or music. But in preschool and lower grade elementary children, otitis media is by far the most common cause (see p. 674). Although otitis media is a disease of the middle ear resulting in conductive loss of fluctuating severity, it appears from more recent research that the reoccurrence of otitis media in young children may have a devastating effect on the development of the entire auditory system. Children with persistent or episodic otitis media before age two who demonstrate hearing deficiencies may have permanent impairment in cognitive, language, and emotional development.

The following criteria have been suggested as indications of significant hearing loss in young children:

1. Hearing level of 15 dB or greater
2. Indications of serous otitis media, in a child under 18 months, more than half the time for a period of 6 months
3. Fluctuating hearing levels from 0 to over 15 dB more than half the time for 1 year

EARLY DETECTION OF HEARING LOSS

Early detection and treatment of hearing loss is the key to reducing its damaging effects. All newborns meeting one or more of the following criteria should be tested and followed for the presence of hearing loss.

High-risk criteria

1. History of hereditary childhood hearing impairment
2. Rubella or other intrauterine infections (TORCHES)
3. Defects of ear, nose, throat, or larynx (mal-

PARAMETERS OF STIMULI USED TO TEST HEARING

Intensity levels—"loudness"

Hearing levels (HL) for pure tone hearing testing are measured in *decibels* (dB). Zero dB HL is the threshold at which sounds are normally first detected. The levels used to measure human hearing thresholds range from 0 dB to 110 dB HL. Normal hearing levels for children for all frequencies tested are considered to be 0 to 15 dB.

Pure tone frequencies—"pitch"

Pure tone frequencies are measured in cycles per second or *hertz* (Hz). Hertz refers to the number of vibrations per second that a sound source makes in order to produce each pure tone. The fewer the vibrations per second, the "lower" the frequency—"pitch"; the greater the number of vibrations, the "higher" the frequency. The human ear (fully intact) can usually hear frequencies from 20 Hz (very low) to 20,000 Hz (very high), but hearing tests usually monitor frequencies of 250, 500, 1000, 2000, 4000 and 8000 Hz.

formed, low set, or absent pinnae, cleft lip or palate, including submucous clefts)
4. Birth weight less than 1500 g
5. High serum bilirubin concentrations associated with jaundice that appear in the first 24 hours
6. Exposure to ototoxic drugs for more than 1 week

An infant meeting any of these criteria should be referred for an in-depth audiologic evaluation within the first 2 months of life. Even if hearing seems normal at that time, the child should receive subsequent regularly scheduled hearing evaluations. Regular evaluations are important because many genetically related hearing impairments and hearing losses resulting from ototoxic drug therapy may not appear until some time after birth.

Today audiometric evaluation can begin in the neonatal nursery. Audiometric procedures that allow for the testing of very young children and children previously thought untestable include: (1) the auditory brainstem evoked response (ABER) test, which objectively measures brain stem neural responses to auditory stimulation in relaxed or sleeping subjects (cortical evoked responses to auditory stimulation can also be recorded; however, this must be done with an awake and coopera-

tive subject); (2) the crib-o-gram, which is a completely automated crib assembly designed for signal presentation and recording of infant response; and (3) the impedance test battery, which objectively measures tympanic membrane mobility, middle ear pressure, eustachian tube patency, and the presence of a functioning acoustic reflex.

Also included in the test battery are the more traditional behavioral tests of sensitivity to pure tones (see the box above), calibrated noises, and speech, and tests of understanding of speech, all of which require the voluntary participation of the subject. Reflex responses to sound and classic conditioning methods are used to obtain this information from young children.

With previously undiagnosed or newly developing hearing impairment, certain child behaviors may alert the observant nurse to the presence of peripheral or central hearing dysfunction. Examples of these are as follows:
1. Better responses in quiet than in noisy environments
2. Difficulty following verbal instructions unless accompanied by visual demonstrations
3. Inadequate vocabulary
4. Defective sentence structure
5. Problems maintaining concentration

6. Social isolation
7. Inadequate reading or spelling
8. Poor reading comprehension
9. Discrepancy between achievement level and potential for learning
10. Significant discrepancy between verbal and performance IQ scores

Peripheral hearing loss is commonly measured using pure tones. Each pure tone has a single frequency of vibration that is perceived as a particular pitch and can be presented to the listener at a variety of levels of intensity or loudness. Presentation of pure tones at different intensity levels to a listener's ears is called the pure tone hearing test. The purpose of this test is to find the intensity level for each frequency at which the listener can "just barely" detect that the tone is present. This hearing level for each pure tone frequency is called the listener's threshold for that tone.

For young children, "mild hearing loss" is considered to be hearing threshold levels of 15 dB or greater for *any one* or all the frequencies considered important for the ability to detect and understand speech (500 Hz, 1000 Hz, 2000 Hz, 4000 Hz). Thresholds of 40 dB to 65 dB HL are moderate losses; 70 dB to 85 dB HL are severe losses; and 90+ dB HL are profound losses. An individual with thresholds of greater than or equal to 90 dB HL for a particular frequency is generally classified as being "deaf" for that frequency.

Before speaking to hearing-impaired children, one should face them directly and obtain their visual attention. This allows them to supplement their limited sound perception with visual cues from your lips. Parents and nurses should take every opportunity to expose these young children to meaningful auditory stimulation to help improve hearing. With abundant and early exposure to meaningful sound, hearing-impaired children have a much better prognosis for maximum utilization of their auditory systems.

The fact that a child has a hearing defect or wears a hearing aid on admission to the hospital is an important nursing observation. If the child is scheduled for surgery, permission should be sought to allow the child to wear the aid until the child is anesthetized in the operating room. The aid should be reapplied as soon as the child has awakened from surgery. Such permission will greatly reduce the fear of the young patient and will facilitate the entire procedure.

It is important for the nurse to remember that she may very well be the first health care professional to suspect the presence of a hearing loss in a child. Sensitivity to the potential of hearing loss and swift and appropriate referral and follow-up could be critical factors in the child's attainment of his full potential.

• • •

This chapter has covered a great deal of information—perhaps too much! It has treated no subject in depth. However, it is hoped that the student has been challenged to do further study of the needs of children with neuromuscular, skeletal, and sensory problems.

CHAPTER 32   Conditions involving the
respiratory and circulatory systems

If one speaks of the respiratory system without mentioning the circulatory system, only part of an important story is told, because these two body systems are intimately related. One might say that the respiratory system begins and ends a story, but the circulatory system contributes the bulky middle chapters. To put it another way, the respiratory system is responsible for so-called *external respiration,* whereas the circulatory system includes in its duties responsibility for *internal respiration.*

For this reason pediatric disorders of the respiratory and circulatory systems are considered here in the same general section, although for convenience they will also be studied as separate units. The respiratory system comprises Part 1 and the circulatory system Part 2 of this chapter.

KEY VOCABULARY

A brief reexamination of basic terminology used in describing respiratory and circulatory action and problems may be helpful:

anemia Condition in which hemoglobin in the blood is reduced.

apnea Absence of breathing.

atelectasis Airless segment of lung; collapse of lung.

bronchiectasis Abnormal dilatation of the bronchi in response to inflammation, which, if prolonged, will lead to associated structural changes and a chronic, productive cough.

Cheyne-Stokes respiration Irregular, cyclic breathing characterized by a period of increasing respiratory action followed by an interval of apnea.

dyspnea Difficult breathing.

edema Abnormal, excessive amount of fluid within the body tissues.

emphysema Abnormal dilatation and loss of elasticity of the microscopic air sacs, or alveoli, of the lung.

empyema Collection of pus in a body cavity, especially the pleural cavity.

eupnea Normal breathing.

leukocytosis Excessive increase in the number of white blood cells circulating in the blood.

orthopnea Condition in which breathing is possible by the patient only when in a standing or sitting position.

pneumothorax Abnormal collection of air or gas in the pleural cavity.

remission Lessening of severity or abatement of symptoms.

stenosis Abnormal narrowing of a passage or opening.

Part 1: The respiratory system

In conjunction with the study of disorders of the respiratory system, the student should review Chapter 27, which briefly outlines the basic anatomy and physiology of the respiratory system and discusses methods of aiding respiration and oxygenation.

Respiratory difficulties (such as respiratory distress syndrome, tracheoesophageal fistula, and diaphragmatic hernia) that are particularly associated with the newborn period are discussed in Chapters

660

14 and 15. In this presentation of respiratory pathology we will begin with a brief anatomic review followed by a consideration of those common problems affecting children in various stages of development.

ANATOMIC REVIEW

THE NOSE

The nose is an extremely interesting structure; although for some people it may not be a cosmetic asset, it performs certain important functions. First of all, it prepares air for entry into the interior of the body. It filters, warms, and moistens the air. Human beings may also breathe through their open mouths, and, except during the period of infancy, they do so fairly often. However, large amounts of air that enter the throat through the mouth are not properly warmed to body temperature or 100% humidified. The nose is also involved in the identification of different odors, because the olfactory nerve endings are located within the nasal cavity. Many of the finer perceptions of the palate are influenced by the sensitivity of these nerves. Consider how uninteresting food seems when one has a cold and the proper ventilation of the nose is disturbed. A normal nose is also necessary for proper vocal resonance.

THE PHARYNX AND TRACHEA

The pharynx is a passageway shared by both the respiratory and digestive systems. It extends from the back of the nasal cavity down past the posterior portion of the oral cavity to the level of the larynx and exophagus. Consequently the pharynx is divided descriptively into three parts: nasal, oral, and hypopharyngeal. The larynx and trachea extending from the hypopharynx complete the upper respiratory system.

THE LOWER RESPIRATORY TRACT

The lower respiratory tract is usually considered to include the bronchi, bronchioles, alveoli, which form the tissues of the lungs, and pleurae, or coverings of the lungs. Infectious conditions involving these structures are, for the most part, more difficult to cure and more threatening to general health than those involving the passages of the upper respiratory system.

RESPIRATORY DISORDERS

The infant

BRONCHIOLITIS

Bronchiolitis is a viral respiratory illness with clinical manifestations attributed to inflammatory narrowing of the small airways. The bronchioles are partially or completely obstructed as a result of mucosal swelling and exudate. The condition is more common in young infants and is seldom seen in children over 2 years of age.

Bronchiolitis begins as a simple cold. After a few days the infant develops a low-grade fever, shallow, rapid respirations, a cough, and an expiratory wheeze. Air can usually enter the bronchioles, but expiratory narrowing causes it to be trapped distal to the obstruction. Suprasternal and subcostal retractions are noted on inspiration. The infant is fatigued, irritable, anxious, and unable to eat or sleep. In severe cases some infants may even become cyanotic.

Some physicians feel that a trial of bronchodilator therapy is warranted in severe cases, but in most cases of pure bronchiolitis, it is not effective. Intravenous aminophylline, subcutaneous epinephrine or aerosol therapy with isoetharine can be used once a trial of bronchodilator therapy is decided. If benefit is achieved, this therapy is continued.

Acute bronchiolitis in infants presents a frightening picture. Parents feel helpless, anxious, and actually fear that the life of their child is in jeopardy. Fortunately mortality is very low, and the most severe period lasts only a few days. Recovery is almost always complete within 2 weeks. This information is most welcome by the worried parents.

Their questions should be answered simply, and they are encouraged to stay at the crib side. The infant should be placed in an atmosphere of cool mist and oxygen. Color, respirations, and pulse need close observation. Rest, oxygen, and hydration are most important. Nasal suctioning is usually necessary before feeding. Fluids should be urged frequently and in small amounts.

PNEUMONIA

Any inflammation of the lung parenchyma is called pneumonia. Many microbiologic agents as well as certain noninfectious agents and conditions are known to cause pneumonia. The anatomic and pathologic changes may involve the lobar, lobular, interstitial, or bronchial areas. Pneumonia, most commonly seen in infants and young children, is a potentially grave condition, and one of the major causes of mortality in the age group of 1 to 14 years. Early recognition and prompt treatment spare lengthy hospitalization and reduce the incidence of complications. Common causes of pneumonias in infants and children are:

I. Primary pneumonias (no underlying predisposing condition diagnosed)
  A. Bacterial
    1. Pneumococcal
    2. Staphylococcal
    3. Streptococcal
    4. *Haemophilus influenzae*
  B. Nonbacterial
    1. Viral
    2. *Mycoplasma*
II. Secondary pneumonias (other predisposing conditions diagnosed)
  A. Hypostatic—caused by stasis of respiratory secretions resulting from lack of adequate respiration
  B. Asthmatic—caused by narrowed airways and increased mucus
  C. Associated with cystic fibrosis—caused by the presence of viscid respiratory secretions
  D. Aspiration pneumonias—involve accidental inhalation of

1. Hydrocarbons—petroleum distillates such as gasoline and furniture polish
2. Foreign bodies—popcorn, peanuts, buttons, and other objects
3. Gastric contents—associated with gastroesophageal reflux (GER) and other congenital anomalies of the esophagus or trachea

Signs and symptoms

The onset and clinical manifestations of pneumonia vary with the age of the child and the etiologic agent. The disease occurs most frequently in winter and spring. Bacterial pneumonias are often preceded by a viral upper respiratory tract infection, which alters the defense mechanisms of the lower respiratory tract. The classic signs and symptoms are fever, anorexia, listlessness, and cough. At first the cough is wet and loose, but soon it becomes dry and painful. The pain associated with lower lobe pneumonia is frequently referred to the abdomen. For this reason a chest x-ray examination of young children with possible appendicitis should be done to rule out pneumonia before they are sent to surgery. In the young child the temperature mounts rapidly, and seizures frequently occur. Respirations become rapid and shallow and are accompanied by flaring of the nostrils, grunting, and retractions. The pulse rate is extremely rapid (it may be doubled). Meningeal irritation such as stiff neck is sometimes present with upper lobe pneumonia, and a spinal tap is necessary to rule out coexisting meningitis. Cyanosis coupled with a rapid, weak pulse is always a grave sign. Since proper therapy depends on knowledge of the causative agents, the common pneumonias will be discussed according to their cause.

Types

Bacterial primary pneumonias. Pneumococcal pneumonia is the most common type encountered in infants and young children. Typically, after symptoms of a mild cold, the infant suddenly refuses his milk or formula and becomes listless. The temperature rises rapidly, and respiratory distress is soon apparent. Fortunately, the pneumo-coccus is responsive to antibiotic therapy. A good response to penicillin usually takes place within 24 to 48 hours in uncomplicated cases. Response to therapy is delayed in those cases that are complicated by fluid in the pleural space (pleural effusion), empyema, otitis media, or meningitis.

Staphylococcal pneumonia is the most serious of the pneumonias in infancy. It may follow an upper respiratory tract infection, or it may spread to the lungs by way of the bloodstream from a staphylococcal infection elsewhere in the body. Unless recognized and treated early, the disease characteristically progresses rapidly, causing severe respiratory distress, and may be associated with the formation of abscesses and air cysts (pneumatoceles). Antibiotic therapy with methicillin or oxacillin is continued for a few weeks. Isolation technique is observed. Pneumothorax is common and is treated with continuous closed-suction drainage. Mortality is high in untreated infants.

Streptococcal pneumonia is more common in young children than in infants. It is usually preceded by a viral infection such as rubeola, rubella, or varicella. The onset of chills and pleuritic pain may be sudden, or the pneumonia may start with a gradual rise in temperature, accompanied by cough. Streptococci cause an interstitial type of pneumonia, and occasionally abscesses and pneumatoceles can develop. Empyema usually requires closed-suction drainage. Penicillin G is the antibiotic of choice and is highly effective.

Pneumonia caused by type B *Haemophilus influenzae* is a serious disease. The onset of illness is insidious, and the clinical course may be prolonged over several weeks. Infants and children under 5 years of age are most often affected and seem susceptible to bacteremia and empyema. A prolonged, pertussis-like cough sometimes accompanies this type of pneumonia. To prevent serious complications, chloramphenicol is given in large doses as soon as the disease is diagnosed and continued until the sensitivity is known.

Nonbacterial primary pneumonias. *Viral pneumonia* can be caused by almost any type of virus. A low-grade fever and coryza precede this interstitial pneumonia, which appears suddenly with the onset of tachypnea and a nonproductive, tight cough. Treatment is symptomatic, since antibiotics are of no value unless secondary bacterial complications occur.

Mycoplasma pneumonia is an atypical pneumonia caused by a pathogenic "filterable" microorganism known as *Mycoplasma pneumoniae* (Eaton agent). It is a tiny, free-living microorganism that has properties between those of bacteria and viruses. Infection usually results in a self-limited, interstitial pneumonia. Mycoplasma pneumonia occurs most commonly in the adolescent. The onset is abrupt and symptoms include fever, headache, malaise, chills, and a characteristic dry, hacking cough. Later the cough becomes productive, sometimes producing blood-streaked mucus. Erythromycin is the antibiotic of choice in treating this type of pneumonia in children.

Secondary aspiration pneumonias. Infants and children have been known to aspirate not only their formula but all kinds of food, poisons, and objects. The right upper lobe is frequently involved. Mucosal swelling and obstruction may occur. Symptoms vary depending on the child, the substance, and the amount aspirated. Treatment is supportive and aimed at preventing intercurrent infections. Of course, prevention of these incidents is the best therapy.

Recently clinical investigators have discovered that infants and young children with gastroesophageal reflux (GER) can develop pneumonias as a result of aspiration of gastric content, which is very toxic to the airways and alveoli. In mild cases, a conservative regimen with thickening of the formula with rice cereal and placing the child in an upright position 1 to 2 hours after feedings may be effective. However, in severe cases a surgical intervention such as fundoplication (in which a valvelike mechanism is created by wrapping the fundus of the stomach around the distal esophagus, reducing reflux) is necessary. Aspiration of gastric content can also occur in tracheoesophageal fistula and in children with neurologic deficit.

Aspiration of petroleum distillates such as kerosene, gasoline, lighter fluid, and furniture polishes causes a very severe chemical pneumonitis, characterized by edema and inflammation. Some petroleum distillates are absorbed from the intestines and then excreted through the lungs. Treatment is symptomatic and may include steroids to reduce inflammatory changes or antibiotics to combat secondary infections.

A number of foreign bodies, including seeds, coins, nuts, popcorn, safety pins, and bones, have been removed from the respiratory passages of young children. (Young children must not eat peanuts or popcorn because of this common problem.) Foreign bodies inhaled into the lungs will occlude the bronchi, causing atelectasis or hyperinflation. The young child will manifest dyspnea, cyanosis, and asymmetric respirations. Incomplete obstruction causes wheezing, and, if untreated, fever and cough-producing purulent sputum soon develop. Delay in removal of the foreign object by bronchoscopy seriously alters the prognosis. Usually the foreign body becomes embedded, injuring the tissues and causing infection. Permanent damage to the area involved follows prolonged atelectasis.

Diagnosis of the pneumonias

A high white blood cell count (WBC), over 10,000, with increased polymorphonuclear cells and a shift to young forms (bands), is suggestive of bacterial infections. A low WBC (5,000 or less) is more typical of viral infections in general; therefore a differential white blood cell count is routinely requested on these patients. Blood cultures obtained before antibiotic therapy is initiated are very helpful in the identification of specific organisms, especially when septicemia is present. Nasopharyngeal cultures are not of great value, since pneumococci, streptococci, *H. influenzae,* and staphylococci can be isolated from healthy children. Tracheal cultures obtained by suction techniques are more helpful in identification of organisms. X-ray films are perhaps the most valuable diagnostic tool in evaluating the extent or type of the pneumonia. Bronchoscopy (visualization of the tracheobronchial tree) may be performed when

other procedures have failed to make an adequate diagnosis of the problem. Fluid or tissue may be removed by this method for a culture or cytology studies. Lung biopsy is sometimes necessary when protracted pulmonary disease cannot be explained by other means.

Treatment and supportive nursing care

Specific therapy is important in the treatment of pneumonia. Differentiating viral and bacterial infections initially is difficult. Since pneumococcal pneumonia is the most common pneumonia seen in infants and young children, therapy for all pneumonias typically is begun with penicillin G. Later, when the cause of the pneumonia is established, a specific drug can be given. Supportive care is as important as antibiotic therapy in lessening the severity of the child's illness. Fluids are encouraged, and acetaminophen or aspirin is given for fever. Rest in bed is recommended during the febrile stage. Humidification and increased amounts of fluid are necessary for liquefaction of bronchial secretions. Saturated solution of potassium iodide (SSKI) or guaifenesin syrup (Robitussin) may help loosen secretions and initiate a productive cough. In general cough suppressants such as codeine are not recommended in pneumonia because a valuable mechanism used to help clear the bronchial tree would be lost. Respiratory therapies are important in the hospital setting. Bronchial drainage is carried out three or four times daily (before meals and at bedtime). Viscid secretions will not drain from the bronchi by gravity alone, but deep breathing, reinforced coughing, and respiratory therapy techniques such as squeezing, cupping, and vibration will assist in their removal. Oxygen administration is used for children with hypoxia.

When the child's appetite improves, a nutritious diet of foods that are appealing should be offered. Before feeding an infant, the nurse should remove nasal secretions. One or two drops of saline solution may be ordered, followed by gentle suctioning. A restless infant who cannot breathe will not eat.

Nursing care involves careful observation of

respiratory patterns, pulse, color, and the general condition of the patient. Observance of the attending physician's positioning orders and frequent modification of body position within the prescribed limits are also important. Patients often breathe better with their heads and chests elevated; babies are often placed in infant seats. Isolation techniques are observed, mainly for contagious conditions such as staphylococcal pneumonia. Convalescence should not be rushed; adequate time for recuperation is very important to allow the child to regain strength and weight.

When a child with pneumonia is treated at home or on an outpatient basis, the parents should be carefully instructed about the therapeutic and nursing measures. They should understand that medicines must be taken on time and in the correct amount. In general young children should be cared for by their parents in the familiar, comforting environment of their own homes. Nevertheless, hospitalization may be advisable during the first 2 or 3 days of illness to provide inhalation therapy and parenteral administration of drugs and fluid. Infants who are under 6 months of age and have pneumonia are always hospitalized. Other children are hospitalized if they become too sick to take fluids, if they require intensive supportive measures (such as intravenous or oxygen therapy or surgical drainage) because of their diagnosis or condition, or if the family cannot or does not adequately care for them.

Although the diagnosis of pneumonia does not produce the same alarm today that it once did in the hearts and minds of parents, it is still a potential threat to the life and future health of the child. Patients suffering from this disease must be frequently evaluated and expertly nursed.

CYSTIC FIBROSIS (MUCOVISCIDOSIS)

Cystic fibrosis (CF) is a hereditary, multisystem disorder in which generalized dysfunction of the exocrine glands occurs, especially involving the mucous and sweat glands. It is usually characterized by the triad of chronic, severe pulmonary disease, pancreatic insufficiency, and abnormally high concentrations of electrolytes in the sweat.

Cystic fibrosis is genetically transmitted as an autosomal recessive trait, and at the present time no reliable way exists to identify individual parents carrying the gene before the disease manifests itself in their offspring. No clinically available method will detect the presence of the disease in an unborn child. If one child has the disease, the risk for each subsequent pregnancy is one in four. That is, each conception has the same 25% chance of producing an affected child (see p. 304 for genetic discussion). The incidence of cystic fibrosis in the United States is one per 1,600 to 2,000 live births. Boys and girls appear to be equally involved. Five percent of the white population and less than 1% of the black population are estimated to be genetic carriers of this hidden trait. Although the survival rate is steadily improving, cystic fibrosis remains a serious condition. Couples who have a child with cystic fibrosis should be made aware of the genetic implications of the disease. (See Fig. 32-1).

Symptoms

Clinical expression of the disease varies because of individual variation in age at onset and severity of involvement of the various organs and systems. However, the altered function of the exocrine glands leads to clinical manifestations, primarily in the respiratory and digestive systems.

Almost all patients with cystic fibrosis have some degree of chronic pulmonary disease. The degree of pulmonary involvement and rate of progression usually determine the prognosis. Involvement occurs through a progressive sequence of events that are experienced by all patients sooner or later. Secretions of the mucus-producing glands become extremely thick and tenacious in the bronchi and bronchioles, causing coughing, wheezing, respiratory obstruction, emphysema, and, frequently, infection. As a result the defense in the lungs against microbes is severely compromised. In severe cases the chronic respiratory disease causes a barrel-like chest deformity, cyanosis, and clubbing of the fingers and toes. As hypoxemia and secondary pulmonary arterial hypertension develop, dilatation of the right side of the heart and thickening of the right ventricular wall will occur. This

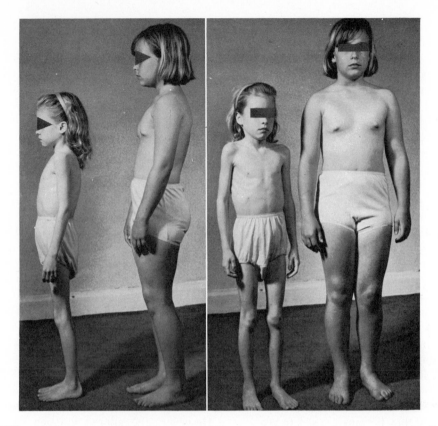

FIG. 32-1   Both these girls are 10 years old. The youngster on the left demonstrates the effects of severe cystic fibrosis.

process can, when untreated, result in heart failure and death. Cardiac disease secondary to pulmonary disease is termed "cor pulmonale" (Fig. 32-2).

Approximately 85% of patients with cystic fibrosis have digestive system problems. Since the pancreatic digestive enzymes may be reduced or absent, foodstuffs (fats and proteins especially) may be poorly digested and assimilated. As a result the infant or child fails to thrive. As much of the food eaten does not undergo the normal process of digestion and assimilation, the child will pass large amounts of feces and develop a protuberant abdomen. This bulky stool has a foul smell and the odor is caused by impaired digestion of fats.

In a small percentage of cases (about 10%), the disease is recognized in the newborn nursery because of the detection of meconium ileus. In this condition the meconium, or stool formed in utero by the newborn infant, is even more thick and sticky than normal meconium because of the absence or reduction of normal pancreatic digestive enzymes. The abnormal stool sticks to the walls of the ileum like paste and obstructs the lower digestive tract. The obstructed intestine becomes distended, and abdominal distention, or bloating, is noted, and no passage of stool occurs. Vomiting and dehydration may ensue. Any newborn infant who does not pass stool within 24 hours after birth should be carefully evaluated and examined for possible obstruction. (See p. 716 for management.)

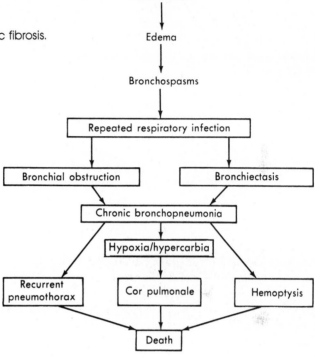

Abnormal thick secretions and impaired ciliary function in respiratory tract

Inflammation

Edema

Bronchospasms

Repeated respiratory infection

Bronchial obstruction

Bronchiectasis

Chronic bronchopneumonia

Hypoxia/hypercarbia

Recurrent pneumothorax

Cor pulmonale

Hemoptysis

Death

FIG. 32-2

Pathologic sequence characteristic of cystic fibrosis.

Other clinical conditions in infancy that indicate the possibility of cystic fibrosis include obstructive jaundice, hypoproteinemia, prolonged bronchiolitis, and rectal prolapse.

Diagnosis

A high degree of clinical suspicion is usually the first step in the diagnosis of cystic fibrosis. Infants and children who suffer from recurrent respiratory tract infections or fail to thrive should be especially evaluated. The diagnosis is confirmed by laboratory evidence of abnormally elevated sweat chloride levels. Children with cystic fibrosis will have a positive sweat test reaction from birth if enough sweat (50 to 100 mg) can be collected. A positive reaction implies an elevation of the concentration of chloride above 60 mEq/L. This feature is so pro-

nounced that mothers have noted that their affected children seem to have a "salty taste" when they are kissed.

The quantitative sweat test by pilocarpine iontophoresis is definitive for confirming the diagnosis of cystic fibrosis at all ages. Because of the seriousness of the disease and to ensure reliability, at least two tests should be done.

When the diagnosis has been established, further tests may be performed to determine the extent of system involvement and to establish a baseline for future assessment of treatment and disease progress. Chest x-ray examinations and pulmonary function tests are done to assess respiratory involvement. Abdominal x-ray examinations, stool analysis, and pancreatic function tests are done to assess gastrointestinal involvement.

Treatment

Treatment is directed toward the organs involved and designed to meet the needs of the individual patient. Since the chief cause of death in patients with cystic fibrosis is directly related to the degree of lung involvement, maximal therapeutic efforts are directed to the lungs (Table 32-1). Thick mucus obstructing the lung leads to recurrent pulmonary infection and tissue damage. Early in the course of the disease, the mucus that accumulates in the bronchi and bronchioles is so viscid that the cilia are unable to expel it. As the mucus stagnates, it becomes contaminated, usually by *Staphylococcus aureus* and *Pseudomonas aeruginosa*. Resultant infection intensifies mucus production, and the accumulation leads to airway obstruction.

Control of pulmonary infection requires the use of appropriate antibiotics and adequate drainage of bronchial secretions by respiratory therapy. During sleep some children still use a fine mist environment but clinical investigations have failed to demonstrate any beneficial effect. The use of a continuing home pulmonary care program from the time of diagnosis to prevent progression and complications as much as possible has improved the life expectancy of children with cystic fibrosis. Children with advanced and steadily increasing pulmonary disease or severe pulmonary infections usually have to be hospitalized for intensive parenteral antibiotic therapy. However, intravenous administration of antibiotics to inpatients and outpatients with acute and chronic infection can be accomplished by use of the heparin lock IV. In fact, many hospitalizations now can be avoided by teaching selected children or parents this convenient method of parenteral antibiotic therapy. The heparin lock IV consists of a butterfly scalp vein needle attached to a small plastic tube that is sealed by a rubber cap in such a way as to protect sterility and patency. It facilitates frequent high intravenous doses of antibiotics without limiting activity. The patient can move about freely with only the lock in place, and the other equipment needed for the intravenous administration of drugs remains at the bedside until the next dose is due. Postural drain-

TABLE 32-1 PULMONARY THERAPY

Treatment	Purpose
Intermittent aerosol therapy	To deliver medications and water to the lower respiratory tract
Antibiotic therapy	To treat infection and minimize progression of infection
Chest physical therapy	To facilitate the removal of secretions and prevent mucus accumulation
Breathing exercises	To establish and maintain a good breathing pattern

age and percussion treatments vital in combating these infections can be more effectively performed. For details of heparin lock IV maintenance, see p. 458.

Nutrition

Maintaining nutritional goals becomes increasingly difficult as the disease progresses. However, initially the aim is to encourage 100% of the recommended dietary allowance (for age) plus extra calories to make up for the calories lost because of malabsorption. Pancreatic insufficiency limits the patient's capacity for digesting fats and proteins. The child usually has an eager appetite; however, because he is unable to use much of the food he eats (and respiratory complications may interfere with nutrition), his arms and legs are characteristically spindly, his buttocks are emaciated, and his growth is retarded (Fig. 32-1). Fortunately the digestive problems usually improve with the addition of commercial preparations of pancreatic enzymes given with each meal. A major advance in this area is the enteric-coated enzyme, Pancrease, which allows for delivery of predictable levels of enzymes to the duodenum at the same time as food. The enzymes are taken by mouth with meals; the dosage varies, depending on the amount of food, the kind of food (particular fat content), and the degree of pancreatic insufficiency. The goal of pancreatic enzyme therapy is to increase intestinal absorption of foodstuff and allow the patient as nearly normal a diet as possible while decreasing the number of bulky, foul-smelling, loose stools. Fat restriction is generally unnecessary, with the exception of the fat load of whole milk and excessive grease in food. Children should be encouraged to use skim or 2% milk rather than homogenized milk.

Medium-chain triglycerides (MCTs) are more easily absorbed than other fats and provide an important source of calories. The MCT oil enables the preparation and digestion of fried foods, salad dressings, and mayonnaise. The diet should also be supplemented with twice the recommended daily dose of vitamins, prepared in such a way that they can be combined with water (water-miscible) because of malabsorption of the fat-soluble vitamins in cystic fibrosis. The water-miscible vitamins make supplementation of vitamins A, D, and K accessible to the patient. Supplementary vitamin K is recommended, especially for infants, to prevent blood clotting problems. In hot weather extra salt intake is necessary because of the large amounts lost in the perspiration. The prescribed amount can be incorporated in the preparation of food and need not be given separately. Heat prostration caused by salt depletion is a real danger to these children, especially on hot summer days and during periods of exertion. If excessive sweating is anticipated, sodium chloride intake should be increased.

Cystic fibrosis centers

Since the disease is chronic, and many organs and systems are involved, care is complex and requires a team effort to coordinate the services of many specialists. Comprehensive, coordinated services are the key to good management, and all children with cystic fibrosis should be referred to a cystic fibrosis center, where a team of experts in all aspects of the disease can design an individualized treatment plan. In addition to a specific treatment plan that includes instructions on medication, diet, and exercise, the patient and family are trained in techniques of postural drainage. Cystic fibrosis centers can also provide initial and continuing psy-

chologic, psychosocial, genetic, and vocational counseling.

Nursing care

Nursing care entails a careful observation of the dietary intake and its effect on the child and on elimination. Every effort should be made to offer a variety in the meals within the limitations imposed and to make eating a pleasant experience.

Provision for frequent changes in position to prevent pneumonia and reduce skin problems is an important consideration in sick, malnourished patients with cystic fibrosis. Some of these children are very emaciated, and the skin over bony prominences is in special need of care. The rectal area must be meticulously cleaned. Rectal prolapse may be a complication occasionally. A soothing, local ointment may prevent irritation from the bulky stools. Any material soiled by feces should be removed immediately from the child's room. Appropriate air fresheners may be useful. Stools should always be described regarding their size, color, consistency, and odor.

The observation and report of respiratory distress is, of course, of paramount importance. Every effort should be made to protect the child from persons with any type of respiratory tract infection.

Because of the chronic nature of the disease, the severe strain it may place on the family finances, and the psychologic needs of the child, home care is recommended, except when the child's condition is such that appropriate care can only be provided through hospitalization. Parents may need much counseling and practical assistance to help meet their child's social and emotional requirements as well as physical needs. They also must be cautioned against becoming so preoccupied with the sick child that the needs of other family members are continually neglected.

Early diagnosis and improved methods of therapy have reduced the morbidity and greatly increased the longevity of children with cystic fibrosis. These children now have a greater than 50% chance of living past the second decade.

Only very rarely will a young man with cystic

fibrosis be fertile, since the same mechanisms that typically obstruct other glandular ducts of the body probably interfere with sperm transport.

Female patients have borne children, but their ability to conceive seems to be below normal because cervical mucus is abnormal.

The nurse caring for the child with cystic fibrosis must realize the strain under which the parents may be operating and their feelings of fatigue and frustration. Many families have lost other children because of this disease and have traveled almost the same road to final farewells before. Such a journey is no easier just because some of the scenery may be familiar.

The toddler

CROUP (LARYNGOTRACHEOBRONCHITIS)

Acute obstructive subglottic laryngitis, commonly known as croup, is a viral respiratory disease that involves the larynx, trachea, and bronchi. Mild to severe forms of laryngotracheobronchitis (LTB) typically occur in children between 6 months and 3 years of age during cold weather. Croup is characterized by a sudden onset of inspiratory stridor, hoarseness, and a barklike cough following a 1- to 3-day history of a "cold." These manifestations are the result of inflammatory edema of the vocal cords and subglottic area, causing varying degrees of laryngeal obstruction. Sometimes, spasm accompanies the process. Most children are awakened without warning in the middle of the night by an acute attack. The child appears extremely anxious and frightened by this respiratory distress. Treatment is symptomatic. High humidity (running hot water in the bathroom) and gentle reassurance are important. If there is spasm, it usually subsides in a few hours with high humidity therapy but may recur for 1 or 2 nights.

A more severe form of croup results when the inflammatory involvement of the trachea and bronchial tree produces a thick, viscous, purulent exudate. Edema and the exudate lead to both inspiratory and expiratory difficulties. As the degree of severity of respiratory distress increases, suprasternal, intercostal, and substernal retractions occur. The child becomes hypoxic, restless, and desperately anxious. Impending suffocation is a real threat and a terrifying experience for both the child and the parents. This child needs immediate medical management and possible endotracheal intubation or tracheostomy.

During the admission procedure, every effort should be made to avoid aggravation of respiratory distress. The parents should remain at the crib side as the child is gently and calmly placed in an atmosphere of high humidity with oxygen. Maximum humidification is best accomplished with cool mist in the tent. The moist vapor will help allay irritation of the mucosa and promote liquefaction of the thick secretions. Clear fluids are encouraged if the respiratory distress is not very severe and are also important in mobilizing respiratory exudate. Refusal to take fluids orally or severe respiratory distress necessitates intravenous therapy.

Increased pulse rate, restlessness, severe stridor, and use of the accessory muscles for breathing must be reported immediately. If the signs and symptoms of acute airway obstruction increase, emergency airway intervention must be considered before the child is exhausted. This is achieved in most hospitals by the insertion of an endotracheal tube or tracheostomy. In recent years, endotracheal intubation has become the preferred method. Arterial or arterialized capillary blood gases are most helpful in assessing the clinical situation and determining the need for emergency airway intervention. Unfortunately this procedure may upset the child to such a degree that the child can be more hypoxic during the blood drawing.

Nebulized racemic epinephrine (Vaponefrin) has been used with success in many cases of LTB. At first the child struggles against the aerosol, but after a short time the child relaxes and the labored breathing subsides as the therapy is continued over 10 to 15 minutes. The procedure is repeated if necessary in 3 to 4 hours. Racemic epinephrine is used for its topical vasoconstrictive effect, resulting in decreased mucosal edema. This treatment has been found to be extremely helpful in providing

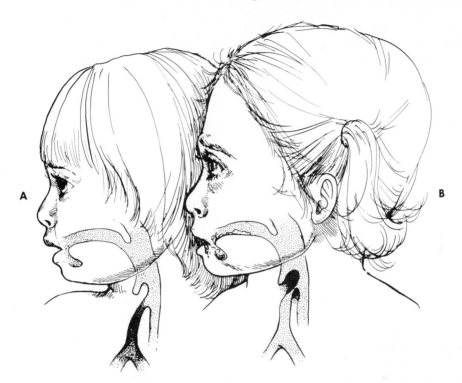

FIG. 32-3   Anatomic difference between acute subglottic and acute supraglottic obstruction. **A,** Laryngotracheobronchitis (LTB), an acute inflammation particularly involving the subglottic area of the larynx, trachea, and bronchial tree, most commonly occurring in the toddler. **B,** Epiglottitis, an acute inflammatory swelling involving the structures above the opening of the trachea (glottis), most often seen in the preschooler.

immediate, temporary improvement in patients with croup. However, the obstruction can recur in 1 to 2 hours as a result of a rebound phenomenon in severe cases. Therefore, severe cases should be observed closely for recurrence even after a remarkable improvement.

Acute LTB should not be confused with epiglottitis (acute supraglottic laryngitis), a most serious acute airway problem that may lead to complete respiratory obstruction and death in several hours (Fig. 32-3).

FOREIGN BODIES IN THE NOSE OR THROAT

Children frequently push objects other than their fingers into the nasal cavity, probably as the result of natural curiosity. If the object does not spontaneously drop out or is not dislodged by sneezing and the episode is not reported by the child, it may be indicated by a bloody or purulent, foul nasal discharge originating from one nostril only. Such a discharge should make one suspect the presence of a foreign body. Removal of such an object should be attempted only by a physician who has the necessary instruments.

If a child is discovered choking, but still is conscious and able to cough, he should be encouraged to cough. If the child develops complete obstruction, four short, controlled blows on the back with the hand may dislodge the object. If the problem still persists, CPR should be initiated. If respiratory distress continues, the child should be seen immediately by a physician who may have to schedule a chest x-ray examination and perform a bronchoscopy. For discussion of aspiration pneumonia see p. 663 and for emergency CPR procedures see p. 522.

BRONCHITIS

Bronchitis is most often caused by the same virus that has invaded other areas of the respiratory tract. Bronchitis is usually preceded by an upper respiratory tract infection and is a common problem in toddlers. It may remain mild or become progressively severe, leading to pneumonia. A disturbing productive cough appears as the disease develops. Paroxysms may occur, particularly when the position of the child is altered, such as in the morning on rising or when first lying in bed after having sat for a period. Vomiting as a result of gagging when the secretions are thick is not uncommon. Cool moisture is sometimes helpful. A generous intake of fluids will thin bronchial secretions, and aspirin or acetaminophen (Tylenol) may be necessary to lessen discomfort or fever. Unless the condition worsens, acute bronchitis is generally a self-limited infection that improves spontaneously in a few days.

The preschool child

EPIGLOTTITIS

Acute obstructive supraglottic laryngitis, commonly known as epiglottitis, is usually caused by the *H. influenzae* type b bacteria. It is characterized by acute respiratory distress, high temperature, difficulty in swallowing, drooling, and a "cherry red" epiglottis on physical examination. The signs and symptoms of supraglottic obstruction result from inflammatory edema of the epiglottis. Children between 3 and 7 years of age are most frequently affected. The conditions are usually seen in the winter months, and the onset is sudden. The child first complains of a severe sore throat and difficulty in swallowing (dysphagia). Soon the child is anxious, unable to eat or drink, prostrated, in a toxic condition, and drooling. Rap-

idly increasing dyspnea and drooling are the most important signs of impending disaster. Once the diagnosis is made, one should not be lulled into hopeful, watchful waiting. This child needs to have his airway secured, either by endotracheal tube or tracheostomy. Endotracheal intubation or tracheostomy should not be deferred in the hope that it will not be necessary. Epiglottitis can lead to complete respiratory obstruction and death in just a few hours. It is important not to unduly disturb the child or to separate the child from his parents. The diagnosis is confirmed by visualization of the inflamed epiglottis or by a lateral neck x-ray film, and the child is moved from the emergency room to the operating room, where an elective endotracheal intubation or tracheostomy can be performed in an ideal setting. Intravenous therapy with ampicillin and/or chloramphenicol and fluids is given. After the airways are secured, arterial blood gases are assessed to assure adequate respirations. It is essential that warm mist with or without oxygen is administered through the artificial airways by a T-piece or tracheostomy collar. The child is then placed in a mist tent and returned to the pediatric intensive care unit where an experienced staff can give constant care. No child should die from epiglottitis when it is diagnosed and treated promptly.

EPISTAXIS

Bleeding from the nose is a common disorder of childhood, especially in boys from 4 to 10 years of age. On the anterior portion of the nasal septum called Kiesselbach's area can be found a fragile network of capillaries subject to drying and multiple minor injuries. Traumas such as nose picking and nose rubbing, forceful blowing, and insertion of foreign bodies are the usual causes of bleeding.

Placing the child in a sitting position with the head tilted forward while compressing the nares with the thumb and forefinger is often sufficient to facilitate clot formation and stop the bleeding. This posture also prevents blood from dripping down the posterior pharynx, possibly leading to aspiration. Ice packs to the nasal area or to the back of the neck are of little or no value. If bleeding is persistent, an anterior nasal pack consisting of ½ inch of petrolatum-impregnated gauze or an application of agents such as aqueous epinephrine solution (1:1000) or thrombin may be useful.

Any condition that contributes to vascular congestion of the nasal mucosa, such as nasal allergy or sinusitis, increases the frequency of epistaxis. Bleeding from the posterior region of the nasal cavity is uncommon. At times such nosebleeds may be a symptom of underlying blood dyscrasias such as purpura, leukemia, or conditions associated with a rise in blood pressure. Frequent nosebleeds may or may not be significant. Parental fears can best be allayed by not only stopping the bleeding but also identifying and treating the underlying causes of the disorder.

DEVIATION OF THE SEPTUM

In some instances the cartilaginous wall, or septum, that divides the nose into two lateral chambers does not occupy the midline. It may deviate toward one side or another as the result of natural development or, more commonly, as an aftermath of trauma. This may indirectly cause occlusion of a nostril and difficult breathing, particularly when the nose is inflamed. This structural anomaly may be corrected surgically by an operation called a submucous resection. To prevent external nasal deformity resulting from the surgery, it is usually not performed until adolescence.

ACUTE NASOPHARYNGITIS (ACUTE CORYZA, COMMON COLD)

The so-called common cold has plagued humanity for countless years, and since no specific preventive or treatment has yet been discovered, it will probably be with us to cause consternation for at least several more. Preschool and young school-age children average approximately six colds a year. The common cold is probably caused by several viral organisms that primarily attack the nose and throat. Symptoms include a dry, scratchy, sore, inflamed pharynx and an inflamed nasal mucosa, which produces a clear mucoid nasal discharge that later becomes thick and purulent. These local symptoms are often accompanied by headache, muscular pains, general malaise, and fever. As the viral infection continues, complications often arise from the intrusion of pathogenic bacteria, which may prolong the congestion and promote the extension of the inflammation to the middle ear, sinuses, larynx, trachea, and even to the bronchi and lungs. It is mainly the possibility of extension that makes the common cold a potentially dangerous condition.

A common cold is probably contagious for a number of hours before symptoms are observed by the patient. It is now believed that the cold sufferer remains contagious for about 8 hours after the onset of visible signs. Contamination by spread of droplets is most common. It is very important to protect infants from exposure to colds, because they are affected more seriously than older children. An infant may have a high temperature of 104° F (40° C), and febrile convulsions are possible. Ears are almost always affected. Nasal congestion causes difficulties in breathing, nursing, and eating. It is impossible to prevent a child from ever having a cold, but everything possible should be done to protect a baby.

Since nasopharyngitis is entirely caused by viruses, no specific therapy is recommended. Supportive treatment consists of rest, relative isolation, increased fluid intake, and a bland, soft diet is desired. Nasal obstruction in infants can be partially relieved by humidification or instillation of 1 or 2 drops of physiologic saline solution in each nostril, followed by gentle suction with an infant's nasal (or ear) syringe. Phenylephrine (Neo-Synephrine) hydrochloride nose drops (⅛% for infants and ¼% for older children) may also relieve nasal symptoms. Nasal vasoconstrictors should not be used for more than 3 or 4 days because of "rebound phenomena." (When the use of such vasoconstrictors has been prolonged and is suddenly stopped, secretion greatly increases, or "rebounds.")

Mild systemic symptoms and fever may be relieved by proper dosage of aspirin or nonsalicylate acetaminophen (Tylenol or Tempra). Aspirin can be extremely dangerous to a child whose intake of fluids has declined significantly. Remember, both the amount of aspirin given and the interval and duration of treatment must always be considered. Many children suffer from salicylate poisoning every year! A rule of thumb a nurse may want to remember is that a child of average weight should be given only 1 grain (60 mg) of aspirin per year of age up to 5 grains and should not be given aspirin more than five times at 4-hour intervals without medical consultation. Dosages for babies under 1 year of age must be very carefully determined. Children over 5 years of age but less than 12 years of age may usually be given 5 grains at a time if administration is not repeated more often than every 4 to 6 hours for a brief period.

To protect the nares of upper lip from excoriation caused by the fairly constant nasal discharge, cold cream or petrolatum may be applied. Antibiotics are indicated in viral infections when secondary bacterial invaders become a problem.

SINUSITIS

Acute sinusitis is often precipitated by an upper respiratory infection. Headache and a mucopurulent discharge from one or both nostrils, cough, and a diffusely red pharynx with mucopurulent discharge clinging to the posterior wall are indications that bacteria have invaded the sinuses. Improved ventilation and drainage are primary goals in the treatment. Hot compresses over the painful areas and increased humidification will provide some comfort. Pain and fever are lessened by use of acetaminophen or aspirin. Instillation of nasal vasoconstrictors, preferably by spray, are helpful in shrinking the nasal mucosa and opening the airways. Each nostril should be sprayed once while the child is in a sitting position. About 3 to 5 minutes later, the spraying should be repeated to reach the posterior part of the nose. Oral decongestants such as pseudoephedrine hydrochloride (sudafed), Triaminic, or Actifed may be useful when local therapy is difficult. Although most acute sinus infections are self-limiting, appropriate antibiotic therapy (culture sensitive) will shorten the course of illness and prevent any further complications.

OTITIS MEDIA

Otitis media, or inflammation of the middle ear, is a common, difficult problem related to malfunction of the eustachian tube which connects the middle ear to the nasopharynx. (Fig. 32-4, A). Normally this tube protects the middle ear from nasopharyngeal secretions, provides drainage of secretions produced within the middle ear into the nasopharynx, and equalizes the air pressure in the middle ear with that of the atmosphere. Persistent obstruction of the eustachian tube caused by infection, allergy, and enlarged adenoids will eventually lead to middle ear disease.

Acute otitis media is a common complication of upper respiratory tract infection in young children. Respiratory mucosa damaged by viral infection is readily colonized by pneumococci, *H. influenzae*, and group A beta-hemolytic streptococci. Bacteria usually gain access to the middle ear by way of the eustachian tube. Purulent fluid accumulates in the middle ear, causing severe pain, fever, and irritability. When the eustachian tube becomes inflamed, it may swell shut, and the purulent material produced by the infection builds up within the middle ear, causing earache, ringing of the ears, elevated temperature, occasional vomiting, and perhaps spontaneous rupture of the eardrum that may result in a "running ear."

Infants are especially susceptible to otitis media and may announce their discomfort by crying, fussy behavior, or pulling at the affected ear. Definitive diagnosis can be made only by visualization of the tympanic membrane and adjacent structures. Antibiotics are the mainstay of therapy. A successful outcome depends in large measure on early treatment. Parents should be encouraged to notify the pediatrician promptly when the child has an earache. Aspirin, acetaminophen, and Auralgan eardrops may be given for pain, although it usually subsides in 4 to 5 hours after antibiotic therapy has been initiated. Antihistamines and decongestants are often prescribed for the first 5 days in an attempt to clear nasal pharyngitis and inflammation of the eustachian tubes.

Specific antibiotic therapy is effective in the prevention of such complications as mastoiditis, men-

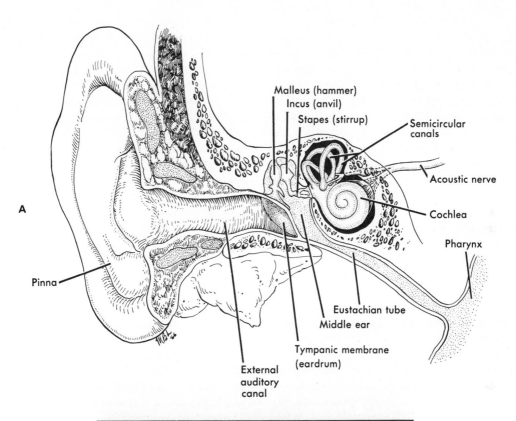

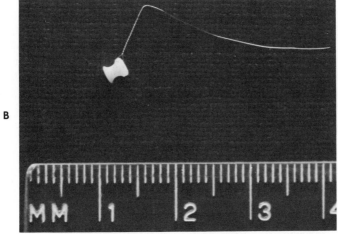

FIG. 32-4   **A,** Basic anatomy of the ear. **B,** A tympanostomy ventilating tube.

ingitis, and the incidence of eardrum perforation. Amoxicillin and trimethoprim-sulfamethoxazole (Septra) are effective against both gram-positive and gram-negative bacteria, and either drug can be used alone. Widely accepted is combined therapy, such as erythromycin or penicillin with sulfisoxazole. Therapy should be continued for at least 10 days. The nurse must forewarn parents that a follow-up visit to the physician is essential. The child's ear must be inspected and evaluated after 10 days of treatment, since the appearance of the eardrum dictates the duration of therapy. No child is considered cured until the signs of middle ear disease have been resolved. Partially treated otitis media is a major cause of meningitis in young children.

In the past a myringotomy (surgical incision of the eardrum) was commonly done to relieve pressure and evacuate fluid. Since most children respond well to antibiotic therapy, myringotomies are now usually reserved for those few patients whose improvement at follow-up examination has not been satisfactory.

Serous otitis media. Recurrent attacks of acute otitis media characteristically precede serous, or "secretory," otitis media, a sterile middle ear effusion. The fluid varies greatly in its viscosity. When it is very thick, the condition is called "glue ear." Serous otitis is the most common complication of acute otitis media, and since no significant symptoms are present, the development of a conductive hearing loss is a real possibility. Unless definitive measures are instituted to open the eustachian tube, permanent hearing loss may result. Learning difficulties often signal such a hearing loss in school-age children. Children with conductive hearing loss caused by serous otitis media should be referred to an otologist. Surgical drainage (myringotomy) is often necessary. The aspirated fluid is cultured, and specific antibiotic therapy may be started. Placement of tiny middle-ear ventilating tubes through the eardrum seems to be the best treatment for serous otitis media (Fig. 32-4, B). The success of tympanostomy tubes is most likely related to improvement of mucous drainage from the middle ear into the nasopharynx. Children should not swim or get water into their ears while the tubes are in place because the infection may extend.

The most important aspect of long-term management is to relieve the basic cause. Allergies must be investigated and treated, and hypertrophied adenoids must be removed if they truly are obstructing the eustachian tube. A significant advance in the identification of middle ear disease has come with the use of the electroacoustic impedance bridge. A small probe in a rubber cuff is placed in the external canal and attached to the impedance meter. A tympanogram, which reflects the dynamics of the entire tympanic membrane—middle ear and eustachian tube system, is produced. For detecting otitis media and common conductive defects in children, tympanometry is far more reliable than otoscopic examination. Tympanometry is a simple procedure that can be easily carried out in a short time by nonprofessional personnel.

Hygiene of the ear. In some instances damage to the ear may follow ill-advised probing of the external auditory canal with implements such as hairpins and matchsticks. It is wise to follow the old saying, "Never put anything in your ear except your elbow." The outer auditory canal should be cleaned only by using a washcloth or a tightly rolled piece of cotton. If a collection of hardened wax, or cerumen, is suspected, the ear should be examined, and a physician or nurse trained in the technique of irrigating the ears should carry out the procedure.

Any body opening seems to offer a challenge to some children. Boys and girls will occasionally push foreign bodies into the external ear canal. When foreign bodies are detected, they should be removed by a physician because the general public has neither the knowledge, skill, nor instruments necessary to perform such a task. An irrigation should never be attempted before the child is taken to a physician. If the object is made of vegetable matter, it will swell with the liquid and become more difficult to extract.

The school-age child

ADENOIDS AND TONSILS

Located on the pharynx are several structures of particular interest to the pediatric nurse. Situated in the nasal pharynx are the pharyngeal tonsils, more often called the adenoids. Farther down on the lateral walls of the oral pharynx are the palatine, or faucial, tonsils, which are the structures indicated when one whispers, "I've just had my tonsils out." These two kinds of tonsils are composed mainly of lymphoid tissue and play a role in the formation of immunoglobulins. In addition they act as a respiratory tract defense mechanism by filtering microbes, thereby helping to prevent microbial invasion of the lower tract. These lymphoid tissues serve a useful purpose and should be preserved unless the problems caused by their continued presence outweigh their possible usefulness. The tonsils and adenoids are present at birth and achieve their maximum growth by 5 years of age. Significantly, at 2 years the tonsils are normally large, and the adenoids occupy one half of the nasopharyngeal cavity. The peak of adenoid size is reached by puberty, after which they cease to grow and begin to shrink. When adenoids are removed in very young children, they usually regrow. In the past the tonsils and adenoids were thought to be the cause of many ills and were removed without too much hesitation. However, much disillusionment has resulted from the failure of surgery to achieve expected results. Moreover, this lightly regarded "minor" procedure has taken the lives of many children. In the United States alone reliable evidence shows that over 200 deaths a year result from cardiac arrest, hemorrhage, and infection that follow tonsillectomy.

Indications for removal

Because the adenoids are located close to the opening of the eustachian, or auditory, tube, enlarged adenoids may also be an underlying cause of frequent middle ear infections, or otitis media. The eustachian tube is more horizontal, broader, and shorter in infants and young children than it is in adults; thus ascending ear infections are fairly common.

Indications for adenoidectomy are obstructive adenoids with recurrent acute purulent otitis media and chronic serous otitis media with conductive hearing loss. Children with the latter condition require surgical drainage to remove the fluid and placement of tympanostomy tubes in the eardrum to promote ventilation and to prevent reaccumulation of fluid.

Tonsillectomy need not be done with adenoidectomy, since these are two independent procedures with very different indications. The best results from tonsillectomy are obtained when the symptoms have been clearly referable to the tonsils and not to ills such as frequent colds, sore throat, poor appetite, failure to gain weight, postnasal drip, or allergies. Definite indications for tonsillectomy include history of peritonsillar abscess (to prevent a second attack), chronic recurrent group A beta-hemolytic streptococcal tonsillitis (culture proved), and hypertrophied tonsils that are causing chronic airway obstruction and pulmonary hypertension.

Tonsillectomies and adenoidectomies (T and A surgery) are delayed as long as possible so that children under 4 years of age will not have to be admitted to the hospital and subjected to the psychologic stresses that this experience may bring them.

Contraindications and postponements

T and A surgery is contraindicated in those children who have hematologic conditions, such as hemophilia, leukemia, aplastic anemia, or purpura. Routine laboratory screening of candidates for this surgery is particularly important to discover the potential postoperative "bleeder." Bleeding and clotting times and prothrombin levels may indicate need for specific treatment or operative delay. Vitamin K is administered for prothrombin deficiencies. Even when severe systemic disorders such as diabetes and cardiac or renal disease are problems, surgery usually can be safely managed if a real need exists. However, T and A surgery is

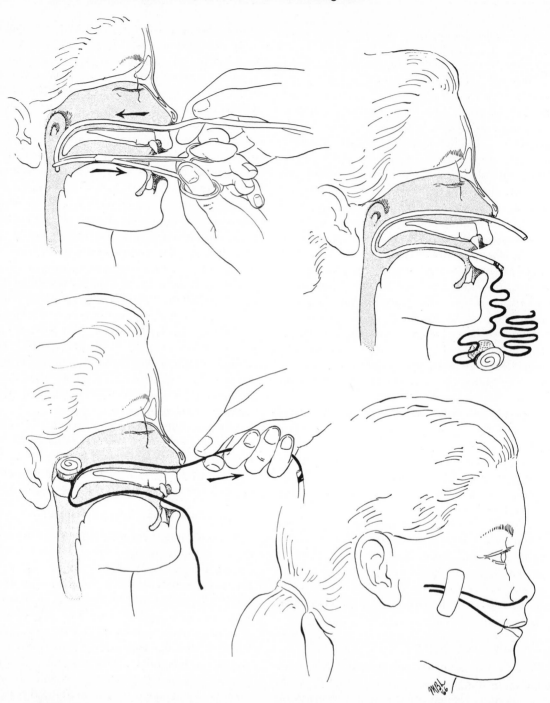

FIG. 32-5   Insertion of a postnasal pack to stop bleeding from the adenoid area.

always postponed if any child is beginning to have an upper respiratory tract infection.

Because of the numerous blood vessels in the operative area and the character of the procedure, the most frequent complication of either tonsillectomy or adenoidectomy is hemorrhage. For this reason the nurse should especially watch for symptoms of excessive bleeding and shock. Children who have their tonsils or adenoids removed remain in the hospital for 24 hours after surgery so that close observation can be maintained and any needed emergency measures quickly carried out. If bleeding occurs, it usually will be within the first 24 hours following surgery. The physician must be called to the bedside to evaluate the seriousness of the situation and try to locate the source of bleeding. Minor bleeding will usually stop when any associated clot, which inadequately obstructs the bleeding yet impedes is constriction, is removed gently by suction, and a sponge moistened with lidocaine hydrochloride (Xylocaine) and epinephrine is held firmly against the area for a few minutes. In the event of major hemorrhage from the tonsillar fossae, or bed, reanesthetizing and resuturing may be necessary. Bleeding from the adenoid area is more common. Again, any clot must first be removed, and if the bleeding does not stop, a postnasal pack or Foley-type catheter with inflatable bag can be inserted to remain in place until the next day (Fig. 32-5). Transfusions may be required if bleeding continues.

Postoperative care

Since the advent and use of recovery rooms, the burden of the immediate postoperative care of the surgical patient carried by the "floor" staff nurse has been lightened. However, it has not been eliminated. After having been gently suctioned and observed for immediate signs of cardiorespiratory distress, the T and A patient returns from the recovery room to the unit. The child is best positioned on the side with the anterior chest at a 45-degree angle with the bed to facilitate oronasal drainage, prevent aspiration, and provide easier observation. The nurse frequently checks pulse

and respirations. She notes the child's level of consciousness and any pronounced restlessness. She observes the skin for color and moisture. She carefully evaluates the amount and kind of oronasal drainage, always asking herself: "Is it profuse? Is it a constant drip or ooze? Is the child swallowing frequently, perhaps swallowing the blood? Does the child need suctioning? Approximately how many tissues have been used? What is the color of the discharge?" Persistent, bright red drainage indicates active bleeding. Sometimes it is difficult for a student nurse to evaluate the amount of bleeding considered normal after T and A surgery. She should never feel apologetic for asking a more experienced nurse to help her judge the condition of her patient. Unless special indications develop, blood pressure is not routinely determined on a young child after T and A surgery.

As soon as patients are conscious and responding, they should be given sips of water to ascertain their tolerance of oral fluids. The early introduction of clear, bland fluids helps prevent dehydration and elevated temperature. It also eventually helps to ease the sore throat. By the second day the child is ready for a soft, bland diet. The incidence of postoperative nausea has been greatly reduced through the use of anesthetics other than ether.

Discharge planning should include written instructions for care. Parents and child should be told that his throat will be decreasingly sore for several days. Complaints of earache (referred pain from the throat) are common. Acetaminophen may be prescribed for this discomfort. The child should be told not to blow his nose forcefully. A soft, bland diet should be continued for several days. The child should be encouraged to drink and eat and open his mouth widely. Fluids and food should be given at room temperature. Crisp or hard foods such as popcorn and dry crackers as well as acid foods such as pickles, oranges, grapefruit, and tomatoes should be avoided. About 3 or 4 days after surgery children may eat whatever they wish.

Children should rest and be kept quiet for the first days at home. They may go outside on the third or fourth day and may resume their usual activities after 1 week. School-age children are allowed to return to school at the end of 2 weeks, provided there are no infectious diseases among the children in their class.

Signs and symptoms that should be reported promptly by the parents to the physician include fresh bleeding, fever, chest pain, or persistant cough. As already stated, the most common post-operative complication is hemorrhage. Parents should understand that occasional blood-streaked nasal or oral mucus is normal during the first 2 days; but if increased bleeding should occur, the child must be returned to the hospital promptly (if possible, without causing the child anxiety) for easier and more rapid care. No surgery is without risk. T and A surgery is not a minor operation, nor is it the answer for all ear, nose, and throat problems. It is, however, an effective therapeutic procedure for selected patients.

STREPTOCOCCAL PHARYNGITIS (STREP THROAT)

Occasionally a severe pharyngitis develops from an infection by the group A beta-hemolytic strep-tococcus. Such a condition is commonly called a "strep throat." Streptococcal pharyngitis is uncommon before 2 years of age and almost nonexistent in children less than 1 year of age. Classically, it has a sudden onset, and the child has a high temperature, severe sore throat, tender cervical lymph nodes, exudate, a beefy, red pharynx, and petechiae on the soft palate. Unfortunately strep throat cannot be diagnosed from clinical findings alone, since the same clinical manifestations accompany viral infections. The demonstration of the group A beta-hemolytic streptococcal organism by means of a throat culture is therefore essential for an accurate diagnosis. Since rheumatic fever, heart disease, and glomerulonephritis follow untreated streptococcal infections in a significant number of children, all patients coming to the physician with pharyngeal inflammations should have routine throat cultures taken. The patient's telephone number should be written on the laboratory slip, and those whose culture reveals a beta-hemolytic streptococcus should be notified and treated.

While awaiting culture results, patients may be treated symptomatically with saline gargles, lozenges, and aspirin or acetaminophen. The 48-hour delay in starting antibiotic therapy does not increase the incidence of rheumatic fever or glomerulonephritis but is thought to be beneficial in that it gives the patient time to develop an antibody response, which will help prevent future infections by that particular strain of streptococcus. If time is taken to explain this to the patient or the parents, they are most grateful. The patient who is in a toxic state and has physical findings suggesting streptococcal pharyngitis may be given antibiotics immediately, but controlled studies have shown that the speed at which the patient recovers is not appreciably influenced by such treatment. The reason for treating streptococcal pharyngitis with antibiotics is not for a more rapid recovery but for the prevention of complications. Numerous studies have shown that this can be done if the child is treated within 7 days of the onset of the illness. The American Heart Association recommends that streptococcal infections be treated for a period of 10 days with penicillin (or erythromycin if the child is allergic to penicillin). Streptococcal organisms are extremely sensitive to an oral course of penicillin, but since many patients stop their medication prematurely, one intramuscular injection of benzathine penicillin G has been recommended as the treatment of choice. It is also advisable to take throat cultures of asymptomatic family contacts.

RESPIRATORY DISEASE RESULTING FROM ALLERGY

About 22 million Americans (one in ten) suffer from sort of allergy. Approximately 75% of these have hay fever, asthma, or both. Allergy is the leading chronic disease in children.

The word "allergy" describes an unfavorable reaction in some portion of the body to a normally harmless substance from the outside environment. These substances may be taken into the body through the nose and lungs (pollens, mold spores, animal danders, and house dust), through the mouth (foods and drugs), or through the skin (wool, insect bites or stings, and injections). A substance that can produce an allergic reaction is called an *allergen*, but the reaction occurs only in a person sensitive to that substance.

The tendency to become sensitive, or allergic, to some otherwise harmless substance is usually inherited. People vary greatly not only in their susceptibility to allergic diseases, but also in the kind of allergic diseases they have. The organs or tissues in which the allergic reactions occur (lungs, asthma; nose, rhinitis; eyes, conjunctivitis; skin, eczema, urticaria, or hives; gastrointestinal tract, diarrhea) may change during an individual's lifetime. These organs are frequently referred to as target or shock organs.

The development of allergic sensitivity to a particular substance depends on exposure to that substance as well as the *amount* and *frequency* of such an exposure. An infant who has developed a sensitivity to cow's milk may exhibit this tendency shortly after birth. Throughout life individuals may develop new sensitivities as they undergo new exposures. The previous sensitivities may remain or may gradually be lost. Although one inherits the tendency to become sensitive to a substance, the allergic response develops only *after* exposure to that substance. This exposure can happen in utero. Sensitization may follow the first exposure or may not occur until after repeated exposures. Penicillin allergy is a well-known example of the latter phenomenon.

A general outline of the allergic process follows:

1. A person contacts a substance and produces sensitizing antibodies (such as immunoglobulin E) to that material.
2. These antibodies are then deposited on special cells (mast cells and basophils) in the body.
3. The allergen (substance to which a person is sensitive or allergic) contacts the antibody E attached to these cells in a subsequent exposure.
4. A reaction occurs whereby chemicals, or "allergic mediators" such as histamine, are released from these cells and cause the symptoms of allergy.

Diagnosis of allergy

The best way to find the sources of allergic symptoms is by a carefully taken history of what exposures preceded each attack and what avoidance preceded each attack-free period. Another way in which allergens may be detected is through skin tests. When the test allergen meets antibodies sensitive to that substance in the skin, the chemical mediators are released, resulting in a positive reaction that resembles a mosquito bite. Tests that indicate inhaled allergens are reliable and commonly agree with the patient's symptoms. Although they can be helpful, skin tests cannot always determine a food allergy. Therefore different trial diets are sometimes suggested to further evaluate foods as the source of the patient's symptoms.

Treatment of allergy

The best way to treat allergy is to prevent it by separating the patient from the allergen. For example, a fur-bearing pet should not be kept in a home with a person having a history of allergic problems. Dust in a patient's bedroom could be minimized by removing cloth draperies, fiber rugs, and using special hypoallergenic pillows and nonporous mattress encasements. The amount of relief from symptoms is in direct proportion to the amount that the exposure is decreased. A second method of treatment consists of immunizing patients to their allergens by injections of these substances in gradually increasing amounts. This regimen is used when allergens (such as pollens) cannot be adequately avoided. The process is called desensitization, hyposensitization, or immunotherapy.

Medications of various types are also employed for relief of symptoms. To be effective for this purpose, medication is often prescribed on a regular daily basis. Regular maintenance doses of medication should be taken as long as objective evidence exists of a symptomatic allergic state. Antihistamines such as tripelennamine hydrochloride (Pyribenzamine) and chlorpheniramine maleate (Chlor-Trimeton maleate and Teldrin) are often effective for the control of allergic rhinitis. They may be combined with a decongestant such as pseudoephedrine (Drixoral). The xanthine drugs theophylline and aminophylline are most valuable in counteracting bronchospasm in asthma. Epinephrine is a rapid-acting, injectable bronchodilator and vasoconstrictor and is the most useful drug for the relief of anaphylactic shock, acute asthma, hives, or edema. More used in chronic asthma are the purely beta-adrenergic sympathomimetic agents such as metaproterenol, terbutaline, and albuterol. The symptom threshold can be increased with various bronchodilator combinations of theophylline and beta agents. However, such useful combinations often increase the side effects of these drugs. Another asthma medication is cromolyn sodium (Intal). It is used prophylactically and as an adjunct in the treatment and control of chronic asthma. It is administered in powder form by direct inhalation into the bronchial tree. Symptomatic improvements can occur without significant side effects. Often exercise tolerance is increased. However, there may be a continued need for bronchodilators, although the dose can be decreased. Follow-up care is important.

Corticosteroids are the most potent group of asthma medications. In addition, they are effective anti-inflammatory agents in all allergic diseases. Their main drawback is that they almost universally have multisystem major adverse side effects when taken over a prolonged period orally or parenterally. These negative effects can be lessened by administering the total dose required for symptom control in the form of prednisone on alternating mornings rather than in a daily regimen. Substantial reduction in these untoward generalized responses occurs with the topical application of the steroid medication—using aerosols for asthma and rhinitis, and drops, creams, and ointments for conjunctivitis and eczema.

Rhinitis is one of the most common allergic manifestations in children. It is characterized by sneezing, a profuse, watery nasal discharge, swelling and itching of the nasal mucosa, and often conjunctivitis. Allergic nasal obstruction is very unpleasant for the child, parents, and teacher. Frequently it leads to constant mouth breathing, snoring, abnormal midface development with associated orthodontic problems, and a nasal voice. Associated problems

are sinusitis and otitis media. Allergic rhinitis is commonly classified as seasonal (hay fever) or nonseasonal (perennial). Seasonal allergic rhinitis results most often from plant pollen sensitivity. House dust, animal danders, mold spores, and foods, in addition, are causes of nonseasonal allergic rhinitis in children. A careful history, physical examination, laboratory aids (such as nasal cytology to identify increased eosinophil counts), and skin testing are all important etiologic diagnostic measures. Treatment depends on the results of the diagnostic procedures. When the specific cause can be determined, the allergen is removed if possible.

The antihistaminic drugs are fairly successful in treating some patients with seasonal allergic rhinitis, even though innumerable airborne substances are potentially sensitizing. When it is impossible or impractical to eliminate the causative allergen or control the body's response to its presence, hyposensitization should be considered. Most children with severe allergic rhinitis will require specific treatment.

ASTHMA

Asthma is the most common major allergic manifestation in childhood. It involves from 1% to 2% of all children. Asthma accounts for 23% of school absenteeism, and in the United States causes numerous deaths annually. It is characterized by difficulty in breathing as the result of spasm of the small bronchi, obstructive edema of the bronchial mucosa, and the production of tenacious secretions, all of which tend to obstruct air exchange (Fig. 32-6). More difficulty is experienced in exhaling than inhaling. A pronounced expiratory wheeze is usually present. Rapid, shallow respirations are characteristic. Milder obstruction is frequently manifested by nocturnal or exertional coughing.

Asthma is the result of hyperreactivity of the bronchial airway. The lungs are clinically referred to as "twitchy." Although often the spasm, edema, and mucus that create this reversible obstruction are caused by an allergic reaction, many nonimmunologic precipitants can also initiate or compound the problem. These include infections, irritants,

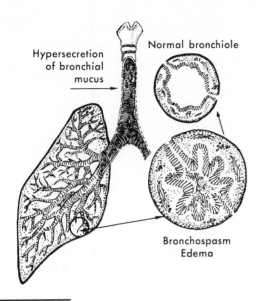

FIG. 32-6

The cardinal anatomic changes in asthma occur at the bronchiole level. Bronchospasm, edema, and hypersecretions of mucus cause severe dyspnea and wheezing.

exercise, emotional stress, cold air, and weather changes. The clinical course of asthma therefore varies in different children as a result of its being such a multifactorial process.

Treatment of asthma

The treatment of asthma is usually divided into (1) specific measures, such as elimination of offending allergens and specific desensitization; and (2) nonspecific measures, which include drugs, fluids, and supportive treatment.

Acute attacks of asthma may occur at any time and are related to multiple factors. There may be no single cause. Children exhibit symptoms when they reach a certain level or threshold of exposure to certain offenders. The cardinal feature is airway obstruction; patients' shoulders are hunched, their thoracic soft tissues retract as they inspire, and their accessory muscles of respiration bulge with the effort of breathing. Their respiratory rates will be initially increased, but may be normal or

decreased if the obstruction is very severe, and their breathing will be punctuated by spasms of coughing and audible wheezes. These children are diaphoretic, restless, and fatigued. Difficulty in breathing always produces anxiety, and the patients' anxiety and that of their parents tend to compound the respiratory problems.

Treatment of acute attacks of asthma usually includes the administration of epinephrine (Adrenalin) by injection and then inhalation therapy with isoetharine, or metaproterenol. Epinephrine suspension (Sus-Phrine) is often used to achieve more lasting effects. Adequate fluid intake is very important. Following the acute phase, postural drainage after inhalation therapy is highly effective in assisting removal of bronchial secretions or mucous plugs.

A life-threatening situation, *status asthmaticus*, exists when the patient does not clear after three consecutive doses of epenephrine 1:1,000, given at 20- to 30-minute intervals. These children are critically ill and must be hospitalized.

Children with status asthmaticus need fluids. They may be dehydrated because they have been too ill to eat or drink and have lost fluids by hyperventilating, coughing, and perspiring. Vomiting also adds to the child's dehydrated state. Intravenous administration of fluids is started immediately to correct the fluid imbalance, maintain liquefied bronchial secretions, and serve as a vehicle for important medications. The nurse should carefully check the amount and time prescribed to prevent overhydration.

Thereafter, aminophylline, a highly effective bronchodilator, is given intravenously over a 15- to 30-minute period and then at 4- to 6-hour intervals or as a maintenance drip after a loading bolus. Signs of aminophylline intoxication include restlessness, irritability, vomiting, and abdominal pain and should not be confused with increased severity of the asthmatic attack. Theophylline levels should be monitored and kept within the therapeutic range of 10 to 20 $\mu g/ml$.

Parents should be encouraged to stay at the child's bedside. They need to see what is happening to their child as well as receive explanations of what is being done. Isoetharine (Bronkosol), or metaproterenol (Metaprel or Alupent) by inhalation are effective in further relieving bronchospasm and dyspnea in children. They are given promptly to all cooperative children 15 minutes after infusion of aminophylline every 4 to 6 hours.

This may be followed by chest physical therapy consisting of vibration, clapping, and coughing in various positions. Chest physical therapy and postural drainage are ordered as soon as the acute phase subsides. It is a significant therapeutic aid for children whose excessive mucus is a problem. It is most effectively performed after bronchodilatation is obtained from aminophylline and the aerosol treatment. Hydrocortisone sodium succinate (Solu-Cortef) or methylprednisolone (Solu-Medrol) is given intravenously to children who do not respond to bronchodilators, who have recently had corticosteroids, or who are receiving maintenance doses of steroids. It is important to note that the therapeutic effect of hydrocortisone sodium succinate is often not seen until 12 hours (and frequently longer) after administration. If the patient improves, corticosteroids may be stopped abruptly after a *short* course. Long-term use of steroids is not recommended because of the serious side effects, which include growth suppression, masking of infection, and osteoporosis. Antibiotics are indicated in the presence of bacterial infection. However, asthmatic flareups are more often associated with viral infections; in these cases antibiotics are not helpful. Oxygen is given to relieve hypoxemia. Since cyanosis is an unreliable sign of hypoxia, arterial blood gas levels should be determined and observed carefully. Oxygen is ordered when the arterial P_{O_2} is less than 70 mm Hg. Sodium bicarbonate administered intravenously may be needed to correct acidosis.

The nurse who is caring for the child with status asthmaticus must constantly but calmly evaluate the progress and changes that occur. Although most children demonstrate significant improvement after administration of aminophylline, inhalation therapy, and intravenous fluids, others do not respond for 12 to 24 hours. During this time, steroids, sodium bicarbonate, antibiotics, and oxygen may be added to their therapeutic regimen. The foregoing measures are usually effective in time. Radiographic studies are most helpful in defining the precise difficulty when management of severe, acute asthma presents a problem. Atelectasis, with or without pneumonia, mucous plugs in the bronchi, and spontaneous pneumothorax account for the major complications and must be treated separately. However, sometimes response is not satisfactory: labored breathing persists, the child becomes exhausted and incoherent and no longer coughs or wheezes, and inspiratory retractions and cyanosis increase. These are the clinical signs of impending respiratory failure. Blood gas determinations exhibit a decreasing level of oxygen, rising carbon dioxide retention, and acidosis.

This situation might be reversed if the danger is recognized and the child is moved to the intensive care unit where adequate equipment and personnel experienced with the grave complication are available. Delivery of 100% humidified oxygen, infusion of isoproterenol and sodium bicarbonate, and mechanical ventilation are necessary measures that must be offered if the child's life is to be saved.

Part 2: Circulatory disorders

This section introduces the student to some of the more common pediatric problems involving the heart and its vessels and circulating blood (Fig. 32-7). Although some of the frequently encountered congenital heart defects were briefly described in Chapter 14, no mention was made of the surgical possibilities of repair of such defects or the nursing care of the cardiac patient. The following paragraphs will supply these omissions.

Varied abnormalities of the heart and large blood vessels may occur. Some cause little inconvenience. Others are incompatible with life or produce severe problems.

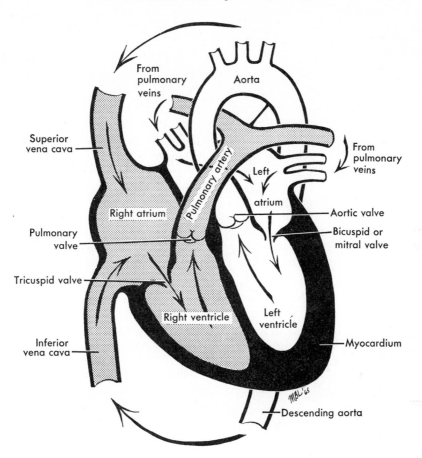

From
pulmonary
veins

Aorta

Superior
vena cava

From
pulmonary
veins

Pulmonary artery

Left

Right atrium

atrium

Aortic valve

Pulmonary
valve

Bicuspid or
mitral valve

Tricuspid valve

Left
ventricle

Right ventricle

Inferior
vena cava

Myocardium

Descending aorta

FIG. 32-7   Structure and circulation of the normal heart. The shaded area represents blood with low oxygen content.

DIAGNOSTIC PROCEDURES

To evaluate heart function and detect cardiac abnormalities, an accurate history of the patient's complaints is sought, a complete physical examination is carried out, and various tests and specialized procedures are ordered.

Common noninvasive tests include observation of the shape and action of the heart and great blood vessels by *fluoroscopy*, permanent recording of the size and shape of the heart by *x-ray examination*, external pulse and heart sound recordings by *phonocardiography*, tests of the activity of the heart by *electrocardiography*, and sonar recordings *(echocardiography)*.

Laboratory tests of special significance include a complete blood cell count and hematocrit and hemoglobin determinations. Patients with a cyanotic type of heart disease may have either an excessive amount of circulating red blood cells (polycythemia) manufactured in an attempt to deliver more oxygen to the deprived body cells or may suffer from anemia. If polycythemia is present, the blood thickens and circulation slows down, occasionally causing the development of abnormal clots in the bloodstream—always a dangerous situation.

A special procedure called "angiography" is occasionally arranged. It involves the injection of a contrast medium into the circulation and observation of its flow by x-ray examination or fluoroscopy. When a contrast medium is injected directly into a heart chamber, it is termed "angiocardiography." Such visualization of the aorta is termed "aortography." Special procedures may also include the performance of right or left side of the heart catheterizations, which are concerned with the introduction of a small catheter, seen by fluoroscopy, into a vein or artery and its gentle manipulation into various chambers of the heart as well as large associated vessels. This procedure is done on an anesthetized or sedated patient and, although it is not without risk, yields considerable information. If possible, children are sedated, not anesthetized, so that they can cooperate consciously during the procedure. It reveals the pressure in various areas of the cardiocirculatory system and the amount of oxygen in the blood at different sites. The presence of abnormal openings may be demonstrated by direct passage of the small catheter through the defects or by evaluation of oxygenation patterns.

Children returning to the nursing unit after cardiac catheterization should be treated as post-operative patients. Vital signs—pulse, respirations, and blood pressure—should be noted every 20 minutes until stable. Children should have blood pressure determinations on the arm that is not used for the catheter insertion. A mist tent or oxygen mask should be in readiness as ordered or indicated. Any dressing applied should be noted and observed. It is important to note skin color and temperature and character of the pulse in the extremity catheterized, as this may detect blood vessel occlusion resulting from thrombus formation.

The infant

CONGENITAL ANOMALIES OF THE HEART AND GREAT VESSELS

About 30,000 infants are born with recognizable heart disease every year in the United States. Formerly, about half of these infants would die within 6 months. Today, early diagnosis and treatment

(through palliative or curative surgery) are effective in approximately 90% of cases.

Congenital heart disease refers to a structural abnormality present in the circulation at birth. These defects create at least three problems related to blood flow within the heart and circulatory system. A *volume overload* occurs when more blood than normal enters a ventricle. A *pressure overload* occurs when the outflow of blood is impeded or obstructed. Ventricular hypertrophy and finally congestive heart failure may result. *Desaturation,* low oxygen content of circulating arterial blood, occurs when unoxygenated blood returning from the body mixes with the oxygenated blood returning from the lungs. Acidosis may occur as the result of poor oxygenation of the various organs. Acidosis leads to decreased cardiac performance and still more acidosis. Some congenital anomalies of the heart illustrate all three types of blood flow problems. Early diagnosis and treatment are important. (See Fig. 32-8.)

Signs and symptoms

Infants with serious congenital heart disease often manifest common signs and symptoms that reflect the underlying anomaly. *Cyanosis*—blueness of the lips, nail beds, and mucosal surfaces—may be caused by shunting of unoxygenated blood into the left side of the heart, or it may be associated with pulmonary edema. *Tachypnea* is defined as an excessive resting respiratory rate, 45 breaths per minute in the full-term infant or over 60 breaths per minute in the premature infant. Retractions and flaring of the nares occur with each breath. Rapid breathing is a response to heart failure or low oxygen content in the blood and is often precipitated by mild exercise. *Tachycardia,* an excessively rapid heart rate, may be difficult to evaluate in the infant, particularly if the child is moving and crying. A heart rate greater than 180 beats per minute when the infant is at rest is significant and should be reported at once, since infants quickly develop cardiac decompensation (inability to maintain the necessary blood flow). *Effort intolerance* is chiefly manifested by feeding

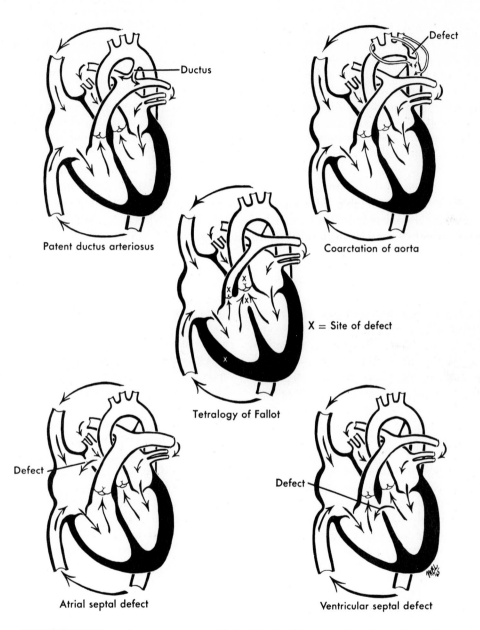

Patent ductus arteriosus

Coarctation of aorta

Tetralogy of Fallot

X = Site of defect

Atrial septal defect

Ventricular septal defect

FIG. 32-8   Common congenital defects of the heart and great vessels.

problems. The infant will usually start feedings eagerly but soon becomes fussy and fatigued and stops feeding. The cycle is often repeated, but the infant seldom finishes a bottle. *Failure to thrive* is also common. Episodes of congestive heart failure and intercurrent pulmonary infection are frequent causes of retarded growth. *Murmurs*, or abnormal heart sounds, occur when flow of blood across a defect is turbulent or when valvular surfaces are irregular. They are the most commonly detected physical findings associated with congenital cardiac defects in infants.

Congestive heart failure (CHF) occurs when the heart can no longer pump blood sufficiently to meet the body's needs. When infants develop CHF in the early months of life, it is usually secondary to structural defects, which produce a pressure or volume overload. In an effort to preserve cardiac output and accommodate the larger volume of residual blood, cardiac dilatation occurs. CHF is typically recognized by a combination of tachypnea and tachycardia associated with hepatomegaly caused by circulatory congestion. The development of CHF warrants prompt cardiac consultation and diagnostic studies. Frequently, surgery offers the only chance of life.

Left-to-right shunts (acyanotic)

Patent ductus arteriosus (PDA). Patent means "open." The condition called patent ductus arteriosus refers to a holdover from the fetal circulation pattern. Review Fig. 4-4. You will remember that the ductus arteriosus is a short blood vessel that connects the pulmonary artery with the aorta, making it unnecessary for the blood circulating through the pulmonary artery to continue on to the nonfunctioning lungs of the fetus. Normally this arterial duct closes soon after birth and within a few weeks becomes a ligament.

If the ductus arteriosus does not close, the higher blood pressure in the aorta, which results after birth, forces well-oxygenated blood from the aorta back into the pulmonary circulation for a return trip to the lungs. This puts an abnormal work load on the left ventricle and may cause a significant elevation of the blood pressure in the pulmonary

circulation. The growth of children suffering from this defect may be impaired if the duct remains large. They may suffer from dyspnea when they are active, and without appropriate treatment their life expectancy is often reduced. The defect does not characteristically produce cyanosis unless pressures in the aorta and pulmonary artery are changed as the result of excessive pulmonary blood flow, which may increase pulmonary vascular resistance. Some premature babies with respiratory distress syndrome have delayed, spontaneous closure of the ductus or may reopen their ductus as a response to poor oxygenation in the lungs. Often this prevents weaning the baby from a mechanical ventilator unless the ductus is closed by drugs or ligation.

Diagnosis is usually made on the basis of several findings. The detection of a continuous murmur or an abnormal sound accompanying heart action is only one. A "thrill" may be noted; the word "thrill" in this case refers to a vibration felt over the cardiac area. Blood pressure determinations may reveal a wide range between the systolic and diastolic readings—termed a "wide pulse pressure." The appearance and stamina of the patient are noted. The patent duct may be visualized by echocardiography, aortography, or by direct passage of a small catheter through the duct during fluoroscopy.

This condition may be treated surgically, usually with excellent results. The duct is tied off (ligated) or divided. Drugs that inhibit the synthesis of prostaglandins by the body's tissues are being used in premature infants to close the ductus; they have no effect in older patients.

Atrial septal defect (ASD). An abnormal opening in the wall, or septum, that separates the right and left atria may be the result of the persistence of the foramen ovale, which during fetal life shunts some of the blood from the right to the left side of the heart. It may also be caused by the presence of a septal opening unassociated with normal fetal circulation. Cyanosis does not characteristically occur, since the blood pressure is higher in the left heart and unoxygenated blood does not enter the systemic circulation. However, if some other abnormality is present (for example, pulmonary valve stenosis), right-to-left flow may occur, and cyanosis may result. Children with ASD usually have an overworked right side of the heart and congested pulmonary circulation because the extra flow through the defect reaches the lungs by way of the right ventricle. They may demonstrate cardiac enlargement, a systolic murmur, decreased resistance to respiratory tract infections, lowered exercise tolerance, and physical underdevelopment. A decision to attempt surgical correction is based on the condition of the individual child. If the shunt is quite small, patients do well without operative intervention. Surgery itself presents a minimal risk. During surgery the defect is either repaired by direct closure with sutures only or by the incorporation of a plastic patch into the repair. The patch is eventually penetrated by growing heart fibers and becomes part of the septum.

Ventricular septal defect (VSD). The presence of an opening between the two ventricles is always an abnormality, whether it occurs in the fetus or newborn infant. How seriously such an opening may disturb normal heart function depends on the position and size of the defect and the presence of other abnormalities in the heart or large vessels leaving the heart. If a large defect is found in the membranous portion of the septum, symptoms are usually severe. The blood generally travels through the opening from the left to the right ventricle. However, in some cases the shunt may reverse as resistance in the pulmonary arterial bed increases and the pressure in the right side of the heart mounts. Diagnosis is made on the basis of clinical symptoms, a characteristic heart murmur, and the results of x-ray examination, electrocardiograms, echocardiography, and cardiac catheterization. Specific treatment may be recommended for the individual child and consists of surgical repair by open heart surgery similar to that employed for ASD. Surgical risk is somewhat increased with VSD repair.

Right-to-left shunts (cyanotic)

Tetralogy of Fallot. The word element "tetra" means "four." Tetralogy of Fallot is a heart condition that is characterized by the presence of four

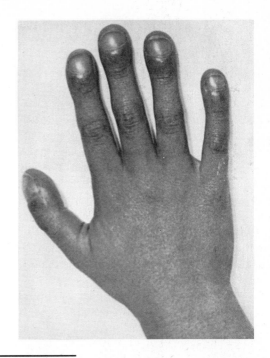

FIG. 32-9

When the ends of the fingers become wide and thick, they are termed "clubbed." These fingers are also very cyanotic.

Courtesy Naval Regional Medical Center, San Diego, Calif.

classic features: an interventricular septal defect, a narrowing of the opening of the outflow tract of the right ventricle (pulmonary stenosis), an aorta situated above the septal defect (overriding aorta), and an enlarged, thickened right ventricular wall (right ventricular hypertrophy). Because the narrowed outflow of the right ventricle causes the pressure to rise in that chamber, hypertrophy of the right heart wall results, and the shunt of blood through the septal defect goes from right to left, usually causing considerable cyanosis. The infant suffering from tetralogy of Fallot has been called a "blue baby." The moderately to severely affected young child with this diagnosis typically has blue lips and nail beds and a dusky-tinted skin, which becomes more cyanotic on exertion. Clubbing of the fingers and toes is often a feature (Fig. 32-9). Thrill and chest

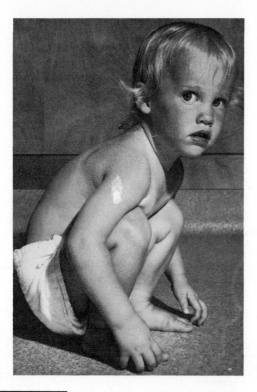

FIG. 32-10

The squatting position improves the oxygenation of some children with congenital heart defects.

deformity may be noted. A child may have hypoxemic spells of respiratory distress, deep cyanosis, loss of consciousness, and convulsions. These children are small for their age. When young children with cyanotic heart disease are fatigued, they often squat (Fig. 32-10). This position lessens the right-to-left flow of unoxygenated blood across the ventricular septal defect, traps desaturated blood in the lower extremities, and improves oxygenation.

Management of hypoxemic spells may be difficult and complex. Initially, when the infant is *excitable*, with respiratory distress, one may use a knee-chest position and administer oxygen. Morphine may be used for sedation. If the infant is flaccid or unconscious, morphine is contraindicated. If metabolic acidosis occurs, sodium bicarbonate may be given intravenously. If these measures fail, phenylephrine (Neo-Synephrine) or propranolol may be administered intravenously with proper monitoring of vital signs.

Diagnosis depends on clinical manifestations, x-ray examinations, electrocardiograms, echocardiograms, angiocardiograms, and cardiac catheterizations. Treatment may be medical or surgical, depending on the condition of the patient. In very blue newborns with tetralogy of Fallot, prostaglandin E_1 is given intravenously to dilate the ductus arteriosus, thereby increasing the flow of blood to the lungs and improving the supply of oxygen to the body's tissues. This drug treatment may be lifesaving and must be followed by surgery. Before open heart surgery was available, surgical techniques were devised to improve the pulmonary circulation by creating an artificial ductus arteriosus, which would recirculate poorly oxygenated blood to the lungs for oxygen enrichment. The Blalock-Taussig operation and the Waterston operation are such techniques. This type of palliative surgery is still useful when the child is considered too small for total correction but is having life-threatening hypoxemic spells. Now open heart surgery with total correction is preferred, because the sources of difficulty may be viewed and repaired directly. Without surgical intervention the typical patient with tetralogy of Fallot faces a brief future.

Complete transposition of the great vessels. Transposition of the great vessels is a serious cyanotic congenital heart defect. In this condition the pulmonary artery originates from the left ventricle, whereas the aorta arises from the right ventricle. Life is possible as long as the foramen ovale or ductus arteriosus remains open or an interventricular septal defect exists. Prominent features are extreme cyanosis and congestive heart failure. Diagnosis is made on the basis of electrocardiogram, x-ray examination, echocardiogram, angiocardiogram, and cardiac catheterization. A palliative surgical procedure (Blalock-Hanlon operation) to create or enlarge an ASD is occasionally required to prolong life. Usually a special balloon catheter (balloon septostomy) is used to create or enlarge an ASD without the risk of palliative surgery. Total correction is possible by switching the venous inflows to the heart. In the Mustard procedure, a "baffle," or partition made of pericardium, is placed in such a manner as to redirect the pulmonary venous return within the left atrium to the right ventricle and the systemic return to the left ventricle. Immediate results have been excellent, with an overall mortality of less than 10% in patients without additional complicating cardiac anomalies.

Obstructive lesions

Pulmonary stenosis. The pulmonary artery carries poorly oxygenated blood from the right ventricle through the pulmonary valve to the lungs, where it is reoxygenated. Narrowing of the valve itself or the areas immediately above or below it causes obstruction to the right ventricular outflow. The condition may be so mild that the infant has no symptoms, or it may be so severe that the infant is dyspneic, has effort intolerance, severe cyanosis, and congestive heart failure. A loud murmur is heard. The condition is diagnosed by electrocardiogram, x-ray film, and cardiac catheterization. Open heart surgical repair is indicated if the right ventricular pressure is high. An incision in the pulmonary artery exposes the dome-shaped valvular stenosis, which is then incised (pulmonary valvotomy). If the primary obstruction is below the valve, the obstructing muscle can be resected. The results of this operation are usually excellent, and the risk is low, except in the case of the infant.

Coarctation of the aorta. The aorta is the largest blood vessel in the body. As it leaves the heart it normally arches to the left. The coronary arteries and three major vessels sprout from the aortic arch before it starts its descent into the lower thorax and abdomen. These are the innominate, left carotid, and left subclavian arteries, which supply the head and upper extremities with oxygenated blood. The ductus arteriosus joins the aorta in the general area of the left subclavian artery before normal postnatal circulation develops. Sometimes the aorta is abnormally narrowed in the area of the arch, usually involving the segment just past the subclavian artery. Often smaller "collateral" vessels (usually branches of the subclavian and intercostal arteries) develop and bypass the narrowed portion to help supply circulation to the lower extremities. The narrowing of the aorta is often called "coarctation," since a narrowed figure results when two arcs are drawn side by side, like two Cs back to back. The symptoms resulting depend on the severity and location of the coarctation and whether any other cardiac or blood vessel abnormalities exist.

The presence of coarctation is suspected when there are forceful arterial pulses in the upper extremities but weak or absent pulses in the lower extremities and a systolic murmur is heard. Severe coarctation in the infant, especially if associated with another congenital heart anomaly, may precipitate profound congestive heart failure and require surgical intervention. The older patient may have few complaints, although occasionally headache, leg cramps, excessive fatigue, and frequent nosebleeds may be reported. Diagnosis is confirmed by blood pressure measurements, x-ray examination, electrocardiogram, and aortogram.

Without appropriate treatment the life span is often shortened because of the onset of complications such as hypertension, cerebral hemorrhage, subacute bacterial endocarditis, or heart failure.

Definitive treatment is surgical. The narrowed portion may be cut out and the adjoining normal-sized segments sewed together. Occasionally the repair involves the insertion of a prosthesis or the use of the subclavian artery to widen the aorta.

CARDIAC SURGERY

Assuming that facilities and skilled physicians are available, surgical treatment of large blood vessel or heart defects depends on the extent of incapacity suffered by the patient, the possibility of a satisfactory repair, and the risk involved. Surgery on the aorta, pulmonary artery, or other associated blood vessels is similar in some respects to heart surgery. However, when the malformations exist in the interior of the heart and cardiac circulation must be interrupted, the difficulty of the procedure and the risk to the patient increase significantly. A heart-lung machine was introduced in 1955. Prior to that time it was impossible to discontinue the beating of the heart long enough to make a lengthy repair without seriously depriving some vital structure (for example, the brain or kidneys) of carbon dioxide–oxygen exchange and thus causing tissue damage.

The heart-lung machine receives blood from the patient's venous circulation through tubes inserted into the inferior and superior venae cavae. It removes the carbon dioxide, instills oxygen, regulates blood temperature, and pumps the blood back into the systemic circulation in most cases by way of the aorta or femoral artery (called a cardiopulmonary bypass). Needless to say, this is a highly complex procedure, requiring a team of skilled physicians, nurses, and technicians.

A patient with a congenital heart defect may undergo surgery as an infant, toddler, or child. To simplify organization, the following discussion will include more than the treatment and nursing care of the infant in its scope. Any child who is to have any type of surgery must be carefully prepared for the event. This is especially true in the case of scheduled chest or heart surgery because of the seriousness of the operation and the many procedures that must be carried out that require the trust and cooperation of the child to achieve optimum results.

Preparation of the child presupposes that the parents are prepared. This does not mean that the parents must feel totally calm and serene or that they and their child must know all the details of the procedure. The former would be unnatural; the latter would be both impossible and undesirable, probably causing many more anxieties than it would ease. How much the child is told will depend on age, expressed concerns, and intellect. How much the parents are told will depend on their expressed concerns, intellects, and familiarity with the sciences involved. Whatever information is given, however simple, should be truthful.

Children who are scheduled for heart surgery are usually admitted to the hospital several days in advance of the procedure to enable them to learn about the hospital, to become acquainted with some of the nurses who will be caring for them, and to be introduced to some of the equipment and techniques that will be used after surgery. This preliminary period is also used as an opportunity to evaluate the child. It is a time when the child's general condition may be observed and nutritional needs noted and, as far as possible, met. Weight is recorded each morning; scheduled blood pressure, respiration, and pulse checks are particularly important. The nurses should be alert for and should report any signs of fever, respiratory tract infection or rash, which may indicate the presence of other diseases. Such signs may necessitate a postponement of surgery.

It is usually very helpful to demonstrate some of he equipment that will be used with the child before its use under more stressful conditions is needed. Children may be shown an oxygen tent with humidifier and may get inside to see how the "small house" feels. They may "practice" taking their breathing exercises with the intermittent positive pressure machine or learn how to cough with the nurse holding their chests. Explanations should be calm, factual, and geared to the child's level of understanding. Play therapy techniques are often helpful in explaining anticipated events to the child.

TREATMENT AND NURSING CARE OF THE CARDIAC PATIENT
Postoperative nursing care

The postoperative nursing care of open heart surgery patients is a nursing specialty in itself. A patient usually remains in the intensive care unit for several days. While the child is in the intensive care unit his condition is usually monitored by machines that graphically record heart action, arterial and venous blood pressures, respirations, and temperature. In some cases heartbeat may be stimulated by the use of a mechanical pacemaker. The rate and quality of respirations are evaluated; the color and feel of the skin are noted. Chest suction is maintained to prevent a buildup of fluid or air in the thorax, causing respiratory distress and atelectasis. Humidified oxygen is often administered by an oxygen tent or mask. The urinary catheter is checked often to determine kidney output. Intravenous fluids and blood transfusions are calculated and maintained according to order. Wound drainage and dressings must be checked. Turning and encouraging the patient to cough are extremely important. Intermittent positive pressure may be prescribed. Tracheal as well as nasopharyngeal suctioning may be ordered. Some patients may have temporary tracheostomies. Initially the patient's temperature may be subnormal, but later temperature-reducing procedures may be necessary, including the use of the hypothermia blanket. A relatively high temperature after open heart surgery is fairly common. In some cases it may be caused by a reaction to the massive blood transfusion received. However, the possibility of infection must not be discounted when a patient's temperature rises abnormally.

Continuing care

The patient needs constant, expert nursing observation and care. Many important nursing evaluations must be made during this critical postoperative interval. Caring for this type of patient in the immediate postoperative period is not within the scope of the vocational nurse. However, at times she may be called on to "lend a careful hand," with supervision, during a treatment or to help change the patient's position, depending on the child's needs and condition. The vocational nurse should know how important it is that the chest tubes remain intact and the drainage bottles and suction machine remain undisturbed. The bottles containing drainage from the chest should always be maintained lower than the lowest level of the child's chest to prevent backflow. To avoid backflow, the bottles should be fastened to the floor or to a correctly positioned holder. In the event that a chest bottle should break or the tube should become disconnected, the part of the tube coming from the patient's chest must be immediately clamped off near the chest wall to prevent pneumo-

thorax. Symptoms of pneumothorax include cyanosis, dyspnea, and chest pain.

As the patient's condition improves, chest suction will be discontinued and the tubes removed. If temporary heart pacing wires were attached to the heart during the operation, they will be withdrawn if the heart rhythm is normal. As the patient's condition becomes stable, the child may be assigned to the care of a licensed vocational nurse under the supervision of a registered nurse. The nurse should know that the child is usually weighed while undressed each morning before breakfast to determine fluid retention. The child may be on a diet that limits sodium and carefully spaces a certain maximum oral fluid intake. The patient's pulse and respirations should be noted and recorded before and after any new activity. During periods of ambulation the child should be carefully evaluated for fatigue and given periods of rest as respirations, pulse, and color dictate. The pulse of these young children and infants is always taken over the heart with a stethoscope—that is, apically for 1 minute. This technique requires training, since there are normally two sounds to each cardiac cycle. Older children may have radial pulse determinations for 1 minute. The quality as well as the rate should be noted. Occasionally apical-radial pulse determinations will be ordered. These pulse rates are taken simultaneously and then compared; they may be written 110A/100R. There may be more apical beats than radial beats (pulse deficit), but there is never an excess of radial beats! Blood pressure determinations are routinely made with the patient's pulse and respiration at scheduled intervals. Care must be taken in the selection of the size of cuff—it should cover two thirds of the distance from the shoulder to the elbow, or be 20% wider than the diameter of the patient's arm. Ambulation and activity privileges will be gradually increased. Many times conferences must be arranged with physician-nurse-parent participation to help parents adjust to the new capabilities of their children and avoid the hazards of overprotection. Help regarding school responsibilities to be assumed and even vocational planning may be sought.

Nonsurgical treatment and care

Sometimes patients' cardiac problems cannot be helped by surgery, or they have to wait until they are in better condition or older before surgery is attempted. In these cases the children are treated by medicines, planned diets, and general health supervision. The nurse should be aware of the types of medications the child is receiving and the expected accomplishments, side effects, and toxic reactions of these medications. Sodium restriction is common. Often patients with cardiac defects must be weighed daily, and accurate intake and output records are maintained. Signs of developing heart failure, cardiac irregularities, or possible respiratory tract infection should be promptly reported. Limitations of activity may be necessary, although many pediatric patients with congenital cardiac defects automatically limit themselves to only the activity they can best tolerate. Quiet play is often more restful than enforced, resented "complete bed rest." The child who must be in an oxygen tent or who demonstrates susceptibility to fatigue should be disturbed as little as possible, and when the child is disturbed, several procedures should be carried out at the same time to allow relatively long uninterrupted periods of sleep or rest (for example, temperature, pulse, respirations, and blood pressure determinations, offering fluids, changing the child's gown or diapers, and shifting position). Changes of position are important in preventing hypostatic pneumonia and skin breakdown. However, no *vigorous* back rubs should be performed on a patient with a cardiac defect. Proper positioning will help to ward off contractures and other deformities and will assist proper body function.

POSSIBLE COMPLICATIONS OF CONGENITAL CARDIAC DEFECTS

Cardiac decompensation—congestive heart failure (CHF)

Certain complications that may develop in patients with congenital heart defects before, during, or after surgery should be mentioned. Probably the most common is the failure of the heart to continue the circulation of the blood in sufficient volume to meet body needs and prevent abnormal congestion of the blood in certain areas. Sometimes the heart can maintain an adequate blood flow by gradually increasing its size or altering its rate. If this occurs, the heart is said to be in *compensation*. If the heart cannot maintain the necessary blood flow, it is said to be in *decompensation*, or failure. Cardiac failure in infants, whatever the cause, is always a medical emergency.

Pulmonary congestion resulting from the inability of the left ventricle to pump effectively is characterized by pooling of blood in the lung capilaries, causing coughing and dyspnea. Blood-tinged froth may be expectorated. Acute pulmonary edema is a grave emergency. Immediate action is necessary! The following measures may be life saving: placement of the infant in a sitting position, administration of oxygen by a ventilator, and possibly parenteral morphine, digitalis, and diuretics.

Congestion of blood in the sytemic venous system as the result of inefficient right ventricular contraction may cause nausea and vomiting, enlargement of the liver, and edema. In infants edema is often best detected by a weight gain. Cyanosis, tachypnea, dyspnea, and tachycardia are major indications for diagnostic studies. But studies are usually undertaken only after congestive heart failure is controlled, since the baby becomes fatigued by the work of breathing and may have an annoying cough and therefore has difficulty eating and sleeping. Prompt treatment with digoxin, oxygen, and diuretics will decrease heart and respiratory rate and improve color, appetite, and disposition. Digoxin slows and strengthens the heartbeat and induces diuresis. A digitalizing dose (high dose) is given over a period of 16 hours, and a maintenance dose of 10% of the digitalizing dose is usually given every 12 hours. However, digoxin should be withheld and the physician notified if the apical pulse rate in the infant is less than 100 beats per minute. Signs and symptoms of toxicity include anorexia, vomiting, and excessive slowing or irregularity of the pulse rate. Diuretics especially help in relieving the pulmonary congestion that accompanies congestive heart failure if response to other forms of treatment is insufficient.

Nursing measures center around making infants more comfortable and conserving their energy. A sitting position in a cool, humidified oxygen tent is beneficial. Early feeding with soft nipples and allowing for frequent rest periods will reduce fatigue. Uninterrupted sleep should be encouraged by bathing infants when they are awake and only when absolutely necessary. The recording of accurate, current vital signs, intake and output determinations, and weight is critical. As soon as the child's condition is stable, the child is prepared for surgery or discharge until a surgery appointment can be made. The parents should be increasingly involved in care while their child is hospitalized so that they are not unprepared when the child goes home. The help of a public health nurse or hospital home visitor can be very valuable in this setting.

Subacute bacterial endocarditis

Any damage to cardiac tissue or a congenital heart or blood vessel anomaly may set the stage for inflammation of the lining of the heart (endocarditis) and arteries (endarteritis). The inflammation usually results from a blood-borne infection, originating at some other body site. It may have its onset after surgical procedures such as dental extraction, tonsillectomy, or adenoidectomy, or it may be spread from an abscess or infection elsewhere in the body. Signs and symptoms include temperature elevation, weight loss, fatigue, anemia, leukocytosis, the presence of petechiae, an enlarged spleen, and perhaps even partial paralysis or other central nervous system symptoms caused by the presence of emboli in the brain that originated in the inflamed heart tissue. Prophylactic antibiotics must be prescribed before and during certain procedures that may introduce bacteria into the bloodstream.

Cerebral thrombosis

Cerebral thrombosis may develop when an excess of circulating red blood cells is called into action to increase the oxygen-carrying capacity of the blood. Dehydration may result in a thicker, slower-moving fluid in the blood vessels. Clots, or thrombi, may form, and a cerebral vascular accident may take place. Maintenance of adequate fluid intake, the use of oxygen to relieve episodes of cyanosis, and possibly the cautious use of anticoagulants in patients likely to develop such a complication are suggested means of reducing the risk.

DISORDERS OF THE BLOOD AND BLOOD-FORMING ORGANS

The entire cardiovascular apparatus (heart and blood vessels) is designed so that nutrients, hormones, and oxygen reach the individual body tissue cells and waste products from those cells are properly transported for elimination by the kidneys, lungs, or skin. To do this efficiently, the circulating fluid within the cardiovascular system—the blood—contains many substances. Of particular interest are the three types of structures called the "formed elements." The red blood cells, or *erythrocytes*, help transport oxygen and carbon dioxide in the blood to and from the lungs. The white blood cells, or *leukocytes*, and antibodies of various types help protect the bloodstream and surrounding body tissues from the intrusion of disease-producing microorgansims and foreign proteins. The platelets, or *thrombocytes* assist in the formation of clots to repair any leak in a damaged blood vessel. However, any lack or defect in the normal makeup of the blood is likely to cause symptoms of disease. It is impossible and of little practical nursing value to describe within the pages of this text all the various problems that may occur when the blood is abnormal. However, four kinds of disorders that are seen with some frequency on the pediatric service will be briefly discussed. They are the *anemias, hemophilias, leukemias,* and *purpuras*.

The anemias

When the term "anemia" is used, it indicates a condition in which the total hemoglobin content of the blood is abnormally reduced, either because of lack of sufficient hemoglobin in the red blood cells or lack of red blood cells. Hemoglobin is the substance in the red blood cells necessary for the normal transport of oxygen to the body cells. The most common cause of anemia in children is iron deficiency. Another anemia that has received much attention is sickle cell disease.

Iron-deficiency anemia. The most common type of anemia in the world, found especially in the pediatric population, is iron-deficiency anemia. Pallor, irritability, anorexia, and listlessness direct attention to this disorder. The anemia is usually discovered secondarily to the problem that brought the child and his parent to the physician. Hemoglobin concentrations of less than 11 g/100 ml and a hematocrit level of less than 33% in a healthy infant strongly suggest iron deficiency. Insufficient iron for synthesis of hemoglobin is the cause of this problem. Children under 3 years of age and adolescent girls have the highest incidence of this disorder. The major cause of iron-deficiency anemia is insufficient dietary intake of iron to meet the demands of body growth (especially of low birth weight and premature infants and adolescents). Infants with iron deficiency commonly have a diet of large amounts of cow's milk, which is low in iron. Causes of anemia other than dietary deficiency include (1) acute or chronic blood loss, and (2) impaired absorption (severe prolonged diarrhea). Treatment consists of oral administration of iron preparations, preferably ferrous iron, a revision of diet to include iron-rich foods (muscle meats, liver, eggs, wheat, green leafy vegetables), and if the condition is particularly severe or unresponsive as a result of parental failure to provide the items above, intramuscular injections of iron-dextran complex may be ordered. Packed red cells are rarely given. Since the highest incidence of iron-deficiency anemia is in infancy (6 to 18 months), the best and cheapest preventive measure against this form of anemia would be the widespread use of iron-fortified formulas during the entire first year of life in bottle-fed infants. It is possible that the use of such formulas would essentially eliminate all iron-deficiency anemia in preschool children. According to some experts this would improve

growth, learning, and resistance to disease.

Sickle cell disease. Sickle cell disease is a collective term that embraces several hereditary disorders whose clinical and laboratory features are related to the presence of sickle hemoglobin (Hb S) in red cells. Although a few cases have been reported in the white race, sickle cell disease is found primarily in blacks. About 75,000 black Americans have the disease. Chronic illness of increasing severity and reduction of life span result from hemolytic anemia with its intermittent crises.

The sickling abnormality is attributed to a mutant gene that is responsible for the synthesis of a type of hemoglobin different from normal. The abnormal change in the shape of the red blood cell from a biconcave disk to a crescent, or sicklelike, shape becomes apparent following exposure to low oxygen tensions or low pH. The basic defect in sickle hemoglobin is in the alteration of only one amino acid of the 574 that make up normal hemoglobin. This single change is responsible for all the clinical manifestations of sickle cell disease!

Sickle cell anemia. Every person possesses a pair of genes that governs the synthesis of hemoglobin. One gene is inherited from each parent. Sickle cell anemia (SCA) is expressed in those persons who receive the mutant sickle cell gene from both parents (homozygous inheritance, SS). (See Fig. 32-11).

Sickle cell trait (SCT). The sickle cell trait is probably the most common defect in hemoglobin found in the United States. It is present in those persons who have received a Hb S gene from one parent and a normal Hb A gene from the other parent (heterozygous inheritance, AS). (See Fig. 32-12). The most important consideration in SCT is the genetic risk of SCA for the offspring. Although persons with SCT have as much as 40% Hb S under normal conditions, no clinical signs of disease or hemoglobin abnormalities are typically present. Rarely someone with sickle cell trait will manifest symptoms of stress when exercising strenuously or traveling at high altitudes in nonpressurized airplanes. SCT confers some degree of protection against the lethal effects of malaria, which may

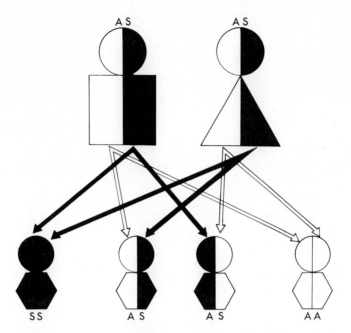

FIG. 32-11
Sickle cell anemia (homozygous inheritance) When both parents carry a sickle cell gene (AS), the possibilities for inheritance in offspring are: one child in four will inherit sickle cell anemia (SS); two children in four will inherit sickle cell trait (AS); one child in four will be normal (AA).

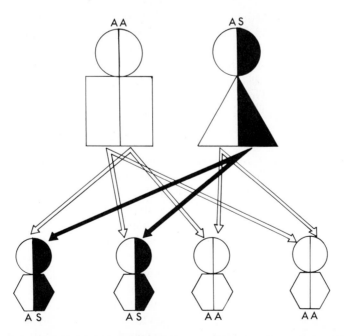

FIG. 32-12
Sickle cell trait (heterozygous inheritance). When only one parent is a carrier of the sickle cell gene (AS), possibilities for inheritance in offspring are: two children in four will be normal (AA); two children in four will carry sickle cell trait (AS).

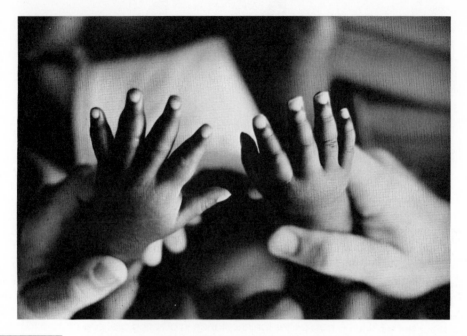

FIG. 32-13   Dactylitis—swelling of the hand—sickle cell interference in the circulation.

Courtesy of CDR Alton L. Lightsey, MC, USN, Naval Regional Medical Center, San Diego, Calif.

account for the major distribution of Hb S in Central Africa and the very fact that SCA exists. The presence of a gene for another abnormal type of hemoglobin, or the gene for thalassemia, should be suspected in a child with sickle cell disease when the blood of only one of the parents shows the sickle trait.

Young infants are usually spared the severe symptoms of SCA because of the temporary presence of fetal hemoglobin (Hb F). Hb F is gradually replaced with the Hb S. As the proportion of Hb S increases, the symptoms of anemia may appear— usually when the baby is between 6 and 12 months of age.

Hemolytic anemia. This anemia is caused by intravascular sickling that occurs diffusely throughout the body. Sickling red cells often form spontaneously during venous circulation when the red blood cells give up oxygen to the tissues. They also form when there are changes in pH or electrolyte balance associated with infection, acidosis, or

dehydration. The body acts quickly to remove these abnormal sickled cells from the bloodstream, and this causes the severe degree of anemia that occurs.

Vasoocclusive crisis. The exact events leading to the onset of painful crises are not clearly known. Many of these crises are preceded by infections. The basis of the painful crisis appears to be occlusion of blood vessels by sickled red cells. This interferes with normal tissue blood supply, resulting in subsequent cellular death and damage of the organs involved. Before an individual reaches 2 years of age, dactylitis or the "hand-foot" syndrome commonly occurs (Fig. 32-13). The symmetric painful swelling of the hands and feet results from interference with circulation to the metacarpals and metatarsals. If the child's pain is not too severe, increased fluids, application of warmth, and acetaminophen will relieve the pain. In other children the pain may be unbearable and can be relieved only by stronger analgesics. Occlusive episodes after the first or second year of life most frequently occur during the preschool period. Episodes of acute abdominal pain may be severe, accompanied by fever, muscle spasm, nausea, vomiting, and leukocytosis.

Sequestration crisis. A crisis associated with shock is called "acute splenic sequestration crisis" (ASSC). The mother notes a rather sudden increase in pallor accompanied by abdominal distention and thirst. By the time these children arrive at the hospital, they have become notably dyspneic and weak. Left-sided abdominal (splenic) pain is present, and the pulse and respirations are elevated. Prompt diagnosis and treatment are essential to assure survival. Transfusions of packed erythrocytes and plasma expanders should be started immediately on admission. The nurse who recognizes the situation should hasten the admission procedure but be sure to check the child's weight and height accurately. It is imperative to take blood specimens and urine samples immediately and to have ready special equipment for transfusions. Since reduced oxygenation increases sickling, an atmosphere of well-humidified oxygen may be used. The nurse also must keep in mind that parents often fear censure or reproach by those in authority and, in their effort to gain approval, may hide their feelings or hold back information regarding the child. The nurse must give these parents every opportunity to examine their feelings about themselves and the child. She should listen carefully as she works with and encourages the parents, since if she is to really help the child, she must first help them. Because of the rapidity with which a sequestration crisis can occur (and even recur) and its threat of fatality, splenectomy may be performed.

Aplastic crisis. Since children with SCA have a continuing hemolytic anemia, they must produce increased numbers of new red blood cells each day. Conditions that suppress the bone marrow production of red blood cells can lead to a life-threatening anemia termed "aplastic crisis." This commonly occurs following infections or as a result of a deficiency of materials needed to produce red blood cells (for example, iron or folic acid). Treatment for aplastic crisis involves transfusions of packed red cells untils the cause of the decreased production can be determined and corrected.

Infections. Children with SCA develop irreversible damage to the spleen after numerous occlusive crises involving this organ. Since a normal spleen is needed to fight certain bacterial infections, children with SCA do not handle these infections well. Pneumoccocal infection, which often complicates upper respiratory infections, has been a leading cause of death in children with SCA. Prompt diagnosis and aggressive antibiotic therapy is essential for these children. Parents should be instructed in the early signs and symptoms of infection, and children should have immediate access to medical care. All children with SCA should receive immunization with the pneumococcal vaccine, which has been shown to be protective against the common strains of pneumococcus.

The therapy for SCA and its frequent crises remains one of the major clinical problems in pediatric hematology. There is no cure for SCA or even a completely satisfactory treatment for its crises.

Detection of sickle hemoglobin and counseling. Screening programs for SCA or SCT should not be set up unless genetic counseling service can be provided to those found to carry the trait. Otherwise, the benefits of the screening are largely lost, and anguish may be created over an essentially benign condition. Screening programs must incorporate meaningful education about the nature of SCA and its mode of inheritance as well as individual counseling. In mass screening, Sickledex (sickle-turbidity tube test) or the sickle cell slide test is adequate, but positive reactions must be followed by hemoglobin electrophoresis to confirm results. Newborn infants may be screened in the hospital for both the condition and the trait. Such hospital programs facilitate optimal infant care and early diagnosis of crises and provide counseling for the parents.

Nursing care. The nursing care of children with anemia, whatever its basic cause, must take into account the excessive fatigue experienced by most of these boys and girls. Their energy must be conserved. They especially need help and encouragement to build good habits in nutrition. Frequent, small feedings are more successful than large, infrequent meals. The enlarged liver and spleen and tender muscles of some of these patients all demand gentle care. Attention to signs of bleeding (external or internal) is important. Signs of jaundice, increased pallor, increased lethargy, or irritability should be reported. Patients receiving blood transfusions should be carefully observed and protected against possible infiltration of the blood (a potentially serious event). Signs of toxic reactions, complaints of chest or back pain, itching hives, or elevated temperature with or without chills should be noted and reported early. The rate of administration should be closely watched to be sure that the circulatory system is not overloaded.

The hemophilias

Hemophilia A—factor VIII deficiency. Classic hemophilia, antihemophilic globulin (AHG), or factor VIII, deficiency, is an uncommon but not rare disorder involving a defect in the clotting mechanism of the blood. Hemophilia results from a defect in a gene in the X chromosome concerned with blood clotting. It is a sex-linked, recessive condition confined almost exclusively to males and may pass from one generation to another from a carrier mother to her son. A male receives only one X, from his mother, which impairs his blood-clotting process. Since the female receives two X chromosomes, one normal gene will ensure normal blood clotting. A girl will inherit the condition only if her father is a hemophiliac and her mother is a carrier. Because of its hereditary feature, it has figured prominently in the history of royal families and has been called the disease of kings.

The defect in clot formation is caused by the lack of antihemophilic globulin, or factor VIII, in the blood plasma. A wide range of factor VIII values (50% to 200%) exists, but in most healthy individuals the average is 100%. A severe hemophiliac has less than 1% of factor VIII. These patients are susceptible to spontaneous, unprovoked hemorrhage. Moderate hemophiliacs have from 2% to 5% of fac-

tor VIII and may bleed excessively with minor trauma. Mild hemophiliacs have 10% to 20% of factor VIII and may, with care, live free of bleeding episodes. Surgical procedures, dental extractions, and even the normal rough-and-tumble existence of young boys are especially hazardous for a hemophilic patient.

Current treatment consists of administration of factor VIII concentrate in an amount necessary to control hemorrhage. However, protection afforded from one infusion rapidly disappears, because the concentration of factor VIII falls to one half of its original level in 8 to 10 hours. Because of this, it may be necessary to repeat administration of factor VIII within 10 hours if bleeding continues. The precise level of factor VIII needed to control bleeding is not known, but the amount of factor VIII given should be related to the seriousness of the bleeding. In central nervous system bleeding, the goal is to maintain 100% factor VIII activity until the site of bleeding is completely healed. In joint bleeding, 50% factor VIII activity is usually sufficient for optimal results. The combination of immobilization and a level of 10% to 20% is usually adequate to control soft tissue bleeding. Efforts to control bleeding by using local measures (pressure, cold, or applications of thrombin) should be attempted, if possible. Some cities have hemophilia centers that are prepared to render intravenous therapy to these patients on an outpatient basis. Some patients are being taught to administer the concentrate to themselves.

Factor VIII inhibitors. A small number (about 5%) of patients with classic hemophilia develop inhibitors (antibodies that block factor VIII). The presence of a circulating inhibitor is usually detected by the lack of response to a dose of factor VIII that normally would control the bleeding. Inhibitors may develop in young children after a few exposures to factor VIII, but no evidence shows that the inhibitors are related to the number of transfusions a patient receives. Without exposure to plasma products, the amount of inhibitor may gradually decrease, and factor VIII can then be given again with temporary benefit. Effective control of bleeding in patients is very difficult when the inhibitor is circulating.

Hemophilia B—factor IX deficiency (Christmas disease). Factor IX plasma thromboplastic component (PTC) deficiency accounts for about 15% of patients with hemophilia. The causes and symptoms are similar to those of hemophilia A. A factor IX concentrate has become available for treatment and is used in the same manner as factor VIII.

Hemophilia C—factor XI deficiency. Factor XI plasma thromboplastin antecedent (PTA) deficiency differs from hemophilias A and B. It is usually a mild disorder and may appear in either boys or girls as the result of an autosomal recessive trait in which bleeding occurs only in the homozygote. Bleeding episodes in factor XI deficiency are best treated with infusions of fresh plasma. The nursing care of all patients with bleeding problems is similar except that the type of intravenous therapy ordered will differ, depending on the kind of replacement needed.

The parents of a patient with hemophilia are under considerable strain. They must constantly observe the environment of their adventuresome toddler or growing boy. With the help of their attending physician, they must progressively educate the child to make choices in activity with consideration for the degree of hazard it may entail. They do not want to make their son a psychologic cripple, unable to live an interesting, creative life, nor do they want him to be a reckless rebel.

Supervision and nursing care. The nursing care of children with hemophilia must emphasize prevention. The sides of infants' cribs should be padded. Toddlers should be denied toys and objects with sharp edges or objects that are easily broken. Rubber toys are very satisfactory for play. Children learning to walk may be fitted with kneepads. Bleeding into the joints may produce considerable pain and deformity. Every effort should be made to prevent stiffening of the joint and loss of function. The nurse must provide her charge with interesting but safe diversion and watch for any signs of increasing bruises or internal or external blood loss. She must observe the child for untoward reaction during transfusion and check whether the intravenous infusion is flowing as ordered. Her care must be gentle and thoughtful.

Home care program. Currently patients are being taught to self-administer replacement factors at home. It has been demonstrated and proved that prompt treatment at home can reduce the amount of factor needed, and can save the patient time-consuming trips and hospital costs. In addition, early treatment of bleeding episodes has been shown to prevent the crippling complications caused by recurrent spontaneous bleeding into the joints.

In an effort to accomplish the goal, selected patients or their parents are being instructed to administer cryoprecipitate and plasma concentrates as necessary at home. Whenever therapy becomes necessary to control minor bleeding episodes, the physician is contacted for advice about the proper dosage. Antihistamines and steroids are kept on hand to be taken by the patient if a transfusion reaction occurs.

Nurses often follow the progress of the patient at home, instructing the family about the importance of accurate records and emphasizing the need for periodic outpatient physical evaluations. The home care program spares patients the expense of frequent hospital visits and the burden of travel and waiting; but most of all, it promotes a more normal life, utilizing the maximum intellectual and social potential of the hemophilic child.

The toddler and preschool child

THE LEUKEMIAS

Although cancer is the leading cause of death from disease in children, and leukemia is the most common childhood malignancy, the outlook can no longer be considered hopeless. Leukemia is a primary malignant disease of the bone marrow characterized by an abnormal increase of immature white blood cells or undifferentiated blast cells. This uncontrolled proliferation of leukemic cells prevents production and development of normal blood cells (hematopoiesis), which leads to infections, anemia, and bleeding. These abnormal white blood cells invade the various tissues of the body, causing pressure symptoms. (For example, infiltration of the bone marrow produces severe pain in bones and joints; mediastinal nodes may cause tracheal compression that in turn causes respiratory difficulty and cough.) The predominating symptoms depend on the area of the body primarily invaded by the leukemic cells. Diagnosis is suspected on the basis of discovery of immature white blood cell forms in the circulating blood. An unequivocal diagnosis is confirmed by microscopic examination of the bone marrow, usually obtained from the posterior iliac crest. At times the number of circulating white blood cells is extremely elevated. Some cases may demonstrate total white blood cell counts of above 100,000 per mm^3. In some children the number of white blood cells in the peripheral circulation is relatively low, and proportionately few immature forms are seen; the disease is said to be *aleukemic*. However, at this time the bone marrow may be packed with abnormal cells.

Incidence

Leukemia is the most common form of cancer in children. A slightly increased incidence occurs in boys, and the peak age of onset in children is 3 to 4 years of age. Certain children have been clearly identified as being at increased risk of developing leukemia (Table 32-2). Although there seems to have been a decline over the past 15 years in the occurrence of acute leukemia, it accounts for almost 32% of the malignant diseases in children under 15 years of age.

Types

There are a number of different types of leukemia classified according to the kind of white cells principally involved and the relative speed of the disease process. The most common leukemic cell observed in pediatric practice is the undifferentiated form called a "blast," or stem cell, a very

TABLE 32-2 INCIDENCE OF LEUKEMIA*

Groups affected	Number affected
Nonwhite American children under 15 years of age	1 in 5,500
White American children under 15 years of age	1 in 3,000
Siblings of leukemic children	1 in 720
Children with Down syndrome	1 in 95
Children exposed to atomic irradiation	1 in 60
Monozygotic twin sibling (with one diagnosed)	1 in 5 (both will get it)

*Peak: white children, 3 to 4 years; nonwhite children, younger.

immature form of white blood cell, usually of the lymphocytic cell line. Acute lymphoblastic leukemia (ALL) accounts for the majority of cases. Acute granulocytic or myelogenous leukemia (AML) accounts for about 20% of cases. This form however, does not respond as favorably as ALL to the anti-leukemic agents presently available.

Signs and symptoms

The signs and symptoms of leukemia may be rather slow and insidious in onset or rapid in their development. These children may complain of fatigue and weakness, and lose weight. They may be pale and bruise easily. Fever, with a persistent respiratory tract infection, is a common complaint. The child's liver and spleen, infiltrated with abnormal cells, may be enlarged. Before the era of modern treatment—total therapy with central nervous system (CNS) prophylaxis—central nervous system involvement developed in approximately 50% of children during the course of their illness. A smaller number of children (8%) initially have central nervous system leukemia at the time of diagnosis. Central nervous system leukemia causes increased intracranial pressure, which is typically manifested by headache, nausea and vomiting, slowed pulse, and elevated blood pressure. The child is highly irritable and tired. Spinal fluid examination confirms the physician's diagnosis.

The course of the disease usually involves several hospitalizations and many trips to the outpatient clinic to receive therapy or to be treated for complications of therapy.

Complete remissions of the disease for extended periods have been induced with specific drug combinations (treatment protocol). The major objectives of chemotherapy are the induction of a complete remission and the maintenance of patients in a state of remission for the longest possible time, with the expectation that a significant percentage of children with ALL (40% to 50%) can be cured of their disease. A complete remission is defined as "restoration to normal health and clinical well-being." Physical and laboratory examinations are negative, blood and bone marrow are considered normal, and all evidence of disease is absent. Best results to date have been achieved with intensive courses of drug combinations and with optimal supportive care, including transfusion of platelets and antibiotic therapy.

Since 1947, when the first brief, temporary remission was induced with aminopterin, antileukemic drug therapy has been greatly improved.

Treatment

Although intensive research continues in an attempt to unravel the origin and development of the disease, there is no doubt that the disease is treatable. In fact, the word "cure" is being used to describe long-term survivors no longer receiving chemotherapy.

Today modern treatment consists of intermittent administration of high does of several drugs in combination (Table 32-3). The duration of remissions has been increased by the addition of prophylactic therapy to the central nervous system by radiation or spinal canal (intrathecal) injections of methotrexate. Use of this therapy has reduced the incidence of central nervous system leukemia from 50% to less than 5%. In an attempt to avoid the immunosuppressive effects of continuous chemotherapy,

the maintenance schedules now being used involve intermittent doses of multiple agents in combination, followed by rest periods without therapy, or moderate daily dose schedules periodically reinforced with "induction" agents. Children with acute leukemia should be referred to specialized centers where optimal opportunity for effective therapy is available.

Complete remissions for long periods have been induced in almost all patients with acute lymphoblastic leukemia. Children in remission must have regular medical supervision, including frequent hematologic studies. Relapse is marked by falling hemoglobin levels, thrombocytopenia, severe decreases in the white blood cells called "neutrophils," and the reappearance of immature or "blast" cells in the blood and bone marrow.

Prognostic factors

The major prognostic determinants in children with acute lymphoblastic leukemia (ALL) are age and white blood cell count at the time of diagnosis. Children between the ages of 2 and 10 years with white blood cell counts of less than 25,000 per mm^3 have the best prognosis. Young infants, older children, and children with white blood cell counts greater than 50,000 per mm^3 have a poor prognosis. The length of the first remission is also considered to be a prognostic indicator of length of survival. The longer the remission endures the more optimistic is the prognosis. In general, chemotherapy for acute lymphoblastic leukemia is discontinued after 3 to 5 years of continuous complete remission. Treatment centers are currently evaluating the time period of maintenance therapy. They indicate that the incidence of relapse after cessation of therapy at 3 years is the same as that which occurs after 5 years of maintenance treatment. Therefore the benefits of two additional years of therapy are controversial. Intensive research ultimately designed to completely control the growth of leukemic cells continues. In the meantime a real effort is being made to develop a long-range therapeutic plan for each patient so that treatment can be large-

TABLE 32-3 DRUGS CURRENTLY USED IN THE TREATMENT OF LEUKEMIA

Agent	Routes of administration	Signs of toxicity
For induction		
Prednisone	Oral	Moon-shaped face, osteoporosis, acne, fluid retention, ulcers, increased susceptibility to infection, personality changes
Vincristine (Oncovin)	IV	Peripheral neuropathy, hair loss
Daunomycin*	IV	Bone marrow depression,† alopecia, nausea, vomiting, oral ulceration, congestive heart failure
L-Asparaginase	IV, IM	Chills, fever, nausea, vomiting, hypersensitivity reactions
Adriamycin	IV	Bone marrow depression,† alopecia, nausea, vomiting, oral ulceration, congestive heart failure
Thioguanine	IV	Bone marrow depression†
Cytarabine (Cytosar)	IV SQ	Bone marrow depression, nausea, vomiting
Amethopterin (methotrexate)	IV Intrathecal	Anorexia, abdominal pain, oral and gastrointestinal tract ulceration, Bone marrow depression, hair loss (rare)
For maintenance		
6-Mercaptopurine	Oral	Bone marrow depression,† nausea, vomiting, oral and gastrointestinal tract ulceration
Amethopterin (methotrexate)	Oral IV Intrathecal	Anorexia, abdominal pain, oral and gastrointestinal tract ulceration, bone marrow depression,† hair loss (rare)
Cyclophosphamide (Cytoxan)	Oral IV	Bone marrow depression,† skin rashes, hair loss, hemorrhagic cystitis, oral ulceration, diarrhea
Cytosine arabinoside (Cytosar or ARA-C)	IV SQ Intrathecal	Bone marrow depression,† nausea, vomiting

*Investigational.
†Bone marrow depression is characterized by leukopenia, thrombocytopenia, and anemia.

ly conducted in cooperation with the physician in the patient's home town.

Supportive care

Platelet transfusions have reduced the number of deaths caused by hemorrhage and increased the opportunity to use effective drugs that depress platelet production. Corticosteroids increase capillary resistance and are useful adjuncts in the control of bleeding. Bleeding from accessible areas is occasionally controlled by the local application of thromboplastin and Gel-foam.

Infection poses the greatest threat to the life of the leukemic child. Although fever may be a result of the primary disease, it is important to search for infection in all patients with an elevated temperature. Cultures should be taken from blood, urine, rectum, throat, and nasopharynx. Drugs used in the control of bacterial infection until cultures are available include oxacillin for staphylococci, streptococci, and pneumococci; ampicillin is used against *Haemophilus influenzae*. Gentamycin, carbenicillin, or both are used against gram-negative organisms such as *Pseudomonas, Escherichia coli,* and *Proteus*. Children who are in relapse are particularly at risk for fungal, viral, and protozoal infections. Oral moniliasis is seen frequently and is treated with oral nystatin (Mycostatin). A susceptible leukemic child who is exposed to chicken pox should receive zoster immune globulin (see p. 609 for availability and use of serum immune globulin). Interstitial pneumonia caused by the protozoal organism *Pneumocystis carinii* is a major cause of illness and death. Trimethoprim-sulfamethoxazole (Septra) is the drug of choice in this condition. Recent studies have shown that daily prophylactic Septra administration will prevent the development of *Pneumocystis carinii* pneumonia. Other methods that are now available in some institutions to assist in the prevention and treatment of infection include granulocyte (white blood cell) transfusions and germ-free environments (laminar-flow rooms). Presently these methods remain investigational, expensive, and not readily available to all patients.

Antileukemic drugs may cause a rapid breakdown in the malignant cells, which in turn raises the uric acid load that must be handled by the kidneys. This increased load, especially coupled with a state of dehydration caused by poor fluid intake and vomiting, causes renal injury. Allopurinol helps accelerate the excretion of uric acid and reduces the risk of kidney stone formation. Parenteral fluid therapy also lessens this risk.

Another side effect of some of the antileukemic drugs is that of alopecia, or hair loss, a nondangerous but distressing development. The child and parent can be consoled by the fact that the hair will grow back.

Children with leukemia who are admitted to the hospital because of recurring symptoms are usually very uncomfortable and irritable. Pressure from the large number of white blood cells infiltrating the various body organs makes them sore. They usually do not like to be moved, although changes in position are necessary to avoid respiratory tract infection and skin breakdown. Their lowered platelet counts lead to easy bruising and spontaneous hemorrhages in many parts of their bodies. Their anemia contributes to their fatigue and pallor. Because of the frequent ulceration of their mucous membranes, oral hygiene must be gentle (Fig. 32-14). Only soft toothbrushes, gauze, or applicators should be used. Mouthwashes of equal amounts of hydrogen peroxide and saline and the application of viscous lidocaine (Xylocaine) before meals are helpful local measures that often provide comfort.

Fever is often present, and measures to reduce temperature elevation (Chapter 28) must be frequently employed. Rectal temperatures are usually contraindicated because of the fear of inducing perirectal abscesses in children with low neutrophil counts. The presence of a member of the family at the bedside at frequent intervals is a great help to the patient, and often the child will respond by taking fluids offered by the parent when all other overtures are refused. The ability to minister to the needs of their child in these trying days is almost always a source of strength to the parents who feel a need to do something for their child. Little routines and special ways of doing things that comfort the child are important to the parent and patient. As much as possible, they should be followed. The nursing staff should not withdraw from the parents, thinking that there is little they can do. Nurses must continue to provide support throughout the illness.

Prognosis

In childhood approximately 97% of the leukemias are acute rather than chronic. Before current methods of treatment were available, the survival time for children with acute leukemia from the time of diagnosis until death was sometimes as brief as 3 to 4 weeks and rarely spanned 6 months. Today, 50% of children with acute lymphoblastic leukemia who get optimal treatment are in uninterrupted remission for at least 5 years. About 40% of

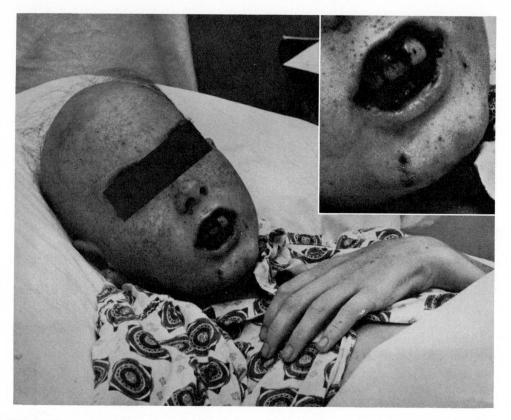

FIG. 32-14   This young boy with leukemia demonstrates the typical mouth lesions. Loss of hair resulted from therapy.

Courtesy Naval Regional Medical Center, San Diego, Calif.

these children will remain in remission indefinitely (Table 32-4).

Because most leukemic children will experience long periods of remission and some indeed will never suffer relapse, maintenance of the family's basic life-style is extremely important. Life should go on in as normal a fashion as possible. Discipline, consistent with developmental age, must be expected and maintained for the affected child just as it is for any sibling. Overly indulgent, permissive treatment usually leads to what become impossible demands, fails to make the child feel any happier or more secure, and often creates resentment, jealousy, and increasing tension within the family.

The child should not be overprotected, and activity limits should be clearly spelled out by the physician. The child should participate in everything physically and mentally feasible that is desirable. Parents should emphasize what the child *can* do. Unless clarified, this one area may cause great dissention between parents. School is "where it's at" for this child. As soon as possible, the child should return to class. Through conferences with the school nurse and teachers involved, guidelines can be established. It is the parent's responsibility to make clear to the school staff from the beginning that special treatment is neither desired nor appreciated.

TABLE 32-4 LIFE EXPECTANCY OF THE CHILD WITH LEUKEMIA

Year	Treatment	Survival in months
Acute lymphoblastic		
1937–1953	Supportive	3–5
1954–1962	Prednisone, 6-mercaptopurine, methotrexate	12
1963–1965	Prednisone, 6-mercaptopurine, vincristine, methotrexate, cyclophosphamide	24
1966–1968	Same drugs used in combination	33+
1969–1982	Total therapy Prednisone, vincristine, 6-mercaptopurine, methotrexate, cyclophosphamide, L-asparaginase, cytarabine (Cytosar) Central nervous system prophylaxis	60 (about 5 years +)
Acute myelogenous		
1982	Daunomycin, thioguanine, vincristine, cytosine, arabinoside, prednisone, cyclophosphamide	6–18

IDIOPATHIC THROMBOCYTOPENIC PURPURA

Idiopathic thrombocytopenic purpura (ITP) is a syndrome of unknown cause characterized by bruises, purpura, and petechiae resulting from a great reduction in the number of platelets (less than 100,000/mm³). A normal circulating platelet count is 250,000/mm³. Each normal thrombocyte has a life span of 8 to 10 days. In ITP the platelet may survive for only hours. Seepage of blood into the mucous membranes, subcutaneous tissues, and skin occurs. Epistaxis is common. A bone marrow sample reveals normal or increased thrombocyte formation, which rules out leukemia, the fear of many parents. ITP occurs in all age groups, with a maximum incidence in the preschool group. About half the number of cases are preceded by a febrile upper respiratory tract infection. In most younger patients the disease runs a benign, self-limited course, and most children experience a spontaneous remission within a period of 6 weeks to 4 months.

Children 10 years of age or over may have a more serious chronic type of ITP. In this age group girls are affected more frequently than boys, and the condition is likely to be associated with bleeding and the presence of an antiplatelet factor in the plasma. Steroids have been employed to help prevent bleeding and to suppress the synthesis of antiplatelet antibodies, but to date their use is questionable. Platelet transfusions have been given to control active bleeding, although platelet survival is short. Splenectomy has been followed by a sustained restoration of platelet numbers in many cases.

During the acute phase, activity should be restricted and the child protected from the risk of increased injury. Children with very low platelet counts should be kept in bed if possible. Salicylates and other drugs that foster bleeding should be avoided, because they may alter platelet function and trigger spontaneous hemorrhage. Other nursing measures include careful observation of the progress of skin lesions and alertness for any signs of internal bleeding. A major complication, and the most serious risk to the child in the early course of the condition, is intracranial hemorrhage.

The school-age child

RHEUMATIC FEVER (Fig. 32-15)

Rheumatic fever is properly classed as a collagen disease, because it affects the connective tissues in the entire body. However, because its most important complication is extensive cardiac damage, it will be discussed here. Although rheumatic fever has dramatically decreased in incidence in this country, it is still a major cause of acquired heart disease.

The mechanism of the disease is not completely known, but it is fairly certain that it is the result of abnormal immune response to a prior infection by group A beta-hemolytic streptococcus, which causes the so-called "strep throat," erysipelas, and scarlet fever. However, rheumatic fever itself is not communicable. It is not understood why some people develop rheumatic fever after beta-hemolytic streptococcus infections, whereas others do not. Rheumatic fever is most commonly found in the school-age child.

Signs and symptoms

The symptoms of rheumatic fever vary. It is a rare patient who exhibits all the possible signs and symptoms (see Jones criteria). The onset of the condition usually occurs about 2 weeks after the streptococcal infection. However, the infection may have been unapparent at the time. The child may complain of leg aches and joint tenderness, which migrates from joint to joint—one time involving a knee, next an ankle, later a wrist (polyarthralgia). These pains occur during the day as well as the night. When the child begins to have migratory, hot, swollen, tender enlarged joints (polyarthritis), the diagnosis is quickly suggested. Salicylates relieve the symptoms, and there is no permanent joint damage. The child may fatigue easily and have a fever. The extent of the fever varies considerably, depending on the severity of the disease. He may also report abdominal pain, believed to be caused by lymph node enlargement. Epistaxis (nosebleed) may occur.

Carditis, or inflammation of the heart, occurs in about 40% to 50% of cases during the initial attack of rheumatic fever. Constant observation for rapid or irregular pulse, heart murmurs, increased heart size, and signs and symptoms of cardiac failure must be carried out. Small inflammatory nodules or growths may form in the heart. Often they interfere with the action of the mitral or aortic valves, making it difficult for the valves to close properly or open sufficiently. Carditis is the most important feature of rheumatic fever. The prognosis of the patient largely rests on the severity of carditis.

Another sign that may occasionally accompany rheumatic fever is the development of painless *subcutaneous nodules* near the occiput, knuckles, knees, elbows, and spine. These nodules appear late in the course of the attack and are usually associated with severe carditis.

Another feature that may be seen at times, especially in preadolescent girls, is Sydenham's *chorea* (known in earlier times as St. Vitus' dance). Chorea may be described as involuntary muscular twitching or movement. It sometimes manifests itself as grimacing. The child may seem exceptionally clumsy and may fail to accomplish muscle tasks involving concentration or fine control. The disorder is characterized by jerky, uncoordinated movements. It may be preceded by a period of emotional instability and behavior problems. It may be so mild as to escape the notice of the casual observer or so severe that it makes normal, daily activities dangerous or impossible. Speech may become slurred and handwriting difficult to decipher.

Still another diagnostic sign of acute rheumatic fever is the appearance of a highly distinctive rash known as *erythema marginatum*. This red-line eruption forms irregular patterns on the trunk and extremities but not on the face. However, it is rarely seen.

Diagnosis is made on the evaluation of the signs and symptoms present plus the reports of several laboratory tests. None of the laboratory tests is specific for rheumatic fever, but when made in conjunction with a clinical evaluation of the patient, they are valuable aids. An increased *blood sedi-*

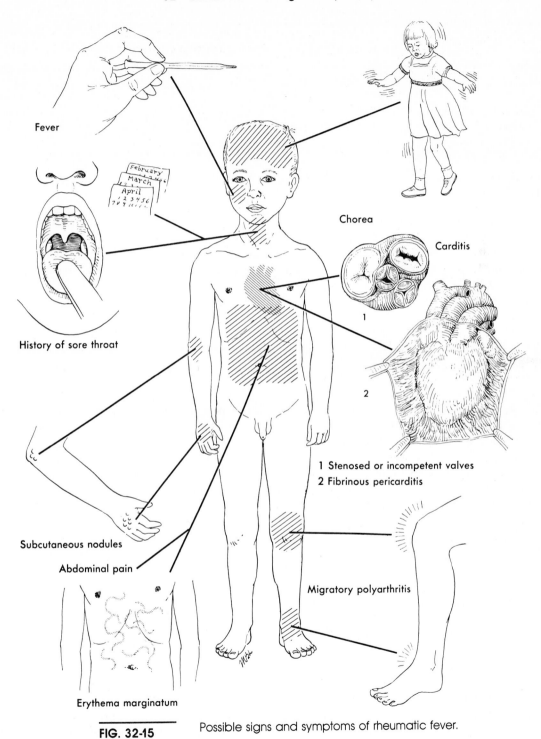

Fever

Chorea

Carditis

History of sore throat

1 Stenosed or incompetent valves
2 Fibrinous pericarditis

Subcutaneous nodules

Abdominal pain

Migratory polyarthritis

Erythema marginatum

FIG. 32-15   Possible signs and symptoms of rheumatic fever.

JONES CRITERIA (REVISED)
FOR GUIDANCE IN THE DIAGNOSIS OF RHEUMATIC FEVER*

Major manifestations

Carditis
Polyarthritis
Chorea
Erythema marginatum
Subcutaneous nodules

Supporting evidence of streptococcal infection

Increased titer of streptococcal antibodies
   ASO (antistreptolysin O)
   Other antibodies
Positive throat culture for Group A streptococcus
Recent scarlet fever

Minor manifestations

Clinical
   Previous rheumatic fever or
      rheumatic heart disease
   Arthralgia
   Fever
Laboratory
   Acute phase reactions:
      erythrocyte sedimentation rate
      C-reactive protein, leukocytosis
Prolonged P-R interval

*The presence of two major criteria, or of one major and two minor criteria, indicates a high probability of the presence of rheumatic fever. Evidence of a preceding streptococcal infection greatly strengthens the possibility of acute rheumatic fever. Its absence should make the diagnosis doubtful (except in Syndenham's chorea or long-standing carditis). From Jones criteria (revised) for guidance in the diagnosis of rheumatic fever, © 1967, American Heart Association. Reprinted with permission.

mentation rate and determination of *C-reactive protein* in the blood indicate the presence of an inflammatory process in the body that may be rheumatic fever. It is also possible to detect, with tests such as the *antistreptolysin O titer*, the presence of antibodies in the blood, formed in response to the invasion of streptococci. But as previously stated, not all beta-hemolytic streptococcal infections cause rheumatic fever. Sometimes a nose and throat culture will return a positive result. Other members of the patient's family should be checked for the presence of a streptococcal infection or the carrier state. Rheumatic fever, because of factors not yet completely determined, has a tendency to run in families.

Treatment

Treatment of rheumatic fever includes the administration of penicillin to eliminate any lingering residual streptococci and prevent a reinfection. Penicillin does not cure the symptoms of rheumatic fever, it only helps prevent further attacks. If the patient is allergic to penicillin, erythromycin may be used to eradicate the streptococcus. Sulfonamides or penicillin is equally useful in preventing reinfections. Aspirin is helpful in controlling the pain of arthritis and lowering the temperature. Prednisone is often used in acute cases of carditis, with the hope of decreasing the possibility of permanent heart valve damage. Prednisone is often lifesaving in overwhelming inflammation involving all the structures of the heart.

Nursing care

The nursing care of the child with rheumatic fever depends on the severity of the disease and the symptoms present. When laboratory tests and clinical features indicate that the disease is active and perhaps progressive, every effort should be made to reduce the work load of the heart by providing emotional and physical rest. However, "doing nothing" is not very restful for most children, especially if they do not really feel very sick. The nurse and the patient's family need a great deal of ingenuity to provide rest that is acceptable and therefore therapeutic for the child. Good observation is essential. The pulse rate is taken for a full minute to determine quality and rhythm. Often the determination of the pulse while the patient is sleeping is requested. The nurse should review the signs and symptoms of rheumatic fever and check her charge for indications of these during her care. Possible signs of cardiac failure are extremely important to report (pp. 694-695). Careful positioning and skin care are necessary.

The child with symptoms of chorea needs special supportive care; careful explanation of the condition to the patients is a necessity. Chorea may appear as the sole symptom of rheumatic disease. In the event of moderate to severe disability, rest, prolonged warm baths under supervision, and tranquilizers may help. Patient nursing care is a must. The condition usually subsides spontaneously in 2 to 3 months.

When the signs of inflammatory activity subside, the electrocardiogram results are favorable, and the pulse rate is within normal limits, the child may be allowed more freedom. However, the child must continue to be carefully evaluated to discover individual tolerance for increased exercise. Because recurrences of the disease are fairly common and the possibility of permanent heart damage increases with each attack, it is imperative that the parents understand the importance of continued medical supervision. To prevent recurrences, the patient should avoid exposure to infections and receive either daily oral or preferably monthly intramuscular, long-acting penicillin therapy.

• • •

The lungs, heart, blood vessels, and blood are separate anatomic entities. However, if one of these entities is disturbed, the others will invariably respond to meet the physiologic needs of the individual. The nurse who recognizes this interdependence is better able to serve the person to whom that deformed heart, inflamed respiratory tract, or abnormal blood belongs.

CHAPTER 33 Conditions involving
digestion and associated metabolism

A well-behaved digestion system can be a source of great pleasure. The digestive system can also initiate considerable distress, depending on its general condition and the amount of dietary discretion its owner employs. This chapter will briefly present the malformations, infestations, infections, and foreign bodies commonly found in the digestive tracts of children (Fig. 33-1). Also, although it is not considered to be basically a digestive problem, a review of diabetes mellitus will be included, since it influences the metabolism of digested glucose and dietary regulation is required. For the convenience of nursing teachers and students, most of the material will be presented according to the age group primarily affected.

ANATOMY AND PHYSIOLOGY

The digestive system is formed by the mouth, esophagus, gastrointestinal tract, and related organs such as the liver, gallbladder, and pancreas. The adult alimentary canal is an unsterile tract of many shapes and turns that, if stretched out for its entire length, would reach about 30 feet. Although in children the size of the alimentary canal may be greatly abbreviated, its importance is not. Hunger is a primary drive, and appetite, its educated twin, is soon acquired. Children may not know all about their digestive tracts, but they know that hunger represents a real need. Parents, rather despairing-

ly, often speak of the "bottomless pit." The digestive tract and its accessory organs serve to reduce foodstuffs (carbohydrates, proteins, and fats) to their smallest working chemical units. These chemical units are then absorbed through the mucous membrane of the intestinal walls and eventually reach the bloodstream to be distributed to the individual cells, providing the body with building materials, heat, and energy. To accomplish this, the digestive system works on food both *mechanically* (through the action of the teeth, tongue, cheeks, and muscular contractions of the tract, called *peristalsis*) and *chemically* (through the activity of various enzymes, emulsifiers, acids, and bacteria, which are normally active in different portions of the tract). The student is invited to review Chapter 18 if more details of the digestive process are desired. Substances not absorbed into the rest of the body by way of the bloodstream or lymphatic system are removed normally by periodic defecation, or bowel movement.

Disorders of the digestive system manifest themselves in several predictable ways. Anorexia, nausea, vomiting, constipation, abdominal distention and pain, diarrhea, and weight loss are common manifestations. The observation of a child's stool is of great importance in pediatrics. The amount, color, consistency, general appearance, and odor of a child's bowel movements can be of real diagnostic significance and aid in evaluating the condition of the digestive tract.

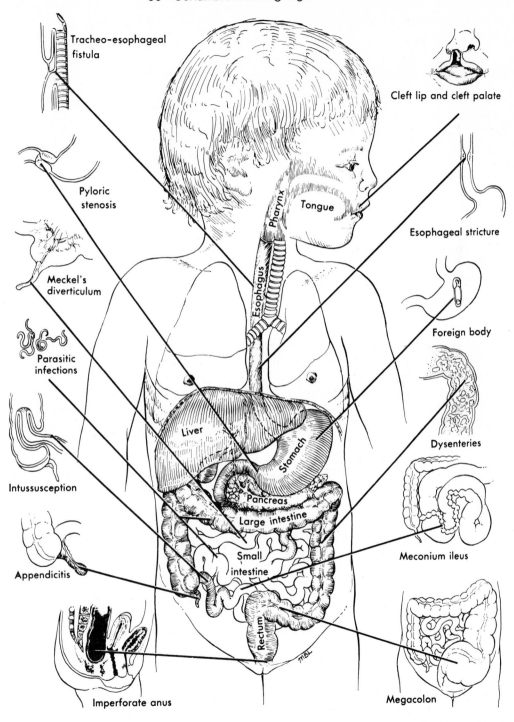

Tracheo-esophageal fistula

Cleft lip and cleft palate

Pyloric stenosis

Esophageal stricture

Meckel's diverticulum

Foreign body

Parasitic infections

Dysenteries

Intussusception

Meconium ileus

Appendicitis

Imperforate anus

Megacolon

Pharynx

Tongue

Esophagus

Liver

Stomach

Pancreas

Large intestine

Small intestine

Rectum

FIG. 33-1   Summary of common pediatric problems involving the digestive system.

KEY VOCABULARY

digestion Process by which food is broken down mechanically and chemically in the gastrointestinal tract and converted into absorbable forms.

endocrine gland Structure producing a hormone that is discharged into the bloodstream.

exocrine gland Structure that produces a secretion that is deposited in a particular area of the body via a duct.

glycosuria Presence of glucose in the urine.

hypoglycemia Deficiency of glucose in the blood.

ileus Obstruction or paralysis of small intestine.

metabolism All energy and material transformations that occur within living cells.

DIGESTIVE AND METABOLIC PROBLEMS

The infant

For a discussion of cleft lip, cleft palate, and esophageal atresia with tracheoesophageal fistula see Chapter 14.

ORAL MONILIASIS

Thrush, or oral moniliasis, mentioned earlier (p. 224) as a possible complication during the newborn period, results from contamination of the infant's oral cavity with vaginal secretion containing *Candida (Monilia) albicans* at the time of birth or from improper hygiene and feeding techniques after birth. White, curdlike plaques appear on the tongue and cheeks and adhere to the surface of the mucous membrane (Fig. 12-3). The mouth may be tender and the desire to eat may be decreased. It may be treated by nystatin (Mycostatin) oral suspension (1 ml) four times a day for 10 days or even the old standby, gentian violet, 1%. All objects that have entered the infected infant's mouth should be adequately sterilized. The condition usually responds well to therapy. Thrush is also a fairly common condition among children receiving long-term, broad-spectrum antibiotic therapy. The antibiotics destroy the normal flora of the alimentary canal and allow the ubiquitous fungus to multiply without competition. Most cases of moniliasis associated with antibiotic therapy resolve when the drug is discontinued.

ESOPHAGEAL STENOSIS

The narrowing of a child's esophagus, esophageal stenosis, may be congenital in origin; however, more often it is posttraumatic. Probably the most common cause is the ingestion of some corrosive substance such as lye, which burns the tissues and produces scarring, leading to stenosis.

Patients usually must undergo periodic esophageal dilatations by catheters. They may need a gastrostomy, or artificial opening into the stomach, because of difficulty in maintaining nutrition. Surgical excision of the narrowed area and joining together of the remaining parts (anastomosis), replacement of the area by a bowel transplant, or esophageal reconstruction using tissue from the greater curvature of the stomach may be undertaken.

CONGENITAL PYLORIC STENOSIS

Abnormal narrowing of the pyloric sphincter, which forms the exit of the stomach, may cause progressive vomiting and malnutrition in the infant (Fig. 33-2). This narrowing is caused by spasm of the sphincter, local edema, and an overgrowth of the circular muscle fibers of the pylorus. The symptoms do not usually begin until the child is approximately 2 to 3 weeks old and rarely have their onset after 2 months of age. This disorder seems to have a slight hereditary tendency and occurs more often in male than in female infants.

At first the vomiting is only occasional. However, if the stenosis is unrelieved, vomiting becomes more frequent, forceful, and projectile. If this situation persists, the child will lose weight and begin to show signs of dehydration, electrolyte imbalance, and malnutrition. The emesis contains no bile, since the opening to the duodenum is too small to allow such staining. Despite the frequent vomiting, the baby continues to have a good appetite and will take fluids when they are offered. The physician makes a diagnosis on the basis of the history, the clinical examination, and x-ray studies that use a contrast medium. A hard, olive-shaped

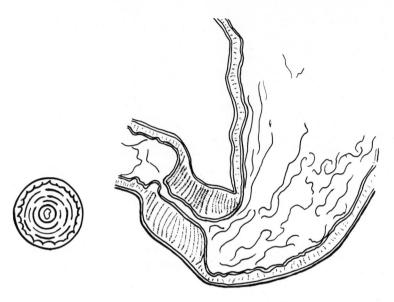

FIG. 33-2   Congenital hypertrophied pyloric stenosis. Abnormal narrowing of the pyloric sphincter—
sagittal and cross-sectional views.

tumor (the hypertrophied pylorus) may be palpated, and visible, left-to-right peristalsis may be noted as the stomach tries to force the swallowed milk or formula into the duodenum. When this effort proves ineffective, the peristaltic waves reverse themselves and emesis results.

In the United States treatment of pyloric stenosis is usually surgical. A nasogastric tube is inserted before surgery to assure that the stomach is empty and to prevent aspiration during the surgery. The procedure is called the Fredet-Ramstedt operation. The surgeon cuts down through the enlarged muscle of the pylorus to the mucous membrane, relieving the constriction. This operation, when performed on infants well prepared for the procedure, is highly successful in relieving the cause of the persistent vomiting. Postoperative care consists of observation of the surgical site or dressing, and careful introduction of glucose water in small amounts as ordered at fairly frequent intervals. The infant should be held at a steep incline while being fed, bubbled well before, during, and after a feeding, and placed in an infant seat or propped on his right side after feedings. When the baby is in the infant seat, gravity aids the drainage of the offered

fluid. Placing the infant on his right side also aids drainage and helps bubbles come to the top of the stomach, where they can be expelled with less formula loss. A side or upright position also helps prevent aspiration. After drinking, the infant should be disturbed as little as possible. It is very important not to overfeed the child. Such a situation leads to possible vomiting and strain on suture lines. If three or four glucose-water feedings are well tolerated, the infant is given progressive amounts of diluted formula, beginning with 30 ml. When 75 ml feedings are reached, the baby is started on his usual formula or begins monitored breast-feeding. If the feedings are retained, the infant is discharged to the care of his parents. This may be as early as the second postoperative day.

MECKEL'S DIVERTICULUM

A structural leftover from embryonic life is the persistence of a pouch on the ileum called Meckel's diverticulum. At one time a duct joined the umbilicus with the intestine and led to the yolk sac, which gave temporary nourishment to the developing fetus. In the course of normal development this duct closes. However, remnants persist in a small percentage of people. Sometimes these remnants cause difficulty. An open tract, capable of discharging the contents of the small bowel onto the abdominal wall, may endure. More often a blind pouch with no connection or only a cord attachment to the umbilicus remains. Occasionally gastric mucosa is found within the pouch. Meckel's diverticulum may ulcerate and hemorrhage. Symptoms similar to those of appendicitis or intestinal obstruction may occur. Frequently its presence is undiagnosed until exploratory surgery reveals the problem. Nursing care is similar to that involving any condition that necessitates exploration of the abdominal cavity.

MECONIUM ILEUS

Obstruction of the small intestine in the newborn infant caused by the presence of exceptionally thick, sticky meconium is called meconium ileus. The meconium is so gummy that it cannot pass normally through the bowel. Obstruction often occurs near the ileocecal junction. This condition always indicates the exocrine disorder, cystic fibrosis of the pancreas, although it is not present in all cases of cystic fibrosis. Meconium ileus results because the pancreas fails to produce the enzymes that normally help liquefy the meconium. (See pp. 665-670 for a discussion of cystic fibrosis.)

Symptoms include bile-stained emesis, abdominal distention, and absence of the normal meconial stool. This is a difficult pediatric problem because of the type of malfunction, the age of the patient, and other aspects of the total disease process. In mild cases the treatment may be medical, with reliance on special enemas that help dissolve or mechanically clear the impaction and on oral administration of pancreatic enzymes. A therapeutic enema of diatrizoate meglumine (Gastrografin) is a promising nonoperative method of relieving the impaction. Intravenous fluid therapy is imperative during this procedure, since diatrizoate meglumine draws fluid and serum from the intravascular compartment into the lumen of the bowel in an effort to release the firm bind of sticky meconium. Many cases, however, require surgery to

clear the obstruction. Resection of the intestine and a temporary ileostomy may be necessary. The child is usually very ill, and the prognosis is guarded.

INTUSSUSCEPTION

A telescoping of adjacent parts of the bowel is called intussusception (Fig. 33-3). When intussusception occurs, it commonly involves the area of the ileocecal valve. Such an abnormal relationship of parts of the intestine may disturb circulation to the involved portions and result in gangrene and perforation as well as obstruction of the bowel. This condition most often affects infants and toddlers. The onset is usually sudden. At first the child may draw up the legs and cry out intermittently. Later the discomfort is intensified by progressive vomiting of bile-stained and even fecal emesis. Stools, at first loose, become scanty and characteristically

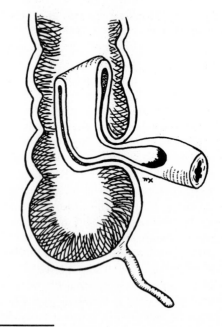

FIG. 33-3

Ileocecal intussusception—a telescoping of adjacent parts of the bowel.

assume the color and consistency of currant jelly, because they are formed at this time largely of mucus and blood. If the condition is unrelieved, the child rapidly becomes prostrate. A high temperature develops, and the child's life is endangered. A favorable prognosis depends on early detection and treatment of the condition.

Diagnosis is made by considering the history, the physical examination, and plain survey films of the abdomen. Treatment of choice in all cases, except those in which peritonitis or frank intestinal obstruction is suspected, is the barium enema. The pressure of the inflowing enema may reduce an intussusception. In some cases reduction comes only after raising the height of the barium or by giving repeated enemas after each evacuation. A small number recur after primary barium enema treatment. When surgery is indicated, the intussusception is identified and usually gently "milked" backward until the telescoping is completely relieved. Resection of the damaged segment of intestine is necessary in other cases.

CONGENITAL MEGACOLON (HIRSCHSPRUNG'S DISEASE OR AGANGLIONIC MEGACOLON)

Classic congenital megacolon, or Hirschsprung's disease, is characterized by lack of normal peristaltic activity in the distal segment of the colon, usually the sigmoid, because of improper *innervation* (lack of the necessary nerve ganglia in the musculature of the affected bowel or lack of coordination between the parasympathetic and sympathetic divisions of the nervous system). It is seen more often in males than in females. Signs and symptoms of congenital megacolon appear early in infancy. constipation, sometimes interrupted by small amounts of stool, progressive abdominal distention, which may be sufficiently severe to cause respiratory embarrassment, anorexia, and occasional vomiting are all indications of the disorder. Pronounced abdominal distention may grossly distort the appearance of the child. Diagnosis is made after a review of the patient's history, palpation and auscultation of the abdomen, rectal examination, x-ray examination, and a rectal biopsy for micro-

scopic examination of the tissue (which is mandatory for the definitive diagnosis). The biopsy is painless and is obtained surgically by securing a small wedge of tissue. Although a rectal biopsy can provide correct diagnosis of congenital megacolon, it may also initiate the serious complication of enterocolitis.

The megacolon may be treated medically or surgically, depending on its severity and its response to conservative measures.

Medical management includes almost daily enemas (usually physiologic saline solution, 2 teaspoons salt to 1 quart water). Tap water enemas are not given, because they are frequently difficult to expel, and therefore water intoxication is a danger. The amount of fluid given at one time is larger than that given nonaffected children of the same age because of the gross distention of the bowel. Digital removal of fecal material from the rectum may be necessary. Stool softeners such as Zymenol or mineral oil may be ordered. The use of drugs that affect the activity of the parasympathetic and sympathetic nervous systems may help obtain more regular bowel movements. A low-residue diet may be helpful in reducing the amount of feces and in keeping the stool soft.

If the condition of the child does not improve sufficiently with medical management, surgical treatment may be elected. The type of procedure done will depend on the age and individual needs of the child. The most satisfactory treatment appears to be an abdominoperineal removal of the abnormal section of bowel with an anastomosis of the remaining normal colon to the anal canal (Swenson's pull-through). A variation of this is the Soave procedure. Afterward, the child is fed parenterally. Gastric suction and an indwelling urinary catheter may be continued for an indefinite period. The anal sphincter may be dilated daily. The presence of bowel sounds and normal stool are eagerly awaited. At times this procedure is inadvisable, and a colostomy is performed.

More common than classic aganglionic megacolon is pseudo-Hirschsprung's disease, which has a psychogenic basis. It does not have an onset in the newborn period; x-ray studies and biopsy studies are negative. Investigation of family living patterns and stresses by qualified personnel is necessary.

COLIC

Although colic is often spoken of as a disease entity, it is not a disease but a symptom. In the dictionary it is defined as "acute abdominal pain." However, when parents and nurses speak of "the colic," they are usually referring to the intermittent abdominal distress in the newborn infant that is fairly common in the early months of life. Fortunately the problem does not always last 3 months, in spite of the frequent use of the phrase "3-month colic." Children and their parents seem to be troubled most in the early evening and night. Babies suddenly draw up their legs on their abdomens, clench their fists, become red in the face, and start to cry. This goes on intermittently as though they were troubled with periodic intestinal cramping. During these episodes they may pass gas by mouth or rectum.

Various explanations for the abdominal discomfort have been advanced. Probably there are multiple causes. Babies troubled with colic tend to have a low birth weight (5 to 7 pounds [2270 to 3180 g]). It may be caused basically by an immaturity of the gastrointestinal system. Most explanations of the pain experienced involve the presence of excessive gas in the digestive tract. Excessive air may result from the following:

1. Poor bottle-feeding techniques, including failure to tip the bottle sufficiently to assure a full nipple at all times, too-rapid feeding, the use of nipples with very small holes, which necessitates considerable suction (and air swallowing) to obtain the formula, and failure to bubble the baby often enough
2. Excessive use of carbohydrate in the formula, which may cause increased fermentation and gas formation
3. A tense, nervous baby fostered by a tense, nervous mother

Attempts to remedy colic consider these possible causes. Various types of bottles and nipples have been marketed as anticolic devices, some of which may merit a try if the baby does not respond to other techniques. Different units using presterilized plastic-bag bottles are available. The physician may recommend a change in formula. Occasionally antispasmodics, tranquilizers, or phenobarbital have been prescribed for both baby and mother with some benefit in a number of cases, but the explanation for improvement is not scientifically proven. It should be remembered that true colic is self-limited and eventually clears in all infants; therefore, reassurance is an integral part of treatment.

An infant will not be hospitalized because of colic alone, but the nurse may care for colicky babies and must realize why feeding techniques are so important. A baby who is not well bubbled will usually eat poorly and is more susceptible to regurgitation, vomiting, and colic.

THE DIARRHEAS

Any diarrheal disease causing profuse fluid loss is a particular threat to the very young person, the very old person, or the debilitated person, regardless of the initial cause of the diarrhea. Subsequent dehydration and electrolyte imbalance is a significant danger. Fortunately, with the improvement in community sanitation and hygiene, the increased availability of refrigeration, and the adoption of the disinfection techniques used in infant formula preparation, infectious types of diarrheas are not as common in the United States today as they were 60 years ago.

The infant who becomes dehydrated because of diarrhea or diarrhea and vomiting is admitted to the hospital. The infant should be weighed and a stool culture obtained immediately.

Diarrheal disease of early childhood is a syndrome, the course of which varies with age, severity, nutritional status, and cause. Some of the common causes of diarrhea include infection, anatomic abnormalities, malabsorption syndromes, and disease outside the gastrointestinal tract. Most acute diarrheas appear to have a viral cause and frequently accompany acute upper respiratory tract infections. Other causes of infectious diarrheas include staphylococci, pathogenic *Escherichia coli*, and

Salmonella and *Shigella* microorganisms, Diarrheal distrubances may also be initiated by injudicious diets or emotional upset.

General nursing care. Whatever the cause, acute diarrheal disorders need immediate treatment. The disturbance in intestinal motility and consequent malabsorption causes dehydration and fluid and electrolyte imbalances. Usually diarrhea subsides when fluid and electrolyte therapy is administered intravenously and oral intake is briefly reduced. Oral intake is restricted to rest the gastrointestinal tract and make it less irritable. Enteric isolation (p. 589) and antibiotic therapy are indicated for treating diarrheas caused by pathogenic *E. coli* and staphylococci and for severe infections caused by salmonella and shigella-type organisms. Daily calculations of the child's fluid intake and output and weight must be accurately recorded. It may be necessary to weigh the infant's diaper to assess output accurately. Because of the frequency of stools, a special medicated ointment may be prescribed to apply after each cleansing of the perirectal area. Of course, the color, consistency, general appearance, and amount of the stool should be regularly noted and recorded. Taking temperatures rectally is contraindicated.

ABDOMINAL HERNIAS

A hernia is an abnormal protrusion of a portion of the contents of a body cavity through a defect in its surrounding wall, commonly causing abnormal swelling or pressure. The general public calls the condition a "rupture." Common in infancy and childhood are inguinal and umbilical hernias. They are usually congenital.

Inguinal hernia

Hernia repair in the inguinal region is a common surgical procedure. Such hernias are found most often in males. They may be unilateral or bilateral and are usually on the right side when unilateral. When the testes originally descend into the scrotum from the abdominal cavity, they are surrounded by a small sac or tube of peritoneum that is continuous with the abdominal lining. Usually this sac soon closes off, making any further communica-

tion with the abdominal cavity impossible. However, occasionally the closure is incomplete or does not take place, and the intestine may slip down the open inguinal canal, causing a swelling in the area. This prolapse of the intestine is not important in itself. However, a possibility exists that the misplaced loop of intestine could become trapped (incarcerated) in the inguinal canal or scrotum, and the circulation to the trapped segment could become impaired (strangulated), causing intestinal obstruction and gangrene of the bowel. Early clinical signs are vomiting and colicky abdominal pain.

Inguinal hernia may also develop in girls. The anatomy is different but parallel. The inguinal canals, which are occupied by the round ligaments, may allow loops of intestine to enter the area of the groin. Only 10% of inguinal hernias involve females.

To prevent incarceration, all inguinal hernias should be corrected soon after diagnosis. In infants and small children up to 2 years of age, the hernia is repaired in a simple procedure (herniotomy). In older children a slightly more complex procedure is used. A surgical incision is made in a natural skin crease where the scar will not be seen. The hernia sac is carefully tied off. For boys an abnormal collection of fluid may be found in the scrotal area surrounding the testes (hydrocele). This fluid is aspirated, and the abnormal peritoneal sac is excised. The child usually tolerates the entire procedure very well, and in most cases no postoperative analgesia is required. A protective spray dressing is applied over the new incision. This allows direct observation of the area.

Diapers are usually not applied in a routine fashion until 24 hours after surgery. One approach to the diaper problem is the use of Stile's dressing (Fig. 33-4). A small bed cradle is placed over the legs of the infant. The diaper is brought upward between the legs and fastened to the frame of the cradle. A long infant gown, securely tied in back, is drawn tightly upward over the frame and also fastened with pins. The cradle is then draped with a small blanket.

Hospitalization for inguinal hernia repair is not

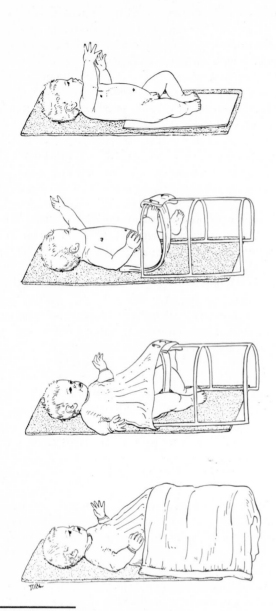

FIG. 33-4

Steps in constructing Stile's dressing. (Be sure that the gown is pulled tightly when attached to the cradle. At times the cradle must be tied to the crib.)

always necessary. A simple hernia repair can be done as an outpatient procedure. Parents are instructed to bring the child to the hospital in a fasting state about 1 hour before the scheduled procedure. The parents remain until the child is taken to the operating room and are present when the child awakes. In 2 to 3 hours and when able to take fluids, the child may be discharged from the hospital. Parents should be reminded to return in 4 days to have the sutures removed from the infant's incision. Older children's sutures are removed on the sixth postoperative day.

Umbilical hernias

Umbilical hernias in infancy are thought to be caused by severe stress to the fresh umbilical wound brought about by crying, coughing, and vomiting. Umbilical hernias often close spontaneously when the child learns to stand and walk and the abdominal muscles are strengthened through use. However, umbilical defects greater than 1.5 cm in diameter in children seldom close spontaneously. (Umbilical hernias are particularly common in black children.) If an umbilical hernia is not closed while the individual is a child, the defect often becomes more serious in pregnant women, and the multiparous woman is subject to the dangerous threat of incarceration. To prevent this serious problem in adulthood, a more aggressive approach is urged. Prophylactic umbilical hernia repair is recommended for all girls over 2 years and all boys over 4 years of age.

IMPERFORATE ANUS

The problem of imperforate anus has already been mentioned in Chapter 14. Fig. 14-15 depicts the common types of the malformation encountered. Usually surgery for correction must be performed very early to avoid complications and assure a better possibility of success. If a male newborn infant has a rectourethral fistula, surgery must be prompt to avoid intestinal obstruction and ascending urinary tract infection. For infant girls with an associated posterior vaginal anus, corrective surgery may be delayed until the child is 4 to 6 months of age.

Whether an abdominal or perineal surgical approach will be necessary depends on the type of defect and the distance of the terminal end of the colon from the perineum. A temporary colostomy may be necessary. After creation or repair of the anorectal area, frequent dilatation of the canal may be ordered.

GALACTOSEMIA

One metabolic defect that has dietary significance and has received considerable attention in the literature recently is *galactosemia*. If this congenital error in the metabolism of the sugar galactose is untreated, it may cause physical and mental retardation, cataracts, enlargement of the liver and spleen, and cirrhosis. The body is unable to change galactose to glucose, a chemical reaction that normally takes place primarily in the liver. An enzyme needed to accomplish the task is deficient or missing. Galactose builds up in the bloodstream and spills over into the urine, where it may be identified by appropriate tests.

Early signs of galactosemia in the infant are vomiting, listlessness, and failure to thrive. These signs are not apparent until at least a week or two after birth. Since galactose is present in milk sugar, it is very important that the defect be diagnosed early and that a milk substitute such as Nutramigen or a meat-base formula be used. Like those of children with phenylketonuria (PKU), the diets of galactosemia patients must be closely supervised to avoid the ingestion of the offending food. Also, like the young patient with PKU, the child with galactosemia may be able to expand dietary horizons gradually after a period of several years on a rigid, restricted regimen.

The toddler and preschool child

FOREIGN BODY INGESTION

Children do not limit their experimental tasting and swallowing to articles that are meant to tempt an appetite or even to indigestible items that might appear delicious. All kinds of objects have gone down the "little red lane." Fortunately most complete the entire journey without incident. One may carefully examine the stool for small round objects that have been ingested. However, sharp or long, angled objects may pose the threat of perforation. If the object is detectable by x-ray examination, it is viewed and periodically watched. If trauma to the tissue seems likely, an operation to retrieve it may be necessary. The abdomen of a child who has swallowed a foreign object should not be palpated. One physician even suggests placing a small sign on the child, cautioning would-be investigators to avoid such maneuvers.

Giving a child large amounts of bread or potato after ingestion of a foreign object is of doubtful value. A laxative should never be given in such circumstances.

PARASITIC INFESTATIONS

All bacteria are parasites; however, when one speaks of *parasitic infestations*, one is usually referring to organisms that are multicellular in their adult form and large enough to be seen with the naked eye. Many kinds of parasites in this category trouble human beings. Many of them are found in abundance in tropical areas of the world and represent tremendous public health problems. This text will mention only those found fairly frequently in the United States: pinworms and roundworms.

Oxyuriasis (pinworm, threadworm, or seatworm infestation)

Although the official name of the pinworm is *Enterobius vermicularis*, the name of the disease this small, white, threadlike worm causes is known as oxyuriasis, or enterobiasis, an extremely common infestation. It does not always produce symptoms and often goes undiagnosed.

The pinworm eggs are ingested or possibly inhaled. Most often children introduce the eggs into their own mouths by their contaminated fingers. Fingers become contaminated by touching objects used by affected children who have not carried out proper toilet hygiene. When the infestation has become established, children may easily reinfect themselves. The eggs are swallowed and hatch in the intestine. They mature in and near the

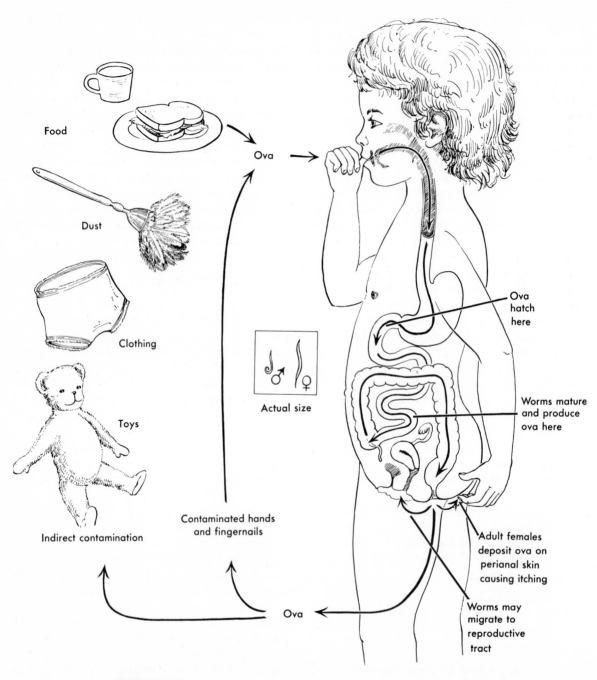

Food

Dust

Clothing

Toys

Indirect contamination

Actual size

Contaminated hands
and fingernails

Ova

Ova

Ova

Ova
hatch
here

Worms mature
and produce
ova here

Adult females
deposit ova on
perianal skin
causing itching

Worms may
migrate to
reproductive
tract

FIG. 33-5   Life cycle of the pinworm *(Enterobius vermicularis).*

cecum. When the adult female worms are ready to lay their eggs, they migrate down the intestinal tract to the anus. During the night the female worms leave the anus and lay their eggs in the folds of the anal sphincter and the perineum. Occasionally the worms may migrate to the vagina and cause a vaginitis in a little girl. All this activity usually causes considerable local irritation and itching. The child usually scratches the area, contaminating the fingers with the eggs laid in the region. In the course of time, fingers travel to the mouth again, and the cycle repeats (Fig. 33-5). The interval between the ingestion of an egg and the appearance of the female pinworm at the anus is approximately 6 to 8 weeks.

Usually mild pinworm infestations cause few symptoms other than anal itching and secondary complications caused by scratching. However, sometimes pinworms may cause anorexia, restlessness, and irritability. Abdominal pain *is not* a part of the clinical picture, despite lay opinion to the contrary. In large infestations, inflammation of the appendix may occur.

Diagnosis is made on the basis of viewing the worms as they emerge from the anus or are inadvertently expelled on the surface of a stool or by the microscopic detection of the eggs. Since the female lays her eggs in the skin folds outside the body of the child, ova are rarely found in the stool. Usually a so-called Scotch tape test is ordered. The night nurse goes to the bedside before the child wakes and shines a light on the rectal region. Sometimes the gravid worms may be seen. She then takes a piece of Scotch tape, which has been fastened "sticky side out" to a tongue blade, and presses it against the rectal area. Some microscopic eggs will adhere to the tape. The tape is then carefully secured to a glass slide "sticky side down" and sent to the laboratory for examination.

In the past when a child was affected, the entire family was treated. Today only the family members who have symptoms are treated, and a more pleasant form of therapy is available. Mebendazole (Vermox), a single-dose, chewable tablet for all ages, is effective in most cases, or pyrvinium pamoate (Pov-

an) may be given in one or two doses. The nurse and parents should know that pyrvinium pamoate colors the stools red, and if the child has an emesis while the medication is still present in the gastrointestinal tract, the emesis may also be reddish.

Other measures must be followed to help ensure a cure. Personal toilet hygiene should be stressed. The necessity for hand washing after using the toilet is not understood by children unless it is taught. Frequent cleansing of the rectogenital area is required. The toilet seat must be cleansed often. Because of the intense itching that may occur at night, an affected child should have very short fingernails. Many children are infested without the nurse's knowledge; therefore it is always good technique to refrain from shaking used bed linen. Instead, it should always be rolled. Waving the child's linens only helps scatter the eggs.

Ascariasis (roundworm infestation)

Ascaris lumbricoides, the worm that causes ascariasis, looks like a pink or white earthworm. It is usually 6 to 15 inches long. The eggs are found in the soil or on objects contaminated by soil containing involved feces. The disease is perpetuated by poor sanitary facilities and poor hygiene practices.

The microscopic egg is swallowed and hatches in the duodenum. The small intermediate stages of the worm (larvae) pass through the wall of the intestine to penetrate the venules or lymphatics. They commonly migrate to the liver, the right side of the heart, and the lungs. The small larvae then penetrate the alveoli and ascend the bronchioles, bronchi, and trachea. On reaching the glottis they are swallowed. These same larvae develop into adult male and female forms in the small intestine. The adult male may be approximately 6 to 10 inches long. The female may be about 8 to 15 inches long and about the diameter of a pencil. The adult worms subsist on the semidigested food in the intestinal canal. Fertilized eggs expelled in feces must undergo a 2- to 3-week period of maturation in the soil before becoming capable of producing disease (Fig. 33-6).

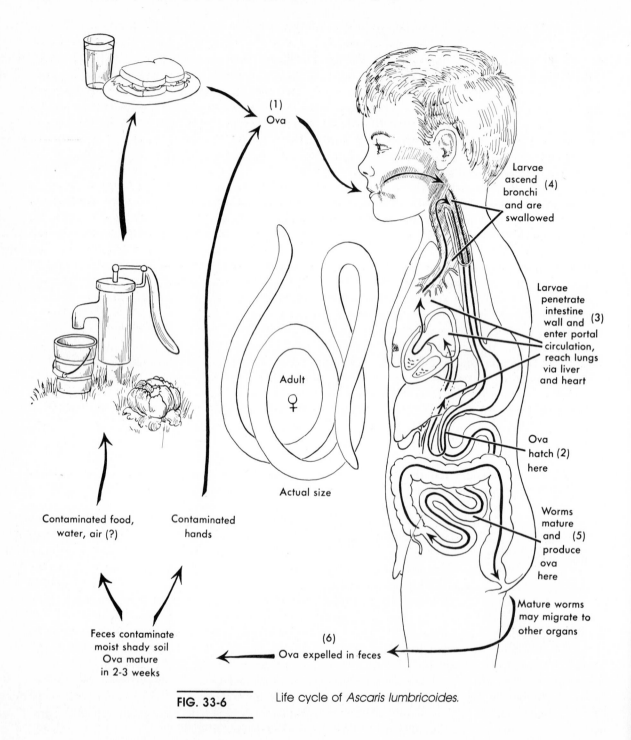

FIG. 33-6   Life cycle of *Ascaris lumbricoides.*

This parasite, because of its migratory habits (even the adult worm may travel up and down the digestive tract, occasionally making an alarming appearance at either end), may cause a variety of symptoms if the infestation is of some intensity. The larval migrations may cause nausea and vomiting or initiate symptoms of pneumonitis or intestinal obstruction. They even may produce perforation. Allergic reactions, skin rash, nervousness, and irritability are not uncommon.

Positive diagnosis is made on the basis of finding the ova in the stool or seeing the worms emerge from the gastrointestinal tract. Treatment by piperazine citrate (Antepar) is effective for *Ascaris* infestation, provided that reinfection caused by poor hygiene practices does not occur. Mebendazole (Vermox) should be used when ascariasis is associated with other worms species. All infected persons must be treated to have successful control of the disease. Public education programs teaching general hygiene are a must. Turning infested topsoil under has also been believed helpful. The prognosis is good unless secondary complications such as pneumonia, intestinal obstruction, or perforation have developed. The outlook then becomes more guarded.

APPENDICITIS

Inflammation caused by local obstruction or infection of the vermiform appendix, located at the base of the cecum, is a common indication for abdominal surgery. However, appendicitis is not always easy to diagnose in young children. Other problems may mimic the condition, and the young child is not often very descriptive regarding general discomfort. Pain may first be felt in the umbilical area. Later it may be localized in the lower right-hand abdominal quadrant. Restlessness, mild constipation or diarrhea, and anorexia followed by nausea and vomiting are often reported. A low-grade fever is characteristic. The white blood cell count is usually elevated. If the inflamed appendix is removed before it has ruptured, recovery is usually prompt and uneventful. However, delay or the use of ill-advised laxatives may result in the rupture of the appendix. Peritonitis may complicate the condition. Recovery is then slower, and the risk to the patient is multiplied considerably. The campaign to educate the public not to give laxatives or enemas to persons complaining of abdominal pain has not yet been won.

The patient with a ruptured appendix, related abscess, or peritonitis is very ill. This individual usually cannot be sent to surgery immediately but must wait until the administration of antibiotics, intravenous fluids, and possible cooling measures are completed so that the patient will be in the best condition possible for the appendectomy. A nasogastric tube is often passed to relieve flatus and prevent vomiting. At the time of the surgery, a drain is usually placed in the abdominal wound, and drainage may be significant. A high Fowler's position is maintained to prevent the spread of infective material in the abdomen. Intravenous feedings are continued for several days postoperatively, and only ice chips or sips of water are allowed by mouth. Intake and output determinations are important. Today, more and more of these patients are recuperating satisfactorily, and the phrase "ruptured appendix" is no longer as dreaded as it was formerly.

The school-age child

DIABETES MELLITUS

Diabetes mellitus is the most common metabolic disorder of children. It is not a true digestive problem, since carbohydrates are reduced to glucose by the digestive system and the glucose is absorbed into the bloodstream. The difficulty arises because the islets of Langerhans in the pancreas fail to produce the hormone insulin. In the absence of effective insulin, utilization of glucose is impaired and hyperglycemia, with its acute and long-term manifestations, results.

About 1 child in 600 of school age has a form of diabetes that requires insulin replacement throughout life. Males and females appear to be equally affected. No correlation with socioeconomic status has been found. Because varied etiologic and pathologic factors cause the different types of hyperglycemia, the term "insulin-dependent diabetes mellitus" (IDDM) is used most commonly to describe the disease exhibited by children and adolescents. In these patients diabetes usually begins before age 15. The young people will eventually demonstrate an absolute deficiency of insulin.

Although diabetes mellitus may manifest itself any time during a person's lifetime, the earlier the disease appears, the earlier complications of the disease will be encountered. During the first year following diagnosis of IDDM, the islets of Langerhans hypertrophy, causing an erratic production of insulin. As the condition progresses, the islets atrophy, finally becoming entirely incapable of insulin production. This is the main difference between IDDM, formerly called "juvenile diabetes," and maturity-onset diabetes in which disturbed carbohydrate metabolism may be the result of many factors which together cause a diminished supply of needed insulin.

Etiologic factors

The exact cause of diabetes mellitus is not known, but inheritance plays an important role. Evidence also indicates that certain environmental factors such as toxins and viral infections may precipitate the condition in susceptible persons. Therefore, it may be hypothesized that a genetic predisposition to developing IDDM exists and that some unknown factor or insult may occur that precipitates the condition resulting in islet destruction.

Pathophysiologic factors

Insulin is important in the metabolism of carbohydrates, fats, and proteins. In insulin-dependent diabetes, glucose is unavailable for cellular metabolism. It cannot be converted to glycogen for storage in the liver and muscles, nor can it be burned properly. Hyperglycemia and other compensatory symptoms occur as glucose utilization by tissue is impaired. When glucose concentration reaches approximately the level of 180 mg/100 ml, glucose spills over into the urine (glycosuria), causing diuresis to occur (polyuria). Large amounts of water and electrolytes are lost, with subsequent dehydration. This is associated with excessive thirst (polydipsia).

When the amount of glucose available is insufficient to provide heat and energy to meet the body's needs, protein and fats are broken down and used to help furnish these necessities. However, metabolism of fat is not complete without the concurrent metabolism of carbohydrate. This incomplete fat metabolism produces ketone bodies (acetone, diacetic acid, and oxybutyric acid) that accumulate abnormally in the blood (ketonemia). Diacetic acid and oxybutyric acid must be neutralized in the body by bases, or alkalies. As the ketones are excreted, sodium, potassium, and neutralizing bases are also lost in the urine. The body's supply of base is depleted, the sensitive electrolyte balance is upset, and metabolic acidosis gradually develops (diabetic ketoacidosis).

Signs and symptoms

The classic clinical symptoms of diabetes are polyuria, dehydration despite polydipsia, and weight loss despite polyphagia. Most children initially have a brief history of lethargy, weakness, and a decrease in weight. Weight loss can be readily explained by the loss of calories as glucose goes into the urine. Improper metabolism of fats and protein also occurs. Unexplained weight loss and polyuria or the resumption of nocturnal enuresis are indications for testing. Glycosuria plus hyperglycemia are diagnostic.

Acute care

The most serious form of this disease is diabetic ketoacidosis (DKA). Severe dehydration, confusion, coma, and even death may occur unless the condition is reversed promptly by insulin and appropriate fluid replacement. DKA is truly a medical emergency requiring the close attention of a physician and a nurse at the bedside.

The goal of initial therapy is to improve circulation. Although insulin replacement is urgent, fluid

TABLE 33-1 INSULINS COMMONLY USED IN THE MANAGEMENT OF CHILDREN WITH INSULIN-DEPENDENT DIABETES MELLITUS (IDDM)

Type of insulin	Appearance	Onset (hours)	Peak (hours)	Duration (hours)
RAPID ACTION—SHORT DURATION				
Regular	Clear	½–1	2–4	6–8
Semilente	Cloudy	½–1	2–4	8–10
INTERMEDIATE ACTION—LONGER DURATION				
Globin	Clear	1–2	6–8	12–14
NPH	Cloudy	1–2	6–8+	12–14
Lente	Cloudy	1–2+	6–12	14–16

and electrolyte replacement is the most important factor in the treatment of DKA because dehydration is often of the magnitude of 10%. An intravenous line is placed and fluids are started immediately. Adequate insulin is administered in small doses by infusion to provide a constant, steady insulin concentration in plasma. When acidosis is corrected (serum bicarbonate of 14 mEq/L or greater), insulin infusion may be discontinued and insulin given subcutaneously. Blood glucose levels are monitored as often as needed by means of the Dextrostix or chem-strips with or without the assistance of a glucometer. Since the urinary output is good a clinitest and acetest can be performed on an hourly basis. Intake and output is carefully plotted, and vital signs—particularly the pulse—should be monitored often, and any significant change should be reported promptly.

Precipitating factors of diabetic ketoacidosis include trauma, infection, pregnancy, vomiting, or emotional stress. This life-threatening condition is now relatively uncommon because of increased recognition of the classic symptoms of diabetes. However, a small number of children demonstrate repeated episodes of DKA, which may represent treatment failure or inadvertent or deliberate error by the patient in the administration of insulin.

Management during the period following control of DKA consists of establishing appropriate nutritional intake while discontinuing intravenous fluids and converting to subcutaneous insulin administration.

Insulin

One of the essentials in the management of the child with diabetes is to provide a dosage of insulin that can effectively cover a 24-hour period. Approximately five types of insulin are available that are commonly used in the management of the child with IDDM. Table 33-1 describes their activity. U-100 insulin, which is 99% pure insulin, is available with special syringes for children. To maintain normal blood glucose levels, twice-a-day injections of a combination of short- and intermediate-acting insulins are often needed. A mixture of two parts NPH insulin and one part regular insulin is given ½ hour before breakfast and ½ hour before the evening meal. (See Fig. 33-7 for sample schedule.) Two thirds of the total dose is given before breakfast, and the remaining one third is given before the evening meal. When both rapid-acting and intermediate-acting insulin are prescribed together, the two insulins should be drawn up in the same syringe and always in the same sequence, so that any residual insulin in the "dead space" remains constant. This ensures greater stability of the patient once a therapeutic dose has been established.

DAILY NUTRITIONAL REQUIREMENTS
This suggested guide should be modified if additional exercise is planned or if the child becomes ill

---

Prepubescent
65 kcal/kg
(30 kcal/lb)

Pubescent and postpubescent
30 kcal/kg
(16 kcal/lb)

Composition of calories
Should supply sufficient calories to meet the needs of exercise, growth and appetite

Carbohydrate	45%	(Avoid sucrose)
Fat	30–40%	(Use polyunsaturated fats)
Protein	15–20%	

Meal plan
Caloric intake should be divided into 3 meals and 2 or 3 snacks based upon the individual's life style and upon the dynamics of insulin

Breakfast	4/18
Midmorning	1/18
Lunch	5/18
Midafternoon	2/18
Dinner	5/18
Bedtime	1/18

Nutritional intake should be evaluated annually to compensate for growth. Referral or consultation with the nutritionist should be made whenever necessary.

The "honeymoon" period

During the initial presentation of IDDM, insulin requirements are 1 U insulin/kg/day, but after stabilization, insulin requirements decline. This period (which lasts for up to 1 year) is characterized by easy control, general well-being, and is known as the "honeymoon" period. During the honeymoon period, glycosuria can usually be completely controlled with administration of a small daily dose of insulin.

When children are being regulated in the hospital, they are often placed on "regular insulin coverage" in addition to the two-dose schedule. Regular insulin has a rapid but relatively brief action. The amount of insulin they receive will depend on the amount of glucose found in their urine at specific times during the day. The sites of injection should be changed each day to prevent atrophy of subcutaneous fat. Children should be taught to keep a record of the daily placement of their insulin. Children 7 and 8 years old often express curiosity about the process of preparing the dosage, and some (who are more dependable and composed) may even be capable of injecting themselves. Children must have considerable practice in preparing dosages with adequate supervision. They also should be taught about the actions of the different insulins to understand the relationship between regular, good dietary habits and insulin injections. Children and their parents need to know when the onset and the peak of the prescribed insulin occur as well as its duration.

At the onset of diabetes or following recovery from ketoacidosis, the total daily dose of insulin should range between 0.5 to 1.0 International Units (IU) of insulin per kilogram of body weight per day. The insulin dose can be kept constant when the child and the parents are taught to anticipate the child's daily activities (exercise) and to vary the nutritional intake to meet changing needs.

Exercise

An integral component of growth and development is exercise, and children with diabetes should be encouraged to participate in any activity they like, including competitive sports. However, exercise decreases insulin requirements by increasing glucose utilization and by allowing a more rapid resorption of insulin from subcutaneous depots. Appropriate adjustments in food intake and insulin dosage must be considered. If exercise is increased

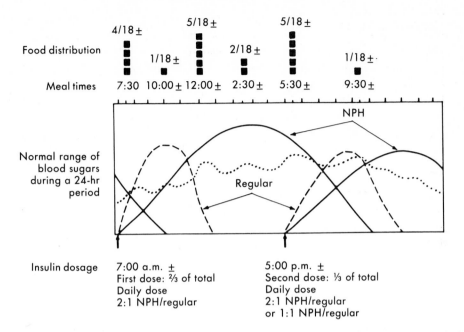

FIG. 33-7   Twenty-four-hour insulin schedule using a 2-dose regimen of regular and NPH insulins.

From Guthrie, R.A., and Guthrie, D.W., Nursing management of diabetes mellitus, ed. 2, St. Louis, 1982, The C.V. Mosby Company.

or decreased, food intake must be adjusted accordingly.

Nutritional intake

The nutritional intake of a child with diabetes should be comparable to that of the healthy nondiabetic child of the same age, sex, weight, and level of activity. Since the amount and type of insulin prescribed depend on caloric intake, regularity of caloric intake for the fixed dose of insulin becomes vital (see Fig. 33-7).

Total calories should be adjusted to meet the individual child's needs in growth, activity, and appetite, including the foods of their own culture, social group, and ethnic background. Because weighing each food imposes rigidity and a burden on the child and family, the American Diabetic Association has prepared a simplified method of calculating food intake based on the concept of food exchanges. Six basic exchanges are listed, and within each exchange a wide variety of foods can be substituted or exchanged. Common foods should be used that can be modified to meet the likes and economic needs of the child and family. Emphasis should be placed on regularity of food intake and on the constancy of carbohydrate intake, avoiding simple sugars (see chart, p. 728).

Insulin-food relationships

In the hospital the patient's nutritional intake is carefully measured to establish a baseline; then, using the urinary glucose spill patterns and the child's appetite, it is modified as needed. No food or liquids should be given, with the exception of water, without a physician's authorization. The patient should be encouraged to eat all the food served on the tray on time. (Before serving a tray, the nursing staff should determine whether the child has received any ordered insulin. The type of insulin the patient receives will dictate when the meal should be served.) The glucose content of any uneaten portion is calculated, and a replacement (usually a drink) that must be finished is sent to the patient. Any inability to eat or emesis should be promptly reported. The way in which the young patient is adhering to the nutritional intake should be carefully reported and recorded. Conferences in which the physician and nutritionist work along with the older child may be arranged and are often profitable. Sometimes when youngsters feel they have made some of the rules, these rules are easier to keep.

Hypoglycemia (insulin-induced hypoglycemia)

Insulin itself may cause problems. Too much insulin may be just as disastrous as too little insulin. A balance between the insulin needed and the insulin available must be maintained to avoid either hyperglycemia or the other extreme known as hypoglycemia (See Fig. 33-8.)

Unlike hyperglycemia, hypoglycemia may develop rapidly, within minutes or hours. The first signs of insulin-induced hypoglycemia are diaphoresis and personality change. This change will take various forms, depending on the patient, but each person usually reacts in a way that is particularly characteristic for that individual. If the condition is not relieved, the patient will develop deep shock, become unconscious, suffer from possible tremors or convulsions, and, if no treatment becomes available, eventually die.

Nurses and patients should be familiar with the early signs of hypoglycemia so that it may be easily counteracted (Fig. 33-8). Children usually learn to recognize their symptoms well. All persons with diabetes should carry some rapidly available source of glucose in the event they feel the beginning of an insulin reaction. A sugar lump followed by a small protein or fat snack is recommended. In the hospital a small glass of orange juice or crackers are usually given. If no improvement is obtained in 15 minutes, additional food should be given. If the child had difficulty taking the necessary oral glucose, an intramuscular or subcutaneous injection of glucagon is ordered. Glucagon activates liver enzymes that break down liver glycogen to produce glucose. It must be remembered that glucagon will

not work in the glycogen-depleted child. The family needs to know that glucagon should be given one time only for each episode, and that the child should be fed immediately. Glucagon is available in 1 mg vials. The usual dose is 0.5 mg (or one-half vial) for children under 3 years of age and 1 mg for children 3 years and over. The intramuscular route is preferred because of more rapid absorption. It usually takes 10 to 20 minutes for glucagon to work. Sometimes intravenous administration by the physician of a 20% to 50% solution of glucose may be required. If the patient has been given a slow-acting, long-duration insulin, response to therapy for hypoglycemia may be slow and treatment more complex. The physician should always be notified of the occurrence of insulin reactions. When a patient complains of symptoms of possible reaction or the nurse is suspicious that such a process is occurring, blood glucose should be evaluated immediately using one of the quick assays. If symptoms of hypoglycemia are present, urine tests usually prove negative for glucose and acetone. At times it may be difficult to determine clinically whether the complaints and appearance of the patient are caused by the lack of glucose or too much glucose in the blood. If no laboratory test is feasible, glucagon or intravenous glucose is often ordered. If the difficulty is caused by insulin reaction, the patient responds. If it is not, no real harm will have been done. Hypoglycemia should be treated promptly. Prolonged, severe hypoglycemia may cause brain damage and subsequent mental deterioration, impaired motor coordination, and, of course, even death.

As can be seen from Fig. 33-8, a number of causes exist for insulin excess and resulting reactions. Probably the most common cause is uncompensated excessive exercise. Exercise causes sugar to be metabolized more effectively and reduces blood glucose levels. Unless insulin dosage is reduced or glucose intake is increased, hypoglycemia is likely in the presence of unplanned exercise. For this reason, it is important for the child with diabetes to have periods of regular exercise suitably spaced after meals and to recognize the possibility

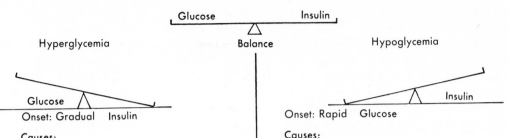

| Hyperglycemia | Balance | Hypoglycemia |

Onset: Gradual   Insulin

Onset: Rapid   Glucose

Causes:

    Infection

    Overeating

    Emotional upset

    Insulin underdose

Causes:

    Uncompensated excess exercise

    Eating too little or too late

    Vomiting

    Insulin overdose

Classical early signs and symptoms:

    Excessive thirst, fluid intake (polydipsia)

    Excessive voiding (polyuria)

    Excessive appetite (polyphagia)

    Weight loss, fatigue, pruritus

Development of ketoacidosis or coma:

    General malaise

    Nausea, vomiting

    Abdominal pain

    Long, deep, labored respirations

    "Apple-pie" breath, red lips

    Dehydration:

        Skin: dry, warm

        Eyeballs: soft, sunken

    Blood pressure low, pulse rapid, thready

    Irritable→Drowsy→Coma→Death

Development of insulin shock:

    Fatigue, weakness, faintness,

        tachycardia, personality change

    Hunger

    Pale clammy skin, diaphoresis

    Lethargy, tremors

    Convulsions → Loss of consciousness → Death

Laboratory findings:

    Glucose in urine (glycosuria)

    Acetone in urine (ketonuria)

    Elevated blood sugar and

        ketone levels

    Low plasma CO_2 and HCO_3 content

    Low blood pH

Laboratory findings:

    No glucose in urine

    No acetone in urine

    Lowered blood sugar (hypoglycemia)

Treatment:

    Regular insulin

    Fluid and electrolyte replacement

    Elimination of any infection

Treatment:

    If conscious: oral CHO, orange juice, sugar

    If unconscious: IM or SQ injections of

        glucagon or IV glucose

FIG. 33-8   Glucose-insulin balance chart.

of needed adjustment to compensate for special activities.

Another cause of hypoglycemia is failure to eat or failure to eat enough or to space the food intake appropriately. Midmorning, midafternoon, and bedtime snacks are essential. The nurse should be sure they are given to the patient and that they are consumed. If the child is nauseated or has an emesis, this should be immediately reported, because this condition may also lead to hypoglycemia. Meals must be served on time; a long delay after the injection of regular insulin also sets the stage for an episode of hypoglycemia.

Difficulties in determining appropriate doses of insulin may also be a source of glucose-insulin imbalance. The patient may not respond to the dosage as expected. Errors in insulin administration resulting in an overdose are also a real possibility. Great care must be taken in reading the orders and in preparing the injection. One strength (U-100) insulin is available in both short-acting and intermediate-acting insulin. When mixing the two types of insulin in the same syringe, the nurse must be sure of her technique.

1. Just enough replacement air must be injected into the bottle of cloudy insulin without dipping the injecting needle into the insulin. The needle is then removed from the bottle.
2. The clear, regular insulin should be withdrawn into the syringe, using the proper scale.
3. The cloudy insulin is then withdrawn into the syringe, using the proper scale.
4. An air bubble is put into the syringe and the syringe rocked back and forth to mix the two types.

This technique must be followed to prevent the conversion of rapid-acting insulin into a longer-acting type by inadvertent injection of intermediate insulin into a vial of regular insulin.

Hyperglycemia

Hyperglycemia, the opposite body condition from hypoglycemia, occurs when the insulin available in the blood is insufficient to metabolize the glucose present.

The most frequent cause for development of hyperglycemia is the onset of infection or illness. Infection greatly intensifies the body's need for insulin, and unless insulin dosage is adjusted, hyperglycemia may result. Prompt and proper attention to even minor infections in the child with diabetes may prevent progression to a serious metabolic disturbance.

Failing to follow the prescribed meal pattern or "snitching sweets" may be a possible problem. It takes a great deal of self-understanding and self-discipline to refrain from eating some of the tempting but forbidden foods available, especially if one feels hungry. Development of self-direction and self-control is paramount for the young child and particularly for the adolescent. Nutritional discipline should be encouraged by allowing the individual to participate in its planning, and possibly making provision for special occasions. With the advent of so many 1-calorie soft drinks, the social lives of teenagers with diabetes mellitus are a bit less strained. However, they should be cautioned that the label "dietetic foods" does not necessarily mean "foods for the diabetic." Children should be made to believe that ultimately the only persons they cheat are themselves when they knowingly choose unwisely or try to falsify urine tests.

Emotional upset also increases the possibility of hyperglycemia. The insulin requirement rises in periods of stress. The emotionally stable child is much easier to regulate with insulin than a child with many emotional problems.

Possible errors in the administration of insulin that can result in an underdose as well as an overdose must be avoided.

The need for insulin progressively increases as the child reaches sexual maturation and adolescence. Failure to increase insulin dosage will lead to the development of hyperglycemia and ketosis. Under these circumstances, the daily dose of insulin may exceed 1.0 IU/kg/day. However, caution must be exercised in preventing rebound hyperglycemia (Somogyi effect).

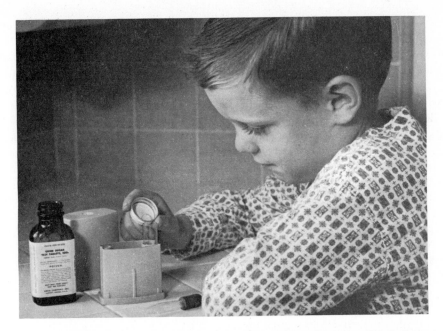

FIG. 33-9   "You're not supposed to touch the tablet with your fingers." Clinitest analysis of urine.

Somogyi phenomenon

Children receiving high doses of insulin, 1.0 to 2.0 IU/kg/day, are likely to experience behavior changes, early morning sweating, restless sleep, or headaches. Other children may be asymptomatic but may rapidly develop glycosuria and ketosis. This is the rebound phenomenon first described by Somogyi (repeated periods of inapparent hypoglycemia followed by rebound hyperglycemia). Treatment for the Somogyi phenomenon is frequent blood glucose checks and gradual reduction of insulin dosage.*

Urine tests

Long before the children are ready to give their own insulin injections, they will be able to test their urine for the presence of glucose and acetone. Several types of tests for glycosuria are available.

They are of varying convenience and expense. In the hospital, Clinitest tablets are usually employed (Fig.33-9), but any of the commercially available preparations are acceptable. Urine analysis for the presence of ketones is also routine. Clinitest using the two-drop method is preferred for children. The mechanics of these various tests are described on pp. 480-481.

Because the type and dosage of insulin must be individualized for each child, all diabetic regimens must use some method for monitoring control. Urine glucose tests serve as useful guides to assess the level of control. Four kinds of urine specimens may be obtained:

1. The fractional quantitative urine glucose method provides an accurate estimation of diabetic control and pinpoints the time of day when control is poor. When the physician orders fractional specimens, the total urine output between testings is saved. Then at the time of the scheduled urine examination, the entire collected volume is mixed,

---

*Somogyi, M.: Exacerabation of diabetes by excess insulin action, Am. J. Med. **26**:169, 1959.

and tests are made on a specimen from the total volume. For example, Johnny is asked to void at 8:00 AM. This voiding is added to the urine collection started the previous night for the period from 8:00 PM (bedtime) until 8:00 AM. The collection is mixed and a small amount of the mixture tested. Then the collection is discarded. The next time Johnny voids, the total voiding is placed in the large, empty, clean collection bottle. If he voids again, this voiding, too, is put in the collection bottle. At 12:00 PM he is asked to void, and the complete voiding is added to the collection. The urine is mixed and a specimen tested. Four such volumes are collected as follows: (1) 8:00 AM to noon; (2) noon to 4:00 PM, (3) 4:00 PM to 8:00 PM, and (4) 8:00 PM to 8:00 AM.

Peak action of the various insulins can be evaluated during these periods. Period 1 reflects AM rapid-acting insulins; period 2 reflects AM intermediate-acting insulin; period 3 reflects PM regular insulin; and period 4 reflects PM dose of an intermediate-acting insulin. Children in "good control" can tolerate a spill of about 20 to 60 g of glucose a day and still maintain normal growth and development. The 24-hour fractional quantitative urine glucose test provides information about the total grams of glucose excreted along with the volume, which helps to assess insulin therapy accurately and enables the physician to make the necessary adjustments.

Periodically the child's clinical course must be evaluated. Parents (or the children themselves) are asked to make several 4-hour urine collections at the same time on different days. Children need not be hospitalized for reevaluation, because urine should be collected on a "typical" day in terms of nutritional intake, exercise, and emotional stress. When these inherent limitations are considered, the pattern of glucose metabolism and insulin-glucose balance derived from the urine test can be profitably used for adjustments in diabetic therapy.

2. A 24-hour urine collection may be ordered while the child is in the hospital. This is a pooling of the four fractional specimens.

3. The single voided specimen method is a modification of the fractional method. Separate specimens are not collected in a container; rather, the urine is retained in the bladder. If the child is able to retain all the urine during the four intervals, this method of quantitative analysis may be more convenient.

4. The qualitative double-voided specimen method is commonly used. The test reflects the blood glucose level at that moment. Urine specimens are usually secured and tested before insulin is given and 30 minutes before scheduled meals (that is, at 7:30 AM, 11:30 AM, 4:30 PM, and bedtime). The patient is asked to void (empty his bladder) at 7:00 AM. Then the child is given a glass of water. A portion of the 7:00 AM specimen is saved but will be discarded later if it is not needed. At 7:30 AM the patient is asked to void again, and a portion of this specimen is tested and reported. The procedure is repeated before lunch, before dinner, and before bedtime. However, practically speaking, it is sometimes difficult for a child to produce the needed urine specimen on schedule. If the second specimen is not forthcoming, the first specimen that was secured (which had not been thrown away) will be tested, reported, and recorded.

Long-term goals and prognosis

Long-term care begins immediately after the initial hospitalization and control of ketoacidosis. The goals of long-term care are: (1) promotion of normal growth and development; (2) maintenance of a high level of metabolic control; (3) instruction of the child (and parent) in the skills of self-care; and (4) development of a happy, useful, and productive citizen.

Advances in the therapeutic use of insulin have provided a reasonably acceptable approach to the treatment of IDDM in children. Vascular disease follows within the second decade after diagnosis. The vascular lesions are of two main types: (1) premature atherosclerosis leading to a high morbidity and mortality from cardiovascular, cerebrovascular, and renal disease; and (2) microangiopathy or peripheral vascular insufficiency (caused by thickening of capillary basement membranes) leading to retinopathy and blindness, progressive renal failure, and various neuropathies. "Poorly controlled" IDDM in children is associated with earlier vascular complications.

Recent advances in the care of children with IDDM indicate that consistent improvement in life expectancy can be accomplished when plasma-glucose levels are maintained as close to normal as possible. To date this is approximated in most children by the split-dose insulin regimen and a multiple feeding plan. However, vascular complications continue to occur in all children sooner or later.

Scientific efforts continue in the search for the exact cause and prevention of diabetes. In the meantime technologic advances in the monitoring of IDDM continue to be sought in an effort to prevent or reduce the long-term complications. Among the most recent developments in the therapeutic regimen is the introduction of practical methods for home blood-glucose monitoring and the use of a portable insulin pump which is designed to mimic the release of insulin by the pancreas. Both developments show promise, but as yet are not suitable for everyone, are costly, and do not provide an easier method of monitoring.

Review of nursing responsibility

The nursing care of the diabetic patient has been discussed throughout this section; however, the following questions should be of assistance in aiding the nurse to organize and evaluate her care of the patient:

1. Insulin requirement. Do you know the type of insulin your patient is receiving and when the patient receives his injections? Do you know how his injections are being rotated?
2. Nutrition. Do you know the amount of calories the physician has prescribed? If a strict diet is ordered (usually the case), have you made sure that your patient has eaten everything or has received a replacement? Do you evaluate his meals for variety and interest?

Do you watch for and limit the possibility of the patient obtaining food not calculated in his diet? Does the patient have a scheduled interval nourishment?

3. Urine testing. Do you know the method to be used? Are you collecting the specimens properly? Where are the results recorded?
4. General hygiene. Is the patient getting as much exercise as possible so that his insulin requirement (because of differences in amounts of exercise taken) will not change greatly on the patient's discharge? Is his skin in good condition? Are there any signs of infection anywhere in the body?
5. Glucose-insulin imbalance. Do you know the signs and symptoms of developing hypoglycemia and hyperglycemia?
6. Patient-parent education and participation. Are you assisting the patient and parents in learning more about the disease and its treatment and control, depending on their level of understanding? Are you helping the patient to develop attitudes of self-control and feelings of achievement and well-being? Does the child keep records of insulin intake, urine tests, and general health? How much is the patient able to participate in his care?
7. What special interests and aspirations does this patient have?
8. What has this patient taught you?

For diabetic patients to become contributing citizens in the community and enjoy life to its maximum, they must understand their disease, accept the limitations it imposes, and learn to function in a relatively independent setting. The alert, intelligent, warm-hearted nurse can do much to help them meet these goals.

It is very helpful for patients with diabetes mellitus to be able to room together. They usually are mutually supportive and learn from one another. (Most of the time such learning is positive and beneficial.) Children with this disorder should be encouraged to participate in school, church, and community activities and not look on their metabolic problem as an excuse for difficult behavior or special privileges. The fact that they have diabetes mellitus should not be hidden. Teachers, schoolmates, and employers should be aware of the presence of the condition. In many states special summer camping experiences are set up for children with this disorder. These 2-week sessions have been of great help to many youngsters.

• • •

A source of much pleasure and occasional pain, the digestive system continually struggles to meet the challenges of unskilled cooks, individual abuse, and emotional stress. Nurses should be able to help prevent or ease some of the difficulties faced by this sensitive body servant. In so doing, they fulfill part of their obligation to the individual whose total well-being is their concern.

CHAPTER 34

Conditions involving
the genitourinary system

URINARY SYSTEM

The urinary system consists of two kidneys, two ureters, the bladder, and the urethra (Fig. 34-1). The primary function of these organs is to excrete metabolic waste products. The kidneys also perform other functions such as the production of renin, which controls blood pressure, and erythropoietin, which stimulates red blood cell synthesis.

To regulate the composition of blood, the kidneys perform the complex task of secreting urine. The ureters, bladder, and urethra are involved in the transportation, storage, and elimination of the urine.

Kidneys

The kidneys are paired organs located on either side of the vertebral column, just above the waistline. They lie outside the peritoneal cavity against the posterior abdominal wall.

In the adult the kidneys are about 4½ inches (11.5 cm) long and 2½ inches (6.4 cm) wide; they are somewhat bean shaped. On the medial border of each kidney is a concave notch called the *hilus*. The renal artery, renal vein, nerves, and ureter join the kidney at the hilus.

When describing the internal structure of the organ, one may speak of two areas: the functioning portion, the *parenchyma*, and the collecting portion, the *pelvis*. A longitudinal section of the kidney reveals that the parenchyma in turn is composed of two parts: an outer portion called the *cortex* and an inner portion called the *medulla*. The pelvis is formed by the expansion of the upper end of the ureter. The pelvis subdivides to form the major and minor *calyces* (singular, calyx).

The parenchyma of each kidney consists of approximately 1 million functional units called *nephrons*. Each nephron has two parts—the glomerulus and the tubule. The glomerulus is a collection of specialized capillaries. The tubule has three main parts—the proximal convoluted tubule, the loop of Henle, and the distal convoluted tubule. Each nephron unit is linked by a connecting segment to the collecting duct, which drains urine into the renal pelvis. The glomeruli and the convoluted tubules are in the cortex. The medulla contains the loop of Henle. The collecting duct begins in the cortex and traverses the medulla.

The kidneys perform the complex task of removing toxic metabolic wastes, such as urea and uric acid, and excessive nontoxic substances, such as water and electrolytes, from the blood. In this way the kidneys regulate the composition and volume of blood. The kidneys also influence blood pressure through complex intermediary mechanisms.

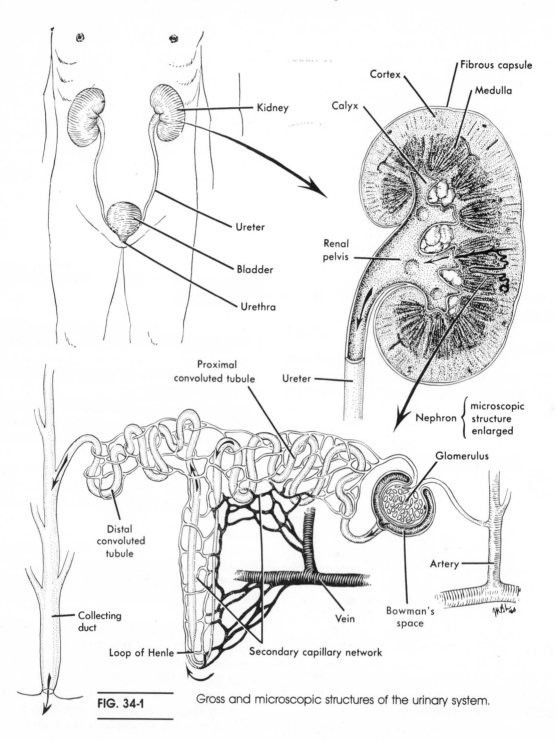

FIG. 34-1   Gross and microscopic structures of the urinary system.

Three processes are involved in the production of urine: filtration, reabsorption, and secretion.

1. *Filtration* occurs in the glomerulus. As blood flows through the lumen of the glomerular capillary, some of the water, salts, and other small molecules are filtered through capillary walls and enter Bowman's space. Blood cells, platelets, and most plasma proteins are not filtered but remain in the capillary lumen because of their large size. The liquid that has passed into Bowman's space is called the filtrate. The filtrate flows down the lumen of the tubule, where it is modified, eventually becoming urine.

2. *Reabsorption* occurs through the walls of the convoluted tubules, the loop of Henle, and the collecting duct. By means of a very complex process, the tubular cells reabsorb water, glucose, electrolytes, and other molecules from the filtrate. This reclamation process is vital to the maintenance of the fluid and electrolyte balance of the body.

3. *Secretion* takes place in the tubules. In the proximal convoluting tubules, penicillin, iodopyracet, phenolsulfonphthalein, and hippuric acid, are among the substances secreted. In the distal convoluting tubule, hydrogen ions and ammonia are secreted in the varying amounts necessary to control and maintain the acid-base balance of the body.

The modified filtrate passes from the distal convoluting tubule into the straight collecting duct where water is reabsorbed. From there it enters the renal pelvis as urine.

In the normal adult approximately 190 liters of filtrate pass through the glomeruli daily. The tubules reclaim about 188.5 liters of filtrate. The remaining filtrate is excreted as urine. The average daily urinary output of urine varies greatly with the size of the child and the fluid intake.

Ureters

In the adult the ureters are small tubes about ⅕ inch (0.5 cm) in diameter and 12 inches (30 cm) in length. (The size varies with age.) The expanded upper end of the ureter collects the urine as it forms, and peristalic waves convey the urine down the ureters and into the bladder. The ureters lie behind the peritoneum and descend from the kidney to the posterior bladder wall. They enter the bladder in an oblique manner, preventing reflux, or the backflow of urine.

Bladder

The bladder is a dome-shaped, hollow, muscular sac that stores urine. It is located directly behind the symphysis pubis. Three layers of smooth muscle form the bladder wall. These three muscular layers are collectively called the *detrusor muscle*. The outlet of the bladder is surrounded by a band of smooth muscle known as the internal sphincter. The bladder outlet and the two ureteral openings outline a triangular area called the *trigone*.

The detrusor muscle is usually relaxed, allowing the bladder to expand as needed to accommodate urine storage. After a certain volume of urine is collected, the urge to void is felt. In the child this urge is usually recognized when the bladder contains approximately 200 ml. The desire to void is recorded by the sensory parasympathetic endings in the detrusor muscle. If the child decides to void, the detrusor muscle contracts, the internal sphincter opens, and urine enters the posterior urethra. Voiding may be postponed, but when the bladder becomes very full, a point is reached at which even the most desperate efforts can no longer retain the urine.

Urethra

The urethra is a small tube that serves as a passageway for the elimination of urine from the bladder. The external opening of the urethra is called the *urethral meatus*.

The urethra is a comparatively short tube in the woman; it is about 1½ inches (3.8 cm) long. In the midportion of the female urethra is a circular striated muscle that forms the external sphincter.

The male urethra is about 8 inches (20 cm) long and also serves as part of the reproductive tract. It is divided into three sections: prostatic, membranous, and penile. The prostatic urethra is about 1 inch (2.54 cm) long and extends from the internal sphincter of the bladder through the prostrate gland to the pelvic floor. The membranous urethra is about ½ inch (1.3 cm) long and lies between the prostatic and penile sections of the urethra; it is surrounded by the external sphincter. The penile urethra is about 6 inches (15 cm) long and extends through the penis, terminating at the urethral meatus.

Urine

Urine is a transparent, amber-colored liquid with a characteristic odor. It is usually acid in reaction. The specific gravity of urine ranges from 1.003 to 1.030. Approximately 95% of urine is water. The remaining 5% consists of wastes from protein metabolism and inorganic components such as sodium and potassium chloride.

The examination of urine is the keystone in diagnosing disorders of the urinary system. A properly collected specimen can yield a wealth of information about renal function and the nature of kidney disorders. Urinalysis also reveals much information about infections and toxic and metabolic disorders.

KEY VOCABULARY Know

anuria Lack of urine formation.
albuminuria Presence of albumin in the urine.
enuresis Bed-wetting at an age when urinary control should be present.
frequency Number of repetitions of a periodic process in a unit of time; when speaking of urinary function, the term implies an abnormal increase in the number of voidings.
hematuria Presence of blood in the urine.
nocturia Excessive urination during the night.

oliguria Diminished amount of urine production with subsequent scanty urination.
polyuria Abnormally increased urinary output.
proteinuria Finding of protein, usually albumin, in the urine.
reflux Return or backward flow (e.g., regurgitation of urine from the bladder into the ureter).
uremia Toxic condition associated with renal insufficiency and the retention in the blood of nitrogenous substances normally excreted by the kidney.

ANOMALIES OF THE GENITOURINARY TRACT

The infant

The embryologic development of the urinary system is closely related to the development of the genital organs in both sexes. Because of this factor, genital and urinary tract deformities will be discussed together. Genitourinary deformities comprise 30% to 40% of all congenital anomalies. Often a deformity of the genitalia is accompanied by a deformity of the upper urinary tract. Deformities are multiple in approximately 20% of cases and often accompany anomalies in other systems (for example, imperforate anus).

Malformations of the genitourinary tract may lead to death. When the anomaly can be recognized early, surgical correction or treatment is lifesaving. This is true because many anomalies are obstructive and lead to hydronephrosis, which ultimately results in renal failure.

External deformities are obvious and readily detected. However, there is little evidence of internal disease unless it is far advanced. The nurse should be aware of this and know the few signals demanding close observation. It is important to note the number and amount of voidings in the newborn infant. Failure to void within the first 24 hours after birth is a danger sign and should be reported to the physician immediately. Abdominal enlargement or swelling in the area of a kidney also warrants immediate attention. Poor urinary stream may be a sign of a pathologic disorder in the genitourinary tract.

The signs and symptoms of urinary problems in older children are more easily detected. Crying on urination, urgent and frequent urination, straining to void, and dribbling all may point to genitourinary system difficulties. Unexplained fever, lassitude, weight loss, and failure to thrive are nondescript symptoms but may relate to advanced disease. Serious kidney infections often run a silent course. It is always wise to investigate any of the preceding signals, since renal failure can be the result of a hidden anomaly.

RENAL AGENESIS

Bilateral renal agenesis is a fatal condition. Autopsy studies have revealed that it is more common in males than in females. Patients with renal agenesis also have pulmonary hypoplasia. Lack of fetal urine causes a severe reduction in amniotic fluid that, in turn, causes the fetal parts to exert pressure on each other for prolonged periods of time, thus interfering with normal growth and development (Potter's syndrome). *Unilateral renal agenesis* is a survivable condition, but the single kidney is more likely to be diseased, since it is often located in the pelvis and associated with other malformations, especially of the ureter.

DOUBLE KIDNEY

Duplication of the kidney and ureter is more common in girls than in boys. The ureters from each double kidney may enter the bladder at different points or may unite to enter the bladder as one ureter. Sometimes the ureter from the upper kidney enters the genitourinary tract ectopically, and may cause incontinence. Duplication of the kidney and ureter is clinically significant only when other anomalies causing obstruction or infection exist.

HORSESHOE KIDNEY

A horseshoe kidney results when the lower ends of both kidneys fuse, forming a single mass shaped like a horseshoe. The kidneys lie closer to the spine and usually lower than separate kidneys do. Horseshoe kidney may be asymptomatic, but complications, especially infection, are common.

POLYCYSTIC KIDNEY

True polycystic disease is always hereditary and always bilateral. Polycystic kidneys are larger than the normal kidneys and sometimes are huge, filling the entire abdomen. They contain innumerable cysts, compressing the parenchyma. Such kidneys are constantly susceptible to infection, obstruction, and stone formation. Treatment can only be palliative. The prognosis varies with the type of polycystic kidneys. Some patients survive only a few months, but others may live into the third or fourth decade.

URETEROCELE

A ureterocele may be described as a ballooning of the lower end of the ureter because of an abnormally narrow ureteral orifice. Ureteroceles are usually unilateral. Double ureters are commonly associated with the anomaly. When an extra ureter is present, the one that enters the bladder normally is often distorted by the enormous ureterocele. As a result it becomes obstructed, and kidney infection may ensue. Treatment consists of excising the redundant portion and reconstructing the orifice so that obstruction is eliminated. If an obstruction does not exist, treatment is symptomatic.

EXSTROPHY OF THE BLADDER

Exstrophy of the bladder, fortunately, is a rare condition. It ranks with the most severe human anomalies. Because of a defect in midline closure associated with incomplete development of the pubic arch, the interior of the bladder lies completely exposed through an opening in the lower abdominal wall. A number of genital anomalies may accompany the defect.

Children who have exstrophy of the bladder become foul smelling because they are constantly soaked in urine. Often the surrounding skin becomes excoriated, causing great pain. Early in life the exposed bladder mucosa becomes inflamed, bleeds readily, and is acutely sensitive. Infection is frequent but can usually be controlled by antibiotic therapy.

Treatment is surgical. An anatomic reconstruction of the bladder is the operation of choice. The

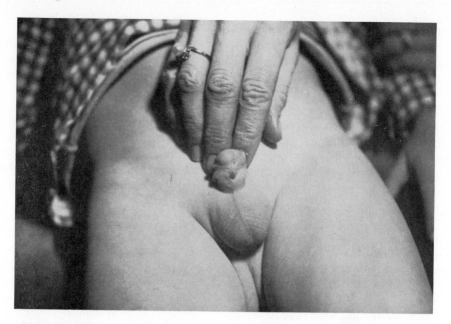

FIG. 34-2   Hypospadias (meatus located on undersurface of penis).
Courtesy Matthew Gleason, M.D., San Diego, Calif.

most desired time for this operation is when children are between 12 and 18 months old, when they
are old enough and strong enough to tolerate a long
operative procedure. After this operation the child
is totally incontinent for a period of years; during
this time the bladder grows sufficiently to make
antireflux operations possible. When the bladder
(vesicle) sphincters are made more complete and
function somewhat normally, efforts can be directed to make the child continent. Dilatation of the
ureter, reflux, and chronic infection often occur
when the child is rendered continent too early.

When the ureters are enlarged or the kidney is
damaged by infection, anatomic reconstruction of
the bladder is contraindicated. Other methods of
diverting the urine, especially ileal bladder or conduit procedures, are employed.

Exstrophy of the bladder is a survivable condition. and the prognosis depends in great measure
on the extent of renal damage resulting from defective drainage and infection.

HYPOSPADIAS

Hypospadias is a common deformity in which
the urethra terminates at some point on the ventral
(under) surface of the penis (Fig. 34-2). The position of the urethra on the penis or perineum will
determine the type of treatment. When the urethra terminates near the glans, a high circumcision
is performed so that the child can learn to direct his
urine stream. Because the prostatic urethra is never involved in hypospadias, the sphincters function
normally and the child has good urinary control.
Often a meatal stricture is associated with varying
degrees of hypospadias. When such a stricture is
recognized, it is easily corrected by dilatation or
meatotomy.

In the more severe types, a cordlike anomaly
may arc the penis downward (chordee). These
more extensive deformities all require surgical
repair to establish normal control of voiding and
make normal reproduction possible later in life.
Boys with severe types of hypospadias should not

be circumcised, since the foreskin is needed in the repair.

Treatment

Operative repair is usually done in two stages before the child enters school. In this way the child avoids severe ridicule and lasting psychologic problems.

The chordee is released early to straighten the penis and allow for normal growth. This is accomplished in the first-stage operation when the child is 2 years of age. When the child is 4 years of age or whenever the amount of local tissue permits, a second-stage operation (urethroplasty) is performed. Various plastic techniques have been employed to correct hypospadias, but the Denis Browne technique seems to be most successful.

The difficulties encountered in achieving a successful result in the correction of hypospadias are considerable. The parents should be well aware that more than one operation is usually required. They should also know that after a successful urethroplasty the penis will show scars and that some penile bowing may remain even though the child is able to urinate normally.

Postoperative care

When surgery is completed, the penis is wrapped in petroleum gauze and then covered with a dry gauze bandage. This helps to prevent postoperative swelling, pain, and bleeding. Unless this precaution is taken, necrosis of the glans may occur. A catheter drains the bladder while the incision is healing. The nurse must observe the patient carefully in order to detect swelling and bleeding.

After the operation the child is kept on his back. A bed cradle helps to prevent pressure on the operative area. Many times Stile's dressing will be used (see Fig. 33-4.)

On the second postoperative day the child may be allowed freedom of movement in his crib, provided the nurse can take time to sit, talk, and play with him. She should attempt to keep his hands busy lest he busy them with his dressing. Parents should be encouraged to stay with their children because they are usually best able to keep them constructively occupied.

EPISPADIAS

When the urethra opens on the dorsal (upper) surface of the penis, the condition is called epispadias. Various degress of epispadias may occur. However, the deformity is uncommon except when associated with exstrophy of the bladder. Treatment is the same as that for hypospadias or exstrophy.

INTERSEXUAL ANOMALIES

A semiemergency exists when simple inspection of the newborn infant's genitalia does not reveal the sex of the child. Chromosome studies are usually helpful in these cases. Exploratory abdominal surgery for gonadal biopsy may also be undertaken to identify the sex of the sexually indeterminate child.

Pseudohermaphroditism

When an individual possesses external genitalia resembling those of one sex and the gonads of the opposing sex, the condition resulting is termed "pseudohermaphroditism." Sometimes a severe hypospadias with undescended testicles or a hypertrophied clitoris and malformed labia cause problems in sex identification. Female pseudohermaphrodites possess ovaries, but their external genitalia mimic those of the male. Such masculinization of the female infant results from an overdeveloped adrenal cortex (congenital adrenal hyperplasia) and subsequent increased production of male sex hormones (androgens) by the adrenal glands. Male pseudohermaphrodites are chromosomal males, but because of some testicular dysfunction or the existence of other problems, sexual ambiguity is present.

Whatever the condition, it should be corrected, but only after the true sex has been determined. Treatment usually consists of corrective plastic procedures on the external genitalia or the administration of appropriate missing hormones.

Hermaphroditism

An extremely rare condition exists when a child possesses gonads and genitalia of both sexes. Prompt attention to this problem lessens the possibilities of serious emotional sequelae. Treatment consists of removing the gonads of one sex. Acceptable female genitalia may often be formed by relatively simple procedures. For this practical reason, when a choice can be made, the male gonad tissues are removed and the child is made female. Conversion of sex should be done as soon as possible so that the individual may have a opportunity for a normal, happy, and successful life.

CRYPTORCHIDISM

Failure of the testes (singular, *testis*) to descend into the scrotum occurs in about 1% to 5% of full-term newborns and more frequently in premature infants. This cryptorchid condition is usually unilateral and frequently associated with an inguinal hernia.

Testicular maldescent is rarely associated with symptoms. It is associated with an increased incidence of testicular injury and torsion. Other concerns are impaired fertility and a possible increased incidence of malignancy in the undescended testis. Though a definite predisposition to malignancy exists with a nonscrotal testis, early surgical correction appears to prevent this.

If spontaneous descent is to occur for a cryptorchid testis, it is usually complete by 1 year of age. If not, human chorionic gonadotropin (HCG) can be helpful as a diagnostic aid. Its use may aid descent, help differentiate between a retractile or a truly cryptorchid testis, or establish the presence or absence of bilateral intra-abdominal testes.

Should the testes not descend spontaneously or in response to HCG, surgical correction, or orchiopexy, is indicated. Though the optimal age for this step is not universally accepted, most pediatric urologists feel it should be done between the ages of 1 and 2 years. Further delay accomplishes little and may result in impaired fertility in the individual or increased danger of eventual testicular malignancy.

Early scrotal placement of the testes or placement of testicular prostheses for congenital absence is important for the child's healthy emotional and social development.

The toddler

INFECTIONS OF THE URINARY TRACT

The diagnosis of urinary tract infection requires demonstration of significant bacteruria, usually over 100,000 bacteria per ml of urine on culture of a properly collected urine specimen. Infection may be confined to the bladder (cystitis) or may spread to the upper urinary tract (pyelonephritis). In patients with pyelonephritis, the kidney may undergo irreversible damage as the result of bacterial invasion. Pyelonephritis may cause hypertension and chronic renal failure. Urinary tract infections are always considered serious and may be difficult to eradicate. Such infections are thought to rank second in frequency only to infections of the respiratory tract.

Etiologic factors

Bacteria usually enter the urinary tract by ascending the urethra. Since the female urethra is shorter than the male urethra, females have a 10 times higher incidence of urinary tract infection than males.

Obstruction of the urinary tract can predispose an individual to urinary tract infection. Sometimes urine actually flows backward from the bladder into the ureters and kidneys during voiding. This abnormality is called vesicoureteral reflux. Reflux will predispose an individual to infection and pyelonephritis.

Incidence

Urinary tract infections are relatively common in children. About 5% of all females will have urinary tract infection during the school-age years.

Anatomical abnormalities of the urinary tract

Most children with proven infection should be screened for anatomical abnormalities of the urinary tract with radiographic procedures. Both an intravenous program and a voiding cystourethrogram are necessary to assess the anatomy of the urinary tract. These studies will detect a wide variety of urinary tract abnormalities, including reflux, obstruction, renal anomalies, and stones. Radiographic studies should be performed when the infected patient is male, regardless of the patient's age. All infected females under 2 years of age and girls with repeated or severe infections must also be screened.

Clinical symptoms

Symptoms vary considerably in urinary tract infections. In children under 3 years of age the onset is likely to be abrupt and severe, accompanied by a high temperature, which may reach 104° F (40° C). Pallor, anorexia, vomiting, diarrhea, and convulsions may occur. These *acute* symptoms usually disappear in a few days with appropriate treatment.

Older children complain of localized discomfort. Sharp or dull pain in the flank or abdominal tenderness is described. Bladder symptoms such as frequent, urgent, and burning urination are also common complaints. In addition to these problems, chills and fever may be present. Some children demonstrate little or no fever, and symptoms suggestive of urinary tract infections may be almost totally lacking.

Some patients whose infections continue for a long period develop chronic pyelonephritis. Chronic pyelonephritis progresses slowly over many years. As the result of continuous low-grade infection, the patient characteristically has a history of recurrent bouts of nonspecific symptoms such as nausea, vomiting, diarrhea, fever, irritability, headache, and transitory urinary abnormalities. Poor general health, anemia, failure to grow, or failure to thrive are typical findings. The child may appear very pale or pasty looking. This condition suggests the late stages of renal damage and the development of uremia. Hypertension frequently appears as the end result of advanced renal scarring and vascular impairment and often accounts for subsequent cerebral hemorrhage or cardiac failure.

Treatment

Urinalysis and culture of a properly collected specimen is the key to successful treatment. Therapy depends primarily on identification of the causative organism and detection and correction of any urinary abnormality. A carefully collected specimen is essential. The genitalia should be washed, rinsed, and then sponged with a 1:750 benzalkonium chloride (Zephiran) solution, and dried with a sterile pad.

A clean, midstream voided specimen is collected and promptly sent to the laboratory for culture and sensitivity studies. If it is impossible to obtain a specimen by such means, a catheterized specimen may be ordered. Prompt therapy is indicated. Sulfonamides or broad-spectrum antibiotics are administered until the laboratory studies are complete. Specific medications are then ordered and continued for a period of at least 10 days to 2 weeks.

The patient should be placed in bed in a cool, quiet environment until the fever has subsided. A tepid sponge bath may also be ordered. Fluids are encouraged to ensure adequate hydration and a good urine output. An accurate account of the fluid intake and urinary output is essential. Although it is not necessary to insert a catheter for accurate output, a check mark is not sufficient for the information needed. An estimation of the amount of diaper saturation is far more valuable. After removing the diaper, the nurse should carefully wash and dry the child's genitalia before applying the clean diaper. This will prevent further contamination and also protect the skin from becoming irritated and excoriated.

An adequate diet is very important, and every attempt should be made to offer food that the child is able to eat and will eat. A good milk intake will supply the needed protein, carbohydrate, fat, and, most of all, water. The parents should be encouraged to visit during feeding time. Parents are best able to understand the sick child's desires, and usually the child is more likely to eat for Mom or Dad. A daily check of weight, blood pressure, and vital signs offers valuable clues in the early detection of complications.

REFLUX

In 20% of children with proven urinary tract infection, urine will reflux from the bladder into the ureters (vesicoureteral reflux) during voiding. This abnormality is detected by a radiographic procedure called a voiding cystourethrogram. Vesicoureteral reflux may be caused by anatomic defects in the urinary tract or by infection alone. Cystoscopy may be helpful in distinguishing between these two causes of reflux. The junction between the bladder and the ureter is only mildly abnormal when reflex is caused by infection. The abnormality will improve if the patient's urine is kept sterile by administration of antibiotics for 6 months. Surgery is usually unnecessary when reflex is caused by infection alone.

Anatomic defects in the connection between the ureter and the bladder or obstruction to urine flow in the urethra may also cause reflux. Patients with anatomic defects generally require surgery. The functional anatomy of the vesicoureteral junction can be improved by surgically reimplanting the distal ureter into the bladder wall.

Nursing care

The general postoperative care of this patient is much the same as for any surgical patient. The nurse should recognize the importance of changing surgical dressings that have become saturated with urine. Urine is an excellent medium for the growth of bacteria. However, the nurse should be aware that some surgical drains may be purposely attached to the dressings, and special care is therefore required. Some physicians wish to change the dressings themselves for this reason. Drainage tubes must be carefully checked for patency. These postoperative patients may return to the nursing area with as many as five urinary catheters, depending on the extent of the surgery (two nephrostomy tubes inserted into the left and right flanks, draining each kidney pelvis, one suprapubic cystotomy tube that empties the bladder of any urine not drained via the nephrostomy tubes, and two ureteral catheters acting as splints for the newly implanted ureters). Drainage from each of the tubes present should be closely observed and

recorded separately. These catheters are never clamped. When the patient is able to be up in a wheelchair, the catheters should be arranged so that they do not kink. The collection bottles must hang below the level of the kidneys, draining freely. Water intake is always encouraged and recorded, particularly in young children, who quickly dehydrate. Dehydration promotes the growth of bacteria.

Pain is commonly associated with this type of surgery. Narcotics should be given as ordered on time! Antispasmodic drugs such as propantheline bromide (Pro-Banthine) or methantheline bromide (Banthine bromide) are also ordered. These drugs usually relieve the immediate postoperative colicky pain.

Reflux associated with renal involvement may also be caused by lower tract congenital obstructions. Unless the obstruction is corrected by reconstructive surgery when indicated, pyelonephritis may progress, leading to severe renal impairment.

Prognosis

When the disease is recognized early and treated properly (long-term antibiotic therapy for infection or surgical removal of obstructions), the prognosis is excellent. Chronic infections present a much more serious and difficult problem because severe renal damage is the ultimate result.

WILMS' TUMOR

Wilms' tumor is one of the most common abdominal neoplasms of childhood. It is a congenital, mixed renal tumor that develops from abnormal embryonic tissue; it rarely occurs bilaterally. Composed of varying ratios of abnormal glomerulotubular structures, connective tissue, muscle and blood vessels the tumor initially grows with the renal capsule. As it grows larger it distorts the kidney in a bizarre manner and may occupy as much as one half of the abdominal cavity. Unfortunately the tumor often invades the renal veins and metastasizes through the bloodstream to vital organs, especially to the lungs. Extension of the tumor through the renal capsule into surrounding tissues may occur and has also been associated with a poor prognosis.

Etiologic factors

Like other forms of cancer, the exact cause of Wilms' tumor is unknown.

Incidence

Wilms' tumor accounts for approximately 7% of all cancer in children. Boys and girls are equally affected. About two thirds of all children with Wilms' tumor are diagnosed before they are 3 years of age. The tumor may be present at birth and is rare after 7 years of age.

Clinical features

The initial manifestation of Wilms' tumor is a mass in the region of the kidney that is usually discovered by the parents in the course of daily care or may be discovered accidentally during a routine examination. As the tumor grows, the child's abdomen becomes very large, and pressure symptoms arise. Constipation, vomiting, abdominal distention, and even dyspnea may occur. Weight loss, pallor, and anemia are common in the late stages. Pain, hematuria, and hypertension are uncommon but, if present, they support the diagnosis of a renal tumor.

Treatment and nursing care

When Wilms' tumor is suspected, both the parent and nurse must be careful not to feel or touch the child's abdomen because handling might cause rupture of the tumor through the renal capsule and metastasis via the bloodstream. Diagnosis is usually confirmed by intravenous pyelography. Occasionally, retrograde pyelography, renal arteriography, or computerized tomography are necessary to evaluate the extent of the tumor. The choice of therapy is guided by the age of the child, extent of the tumor, metastatic considerations, and stage of the disease at the time of diagnosis. Treatment usually consists of prompt radical nephrectomy, radiation therapy, and chemotherapy.

The kidney, tumor, and perirenal fat are removed through a transabdominal approach. Blood transfusions are often given to replace blood lost during the surgical procedure and to correct preexisting anemia. Intravenous administration of fluids is continued for 24 hours. When patients return to the ward, they usually assume a position of comfort. If bleeding occurs, it can easily be detected when pulse rate, respirations, blood pressure, and the child's color are checked often. The dressings should be changed only if necessary, since little or no drainage occurs from the incision.

Actinomycin D has a significant antitumor effect and is particularly useful in the prevention of pulmonary metastases. Vincristine has also been a highly effective drug in the treatment of Wilms' tumor. When both drugs are used in combination, the survival rate is significantly greater. Actinomycin D potentiates radiation and therefore should begin on the first day of therapy. When indicated, courses of combination drug therapy are given at the time of resection, 6 weeks later, and every 3 months for a 15-month period. Side effects from the administration of chemotherapy and radiation therapy include nausea, vomiting, anorexia, malaise, diarrhea and loss of hair. During the interval between medication and x-ray therapy, the child's hair usually grows back. Bone marrow depression, ulceration of the mucous membranes, and peripheral neuropathies are manifestations of acute toxicity associated with the administration of actinomycin D and vincristine. Drug therapy may be temporarily discontinued to allow the child to recover from the toxicity of the treatment.

Complications

The most serious complication in Wilms' tumor is metastasis. Characteristically, Wilms' tumor metastasizes through the blood-stream to the liver, lungs, brain and other vital organs. The tumor may also spread by direct extension or by the lymphatics.

Prognosis

Wilms' tumor is uniformly fatal if not treated and until recently has had high mortality rates despite treatment. However, major therapeutic advances in the last decade relating to the use of surgery, radiation therapy, and combination chemotherapy have led to the current expectation that more than 80% of children with Wilms' tumor can be cured of their disease. Although the prognosis is better when the tumor is discovered early, the use of combined modality therapy offers children with metastatic disease a good chance for cure. Follow-up care includes frequent x-ray examinations of the lungs and other areas of potential tumor involvement and close monitoring of the remaining normal kidney. As the child progresses favorably, less frequent examinations are required, but annual examinations are recommended to follow normal development and to detect any late effects of treatment.

HYPERTENSION AND RENAL DISEASE

Measurement of blood pressure in children can be very difficult. The patient should be as quiet as possible. The blood pressure cuff should cover at least two thirds of the upper arm. Repeated measurements may be required to establish an accurate average reading of the patient. Normal blood pressure is related to age and weight. Technically, high blood pressure, or hypertension, is defined as a blood pressure over two standard deviations above the mean for the age in question. For a child 5 years of age, the upper limit of normal is 110/80.

There are two basic categories of hypertension: borderline hypertension and definite hypertension. Patients with blood pressure over 140/90 are said to have definite hypertension. Patients with blood pressure elevated for age but less than 140/90 have borderline hypertension. Thus, a 5-year-old with a blood pressure of 135/85 would have borderline hypertension.

Investigators are currently collecting data on patients with borderline hypertension. From early studies it appears these patients rarely have a known underlying cause for their hypertension. Borderline hypertension is thus "essential" or idiopathic, and a diagnostic workup is deemed unnecessary. Dietary salt restriction may be recommended for control of borderline hypertension. Use of antihypertensive drugs in these patients is controversial.

Children with definite hypertension usually have an underlying disease causing the hypertension. The most common cause of hypertension in children is renal disease. Renal tumors, renal vascular disease, hydronephrosis, and glomerulonephritis may cause hypertension. Occasionally, excess secretion of catecholamines or aldosterone by a tumor may cause hypertension in a child. Careful diagnostic workups are mandatory in children with definite hypertension.

Patients with definite hypertension are prone to develop target organ disease. Congestive heart failure may occur. Blood vessels may also be damaged. Children with severe hypertension—blood pressure over 160/110—may suddenly develop target organ damage. Common signs and symptoms are headache, visual disturbance, tinnitus, seizures, and coma. Sometimes hemorrhages, exudates, and arterial spasm can be viewed in the retinal vessels with an ophthalmoscope. These changes are called hypertensive retinopathy. Severe symptomatic hypertension is a medical emergency requiring prompt treatment.

Treatment of hypertension depends on its cause. Tumors should be surgically excised. Surgeons can also repair renal artery stenosis and hydronephrosis. In other cases, drugs are effective. Propranolol (Inderal), hydralazine (Apresoline), and diazoxide (Hyperstat) are commonly used drugs. Diuretics also will help lower blood pressure. New agents such as captopril (Capoten) and minoxidil (Loniten) are helpful in severe hypertension. The patient must be carefully monitored for drug side effects. Aggressive medical management is important to lower the risk of stroke and other types of vascular injury.

The preschool child

NEPHROTIC SYNDROME OF CHILDHOOD (MINIMAL CHANGE NEPHROTIC SYNDROME)

Nephrotic syndrome is a chronic renal disease characterized by anasarca (severe generalized edema), heavy proteinuria, low serum albumin levels,

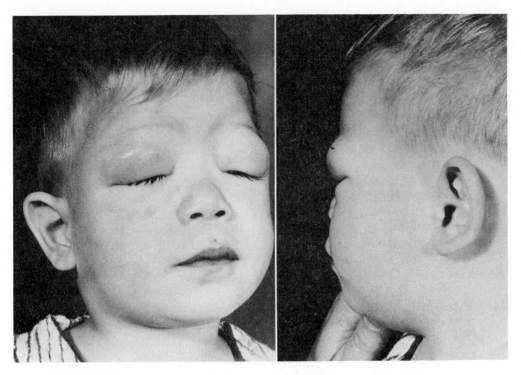

FIG. 34-3   A 2-year-old child with nephrotic syndrome. Progressive periorbital edema.
Courtesy Naval Regional Medical Center, San Diego, Calif.

and high serum cholesterol values. Elevated blood pressure and hematuria are not typical of the disease.

Etiologic factors

In 80% of children with nephrotic syndrome, the renal biopsy shows only minimal abnormalities. This disease is also called lipoid nephrosis, idiopathic nephrotic syndrome of childhood, or minimal change nephrotic syndrome. In these patients the cause of nephrotic syndrome is unknown. In the remaining 20%, renal biopsies may show abnormalities such as glomerulonephritis. These patients will be discussed in the section on chronic glomerulonephritis.

Incidence

The disease seems to be more common in boys than in girls, and occurs most frequently between 2

and 6 years of age. The incidence of nephrotic syndrome in childhood is 7 per 100,000.

Clinical symptoms

The onset of nephrotic syndrome is insidious. Periorbital puffiness may be the first sign. In severe cases, it progresses steadily until the eyes are closed (Fig. 34-3). As the edema increases, the arms, legs, and abdomen reach massive proportions. At the peak of the edema, the child can weigh almost twice as much as usual (Fig. 34-4). Anorexia and varying degrees of diarrhea are commonly found. Discomfort from massive edema causes the child to be irritable and easily fatigued. Anasarca may lead to inadequate ventilation.

Complications

The nephrotic child is vulnerable to infections, probably because of loss of gamma globulin in the

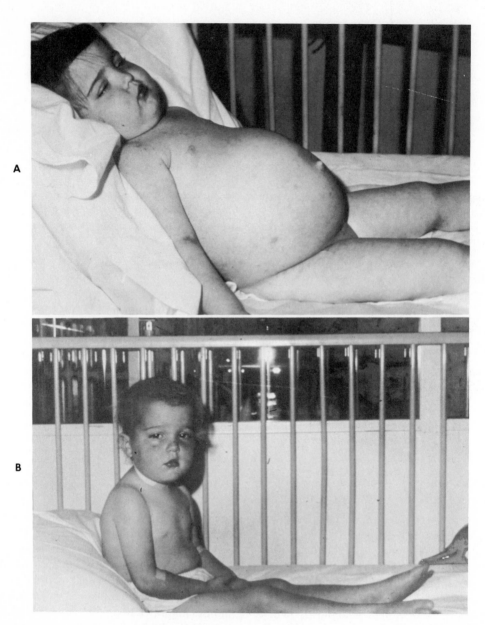

FIG. 34-4   A 2½-year-old child with nephrotic syndrome. **A,** Before therapy. **B,** After therapy.
Courtesy Naval Regional Medical Center, San Diego, Calif.

urine (proteinuria). Bacteremia associated with peritonitis is common. Upper respiratory tract infections are highly dangerous, especially those caused by pneumococci. Infections are the leading cause of death in patients with minimal change nephrotic syndrome.

Treatment and nursing care

The goal of treatment is a child as nearly normal as possible, judged by both clinical well-being and laboratory findings. The aims of nursing care include comforting the patient during the distresses of massive edema, maintaining good nutrition, and preventing intercurrent infections.

If the edema is severe, intravenous albumin and diuretics may be administered to increase urine production immediately. Most patients with minimal change nephrotic syndrome will respond to steroid therapy. Prednisone, 2 mg/kg/day, will reverse the proteinuria, often within 10 to 14 days. When proteinuria ceases, urine output improves, serum albumin normalizes, and edema disappears. During remission the steroid therapy is gradually withdrawn. Some patients will stay in remission on no medication; other patients will require maintenance therapy. Maintenance prednisone is usually given every other day to minimize side effects. Alkylating agents such as cyclophosphamide or chlorambucil may produce a prolonged remission in some patients.

Relapses of nephrotic syndrome are often associated with intercurrent infections, especially those involving the respiratory and urinary tracts. Immediate intensive antibiotic therapy is mandatory if infection arises.

In selecting a hospital room for the nephrotic child, the nurse must remember the child's increased susceptibility to infection. Placing the child in a double room with another child the same age who has nephrotic syndrome is most desirable.

Weighing the child on admission and each morning thereafter is one way of evaluating the amount of edema present. A daily abdominal girth measurement taken in flat position at the level of the umbilicus just after a breath is exhaled is also helpful. If massive edema is present, the child's self-concept is likely to be greatly distorted. It is important for the parents to be reassured and to be given whatever information is necessary about the condition and its outcome so that they in turn can reassure their child. They should particularly realize the seriousness of the disorder, even though the prognosis is now better than ever before.

Massive edema is most uncomfortable. The skin is stretched thin and easily broken. Keeping the child's body dry and clean will help prevent skin infections. Application of powder between skin surfaces and in skin folds is soothing and protective. If the child is not toilet trained, the nurse must take great care to prevent excoriation of the buttocks and genitalia. Medicines are given orally or intravenously but never by the intramuscular or subcutaneous route. Great care must be taken to protect the edematous skin from injury and subsequent secondary infection. Usually the child is most comfortable in a semi-Fowler's position to reduce respiratory embarrassment. This position may also reduce periorbital edema.

Maintenance of good nutrition is essential, because beneath the edema exists a thin, poorly nourished body. The child should be given a well-balanced high-protein diet. Salty foods such as potato chips and pickles should be avoided. Restriction of fluid intake may be necessary to control edema. Allowing the child some choice will encourage appetite and help prevent severe nutritional depletion, which readily occurs.

An accurate account of fluid intake is very important when the output is scanty. Although the nurse may not be able to measure the exact output, she must record approximate amounts each time the child voids.

Bed rest is recommended until diuresis has begun. During the active phase of the disease, the child is usually sluggish and therefore satisfied to be resting most of the time. When massive edema is present, the child is content to rest all the time.

After discharge from the hospital, the child is

periodically examined until the prednisone has been discontinued without any relapses. Although infection is a common complication in these children while they are receiving prednisone, it is not necessary to interfere with their normal home and school activities. If an outbreak of some infectious disease such as chicken pox (varicella) should occur at school, it is wise to have the child remain at home. Any sign of intercurrent infection must be reported to the physician and treated immediately. Some physicians would rather overtreat than risk the child's life to this most common cause of death.

Prognosis

By controlling infection, antibiotic therapy has greatly reduced the death rate of nephrotic patients. About 80% of the children respond to steroid therapy. Eventually, after many years of intermittent treatment, these children usually fully enjoy healthful living with normal kidneys and absence of medication. Progression to end-stage renal disease is unusual.

The school-age child

ACUTE GLOMERULONEPHRITIS (NEPHRITIS, OR BRIGHT'S DISEASE)

Acute glomerulonephritis is an inflammatory disease of the glomeruli affecting both kidneys. The clinical manifestations include gross hematuria, often with cola-colored urine, edema, proteinuria, casts, hypertension, and elevated amounts of nitrogen products in the bloodstream (azotemia).

Etiologic factors

Streptococcal infection is the most common cause of acute glomerulonephritis. The infection precedes the onset of glomerulonephritis by 1 to 3 weeks. Other infectious agents such as pneumococcus, hepatitis virus, or Epstein-Barr virus can also cause acute glomerulonephritis.

Patients with acute glomerulonephritis should be carefully studied to determine the infectious etiology. Since group A streptococcus is the most common cause, streptozyme titer test, antistreptolysin titer test, and direct culture of the pharynx or skin lesions are essential.

Incidence

Glomerulonephritis is common in children, especially between 5 and 10 years of age. It seems to be more common in boys than in girls and is most frequently observed in the late winter months or early spring. This seasonal pattern is related to the peak incidence of streptococcal infections of the upper respiratory tract.

Symptoms

Acute glomerulonephritis is not always recognized because clinical signs and symptoms vary greatly. Microscopic hematuria and proteinuria may be the only signs, or gross hematuria and proteinuria, edema, periorbital puffiness, hypertension, weakness, pallor, anorexia, headache, nausea, and vomiting may be present. Rarely, onset is sudden, with severe symptoms followed by dysfunction of the brain because of hypertension.

Treatment and nursing care

Necessary bed rest is usually welcomed by the child during the acute phase of the disease. Activities may be resumed as soon as gross hematuria has cleared and signs of edema, hypertension, and other urinary abnormalities have subsided.

These children should be separated from other children who have infections (especially of the upper respiratory tract), but complete isolation is not indicated. They should be observed closely for any recurrences of upper respiratory tract infection. Exacerbations rarely occur with new strains of streptococcal organisms. Reinfection by the same nephritogenic strain is generally not possible by virtue of type-specific immunity after infection. Antibiotic therapy is indicated when evidence of infection is present. Prophylactic use of penicillin in the prevention of recurrence of glomerulonephritis is not recommended.

A regular diet without added salt is offered to the

child whose case is uncomplicated. Fluid restriction may be required for some patients. Careful observation of the color and volume of urine serves as a valuable guide in controlling fluid balance. Samples of successive voidings (aliquot urines) may be saved in test tubes, labeled, and placed on a rack for comparison by the physician and nurses. Measurement of fluid intake, urinary output, and daily weight aids recognition of early signs of edema.

Temperature and pulse and respiration rates are checked frequently. Blood pressure should be checked often with the proper size of sphygmomanometer. The cuff should cover two thirds of the upper arm and should be applied smoothly.

Complications

Changes in physical and mental status such as drowsiness, lethargy, double vision, muscular twitching, and convulsions should be reported at once. Complications can be discovered early when the observant nurse is aware of the clues that indicate that all is not well.

Hypertensive encephalopathy. Hypertensive encephalopathy is characterized by irritability, headache, vomiting, and blurred or double vision. Convulsions may also occur. The rise in blood pressure is almost always accompanied by a drop in pulse rate. This complication is caused by lack of proper blood supply to the brain, resulting from vasospasm. It usually responds to antihypertensive drug therapy.

Cardiac decompensation. Cardiac decompensation occurs as a result of severe hypertension and fluid overload. Signs of cardiac involvement are tachycardia, arrhythmia, rapid, difficult breathing, and heart enlargement. Treatment with diuretics and antihypertensive medication should be started immediately. If these measures do not improve the patient's condition, then dialysis should be undertaken. Other measures include rest in the orthopenic position, administration of oxygen, and sedation. Digitalization is not necessary unless severe heart failure ensues. Cardiac involvement is greatly decreased when hypertension is adequately controlled and fluid overload is corrected.

Severe renal failure. Severe renal failure is uncommon in children, although urine production at times may become scanty or absent. Usually this acute situation is transitory and reversible. When an imbalance of fluids and electrolytes persists, peritoneal dialysis or hemodialysis may be needed to control the uremia.

Prognosis

Acute glomerulonephritis is usually a self-limiting condition, and most children recover completely. A few children present a more complex entity with persistent urinary abnormalities and hypertension, which ultimately results in chronic nephritis and death.

CHRONIC GLOMERULONEPHRITIS

Chronic glomerulonephritis is a major cause of kidney failure in children.

Etiologic factors

There are many causes of chronic glomerulonephritis. Systemic infections, hereditary diseases, drugs, and toxins are known causes. Renal biopsy can be helpful in defining the type and the prognosis of nephritis.

Clinical symptoms

Gross hematuria, edema, severe hypertension, and anemia may be initial symptoms. Some patients with glomerulonephritis have nephrotic syndrome. These patients usually differ clinically from patients with minimal change nephrotic syndrome, discussed earlier.

Complications

Hypertension, anemia, growth failure, nephrotic syndrome, and end-stage renal disease are common complications of chronic glomerulonephritis.

Prognosis

The majority of patients, untreated, will develop chronic renal failure and end-stage renal disease (see discussion on p. 754). The onset of end-stage renal disease varies in length from a few months to 10 to 20 years.

Treatment and nursing care

In general chronic glomerulonephritis is difficult to treat; the nephrotic syndrome associated with chronic glomerulonephritis does not improve with oral prednisone therapy. However, recent studies have shown that some forms of glomerulonephritis can be improved with new treatments. Removal of blood plasma, performed by an automated plasma exchange, may improve certain patients. High-dose steroid therapy—methylprednisolone (Solu-Medrol) 30 mg/kg—given intravenously may also improve renal function. Sometimes treatments to reverse the destructive inflammation in the kidney are unsuccessful. These patients develop end-stage renal disease and require kidney transplants or dialysis.

Patients with chronic glomerulonephritis may be hospitalized for a course of treatment or for complications. They should be watched closely for hypertension. Daily weights are critical for estimating fluid balance. Frequently these children are very anxious and will benefit greatly from kind and understanding nursing care. Exposure to infectious illnesses should be avoided.

END-STAGE RENAL DISEASE

The term end-stage renal disease refers to patients with severe failure of the kidney function. This occurs when kidney function, as measured by creatinine clearance, is less than 10% of normal.

Incidence

Each year two to three children per million total population develop end-stage renal disease.

Etiology

Congenital defects, toxins, glomerulonephritis, obstruction of the urinary tract, and pyelonephritis may cause end-stage renal disease.

Symptoms

Patients are lethargic and anorexic. Confusion, seizures, and coma may also be observed. Pallor caused by anemia is often notable. Growth retardation is common.

Treatment and nursing care

There are three treatments for patients with end-stage renal disease: renal transplantation, peritoneal dialysis, and hemodialysis. Each treatment has advantages and disadvantages. Treated with combinations of these courses of care, children with severe renal failure can survive for many years. Almost all these patients attend school and participate in normal activities, with the possible exception of strenuous physical exercise. Nursing care for these patients is very rewarding and challenging.

Enuresis

Enuresis may be defined as involuntary voiding of urine, especially at night (nocturnal enuresis), after 4 years of age. However, there appears to be a rather wide age range associated with the neuromuscular maturation of urinary sphincter control. Children with nocturnal enuresis usually have a normal urinary stream and good daytime bladder control. Enuresis may be primary or acquired. When bladder control has never been achieved, enuresis is said to be primary. If enuresis occurs after control has been achieved for at least 1 year, it is said to be acquired.

About 15% of pediatric patients are evaluated because of this disturbance. Enuresis is very common in childhood, and the condition is more prevalent in boys than in girls.

The exact cause of enuresis in most children is unknown. Psychologic or developmental disorders are found in many patients, but enuresis may also be caused by an anatomic defect or a systemic disease. The most significant step toward solving the problem is an attempt to find the correct cause. Before a psychologic explanation is sought, anatomic abnormalities and organic disease must be ruled out.

Generally daytime wetting (diurnal enuresis) and other urologic symptoms are associated with organic disease. Diabetes mellitus, urinary tract infection, urinary tract anomalies, neurologic defects, and obstructions such as meatal stenosis are often responsible for the condition. Psychologic problems also account for some cases of enuresis. Improper toilet training, an unhappy environment, a poor mother-child relationship, immaturity associated with other infantile habits, and developmental disturbances such as jealousy and insecurity are some psychologic causes of enuresis. Whatever the cause, the correction of enuresis is highly important to both these children and their parents. It enables children to develop normally and to be like their friends, and it offers the parents peace of mind and a healthy child.

Every enuretic patient should have a careful medical history and physical examination performed to determine if renal enlargements, a distended bladder, a constriction of the external urinary meatus, or a neurologic change is present. An extremely careful urinalysis and urine culture are essential. Intravenous urography, cystography, and cystoscopy are sometimes necessary to diagnose organic causes, since sometimes history and physical examination may be entirely within normal limits.

Imipramine hydrochloride (Tofranil) has been found to control the condition completely in some patients. This drug, however, has some potential toxic manifestations. Thus a physician must carefully evaluate the problem before ordering imipramine hydrochloride, and if it is indicated, the child must be carefully watched for side effects. Facial tics have been reported.

A condition often confused with enuresis is an ectopic ureter in a girl in which the ueter empties into the vagina or urethra beyond the sphincter. These children may void normally (from their normal ureters and bladder) but are always wet from constant drainage from the ectopic ureter. Surgery will correct this problem.

Enuresis may also diminish through the use of fairly simple techniques. Giving less fluids in the evening may be helpful to some children. Waking children and taking them to the toilet during the night saves embarrassment to school-age children.

Some children, principally those who have had deep sleep patterns, have benefited from the use of mechanical devices that wake them with lights or alarms when the bed becomes wet. Consistent use of these detectors and the associated programs recommended may encourage lighter sleep, more awareness of bladder filling, and fewer accidents.

Parents should not threaten or punish their children because they wet the bed. This only increases the child's sense of inferiority and failure and may even deter the will to improve. Instead, every effort should be made to assure children that they can overcome the condition if they really want to. Encouragement comes in the form of rewards (for example, being able to go camping or sleep overnight at grandmother's house). Such rewards, together with the child's desire to stay dry, can achieve positive results. Enuretic children without any organic disease or severe psychologic problem usually gradually overcome the condition by age 10 to 12 years.

TORSION OF THE TESTIS

Contraction of the cremaster muscle not only elevates the testis but rotates it outward. Depending on the degree of twisting, torsion of the spermatic cord usually causes severe scrotal pain as the result of an interruption of the blood supply and ensuing necrosis of the testis. Torsion may occur at any age and is not uncommon in the adolescent. It may occur while sleeping, playing games, or jumping into cold water. To preserve the fertility and viability of the testis, prompt diagnosis and action must be taken to relieve the condition. Immediate steps, such as manipulative reduction or surgical intervention to untwist the testis, are necessary to save the organ. Surgical exploration must be done within 6 hours to verify the success of any manipulative attempts to reduce the malrotation. Bilateral orchiopexy (fixation of both testes in the scrotum) is usually performed, since recurrence occurs frequently.

CONDITIONS INVOLVING THE INTEGUMENTARY SYSTEM

Burns

Allyn, P., and Bartlett, R.: Management of the burn patient. In Zschoche, D.A., editor: Mosby's comprehensive review of critical care, ed. 2, St. Louis, 1981, The C.V. Mosby Co.

Bailey, W.C., editor: Pediatric burns, Chicago, 1979, Yearbook Medical Publishers.

Frank, H.: Emergency management of burns. In Warner, C.G., editor: Emergency care: assessment and intervention, ed. 2, St. Louis, 1978, The C.V. Mosby Co.

Kingie, V., and Lau, N.: What to do for the severely burned, RN **43**:46-51, Apr. 1980.

Lushbaugh, M.A.: Critical care of the child with burns, Nurs. Clin. North Am. **16**:635-646, Dec. 1981.

McHugh, M.L., Dimitroff, K., and Dinsmore, N.: Family support group in a burn unit, Am. J. Nurs. **79**:2148-2150, Dec. 1979.

Schumann, L., and Gasfon, S.: Common-sense guide to topical burn therapy, Nurs. '79 **9**:34-39, Mar. 1979.

Severely burned patients: anticipating their emotional needs, Nurs. '80, **10**:46-50, Sept. 1980.

Van Oss, S.: Emergency burn care: those crucial first minutes, RN **45**:44-49, Oct. 1982.

Wooldridge, M., and Surveyer, J.A.: Skin grafting for full-thickness burn injury, Am. J. Nurs. **80**:2000-2004, Nov. 1980.

Common skin problems

Bielan, B.: What that rash really means, RN **42**:58-63, Feb. 1979.

Black skin problems, Am. J. Nurs. **79**:1092-1094, June 1979.

DeLoughery, M.: Sunburn: prevention and treatment, Nurs. Pract. **6**:28-30, May-June 1981.

Fleming, J.W.: Common dermatologic conditions in children, Am. J. Mat. Child Nurs. **6**:346-354, Sept.-Oct. 1981.

Hand, J.: Lice: how to break the news gently, RN **42**:27-29, Nov. 1979.

Hurwitz, S.: Atopic dermatitis, Pediatr. Ann. **11**:237-250, Feb. 1982.

Hurwitz, S.: Update: scabies in childhood, Pediatr. Ann. **11**:226-235, Feb. 1982.

Larrow, L., and Noe, J.: Port-wine stain hemangiomas, Am. J. Nurs. **82**:786-790, May 1982.

Norins, A.L., and Treadwell, P.A.: The management of persistant pediatric skin problems, Pediatr. Clin. North Am. **29**:37-53, Feb. 1982.

Quan, M.A., et al: Treatment of acne vulgaris, J. Fam. Pract. **11**:1029-1035, Dec. 1980.

Rubin, A.: Black skin: how to adjust assessment and care, RN **42**:31-35, Mar. 1979.

Welch, L.B.: Pediculosis at summer camp, Am. J. Nurs. **79**:1073, June 1979.

ISOLATION TECHNIQUE AND COMMUNICABLE CHILDHOOD DISEASES

Infectious diseases

Brown, S.G.: The devastating effects of congenital rubella, Am. J. Mat. Child Nurs. **4**:171-173, May-June 1979.

Bryan, E.M., and Nicholson, E.: Congenital syphilis: a study of physical and biochemical aspects, Clin. Pediatr. **20**:81-87, Feb. 1981.

CDC: Annual summary, 1980, reported morbidity and mortality in the U.S. MMWR **29**:54, Sept. 1981.

CDC: Genital herpes infection, U.S. 1966-1979, MMWR **31**:137-140, 145, Mar. 26, 1982.

CDC: Immune globulins for protection against viral hepatitis, MMWR **30**:421-435, Sept. 4, 1981.

CDC: Syphilis trends in the United States, MMWR **30**:441-443, Sept. 11, 1981.

CDC: Varicella-zoster immune globulin, MMWR **30**:15-16; 21-23, Jan. 23, 1981.

Claypool, J.M.: Rubella protection for maternal child health care providers, Am. J. Mat. Child Nurs. **6**:53-56, Jan.-Feb. 1981.

Gennaros, S.: Listerial infection: nursing care of mother and infant, Am. J. Mat. Child Nurs. **5**:390-392, Nov.-Dec. 1980.

Giese, C.J.D.: Protocol: varicella, Nurse Pract. **6**:10-13, Sept. Oct. 1981.

Grow, D.H.: Reye's syndrome, Nurs. '81 **11**:156-158, Nov. 1981.

Hodes, H.L.: Diphtheria, Pediatr. Clin. North Am. **26:**445-459, May 1979.

Jackson, M.M.: Viral hepatitis, Nurs. Clin. North Am. **15:**729-746, Dec. 1980.

Kinsel, C., Ferguson, K., and Roll, L.J.: Human rabies, Am. J. Nurs. **81:**1174-1179, June 1981.

Massey, K.: Rocky mountain spotted fever: a national disease, Am. J. Mat. Child Nurs. **7:**104-109, Mar.-Apr. 1982.

Potter, S.: Critical infections in the pediatric oncologic patient, Nurs. Clin. North Am. **16:**699-704, Dec. 1981.

Rogers, E.L., and Rogers, M.C.: Fulminant hepatic failure and hepatic encephalopathy, Pediatr. Clin. North Am. **27:**701-703, Aug. 1980.

Sever, J.L.: Congenital rubella: keeping up the fight, Contemp. OB/GYN **9:**137-140, May 1977.

Shetler, M.G., and Bartos, H.: Is it a fungal infection, or VD? RN **44:**66-69, Apr. 1981.

Shurin, S.B.: Infectious mononucleosis, Pediatr. Clin. North Am. **26:**315-326, May 1979.

Spires, R.: Tuberculosis today: the seige isn't over yet, RN **43:**42-47, Aug. 1980.

Stoll, B.J.: Tetanus, Pediatr. Clin. North Am. **26:**415-431, May 1979.

Control of infectious disease

American Academy of Pediatrics: Report of the committee on infectious diseases, ed. 19, Evanston, Ill., 1982, The Academy.

Arking, L.M., and McArthur, B.J., guest editors: Infection, Nurs. Clin. North Am. **16:**(entire volume), Dec. 1980.

Benenson, A.S., editor: Control of communicable diseases in man, ed. 4, Washington, D.C., 1982, American Public Health Assoc.

Feigin, R.D., and Cherry, J.D.: Textbook of pediatric infectious diseases, Philadelphia, 1981, W.B. Saunders Co.

Krugman, S., and Katz, S.L.: Infectious diseases of children, ed. 7, St. Louis, 1981, The C.V. Mosby Co.

Moffett, H.L.: Pediatric infectious diseases, ed. 2, Philadelphia, 1981, J.B. Lippincott Co.

Prevention of hospital-acquired infection

Brandt, S.L., and Benner, P.: Infection control in hospitals: what are the challenges, Am. J. Nurs. **80:**432-434, Mar. 1980.

Hargiss, C.D., and Larson, E.: Guidelines for prevention of hospital-acquired infection, Am. J. Nurs. **81:**2175-2183, Dec. 1981.

Mallison, G.F.: Decontamination, disinfection and sterilization, Nurs. Clin. North Am. **15:**757-768, Dec. 1980.

Meehan, R.M.: Isolation—to be or not to be afraid, Am. J. Mat. Child Nurs. **5:**257-261, July-Aug. 1980.

Nadolny, M.D.: Infection control in hospitals: what does the infection control nurse do? Am. J. Nurs. **80:**430-431, Mar. 1980.

Umpherous, J.H.: Bacterial colonization in neonates with sibling visitation, JOGN Nurs. **9:**73-75, Mar.-Apr. 1980.

CONDITIONS INVOLVING THE NEUROMUSCULAR AND SKELETAL SYSTEMS

General

Brady, M.H.: Lifelong care of the child with Duchenne muscular dystrophy, Am. J. Mat. Child Nurs. **4:**227-230, July-Aug. 1979.

Cantwell, D.P.: The hyperactive child, Pediatr. Nurs. **5:**11-22, Sept.-Oct. 1979.

Chusid, M.J., and Sty, J.R.: Pneumococcal arthritis and osteomyelitis in children, Clin. Pediatr. **20:**105-107, Feb. 1981.

Conway, B.L.: Pediatric neurologic nursing, St. Louis, 1977, The C.V. Mosby Co.

Crossland, S., and Deyerle, W.M.: Compartmental syndromes, Nurs. '80 **10:**51-53, Nov. 1980.

Damon, J., and Taylor, L.F.: Brain tumors in children, Pediatr. Clin. North Am. **15:**99-113, Mar. 1980.

Davis, G.T., and Hill, P.M.: Cerebral palsy, Pediatr. Clin. North Am. **15:**35-50, Mar. 1980.

Friedman, A., and Fleisher, G.: Meningitis: update of recommendations for the neonate, Clin. Pediatr. **19:**395-397, June 1980.

Gaddy, D.S.: Meningitis in the pediatric population, Pediatr. Clin. North Am. **15:**83-97, Mar. 1980.

Gutowicz, L., and Boenning, D.W.: Septic hip in a child, J. Fam. Pract. **12:**841-845, May 1981.

Hausman, K.A.: Critical care of the child with increased intracranial pressure, Nurs. Clin. North Am. **16:**647-656, Dec. 1981.

Leonidas, J.C., et al: Head trauma in children, Pediatrics **69:**139-143, Feb. 1982.

Lupien, A.E.: Head off compartment syndrome before it's too late, RN **43:**38-41, Dec. 1980.

McCarthy, A.M. Chronic headaches in children, Pediatr. Nurs. **8:**88-93, Mar.-Apr. 1982.

McCarthy, P.L., et al: Evaluation of arthritis and arthralgia in the pediatric patient, Clin. Pediatr. **19**:183-190, Mar. 1980.

McElroy, D.B., Davis G.T., guest editors: Nurs. Clin. North Am. **15**:1-127, Mar. 1980.

Miller, B.K.,: How to spot . . . and treat . . . carpal tunnel syndrome . . . early, Nurs. '80, **10**:50-53, Mar. 1980.

Passo, M.H.: Aches and limb pain, Pediatr. Clin. North Am. **29**:209-219, Feb. 1982.

Shinnar, S., and D'Souza, B.J.: The diagnosis and management of headaches in childhood, Pediatr. Clin. North Am. **29**:79-94, Feb. 1982.

Siegel, I.M.: Maintenance of ambulation in Duchenne muscular dystrophy: the role of the orthopedic surgeon, Clin. Pediatr. **19**:383-388, June 1980.

Spruck, M.: Gold therapy for rheumatoid arthritis, Am. J. Nurs. **79**:1246-1248, July 1979.

Stout, J.A., and Gibbs, K.R.: The child undergoing a leg-lengthening procedure, Am. J. Nurs. **81**:1152-1155, June 1981.

Trauner, D.A.: Childhood neurological problems, Chicago, 1979, Yearbook Medical Publishers, Inc.

Wald, E.R., et al: Pitfalls in the diagnosis of acute osteomyelitis by bone scan, Clin. Pediatr. **19**:597-600, Sept. 1980.

Walleck, C.: Head trauma in children, Pediatr. Clin. North Am. **15**:115-127, Mar. 1980.

Hearing and vision

Beauchamp, G.R.: Causes of visual impairment in children, Pediatr. Ann. **9**:13-22, Nov. 1980.

Bergstrom, L.V.: Causes of severe hearing loss in early childhood, Pediatr. Ann. **9**:23-30, Jan. 1980.

Holland, S.H.: 20/20 vision screening, Pediatr. Nurs. **8**:81-87, Mar.-Apr. 1982.

Jones, M.L., and Tippett, T.: Assessing the red eye, Nurs. Pract. **5**:10-15, Jan.-Feb. 1980.

McFarland, W.H., and Simmons, F.B.: The importance of early intervention with severe childhood deafness, Pediatr. Ann. **9**:13-19, Jan. 1980.

Palfrey, J.S.: Selective hearing screening for young children, Clin. Pediatr. **19**:473-477, July 1980.

Poland, R.M.: Methods for detecting hearing impairment in infancy, Pediatr. Ann. **9**:31-32, 37, 39, 43-44, Jan. 1980.

Wassenberg, C.: Common visual disorders in children, Nurs. Clin. North Am. **16**:479-499, Nov. 1981.

Scoliosis

Anderson, B.: The patient with scoliosis: Carole, a girl treated with bracing, Am. J. Nurs. **79**:1592-1597, Aug. 1979.

de Toledo, C.H.; The patient with scoliosis: the defect: classification and detection, Am. J. Nurs. **79**:1588-1591, Aug. 1979.

Micheli, L.J., et al: The patient with scoliosis: surgical management and nursing care, Am. J. Nurs. **79**:1599-1607, Aug. 1979.

The patient with scoliosis: the orthoplast jacket, Am. J. Nurs. **79**;1598, Aug. 1979.

Rutecki, B., and Seligson, D.: Caring for the patient in a halo apparatus, Nurs. '80, **10**:73-77, Oct. 1980.

Schatzinger, L.H., et al: The patient with scoliosis: spinalfusion: emotional stress and adjustment, Am. J. Nurs. **79**:1608-1612, Aug. 1979.

Tibbits, C.W.: Adolescent idiopathic scoliosis, Nurs. Pract. **5**:11-13, 17-20, Mar.-Apr. 1980.

Seizure disorders

Blake, R.L., Jr., et al: After-hours management of febrile children, J. Fam. Pract. **13**:613-617, Oct. 1981.

Coughlin, M.K.: Teaching children about their seizures and medications, Am. J. Mat. Child Nurs. **4**:141-162, May-June 1979.

Mills, M.: When a child has surgery for focal epilepsy, Am. J. Mat. Child Nurs. **7**:304-308, Sept.-Oct. 1982.

Muehl, J.N.: Seizure disorders in children: prevention and care, Am. J. Mat. Child Nurs. **4**:154-160, May-June 1979.

Santilli, N., and Tonelson, S.: Screening for seizures, Pediatr. Nurs. **7**:11-15, Mar.-Apr. 1981.

Surpuse, J.S.: Febrile convulsions: what happens to the infant admitted to the hospital, Clin. Pediatr. **19**:361-362, May 1980.

CONDITIONS INVOLVING THE RESPIRATORY AND CIRCULATORY SYSTEM

General

Barker, G.A.: Current management of croup and epiglottitis, Pediatr. Clin. North Am. **26**:565-579, Aug. 1979.

Davis, H.W., et al: Acute upper airway obstruction: croup and epiglottitis, Pediatr. Clin. North Am. **28:**859-880, Nov. 1981.

Eigen, H.: The clinical evaluation of chronic cough, Pediatr. Clin. North Am. **29:**67-78, Feb. 1982.

Ginsburg, C.M.: Acute mastoiditis in infants and children, Clin. Pediatr. **19:**549-553, Aug. 1980.

Gurwitz, D., et al: Perspectives in cystic fibrosis, Pediatr. Clin. North Am. **26:**603-615, Aug. 1979.

Herbst, J., et al, consultants: Spotting and sustaining patients with cystic fibrosis, Patient Care **16:**16-53, Feb. 28, 1982.

Jarvis, W.R.: A study of beta hemolytic streptococcal pharyngitis in patients with infectious mononucleosis, Clin. Pediatr. **19:**463+, July 1980.

Katznelson, D., and Gross, S.: Familial clustering of tonsillectomies and adenoidectomies, Clin. Pediatr. **19:**276+, Apr. 1980.

Larter, N.: Cystic fibrosis, Am. J. Nurs. **81:**527-532, Mar. 1981.

Levison, H., guest editor: Chest symposium, Pediatr. Clin. North Am. **26:**(entire issue), Aug. 1979.

Mellis, C.M.: Evaluation and treatment of chronic cough in children, Pediatr. Clin. North Am. **26:**553-564, Aug. 1979.

Paradise, J.L.: Tonsillectomy and adenoidectomy, Pediatr. Clin. North Am. **28:**881-892, Nov. 1981.

Passero, M.A., Remor, B., and Solomon, J.: Patient-reported compliance with cystic fibrosis therapy, Clin. Pediatr. **20:**264-268, Apr. 1981.

Pinney, M.: Foreign body aspiration, Am. J. Nurs. **81:**521-522, Mar. 1981.

Pinney, M.: Pneumonia, Am. J. Nurs. **81:**517-518, Mar. 1981.

Simkins, R.: Bronchiolitis, Am. J. Nurs. **81:**514-516, Mar. 1981.

Simkins, R.: Croup and epiglottitis, Am. J. Nurs. **81:**519-520, Mar. 1981.

Twiggs, J.T., et al: Respiratory syncytial virus infection: ten-year follow-up, Clin. Pediatr. **20:**187-190, Mar. 1981.

Zabriskie, J.B. Rheumatic fever: a streptococcal induced autoimmune disease? Pediatr. Ann. **11:**383-296, Apr. 1982.

Asthma and allergy

Balkan, J.A.J.: Allergic rhinitis therapy and the nursing mother, Pediatr. Nurs. **7:**47-49, Mar.-Apr. 1981.

Church, J.A.: Allergic rhinitis: diagnosis and management, Clin. Pediatr. **19:**665-668, Oct. 1980.

Fagin, J., Friedman, R., and Fireman, P.: Allergic rhinitis, Pediatr. Clin. North Am. **28:**797-806, Nov. 1981.

Harmon, A.L., and Harmon, D.C.: Anaphylaxis can mean sudden death anytime, Nurs. '80 **10:**40-43, Oct. 1980.

Hudgel, D.W., and Madson, L.R.: Acute and chronic asthma: a guide to intervention, Am. J. Nurs. **80:**1791-1795, Oct. 1980.

Parker, C.: Food allergies, Am. J. Nurs. **80:**262-265, Feb. 1980.

Simkins, R.: Asthma: reactive airways disease, Am. J. Nurs. **81:**522-524, Mar. 1981.

Walsh, S.: Parents of asthmatic kids (PAK): a successful parent support group, Pediatr. Nurs. **7:**28-29, May-June 1981.

Wieczorek, R.R., and Horner-Rosner, B.: The asthmatic child: preventing and controlling attacks, Am. J. Nurs. **79:**258-262, Feb. 1979.

Wolf, S.I.: Exercise, the asthmatic child, and P.L. 94-142, Pediatr. Nurs. **6:**21-23, Nov.-Dec. 1980.

Congenital heart defects

Gottesfeld, I.B.: The family of the child with congenital heart diseases, Am. J. Mat. Child. Nurs. **4:**101-104, Mar.-Apr. 1979.

Cloutier, J., and Measel, C.P.: Home care for the infant with congenital heart disease, Am. J. Nurs. **82:**100-103, Jan. 1982.

McEvoy, M.: Functional heart murmurs, Nurs. Pract. **6:**34-36, Mar.-Apr. 1981.

NAPNAP Continuing Education Series: Update for pediatric nurses No. 7, Pediatric cardiology, Pediatr. Nurs. **5:**29-38, Jan.-Feb. 1980.

Smith, K.M.: Recognizing cardiac failure in neonates, Am. J. Mat. Child Nurs. **4:**98-100, Mar.-Apr. 1979.

Stafford, M.A., et al: Coarctation of the aorta, Pediatrics **69:**159-163, Feb. 1982.

Malignancies

Dangio, G.J., et al: Results of the second national Wilms' tumor study, Cancer **47:**2302-2311, 1981.

Klopovich, P.: Immunosuppression in the child who has cancer, Am. J. Mat. Child Nurs. **4:**288-292, Sept.-Oct. 1979.

Fochtman, D., and Foley, G.: Nursing care of the child with cancer, Boston, 1982, Little, Brown & Co.

Kobrinsky, N.L., et al: Acute nonlymphocytic leukemia, Pediatr. Clin. North Am. **27**:345-360, May 1980.

Miller, D.R.: Acute lymphoblastic leukemia, Pediatr. Clin. North Am. **27**:269-291, May 1980.

Miser, J.S., et al: Septicemia in childhood malignancy: analysis of 101 consecutive episodes, Clin. Pediatr. **20**:320-323, May 1981.

Nirenberg, A., and Rosea, G.: The day hospital: ambulatory care for the adolescent with cancer, Am. J. Nurs. **79**:500-504, Mar. 1979.

Pochedly, C.: Neuroblastoma, Nurs. Pract. **4**:12-14, 55, Jan.-Feb., 1979.

Wackenhut, J.S., and Barnwell, R.A.: Burkitt's lymphoma, Am. J. Nurs. **79**:1766-1770, Oct. 1979.

Wolf, W.J., and Bancroft, B.: Early detection of childhood malignancies, Pediatr. Nurs. **5**:43-46, Jan.-Feb. 1980.

Diseases of the blood

Buchanan, G.R.: Hemophilia, Pediatr. Clin. North Am. **27**:309-326, May 1980.

Kim, H.C.: Laboratory identification of inherited hemoglobinopathies in children, Clin. Pediatr. **20**:161-171, Mar. 1981.

Lightsey, A.L.: Thrombocytopenia in children, Pediatr. Clin. North Am. **27**:292-308, May 1980.

NAPNAP Continuing Education Series: Update for pediatric nurses No. 8, sickle cell anemia, Pediatr. Nurs. **6**:29-37, Mar.-Apr. 1980.

Oski, F.A., and Stockman, J.A.: Anemia due to inadequate iron sources or poor iron utilization, Pediatr. Clin. North Am. **27**:237-252, May 1980.

Stevens, M.C., et al: Observation on the natural history of doctylitis in homozygous sickle cell disease, Clin. Pediatr. **20**:311-317, May 1981.

Vichinsky, E.P., and Lubin, B.H.: Sickle cell anemia and related hemoglobinopathies, Pediatr. Clin. North Am. **27**:429-447, May 1980.

Understanding and treating hemophilia, Nurs. '80 **10**:72-73, Aug. 1980.

Otitis media

Bluestone, C.D.: Recent advances in the pathogenesis, diagnosis, and management of otitis media, Pediatr. Clin. North Am. **28**:727-755, Nov. 1981.

Bruch, W.M.: Otitis media, Pediatr. Nurs. **5**:9-12, Jan.-Feb. 1979.

McCurdy, J.A., et al: Auditory screening of preschool children with impedance audiometry—a comparison with pure tone audiometry, Clin. Pediatr. **15**:436-441, May 1976.

Sataloff, R.T., and Colton, C.M.: Otitis media: a common childhood infection, Am. J. Nurs. **81**:1480-1483, Aug. 1981.

CONDITIONS INVOLVING DIGESTION AND ASSOCIATED METABOLISM

General

Fitzgerald, J.F., and Clark, J.H.: Chronic diarrhea, Pediatr. Clin. North Am. **29**:221-231, Feb. 1982.

Hyman, P.E., and Ament, M.E.: Acute infectious gastroenteritis in children, Pediatr. Ann. **11**:147-155, Jan. 1982.

John, R.L.: Giardiasis and amebiasis: symptoms, specimens, the counseling you'll need to do. RN **44**:52-57, Apr. 1981.

Jones, J.E.: Identification of intestinal nematodes using the digital rectal examination, J. Fam. Pract. **12**:563-565, Mar. 1981.

Jones, J.E.: Office parasitology, Am. Fam. Physician **86**:90, Aug. 1980.

Jones, J.E.: The royal roundworm—*Ascaris lumbricoides*, J. Fam. Pract. **13**:271-276, Aug. 1981.

Kurfiss-Daniels, D: Positioning as treatment for infant gastroesophageal reflux, Am. J. Nurs. **82**:1535-1537, Oct. 1982.

Raffensperger, J.J.: Swenson's pediatric surgery: Hirschsprung's disease, New York, 1980, Appleton-Century-Crofts.

Raritch, M.M., et al: Pediatric surgery: Hirschsprung's disease, Chicago, 1979, Yearbook Medical Publishers, Inc.

Smith, E.J., Galactosemia: an inborn error of metabolism, Nurs. Pract., **5**:8-9, Mar.-Apr. 1980.

Diabetes

Fredholm, N.Z.: The insulin pump: new method of insulin delivery, Am. J. Nurs. **81**:2024-2026, Nov. 1981.

Ginsberg-Fellner, F.: Insulin-dependent diabetes mellitus, Pediatr. Ann. **9**:24-28, 30-39, Apr. 1980.

Guthrie, D.W., and Guthrie, R.A., editors: Nursing management of diabetes mellitus, ed. 2., St. Louis, 1982, The C.V. Mosby Co.

Hite, A.F., and Humphrey, J.P.: How to spot the vicious cycle of "insulin rebound," RN **42**:44-47, July, 1979.

Matthes, M.L.: Diabetes day care, Am. J. Nurs. **79**:105-106, Jan. 1979.

Simpson, O.W., and Smith M.A.: Lightening the load for parents of children with diabetes, Am. J. Mat. Child Nurs. **4**:295-296, Sept.-Oct. 1979.

Sperling, M.A.: Diabetes mellitus, Clin. Pediatr. **26**:149-169, Feb. 1979.

Stevens, A.D.: Monitoring blood glucose at home—who should do it and how, Am. J. Nurs. **81**:2026-2027, Nov. 1981.

Failure to thrive

Goldbloom, R.B.: Failure to thrive, Pediatr. Clin. North Am. **29**:151-166, Feb. 1982.

Mira, M., and Cairns, G.: Intervention in the interaction of a mother and child with nonorganic failure to thrive, Pediatr. Nurs. **7**:41-45, Mar.-Apr. 1981.

Stephenson, C.W.: Nonorganic failure to thrive, Nurs. Pract. **5**:12-13, May-June 1980.

CONDITIONS INVOLVING THE GENITOURINARY SYSTEM

Common problems

Breen, J.L., et al: Genital tract tumors in children, Pediatr. Clin. North Am. **28**:355-367, May 1981.

Britton, C.V., Blood pressure measurement and hypertension in children, Pediatr. Nurs. **7**:9-17, July-Aug. 1981.

Cippe, B.M.: Ambiguous genitalia and pseudohermaphroditism, Pediatr. Clin. North Am. **26**:91-106, Feb. 1979.

Fonkalsrud, E.W., and Mengel, W.: The undescended testis, cryptorchidism, Chicago, 1981, Yearbook Publishers, Inc.

Gross, S., and Algrim, C.: Teaching young patients—and their families—about home peritoneal dialysis, Nurs. '80 **10**:72-73, Dec. 1980.

Hetrick, A., et al: Nutrition in renal failure: when the patient is a child, Am. J. Nurs. **79**:2152-2154, Dec. 1979.

Mather, D.G.: Ideal conduit surgery: how to help a terrified patient, RN **44**:29-31, Oct. 1981.

Penny, R.: The testis, Clin Pediatr. **26**:107-121, Feb. 1979.

Richards, S.I.: Pelvic examination of children, JOGN Nurs. **10**:208-209, May-June 1981.

Spika, J.S., et al: Serum antibody response to pneumococcal vaccine in children with nephrotic syndrome, Pediatrics, **69**:219-223, Feb. 1982.

Stevens, M.S., and Reinitz, M.: Nursing a child through exstrophic bladder reconstruction surgery, Am. J. Mat. Child Nurs. **5**:265-270, July-Aug. 1980.

Topor, M.: Chronic renal disease in children, Nurs. Clin. North Am. **16**:587-597, Sept. 1981.

Williams, H.A.: Screening for testicular cancer, Pediatr. Nurs. **7**:38-40, Sept.-Oct. 1981.

Urinary tract infections

Bergstein, J.M.: Hematuria, proteinuria, and urinary tract infections, Pediatr. Clin. North Am. **29**:55-66, Feb. 1982.

Fennell, R.S., et al: Urinary tract infections in children: effect of short course antibiotic therapy on recurrence rate in children with previous infections, Clin. Pediatr. **19**:121-124, Feb. 1980.

Lach, P.A., et al: Sexual behavior and urinary tract infection, Nurs. Pract. **5**:27-28, 32, Jan.-Feb. 1980.

McCoy, J.A.: Preliminary diagnosis of urinary tract infection in symptomatic children, Nurs. Pract. **7**:28-33, Jan. 1982.

Stan, J.H.: Urinary tract infections in children, Pediatr. Nurs. **5**:49-52, July-Aug. 1979.

Thomas, C.K.: Childhood urinary tract infection, Pediatr. Nurs. **8**:114-119, Mar.-Apr. 1982.

Enuresis

Ruble, J.A.: Childhood nocturnal enuresis, Am. J. Mat. Child Nurs. **6**:26-31, Jan.-Feb. 1981.

Schmitt, B.D.: Daytime wetting (diurnal enuresis), Pediatr. Clin. North Am. **29**:9-20, Feb. 1982.

Schmitt, B.D., Nocturnal enuresis: an update on treatment, Pediatr. Clin. North Am. **29**:21-36, Feb. 1982.

GENERAL BIBLIOGRAPHY

Aladjem, S., editor: Obstetrical practice, St. Louis, 1980, The C.V. Mosby Co.

Benson, R.C.: Current obstetric and gynecologic diagnosis and treatment, ed. 3, Los Altos, Calif., 1980, Lange Medical Publications.

Blake, F., and Waechter, E.: Nursing care of children, ed. 9, Philadelphia, 1976, J.B. Lippincott Co.

Brunner, L.S., and Suddarth, D.S.: The Lippincott manual of nursing practice, ed. 3, Philadelphia, 1981, J.B. Lippincott Co.

Chow, M., et al: Handbook of pediatric primary care, New York, 1979, John Wiley & Sons, Inc.

Clark, A.L., et al: Childbearing: a nursing perspective, ed. 2., Philadelphia, 1979, F.A. Davis Co.

Conway, B.L.: Pediatric neurological nursing, St. Louis, 1977, The C.V. Mosby Co.

Droske, S.C., and Francis, S.A.: Pediatric diagnostic procedures, New York, 1981, John Wiley & Sons, Inc.

Friedman, M.M.: Family nursing, New York, 1981, Appleton-Century-Crofts.

Gettis, S.S., and Kagan, B.M.: Current pediatric therapy, ed. 8, Philadelphia, 1982, W.B. Saunders Co.

Green, M., and Haggerty, R.J.: Ambulatory pediatrics II, Philadelphia, 1977, W.B. Saunders Co.

Hendren, W.H.: Symposium on pediatric surgery, Surg. Clin. North Am. **56:**245-535 (entire issue), April 1976.

Hughes, J.G.: Synopsis of pediatrics, ed. 5, St. Louis, 1980. The C.V. Mosby Co.

Jacoby, F.G.: Nursing care of the patient with burns, ed. 2, St. Louis, 1976, The C.V. Mosby Co.

Jensen, M.D., Benson, R.C., and Bobak, I.: Maternity care: the nurse and the family, ed. 2, St. Louis, 1981, The C.V. Mosby Co.

Krugman, S., Ward, R., and Katz, S.L.: Infectious diseases of children, ed. 7, St. Louis, 1981, the C.V. Mosby Co.

Leifer, G.: Principles and techniques in pediatric nursing, ed. 4, Philadelphia, 1982, W.B. Saunders Co.

Marlow, D.R.: Textbook of pediatric nursing, ed. 5, Philadelphia, 1977, W.B. Saunders Co.

McFarlane, J., Whitson, B.J., and Hartley, L.M.: Contemporary pediatric nursing—a conceptual approach, New York, 1980, John Wiley & Sons, Inc.

Metheny, N.M., and Snively, W.D.: Nurses' handbook of fluid balance, ed. 2, Philadelphia, 1974, J.B. Lippincott Co.

Moore, M.L.: Realities in childbearing, Philadelphia, 1978, W.B. Saunders Co.

Pillitteri, A.: Child health nursing—care of the growing family, ed. 2, Boston, 1981, Little, Brown & Co.

Pillitteri, A.: Maternal-newborn nursing—care of the growing family, ed. 2, Boston, 1981, Little, Brown & Co.

Pritchard, J.A., and MacDonald, P.C.: Williams' obstetrics, ed. 16, New York, 1980, Appleton-Century-Crofts.

Reeder, S.J., Mastroianni, L., Jr., and Martin, L.L.: Maternity nursing, ed. 14, Philadelphia, 1980, J.B. Lippincott Co.

Report of the Committee on Infectious Diseases, ed. 19, Evanston, Ill., 1982, American Academy of Pediatrics.

Rudolph, A.M., editor: Pediatrics, ed. 16, New York, 1977, Appleton-Century-Crofts.

Scipien, G.M., et al: Comprehensive pediatric nursing, ed. 2, New York, 1981, McGraw-Hill Book Co.

Shirkey, H.C., editor: Pediatric therapy, ed. 6, St. Louis, 1980, The C.V. Mosby Co.

Smith, C.A., editor: The critically ill child, ed. 2, Philadelphia, 1977, W.B. Saunders Co.

Steele, S., editor: Nursing care of the child with long-term illness, ed. 2, New York, 1977, Appleton-Century-Crofts.

Vaughn, V.C., McKay, R.J., and Behrman, N.: Nelson textbook of pediatrics, ed. 10, Philadelphia, 1979, W.B. Saunders Co.

Vestal, K.W.: Pediatric critical care nursing, New York, 1981, John Wiley & Sons, Inc.

Wallace, H.M., et al, editors: Maternal and child health practices, Springfield, Ill., 1973, Charles C Thomas, Publisher.

Whaley, L.F., and Wong, D.L. Essentials of pediatric nursing, St. Louis, 1982, The C.V. Mosby Co.

Williams, S.R. Nutrition and diet therapy, ed. 4, St. Louis, 1981, The C.V. Mosby, Co.

GLOSSARY

Key to pronunciation

ā	āte	à	sofà	ē	ēat	ī	"eye"	ō	ōh	ü	boot
ă	ăs	ä	ärm	ĕ	bĕt	ĭ	ĭt	ŏ	nŏt	ū	"you"
å	åh			er	(ur)her			ò	saw	ŭ	bŭt

abduction (ăb-dŭk′shŭn) Movement away from the midline.

abortion (à-bŏr′shŭn) Termination of a pregnancy before viability; may be spontaneous or induced; definitions of viability may vary.

abrasion (à-brā′zhŭn) Loss of superficial tissue, skin, or mucous membrane because of friction.

abruptio (ăb-rŭp′shē-ō) A tearing away from.

abruptio placentae (plà-sĕn′tē) Premature separation of a normally implanted placenta.

abscess (ăb′sĕs) Focus of suppuration within a tissue; pocket of pus.

abstinence (ab′stĭ-nents) Going without voluntarily; refraining from sexual intercourse.

acetabulum (ăs-ĕ-tăb′ū-lŭm) Rounded cavity on the external surface of the innominate bone that receives the head of the femur.

acidosis (as-ĭ-dō′sis) Abnormal increase in acidity of the blood and tissues.

acinus (ăs′ĭ-nŭs) (pl. acini) Smallest division of a gland, often referring to the mammary glands.

adenoids (ăd′ĕ-noyds) Grouping of lymphoid tissue located on the posterior wall of the nasopharynx (the pharyngeal tonsils).

adnexa (ăd-nĕx′à) Accessory parts of a structure; uterine adnexa—oviducts and ovaries.

afebrile (ā-fĕb′ril) Without fever.

afibrinogenemia (ā-fī″brĭn-ō-jĕ-nē′mĭ-à) Lack of the protein fibrinogen in the blood, causing problems in coagulation.

aggregate (ăg′grē-gāt) Total substances making up a mass.

airway Normal passageway for respired air or a device used to prevent or correct respiratory obstruction.

albinism (ăl′bĭn-ĭsm) Abnormal but nonpathogenic absence of pigment in skin, hair, and eyes.

albumin (ăl-bū′mĭn) One kind of protein.

albuminuria (ăl-bū′-mĭ-nū′rĭ-à) Presence of albumin in the urine.

alignment (à-līn′ment) Arranging in a line.

alimentation (ăl-ĭ-mĕn-tā′shŭn) General process of nourishing the body.

alkalosis (ăl″kà-lō′sĭs) Abnormal increase of alkalinity of the blood and tissues.

allergen (ăl′er-jĕn) Any substance that produces an allergic response.

alveolus (ăl-vē′ō-lŭs) (pl. alve′oli) Little hollow or cavity; the air sac or cell of the lung tissue.

ambient (ăm′bē-ănt) Surrounding

ambivalence (ăm-bĭv′à-lĕnts) Simultaneous feelings of attraction and repulsion, love and hate for a person, object, or action.

amblyopia (ăm-blĭ-ō′pē-à) Reduction or dimness of vision in one eye without apparent associated organic abnormality.

amenorrhea (ā-mĕn-ō-rē′à) Absence of menstruation.

amnesic (ăm-nē′sĭk) Capable of producing amnesia, or loss of memory.

amniocentesis (ăm′nē-ō-sĕn-tē′sĭs) Puncture of the intrauterine amniotic sac usually through the abdominal wall to obtain sample of amniotic fluid.

amniotic (ăm-nē-ŏt′ĭk) Pertaining to the amnion, the innermost of the fetal membranes that secretes the fluid inside the bag of waters.

analgesic (ăn′ăl-jē′sĭk) Capable of producing analgesia, or relief from pain.

analogue (ăn′à-lòg) One of two organs in different species that are similar in function but different in structure.

anaphylactic shock (ăn″à-fĭ-lăk′tĭk) Syndrome that occasionally occurs after the reintroduction of a substance (antigen) into a person or animal previously sensitized to it; characterized by circulatory collapse and shock.

763

anasarca (ăn-à-sär′ka) Severe generalized edema.

anastomosis (ă-năs′tō-mō′sĭs) Natural or surgical joining of blood or lymph vessels, or a surgically created communication between different hollow organs or parts of the same organs.

ancillary (ăn′sĭ-ler-ē) Subordinate or auxiliary.

android (ăn′droyd) Manlike; adjective used to describe a male-type pelvis.

anemia (an-ē′mē-à) Condition in which there is a reduction below normal of hemoglobin in the blood.

anencephalic (ăn-ĕn-sĕf′à-lĭk) Lacking a cerebrum, cerebellum, and part of the cranium.

anesthetic (ăn′ĕs-thĕt′ĭk) Capable of producing anesthesia, that is, complete or partial loss of feeling.

angiocardiography (ăn″jē-ō-cär-dē-ŏg′ră-fē) Injection of contrast material into the pulmonary circulation and observation of its flow by radiography or fluoroscopy.

anion (ăn′ī-àn) Particle of matter (ion) carrying a negative electrical charge.

ankylosis (ăn-kĭ-lō′sĭs) Abnormal immobility and consolidation of a joint.

anomalies (à-nŏm′à-lēz) Deviations from the normal.

anorexia (ăn-à-rĕk′sē-à) Loss of appetite.

anovulatory (ăn-ov′ū-lă-tō″rē) Not accompanied by production and discharge of an ovum.

anoxia (ăn-ŏk′sē-à) Lack of oxygen.

antagonistic (ăn-tăg-à-nĭs′tĭk) Acting with antagonism, that is, in opposition to an agent or principle; counteracting; hostile.

antenatal (ăn-tē-nā′tàl) Before birth; prenatal.

antepartal (ăn-tē-pär′tàl) Before delivery.

anteroposterior (ăn′tĕr-ō-pŏs-tĭr′ē-ur) From front to back.

antiarrhythmic (ăn″tē-à-rĭth′mĭk) Preventing (or effective against) arrhythmia, or irregular cardiac contractions.

antibody (ăn′tĭ-bŏd-ē) Protective protein substance formed by the body in the presence of pathogenic organisms or foreign materials.

antisepsis (ăn″tĭ-sĕp′sĭs) Literally "against infection or decay"; the use of procedures usually involving chemicals (antiseptics) that hinder the growth of microorganisms without necessarily destroying them.

antitoxin (ăn-tĭ-tŏk′sĭn) Protective protein formed by the body in response to the presence of a toxin; a preparation containing antibodies designed to produce passive immunization.

anuria (à-nyur′ē-à) Failure of kidney function; lack of urine formation.

apnea (ăp′nē-à) Absence of respiration, temporary or permanent.

areola (à-rē′ō-là) (pl. areolae) Ring of pigment on the breast surrounding the nipple.

arteriogram (är-tĭr′ē-ō-grăm) X-ray procedure that reveals arterial pathways injected with special contrast materials.

artery (är′ter-ē) Blood vessel that carries blood away from the heart.

arthralgia (ar-thrăl′jĭ-à) Pain in a joint.

arthritis (är-thrī′tĭs) Inflammation of a joint, usually accompanied by pain and frequently by changes in structure.

arthrodesis (är″thrŏd-ē-sĭs) Surgical fusion of a joint performed to gain stability for weight bearing.

arthroplasty (är′thrō-plăs-tē) Surgical formation or reconstruction of a joint.

asepsis (à-sĕp′sĭs) Literally "without infection or decay"; refers to the absence of living disease-producing microorganisms or to procedures that produce such an absence.

asphyxia (ăs-fĭk′sē-à) Lack of oxygen and excessive carbon dioxide buildup in the body resulting from an abnormal gaseous environment or disease.

aspirate (Verb: see aspiration.) Noun: that which is obtained by aspiration.

aspiration (ăs-pĭ-rā′shun) Process of drawing in or out as by suction.

assimilation (a-sĭm-ĕ-lā′shun) Processes whereby the products of digestion change to resemble the chemical substances of the body tissues, first passing through the lacteals and blood vessels.

astrocytoma (ăs-trō-sī-tō′ma) Tumor of the brain tissue.

ataxic (à-tăk′sĭk) Pertaining to ataxia, or the incoordination of the voluntary muscles; one possible result of brain damage.

atelectasis (ăt-ē-lĕk′tà-sĭs) Lack of proper lung expansion; collapsed or airless segment of lung.

athetoid (ăth′ĕ-toyd) Pertaining to athetosis, or the presence of involuntary, purposeless weaving motions of the body or its extremities; one possible result of brain damage.

atopic (ā-tŏp′ĭk) Pertaining to allergic responses, particularly those of a hereditary nature.

atresia (à-trē′zhuh) Lack of a normal opening or canal.

atrium (ā′trē-ŭm) (pl. atria) Cavity or sinus; one of two upper chambers of the heart.

atrophy (ăt′rà-fē) Lack of nourishment; wasting or reduction in size of cells, tissues, organs, or regions of the body.

attenuate (à-tĕn′yoo-āt) To weaken the virulence of; to reduce in force; to make thin.

attitude (ăt′ĭ-tüd) In speaking of fetal position, refers to the degree of flexion of the baby's head and extremities in the uterus.

aura (är′à) Subjective warning of an impending epileptic seizure.

auscultation (aws-kŭl-tā′shŭn) Process of listening for sounds produced in some body cavity.

autoclave (aw-tŏ-clāv) Appliance used to sterilize objects by steam under pressure.

autoimmune (ah′-tŏh-ĭ-mū′n) Production in an organism of reactivity to its own tissues, with appearance of certain clinical and laboratory manifestations.

autonomy (aw-tŏn′ă-mē) State of self-government or self-direction.

autosomal (aw′tŏ-sōhm-ŭl). Having the character of a non-sex-determining chromosome.

autosomes (äw′tŏ-sōhm) All chromosomes except sex-determining X and Y.

bacillus (bà-sĭl′ŭs) (pl. bacilli) Rod-shaped bacterium.

barrier techniques Various forms of isolation.

basophil (bā′sŏ-fĭl) One type of white blood cell.

bilirubin (bĭl-ĭ-rū′bĭn) Orange or yellow pigment in bile; a product of red blood cell destruction; elevated levels in the blood may cause jaundice.

biopsy (bī′ŏp-sē) Procurement of a specimen of tissue for microscopic examination.

blastocyst (blăs′-tŏ-sĭst) Spherical mass consisting of a central cavity surrounded by a single layer of cells produced by the cleavage of the ovum.

booster injection Substance or dose used to renew or increase the effect of a drug or immunizing agent.

bossing Rounded protuberance, particularly on the skull, in the area of the forehead; one possible manifestation of rickets.

bradycardia (brăd″ē-kär′dē-à) Slowness of the heartbeat; in adults, usually a rate of less than 60 beats per minute.

Braxton Hicks (brăx′ton hĭks) *contractions* uterine contractions that occur throughout pregnancy and help enlarge the uterus to accommodate the growing fetus; during the last weeks of pregnancy they may become very noticeable; false labor contractions.

breech (brēch) *birth* Delivery of the child feet or buttocks first.

bronchiectasis (brŏn-kē-ĕk′tà-sĭs) Abnormal dilatation of the bronchi in response to inflammation, which may lead to structural changes and chronic cough.

buffer apparatus or substance serving to neutralize the shock of opposing forces.

bulbar (bŭl′bär) Pertaining to the "bulb," or medulla, of the brain and the cranial nerves.

calcaneus (kăl-kā′nē-ŭs) Heel bone, or os calcis; type of clubfoot in which only the heel touches the ground; patient may walk on inner side of heel.

callus (kăl′ŭs) New bone formation at the site of a healing fracture.

calyx (kā′lĭks) (pl. calyces) Small subdivision of the pelvis of the kidney.

Candida albicans (kăn′dĭ-dà ăl′bĭ-kănz) Formerly called *Monilia albicans*; a yeastlike fungus that may infect various portions of the body, causing a variety of symptoms (e.g., leukorrhea, dermatitis, stomatitis).

cannula (kăn′ū-là) (pl. cannulae) Small tube; large needle sheath used for insertion into a body cavity or tube.

canthus (kăn-thŭs) (pl. canthi) Corner at each side of the eye where the eyelids meet.

caput succedaneum (kă′pŭt sŭk-sē-dā′nē-ŭm) Abnormal collection of fluid under the scalp.

carbohydrate (kăr″bŏ-hī′drāt) a compound of carbon combined with H_2 and O_2 that supplies heat and energy to the body.

cardiovascular (kär-dē-ō-văs′kŭl-är) Pertaining to the heart and blood vessels.

caries (kăr′ēz) Dental decay.

carrier Person or animal capable of transmitting a contagious or hereditary disease but showing no outward sign of the disease.

cast Solid mold usually made of plaster to help protect, position, or immobilize a part; microscopic sediment that has been partially shaped by the kidney tubules; any other body discharge or excretion retaining the shape of a body part that held it.

catalyst (kăt′à-lĭst) Substance that speeds the rate of a chemical reaction without itself being permanently altered by the reaction.

catamenia (kăt-à-mē′nē-à) Menses, or menstruation.

cataract (kăt′à-răkt) Abnormal opacity of the crystalline lens of the eye.

catecholamines (kăt-ē-kōl′à-mēnz) Group of similar compounds that includes dopamine, norepinephrine, and epinephrine.

catheter (kăth′ĕ-ter) Hollow tube for insertion into a cavity or a canal for the purpose of discharging its fluid contents or introducing other substances into it.

cation (kăt′ī-àn) Particle of matter (ion) carrying a positive electrical charge.

cecum (sē′kŭm) Blind pouch that forms the first portion of the large intestine or colon; the attachment for the appendix.

celiac (sē′lē-ăk) *disease* Chronic intestinal indigestion.

cellulitis (sĕl-ū-lī′tĭs) Inflammation of the cellular or connective tissues.

cephalhematoma (sĕf-ăl-hē-mà-tō′mà) Swelling on the head caused by a collection of bloody fluid under the periosteum of the skull as the result of trauma.

cephalic (sĕ-făl′ĭk) Pertaining to the head.

cephalocaudal (sĕf-à-lō-cawd′àl) Moving from the head toward the base of the spine.

cerumen (sĕ-rū′mĕn) Ear wax.

cervical (sĕr′vĭ-kàl) Pertaining to the neck or cervix.

cesarean (sĕz-ăr'ē-ăn) *birth* Abdominal delivery made possible by incising the uterine and abdominal walls.

Chadwick's (chăd'wĭks) *sign* Violet tinge of the cervical and vaginal mucous membranes; a presumptive sign of pregnancy.

chancre (shăng'ker) Craterlike lesion seen in first-stage syphilis.

chemotherapy (kē'mō-thĕr"ă-pē) Application of chemical reagents in the treatment of disease having a specific and toxic effect upon the disease-causing microorganism or malignant process.

Cheyne-Stokes (chān'stōks) *respiration* Irregular, cyclic-type breathing characterized by a period of increasing respiratory action followed by an interval of apnea.

chloasma gravidarum (klō-ăz'mȧ grăv-ĭ-dā'rŭm) Deepening pigmentation of skin during pregnancy, especially of the face; "mask of pregnancy."

chordee (kŏr-dē') Abnormal downward curvature of the penis.

chorea (kō-rē'a) Involuntary muscular twitching or movement.

choriocarcinoma (kō-rĭ-ō-kär-sĭ-nō'mȧ) Rare malignancy associated with hydatidiform mole of pregnancy.

chorion (kō'rĭ-ŏn) Outermost membrane of the growing fertilized egg; one of two membranes that later form the "bag of waters."

chorionic gonadotropin (kō'rē-ŏn-ĭk gŏ-năd'ō-trō'pĭn) Gonad-regulating hormone produced by the outermost tissue covering the fetus in early pregnancy.

chorionic villi (vĭl'ī) Fingerlike tissue projections of chorion on the outer wall of the fertilized egg.

chromosomes (krō'mȧ-sōmz) Microscopic structures seen fairly easily in the nucleus of a cell during its reproduction, which contain the genes or determiners of heredity.

chronicity (krŏn-ĭs'ĭt-ē) State of being chronic.

cisternal (sĭs-tĕr'năl) *puncture* Puncture with a hollow needle between the cervical vertebrae, through the dura mater, into the cisterna at the base of the brain.

clavicle (klăv'ĭ-kȧl) Collarbone.

clitoris (klĭ'tȧ-rĭs) Small, sensitive erectile structure located at the anterior junction of the labia minora.

coagulation (ko-ăg-ye-lā'shun) Process of clotting.

coccus (kŏk'ŭs) (pl. cocci) Spherical-shaped bacterium.

coitus (kō'ĭ-tŭs) Sexual intercourse.

colic (kŏl'ĭk) Intermittent pain caused by spasm of any hollow or tubular soft organ; abdominal cramping fairly common in first 3 months of infancy.

collagen (kŏl'ȧ-jĕn) Protein substance existing in many of the body's connective tissues.

collateral (kȧ-lăt'er-ȧl) Situated at the sides; supplementary, reinforcing.

colostrum (kŏl-ŏs'trŭm) Breast secretion produced by the mother the first few days after childbirth.

colporrhaphy (kŏl-pōr'ă-fē) Surgical repair of the walls of the vagina.

comatose (kō'mȧ-tōs) In a coma, or abnormally deep sleep, caused by illness or injury.

comedo (kŏm'ē-dō) (pl. comedones) Discolored, dried, oily secretion plugging the pores of the skin; blackhead.

comminuted (kŏm'ĭ-nūt-ĕd) Broken into many pieces; comminuted fracture, a crushed bone.

compatible Able to work together; not in opposition; able to be mixed without destructive changes.

compression (kom-presh'un) Squeezing together; state of being pressed together.

conception (kon-sĕp'shŭn) Union of the male sex cell, spermatozoon, and the female sex cell, ovum; fertilization; beginning of a new being.

conduit (kŏn'dü-ĭt) Tube or other device conveying water or other fluid from one region to another.

condyloma (kŏn-dĭ-lō'ma) Wartlike growth usually found near the anus or vulva; the broad, flat form (c. latum) is characteristic of syphilis in its secondary stage.

congenital (kon-jĕn'ĭ-tȧl) Existing at birth.

conjugate (kŏn'jū-gāt) Anteroposterior diameter of the pelvis.

conjunctiva (kŏn-jŭnk-tī'vȧ) Mucous membrane that lines the inner surface of the eyelid and covers the anterior portion of the eye.

contaminated Soiled, stained, touched, or exposed in such a manner that the article in question becomes unsafe to use as intended or without barrier techniques.

continence (kŏnt'ĭ-nĕnts) Control of bladder or bowel function, or self-restraint, especially in regard to sexual intercourse.

contraception (kŏn-trȧ-sĕp'shun) Prevention of the fertilization of an egg or ovum.

contracture (kon-trăk'chur) Permanent contraction of a muscle resulting from spasm or paralysis causing limitation of motion; high resistance to the passive stretch of a muscle.

contusion (kŏn-tū'zhŭn) Injury that does not result in breaking the skin; black-and-blue area; bruise.

convulsion (kon-vŭl'shŭn) Violent, involuntary contraction or series of contractions of muscles.

corium (kō'rĭ-ŭm) Dermis layer of the skin; "true skin."

cor pulmonale (kŏr pŭl-mŏn-ăl'ē) Cardiac enlargement or failure secondary to respiratory disease.

cortex (kŏr'tĕks) Outer or more superficial part of an organ.

coryza (kōrī'zȧ) "Common" head cold.

crepitus (krĕp′ĭ-tŭs) Grating sensation sometimes heard or felt at the site of a fracture; crackling sound heard in certain diseases.

cretinism (krē′tĭn-ĭzm) Infantile hypothyroidism characterized by mental retardation and other disturbances in mental and physical development.

crust (crustation) External protective layer; scab.

cryptorchidism (krĭpt-or′kĭd-ĭzm) Failure of the testicles to descend into the scrotum.

cul-de-sac of Douglas Blind pouch formed by the peritoneal lining of the abdominal cavity located between the uterus and rectum.

curettage (kü-ret′ăj) (uterine) Scraping with a curette to remove uterine contents (as in inevitable, incomplete, or early therapeutic abortion), to obtain specimens for use in diagnosis, or to remove growths (e.g., polyps).

CVA Cerebrovascular accident.

cyanosis (sī-ăn-ō′sĭs) Bluish or grayish coloration of the skin caused by poor oxygenation of the blood.

cystitis (sĭs-tī′tĭs) Inflammation of the urinary bladder.

cystocele (sĭs′tō-sēl) Prolapse of the urinary bladder caused by the weakened tissue wall between the bladder and vagina.

cystourethrogram (sĭs″tō-ū-rēth′rō-gram) X-ray film of the bladder and urethra.

cytology (sī″-tŏl′ō-jē) Study of cells.

cytoplasm (sī′tō-plăz-ŭm) Portion of a cell inside the cell membrane but outside the nucleus.

debilitate (dē-bĭl′ĭ-tāt) To produce weakness; enfeeble.

debridement (dā-brēd-mŏn′) Surgical removal of dead, damaged, or contaminated tissue.

debris (dà-brē) Rubbish; ruins.

decalcification (dē-kăl-sĭ-fĭ-kā′shŭn) Removal of or withdrawal of lime salts from bone.

decidua (dī-sĭd′-ū-ä) Pertaining to endometrium of pregnancy, which is cast off at parturition.

deciduous (dē-sĭd′ū-ŭs) *teeth* Primary or baby teeth.

decubitus (dĕ-kū′bĭ-tŭs) Bedsore.

dehydration (dē-hī-drā′shŭn) Condition in which the body tissues lack normal fluid content.

dentition (dĕn-tĭsh′ŭn) Process or time of teething.

dermatitis (dĕr-mà-tī′tĭs) *venenata* Skin disturbance caused by external irritants.

deterioration (di-tir″′ē-à-rā′shun) Gradually worsening.

detrusor (dē-trü′sor) *muscle* Smooth muscle of the bladder wall.

diaphoresis (dī-ā-fō-rē′sĭs) Profuse sweating.

diaphragmatic (dī-à-frăg-măt′ĭk) *hernia* Protrusion of abdominal contents through an abnormal opening in the diaphragm.

diaphysis (dī-ăf′ĭ-sĭs) Shaft or middle part of a long bone.

diastolic (dī-ăs-tŏl′ĭk) Pertaining to diastole—the blood pressure at the time of greatest cardiac relaxation.

digestion (dī′jĕs′chĕn) Process by which food is broken down mechanically and chemically in the gastrointestinal tract and converted into absorbable forms.

digital (dĭj′ĭ-tàl) Pertaining to the digits; that is, the fingers or toes.

digitalization (dij′-ĭ-tăl-ĭ-zā′shŭn) Administration of digitalis to slow and strengthen the heartbeat (particularly the initial administration of the drug).

dilatation (dĭl-à-tā′shŭn) Expansion of an organ or orifice; dilation.

diploid (dĭp′loyd) Having double the number of chromosomes found in the ova or sperm, the normal chromosome number for body cells.

disorientation (dĭs-ō-rē-ĕn-tā′shŭn) Inability to evaluate properly direction, location, time, surroundings, or personal role.

distal (dĭs′tàl) Farthest from the trunk of the body or from a specific point of reference.

distention (dĭs-tĕn′shŭn) (also distension) Inflation, stretch, ballooning.

diuresis (dī″ū-rē′sĭs) Increased urine output.

diuretic (dī-ū-rĕt′ĭk) Agent that increases the secretion of urine.

diverticulum (dī-ver-tĭk′ū-lŭm) (pl. diverticula) Sac or pouch in the walls of a canal or organ, especially the colon.

ductus arteriosus (dŭk′tŭs är-tēr-ē-ō′sŭs) Short blood vessel located between the pulmonary artery and aorta in the fetus.

ductus deferens (dŭk′tŭs dĕf′ĕr-ĕnz) Excretory duct of the testicle; vas deferens.

dyscrasia (dĭs-krā′zhē-à) Undefined disease, malfunction, or abnormal condition, often used when speaking of abnormalities of the blood.

dysentery (dĭs′ĕn-tĕr-ē) Inflammation of the intestines, especially of the colon, usually characterized by mild to severe diarrhea.

dysmenorrhea (dĭs-mĕn-ō-rē′à) Painful or difficult menstruation.

dyspnea (dĭsp-nē′à) Difficult breathing.

dystocia (dĭs-tō′shà) Difficult labor, particularly difficulty in the mechanics of childbirth.

ecchymosis (ĕk-ĭ-mō′sĭs) Black-and-blue mark caused by hemorrhage into the skin, usually a relatively large area.

eclampsia (ĕ-klămp′sē-à) Toxemia of pregnancy characterized by convulsion of a pregnant or newly delivered patient who classically displays signs of albuminuria, hypertension, and edema; if the patient has these symptoms but has not convulsed, she may be termed "preeclamptic."

ecology (ĭ-kŏl′ȧjī) Interrelationships of organisms and their environment as manifested by natural cycles and rhythms.

ectopic (ĕk-tŏp-ĭk) *pregnancy* Pregnancy that develops in an abnormal place (e.g., in the uterine tube, abdomen, or ovary).

edema (ē-dē′ma) Abnormal, excessive amount of fluid within the body tissues.

edematous (ē-dĕm′ăt-ŭs) Characterized by the presence of edema, that is, an abnormal amount of fluid in the tissues.

effacement (ĕf-ās′mĕnt) (of the cervix) Shortening and thinning of the cervix or neck of the uterus.

efficacious (ef″ȧ-kā′shus) Capable of producing an intended effect.

effleurage (ĕf-lü-rahzh′) Stroking movement used in massage.

effusion (ē-fu′-shun) Escape of fluid into an area.

ejaculation (ē-jăk-ū-lā′shŭn) Ejection of the seminal fluid from the male urethra.

electroencephalogram (ē-lĕk-trō-ĕn-sĕf′ȧ-lō-grăm) Tracing made by an apparatus designed to detect and record brain waves.

electrolyte (ē-lĕk′trō-līt) Substance that, in solution, conducts electric current.

embolus (ĕm′bō-lŭs) (pl. emboli) Foreign substance traveling in the circulatory system, e.g., a blood clot or air.

embryo (ĕm′brē-ō) Unborn young of any creature in an early stage of development when specific identification is difficult with the naked eye.

emesis (ĕm′ē-sĭs) Referring to vomiting or the substance vomited.

emission (ē-mĭsh′ŭn) Discharge (e.g., discharge of semen), especially involuntary.

emphysema (ĕm-fĭ-sē′mȧ) Abnormal dilatation and loss of elasticity of the alveoli or air sacs of the lungs.

empyema (ĕm-pī-ē′mȧ) Collection of pus in a body cavity, especially the pleural cavity.

encephalitis (ĕn-sĕf-a-lī′tĭs) Inflammation of the encephalon, that is, the brain.

encephalopathy (ĕn-sĕf″ȧ-lŏp′ȧ-thē) Any dysfunction of the brain.

endarteritis (ĕnd-är-tĕr-ī′tĭs) Inflammation of the lining of the arteries.

endocarditis (ĕn-dō-kär-dī′tĭs) Inflammation of the lining of the heart.

endocrine (ĕn′dō-krĭn) Pertaining to ductless glands that discharge their secretions (hormones) directly into the bloodstream.

endometritis (ĕn-dō-mē-trī′tĭs) Inflammation of the endometrium, or lining of the uterus.

endotracheal (ĕn′dō-trā′kē-ȧl) Within the trachea.

engagement (ĕn-gāj′mĕnt) In obstetrics, refers to the entrance of the presenting part of the fetus into the true pelvis; the passage of the largest diameter of the presenting part into the true pelvis.

engorgement (ĕn-gōrj′mĕnt) In obstetrics, refers to the swelling of the breasts because of local congestion of the veins and lymphatics associated with lactation.

enteric (en-tĕr′ĭk) Pertaining to the small intestine.

enterobiasis (ĕn″tĕr-ō-bī′a-sĭs) Disease caused by pinworm infestation.

enterostomy (ĕn-tĕr-ŏs′to-mĭ) Surgical opening into the intestine through the abdominal wall.

enuresis (ĕn-ū-rē′sĭs) Bed-wetting at an age when urinary control should be present.

epicanthus (ē-pī-kăn′thŭs) Fold of skin extending from the nose to the median end of the eyebrow, characteristic of the Mongolian race.

epidemiologic (ep′ĭ-dē″mē-o-loj′ĭ-kal) Pertaining to the study of epidemics, their origin and prevention or, more broadly, the origins of any condition.

epididymis (ĕp-ĭ-dĭd′ĭ-mĭs) (pl. epididymides) Small oblong organ, situated on the testis, containing a coiled extension of the tubules of the testis, which eventually joins the vas deferens.

epiphysis (ē-pĭf′ĭ-sĭs) (pl. epiphyses) End of a long bone.

episiotomy (ĭ-pĭz-ē-ŏt′ȧ-mē) Surgical incision extending from the soft tissue of the vaginal opening into the true perineum, performed to protect the perineum from laceration or help hasten the delivery of an infant.

epispadias (ĕp-ĭ-spā′dē-ȧs) Abnormal condition in which the urethral opening is located on the upper (dorsal) surface of the penis.

epistaxis (ĕp-ĭ-stăk′sĭs) Nosebleed.

epithelial (ĕp″ĭ-thē′lē-al) Pertaining to the outermost layer of the skin and/or the lining tissue of hollow organs and inner passages of the body.

equilibrium (ē-kwĭ-lĭb′rē-um) Equal balance, between powers; mental balance; equality of effect.

equinus (ē-kwī′nŭs) Condition characterized by a tiptoe walk affecting one or both feet, often associated with clubfoot.

Erbs' palsy (erbz pawl′zē) Injury to the brachial plexus causing partial paralysis of the arm.

erectile (ē-rĕk′tīl) Capable of becoming erect.

erysipelas (ĕr-ĭ-sĭp′ĕ-lŭs) Acute febrile disease, with localized inflammation and swelling of the skin and subcutaneous tissue accompanied by systemic disturbance of variable degree, caused by a streptococcus.

erythema (ār-ĭ-thē′mȧ) Redness of the skin; characteristic red blotches on the skin of the newborn infant.

erythema marginatum (märj-ĭ-nȧ′tŭm) Rash occasionally seen in cases of rheumatic fever.

erythroblast (ĕ-rĭth'rō-blăst) Immature, inadequate form of red blood cell normally found only in the bone marrow.

erythroblastosis fetalis (ĕ-rith"rō-blăst-ō-sĭs fē-tă'lĭs) Hemolytic disease of the newborn characterized by anemia, jaundice, enlarged liver and spleen, and the presence of erythroblasts circulating in the bloodstream.

erythrocyte (ĕ-rĭth'rō-sīt) Red blood corpuscle or cell.

eschar (ĕs'kär) Thick crusts that may form over burned areas on the body, composed of hardened drainage.

esophageal (ĕ-sŏf"a-jē-ăl) Pertaining to the esophagus, or food tube, leading from the throat to the stomach.

estrogen (ĕs'trō-jĕn) Class name for a female sex hormone; more particularly, the hormonal secretion of the ovary that builds up the lining of the uterus and promotes feminine characteristics.

etiology (ē"tē-ol'ə-jē) Cause of a disease.

eupnea (ūp-nē'à) Normal breathing.

excoriation (ĕks-kō-rī-ā'shŭn) Scraping of the skin's surface through injury.

excrete (ek-skrēt) To separate and eliminate from an organic body.

exocrine (ĕks'ō-krĭn) Term applied to glands whose secretion reaches an epithelial surface either directly or through a duct.

exstrophy (ĕks'trō-fē) Eversion or the turning inside out of a part with or without the abnormal exposure of the part.

exudate (ĕks'ū-dāt) Accumulation of a fluid in a cavity; drainage flowing from one body area to another; drainage from wounds.

fallopian (fă-lō'pī-on) **tubes** Uterine tubes, or oviducts, leading from the uterine cavity toward each ovary.

familial (fă-mĭl'ēăl) Pertaining to or characteristic of a family.

fascia (făsh'ē-à) Fibrous connective tissue found under the skin or covering, supporting, and separating muscles and other organs.

febrile (fĕb'rĕl or fĕb'rĭl) State of being feverish.

fertility (fertile) (fĕr-tĭl'ĭ-tē) Quality of being productive.

fertilization (fĕr-tĭ-lĭ-za'shŭn) Union of male and female sex cells; conception.

fetus (fē'tŭs) Later stages of the developing young of an animal within the uterus or egg when the species is distinguishable by the naked eye.

FHR Fetal heart rate.

fibrinogen (fĭ-brĭn'ō-jĕn) Protein in the blood plasma necessary to coagulation.

fistula (fĭs'tū-là) (pl. fistulae) Abnormal tubelike passageway from a normal body cavity or canal to another body cavity or to the outside of the body.

flaccid (flă'sĭd) Soft, flabby, relaxed; lacking normal tension or tone.

flexion (flĕk'shŭn) Act of being bent.

follicle (fŏl'ĭ-kăl) Small secretory sac or cavity; protective tissue envelope of the female sex cell, or ovum.

fontanel (fŏn'tà-nĕl) Soft spot found between the cranial bones of the skull of an infant, formed where sutures meet or cross.

foramen (fō-rā'mĕn) Small opening.

foramen ovale (ō-vā'lē) Normal opening between the atria in the heart of the fetus.

foreskin (fōr'skĭn) Prepuce, or fold of skin covering the glans penis.

fornix (fōr'nĭx) (pl. fornices) Arch or fold.

fourchette (für-shĕt') Tense band of mucous membrane connecting the posterior ends of the labia minora.

frenulum (frĕn'ū-lŭm) (pl. frenula) Any small fold of mucous membrane or tissue that acts like a bridle; fold of mucous membrane extending from the underside of the tongue to the floor of the mouth at the midline; lower fold of the labia minora that surrounds the clitoris.

frequency (frē'kwĕn-sē) Number of repetitions of a periodic process in a unit of time; when speaking of urinary function, the term implies an abnormal increase in the number of voidings.

FSH Follicle-stimulating hormone.

fulminating (fŭl'mĭ-nā-tĭng) Occurring with great rapidity.

fundus (fŭn'dŭs) (pl. fundi) Part of an organ opposite its opening; top of the uterus.

funic souffle (fū'nĭk sü-făl) Sound sometimes heard over the pregnant uterus having same rate as fetal heartbeat; it may be related to compression of the umbilical cord.

furuncle (fū'rŭng-kăl) Infected hair follicle; a boil.

fusion (fū'shŭn) Process of uniting.

galactosemia (gă-lăk"tō-sē'mē-a) Metabolic condition involving the metabolism of galactose, which may produce mental retardation and other symptoms.

gamete (găm'ēt). Male or female reproductive cell capable of entering into union with each other in the process of fertilization.

gamma globulin (găm'mà glŏb'ū-lĭn) Blood protein fraction containing most of the protective immune antibodies.

gastroenteritis (găs"trō-ĕn-ter-ĭ-tīs) Inflammation of the mucosa of the stomach and intestines.

gastrostomy (găs-trō'sta-mē) Intentional establishment of an opening into the stomach through the abdominal wall, usually for artificial feeding.

gavage (gà-vazh') Feeding through a stomach tube passed either nasally or orally.

gene (jēn) Hereditary determiner located on the chromosomes.

genetics (jĕ-nĕt′ĭks) Study of inheritance or genes.

genitalia (jĕn-ĭ-tal′ē-à) Organs of generation, or reproduction.

gestation (jĕs-tā′shŭn) Period of intrauterine fetal development; pregnancy.

gingivitis (jĭn″jĭ-vī′tĭs) Inflammation of the gums.

glans penis (glănz pē′nĭs) Sensitive portion (tip) of the penis.

glioma (glī-ō′mà) Tumor involving the supportive tissue of the brain or glial cells.

glomerulus (glō-măr′ū-lŭs) (pl. glomeruli) Cluster or coil of connecting capillaries located at the top of the expanded end (Bowman's capsule) of the urinary tubules in the kidney.

glottis (glŏt′ĭs) Opening of the larynx including the associated vocal cords.

glucometer (glū-kŏm′ĕ-tĕr) Portable device used by staff and patients to measure blood glucose.

gluten (glū′tĕn) Protein found in wheat, rye, and oats.

gluteus (glū-tē′us) Any of the three muscles that form the buttocks.

glycosuria (glī-kō-sü′rē-à) Presence of glucose in the urine.

gonadotropic (gō-năd-ō-trō′pĭk) Relating to stimulation of the gonads, that is, the ovaries or testes.

gravida (grăv′ĭ-dà) Pertaining to the number of pregnancies a woman has had; a pregnant woman.

gumma (gŭm′mà) Soft gummy tumor that may develop during third stage of syphilis.

gynecoid (gī′nĕ-coyd or jĭn′ĕ-coyd) Womanlike; typical female pelvis.

gynecomastia (gī-nĕ-kō-măs′tĭ-à or jĭn-ĕ-kō-măs′tĭ′à) Swelling of the newborn or adult male breast tissue.

habilitate (hă-bĭl′ĭ-tāt) Equip for working and for everyday tasks or activities.

hallucination (hă-lū-sĭ-nā′shŭn) False perception having no relation to reality and not accounted for by any external stimuli; may be visual, auditory, olfactory, etc.

Hegar's (hā′gärz) *sign* Softening of the uterine isthmus, the area between the cervix and body of the uterus; a probable sign of pregnancy.

hemangioma (hē-măn-jē-ō′mà) Blood vessel tumor.

hematocrit (hē-măt′à-krĭt) *reading* The percentage of whole blood volume occupied by red blood cells after they have been separated through use of a centrifuge.

hematoma (hē-mă-tō′mà) Tumor composed of blood cells, resulting from tissue injury.

hematuria (hē-mă-tü′rĭ-à) Presence of blood in the urine.

hemoglobin (hē-mō-glō′bĭn) Oxygen-carrying protein pigment found in the red blood cells.

hemolytic (hē-mō-lĭt′ĭk) Pertaining to or causing the breakdown of red blood cells.

hemoptysis (hē-mŏp′tĭ-sĭs) Presence of blood-stained sputum.

hemorrhoid (hĕm′ō-royd) Rectal varicosity; "pile."

heparinized (hĕp′er-rĭn-īzed) Containing heparin employed as an anticoagulant.

hermaphroditism (her-măf′rō-dĭt-ĭsm) Possession by one individual of the gonads and external genitalia of both sexes.

hernia (hĕr′nĭ-à) Rupture; an abnormal protrusion of a portion of the contents of a body cavity because of a defect in its surrounding walls, frequently causing swelling, pressure symptoms, or other complications.

herpes (hĕr′pēz) *simplex* Viral infection characteristically causing an eruption of small, clustered blisters on the skin or mucous membranes.

heterozygous (hĕt″er-ō-zī′gŭs) Having the two members of one or more pairs of genes dissimilar.

homozygate (hō″-mō-zī′gāte) A homozygous individual.

homozygous (hō″mō-zī′gŭs) Having both of a given pair of genes alike.

hordeolum (hŏr-dē′ō-lŭm) Sty or infection involving the eyelash follicle.

hormone (hŏr′mōn) Internal secretions of thyroid gland, pancreas, etc.; chemical substance originating in an organ, gland, or part that is conveyed through the blood to another part of the body, helping to regulate body processes.

Hutchinson's (hŭch′ĭn-sŭnz) *teeth* Notched teeth characteristic of congenital syphilis.

hydatidiform (hī″da-tĭdĭ-fŏrm) *mole* Condition in which the fertilized ovum becomes altered and an abnormal tissue develops instead of a baby and normal placenta.

hydrocele (hī′drō-sēl) Abnormal collection of fluid in the lining tissue (tunica vaginalis) of the testis.

hydrocephalus (hī-drō-sĕf′à-lŭs) Collection of abnormal amounts of cerebrospinal fluid within the cranium, causing enlargement of the immature skull.

hydrophobia (hī-drō-fō-′bē-à) Rabies; fear of water.

hydrotherapy (hī-drō-thĕr′à-pē) Scientific application of water to treat diseases (hot baths, etc.).

hymen (hī′mĕn) Membrane partially covering the vaginal opening; "the maidenhead."

hyperalimentation (hī″per-ăl′ĭ-mĕn-tā′shŭn) Term usually used to describe total parenteral nutrition by vein (TPN).

hypercalcemia (hī-per-kăl-sē′mē-à) Excessive amount of calcium in the blood.

hypercapnia (hī″per-kăp′nē-à) (increased P$_{CO_2}$) Excessive amount of carbon dioxide in the blood.

hyperemesis gravidarum (hī-pĕr-ĕm′ĕ-sīs grăv-ĭ-dā′rŭm) Persistent, exaggerated nausea and vomiting during pregnancy.

hyperextension (hī″pŭr-ĕck-stĕn′shŭn) Overextension of a limb or part for the correction of a physiological problem.

hyperglycemia (hī-pĕr-glī-sē′mē-à) Excessive amount of glucose in the bloodstream.

hyperkalemia (hī-per-kà-lē′mē-ă) Excessive amount of potassium in the blood.

hypernatremia (hī-per-nà-trē′mē-ă) Excessive amount of sodium in the blood.

hypertension (hī-per-tĕn′shŭn) Abnormal elevation of the blood pressure, especially the diastolic pressure.

hypertonic (hī″per-tŏn′ĭk) Excessive or above normal in tone or tension; a solution containing excessive amounts of salts.

hypertrophy (hī-per′trō-fē) Increase in size or bulk; excessive development.

hyperventilation (hī-per-vĕn-tĭl-ā′shŭn) Overbreathing accompanied by a carbon dioxide deficit commonly causing dizziness as well as tingling and numbness in the hands.

hypnotic (hĭp-nŏt′ĭk) Medication that causes sleep.

hypocalcemia (hī-pō-kăl-sē′mē-ă) Abnormally low blood calcium level.

hypogastric (hī-pō-găs′trĭk) Pertaining to lower middle area of the abdomen.

hypoglycemia (hī-pō-glī-sē′mē-à) Deficiency of glucose in the blood.

hypokalemia (hī-pō-kà-lē′mē-à) Deficiency of potassium in the blood.

hyponatremia (hī-pō-nā-trē′mē-à) Deficiency of sodium in the blood.

hypospadias (hī-pō-spā′dē-às) Condition characterized by the abnormal opening of the urethra on the undersurface of the penis.

hypostatic (hī-pō-stăt′ĭk) Pertaining to the settling of a deposit or congestion in an area, caused by lack of proper activity.

hypotension (hī-pō-tĕn′shun) Abnormal decrease of systolic and diastolic blood pressure.

hypothalamus (hī-pō-thăl′à-mŭs) Area of heat control and other body regulation located near the base of the brain.

hypothermia (hī″pō-thur′mē-à) Pertaining to subnormal temperature of the body.

hypovolemia (hī″pō-vō-lē′mē-ă) Diminished blood volume.

hypoxia (hī-pŏks′ē-ă) Lack of adequate amount of oxygen.

hysterotomy (hĭs-tĕr-ŏt′ō-mē) Opening of the uterus; cesarean birth.

icterus (ĭk′tĕr-ŭs) Jaundice; a yellow tint to the skin.

idiopathic (ĭd-ē-ō-păth′ĭk) Adjective meaning that the cause of the condition is unknown.

ileostomy (ĭl″ē-ŏs′tà-mē) Surgical formation of a fistula or artificial anus through the abdominal wall into the ileum, or an ileal pouch created as a part of the Bricker procedure.

ileum (ĭl′ē-ŭm) Lower portion of small intestine.

ileus (il′ē-ŭs) Obstruction or paralysis of small intestine.

iliopectineal (ĭl″ē-ō-pĕk-tīnē-al) *line* Imaginary line dividing the upper or false pelvis from the lower or true pelvis; the linea terminalis forming the brim or inlet of the pelvis.

immunity (ĭ-mū′nĭ-tē) Ability to protect oneself against the development of infectious disease.

immunofluorescent (ĭm″mŭ-nō-floo-ō-rĕs′ĕnt) antibody technique. Detection of antibodies using special proteins labeled with fluorescein to illuminate with fluorescent light source.

immunosuppressive (ĭm″yòò-nō-sŭh-prĕs′ĭv) Capable of interfering with a normal immune response.

impaction (ĭm-păk′shŭn) State of being lodged and retained abnormally in a part or strait; a large accumulation of relatively hard stool in the rectum or colon, difficult to move.

imperforate (ĭm-pĕr′fŏr-āt) Without an opening.

impetigo (ĭm-pĕ-tī′gō) Contagious skin infection caused by coagulase-positive staphylococci or beta-hemolytic streptococci.

implantation (ĭm-plăn-tā′shŭn) Nesting of the fertilized ovum in the wall of the uterus; artificial placement of a substance in the body.

incarcerated (ĭn-kär′sĕr-ā-tĕd) Trapped; confined.

incest (ĭn′sĕst) Sexual intercourse between close relations.

incontinence (ĭn-kŏn′tĭ-nĕnts) Inability to retain urine or feces because of loss of sphincter control.

incubation (ĭn-kū-bā′shŭn) *period* Period of time that must elapse between the infection of an individual at the time of exposure until the appearance of signs and symptoms of the disease; time during which hatching or developing takes place.

inertia (ĭn-ĕr′shà) Sluggishness; absence of activity; resistance to movement or change.

infanticide (ĭn-făn′tĭs-īd) Killing of an infant.

infectious (ĭn-fĕk′shŭs) *disease* Disorders caused by organisms that invade tissue and cause symptoms of illness.

infecund (ĭn′fĕk-ŭnd) Unfruitful; infertile; inability to conceive.

infertile (ĭn-fer′til) Inability of a man or woman to conceive.

infusion (ĭn-fū′zhun) Introduction of a solution into a vein.

inguinal (ĭn-gwĭ-nal) Pertaining to the region of the groin.

inhibitor (ĭn-hĭb-ĭt-er) Agent that curtails or stops certain activity.

insemination (ĭn'sĕm-ĭ-nā-shŭn) (artificial) Injection of semen into the uterine canal by a process unrelated to intercourse.

integumentary (ĭn-tĕg-ū-mĕn'tà-rē) Referring to the integument, that is, the skin, including the hair, nails, oil and sweat glands, and superficial sensory nerve endings.

interstitial (ĭn-tĕr-stĭsh'al) *fluid* Body fluid found outside the bloodstream in the spaces between the tissue cells.

intertrigo (ĭn"ter-trē'gō) Reddened skin eruption produced by friction of adjacent parts; chafing.

intrauterine device (IUD) Object placed into the uterus to avoid pregnancy by perhaps disrupting implantation.

intubation (ĭn"tū-bā'shŭn) Introduction of a tube into a hollow organ or passageway to keep it open.

intussusception (ĭn-tŭs-sŭs-sĕp'shŭn) Telescoping of adjacent parts of the bowel, usually in the ileocecal region.

in utero (ū'tĕr-ō) Inside the uterus.

inversion (ĭn-vĕr'shŭn or ĭn-vĕr'zhŭn) A turning upside down, inside out, or end to end.

involution (ĭn-vō-lū'shŭn) A turning or rolling inward; the reverse of evolution, a term especially used to describe the return of the uterus to approximately its prepregnant size and position after childbirth.

iodophor (ī-ō'dà-fŏr) Antiseptic containing iodine combined with detergent or an agent or carrier that enhances its solubility.

ion (ī'ăn) One or more atoms carrying an electrical charge.

IPPB Intermittent positive pressure breathing device used to help expand the lungs.

irrigation (irr"ĭ-gā'shŭn) Act of cleansing by a stream of water.

ischial (ĭs'kē-al) *spines* Two relatively sharp bony projections protruding into the pelvic outlet from the ischial bones that form the lower lateral border of the pelvis, used in determining the progress of the fetus down the birth canal.

isolation (ī-sō-lā'shŭn) Prevention of direct or indirect contact with a person with a contagious disease during its period of communicability by the observance of certain barrier techniques designed to prevent the spread of illness.

jaundice (jawn'dĭs) Yellow tinge to the skin or sclerae; icterus.

karyotype (kăr'ē-ō-tīp) Total characteristics of the chromosomes of a cell nucleus including number, form, size, and grouping, usually photographed, cut out and arranged on a card for study.

kernicterus (ker-nĭk'ter-ŭs) Yellow staining of the basal ganglia of the brain in the jaundiced newborn infant; a complication of severe hyperbilirubinemia.

ketogenic (kē-tō-jĕn'ĭk) *diet* High-fat, low-carbohydrate diet.

ketone (kē'tōn) *bodies* Group of compounds produced during the oxidation of fatty acids; one example is acetone.

kwashiorkor (kwash-ĭ-ŏr'kŏr) Disease resulting from protein deprivation in infancy and childhood, common in certain parts of Africa.

kyphosis (kī-fō'sĭs) Humpback.

labia majora (lā'bē-à mà-jō-ra) (sing. labium) Two fleshy, haircovered folds located on both sides of the perineal midline, extending from the mons veneris almost to the anus in women.

labia minora (mĭ-nō'ra) Two small folds of tissue covering the vestibule located just under the labia majora in women.

laceration (lăs-er-ā'shŭn) Jagged cut or tear.

lacrimal (lăk'rĭm-al) *glands* Tear glands.

lactation (lăk-tā'shŭn) Process of milk production or the period of breast feeding in mammals.

lactogenic (lăk-tō-jĕn'ĭk) Inducing the secretion of milk (e.g., the lactogenic hormone *prolactin*, or LTH).

lanugo (là-nū'gō) Soft, fine hair on the body of the fetus or newborn.

laparotomy (lăp-a-rŏt'ō-mē) Abdominal operation; surgical opening of the abdomen.

laryngospasm (lăr-ĭng'gō-spă-zŭm) Spasm of the muscles of the larynx.

larynx (lăr'ĭnks) Voice box.

lesion (lē'zhŭn) Any change or irregularity in tissue resulting from disease or injury.

lethargic (lĕth-är'jĭk) Drowsy; sluggish.

leukemia (lū-kē'mē-a) Disease characterized by overproduction of abnormal, immature, white blood cells; "cancer of the blood."

leukocyte (lū'kō-sīt) White blood cell.

leukocytosis (lū-kō-sī-tō'sĭs) Excessive increase in the number of white blood cells circulating in the blood.

leukopenia (lū-kō-pē'nē-à) Abnormal decrease of circulating white blood cells.

leukorrhea (lū-kō-rē'à) White or yellowish cervical or vaginal discharge.

levator ani (lĕ-vā'tōr ă'nē) Major muscle that helps form the pelvic diaphragm or floor.

ligament (lĭg′ă-mĕnt) Strong, fibrous tissue that serves to connect bone to bone or to support an organ.

ligation (lī-gā′shŭn) Closing off by tying, especially arteries, veins, tubes, or ducts.

lightening (līt′ĕn-ĭng) Descent of the fetus into the true pelvis, which lessens pressure on the maternal thorax and abdomen.

linea nigra (lĭn′ē-ă nī′gra) Dark line that develops during pregnancy extending from the pubis to the umbilicus.

lipoids (lĭp′oydz) Fatty-type substances.

lipoprotein (lĭp″ō-prō′tēn) Simple protein combined with a lipid or fatlike substance.

lithotomy (lĭth-ŏt′a-mē) Cutting operation for removal of a calculus, usually a urinary tract stone.

lochia (lō′kē-ă) Vaginal drainage after childbirth.

lordosis (lōr-dō′sĭs) Exaggerated lumbar curvature; swayback.

lues (lū′ēz) Syphilis.

lumbar puncture Needle insertion into the subarachnoid space of the spinal cord between the lumbar vertebrae for diagnosis or therapy.

luteal (lū′tē-ăl) **hormone** Progesterone.

lymphocyte (lĭm′fō-sīt) One kind of white blood cell.

macule (măk′ŭl) Flat spot or stain.

malaise (ma-lāz′) General discomfort, uneasiness.

mandible (măn′dĭ-bŭl) Jawbone.

mastitis (măs-tī′tĭs) Inflammation of the breast.

maternicity (mă-tern-ĭs′-ĭtē) Emotional attachment of mother to infant with bonds of affection.

maturation (măt-ū-rā′shŭn) Process of developing, ripening, or becoming more adult.

meatotomy (mē-ă-tŏt′ō-mē) Incision of the urinary meatus or opening to enlarge the passage.

meatus (mē-ā′tŭs) Passage or opening.

meconium (mē-kō′nē-ŭm) First feces of the fetus or newborn

medium-chain triglycerides (MCT) (trī-glĭs′ŭr·ĭdz) A glycerine ester combined with an acid and distinguished from other triglycerides by having 8 to 10 carbon atoms; easily digested, high-caloric in nature.

medulla (mē-dŭl′ă) Inner portion of an organ (e.g., the medulla of the kidney or adrenal gland).

megacolon (mĕg-ă-kō′lŏn) Abnormally large colon.

megaloblast (mĕg′ă-lō-blăst) Large, early form of red blood cell with a characteristic nuclear pattern, found in the blood where there is vitamin B_{12} or folic acid deficiency.

menarche (mē-năr′kē) First menses, or menstruation, experienced by a girl.

meningitis (mĕn-ĭn-jī′tĭs) Inflammation of the meninges covering the spinal cord or brain.

meningococcemia (mē-nĭn-gō-kŏk-sē′mĭ-ă) Presence of meningococci in the blood.

meningococcic (mē-nĭn-gō-kŏk′sĭk) **meningitis** Cerebrospinal fever.

meningomyelocele (See myelomeningocele.)

menopause (mĕn′ō-pawz) Period that marks the permanent cessation of menstrual activity.

menorrhagia (mĕn-ō-rā′jē-ă) Excessive bleeding at time of the menstrual period.

menses (mĕn′sēz) Menstruation.

menstruation (mĕn-strū-ā′shŭn) Monthly elimination of a bloody vaginal discharge, the portion of the lining of the uterus that had been prepared for the fertilized egg in the event of pregnancy.

mentum (mĕn′tŭm) Chin.

metabolic (mĕt-ă-bŏl′ĭk) Pertaining to the physical and chemical changes that take place within a living organism.

metabolism (mē-tăb′ă-lĭz-ĕm) All energy and material transformations that occur within living cells.

metacarpal (mĕt″ă-kär′păl) Pertaining to one of the five bones of the hand.

metastasis (mē-tăs′tă-sĭs) Spread of a disease (e.g., cancer) from its primary location to secondary locations; the colonizing element.

metrorrhagia (mē-trō-rā′jē-ă) Presence of bloody vaginal discharge between menstrual periods.

microcephaly (mī-krō-sĕf′ă-lē) Failure of the brain to develop to a normal size.

microgram (μg) One one-thousandth of a milligram (μ=mu).

microorganisms (mī-krō-or′găn-ĭzmz) Minute living bodies not perceptible to the naked eye (e.g., bacteria, protozoa).

milia (mĭl′ē-a) (sing. milium) Pinpoint white or yellow dots commonly found on the nose, forehead, and cheeks of newborn babies resulting from nonfunctioning or clogged sebaceous glands.

miliaria rubra (mĭl-ē-ā′rĭ-ă rü′bră) Heat rash; prickly heat.

miscarriage Spontaneous abortion.

mitosis (mī-tō′sĭs) Cellular division where the chromosomes split longitudinally to reproduce an identical tissue cell.

mohel (moy′ĭl) Ordained Jewish circumciser.

molding Shaping of the baby's head as it travels through the birth canal.

Monilia (mō-nĭl′ē-ă) See moniliasis.

moniliasis (mō-nī-lī′ă-sĭs) Yeast infection of the skin or mucous membranes caused by *Candida albicans*, formerly called *Monilia albicans*; commonly found in the vagina; infection of the mouth is termed thrush.

monitrice (mōn′-ă-trīs) A monitor or adviser of a patient, especially during labor and birth.

monocyte (mŏn′ō-sīt) Type of white blood cell.

mortality (mŏr-tăl′ĭ-tē) State of being mortal, subject to death or destined to die; the death rate.

morula (mŏr′ū-là) Mass of dividing cells resembling a mulberry, resulting from the fertilization of an ovum; an early stage of life.

mosaicism (mō-zā′ĭ-cĭzm) Presence of body cells with differing genetic contents in the same individual.

motile (mō′tĭl) Capability of spontaneous movement.

mucosa (mū-kō′sà) Mucous membrane.

mucous (mū′kŭs) (adj.) Secreting or containing mucus; slimy.

mucoviscidosis (mū-cō-vĭs-ĭd-ō′sĭs) Cystic fibrosis of the pancreas; a disease affecting the exocrine glands involving primarily the respiratory and digestive systems.

mucus (mū′kŭs) (n.) Slippery secretion produced by the mucous membranes.

multifactorial Caused by many factors; involving many genes or combinations of genes.

multiform (mŭl′tĭ-form) Having many forms or shapes.

multigravida (mŭl-tĭ-grăv′ĭ-dà) Woman who has had two or more pregnancies.

multipara (mŭl-tĭp′à-ra) Strictly speaking, a woman who has given birth to two or more infants of 500 g or more; however, in the delivery room, a woman in the process of labor with her second child is often called a multipara.

musculature (mŭs′kū-là-tūr) Arrangement and condition of the muscles in the body or its parts.

mutation (myōō-tā′shŭn) Process of change or alteration.

myelin (mī′lĭn) The white fatty sheath that covers some nerves.

myelinization (mī′lĭn-ĭ-zā′shŭn) Process of supplying or accumulating myelin during development, or repair, of nerves.

myelitis (mī-ĕl-ī′tĭs) Inflammation of the spinal cord or bone marrow (osteomyelitis).

myelomeningocele (mī″ĕl-ō-mĕ-nĭng′ō-sēl) Herniation of elements of the spinal cord and the meninges through an abnormal opening in the spine.

myocarditis (mī″ō-kär-dī′tĭs) Inflammation of the muscular tissue of the heart.

myomectomy (mī-ō-mĕk′tō-mē) Removal of a portion of muscle or muscular tissue.

myometrium (mī″ō-mē′trē-ŭm) Muscular layer of the uterus.

myopia (mī-ō′pē-à) Nearsightedness.

myringotomy (mĭr-ĭn-gŏt′ō-mē) Incision into the eardrum.

nebulization (nĕb′ū-là zā′shŭn) Producing spray or mist-like particles from a liquid.

necrosis (nĕk-rō′sĭs) Death of tissue.

neonatal (nē-ō-nā′tàl) Concerning the newborn infant or the first 4 weeks of life after birth.

neoplasm (nē′ō-plă-zŭm) Tumor.

nephron (nĕf′rŏn) Working unit of the kidney; the renal corpuscle and its tubule.

nephrosis (nĕf-rō′sĭs) Renal disease of unknown cause seen in children, characterized by massive edema and albuminuria.

neuropathy (nū-rŏp′ă-thē) Any disease of the nerves.

neutrophil (nū′trō-fĭl) One kind of white blood cell.

nevus (nē′vŭs) (pl. nevi) Mole, pigmented area, or vascular tumor on the skin.

nitrous oxide (nī′trŭs ŏk′sīd) Laughing gas (N_2O).

nocturia (nŏk-tū′rī-a) Excessive urination during the night.

nodule (nŏd′ūl) Small aggregate of cells.

nuchal (nū′kàl) Pertaining to the neck.

nucleus (nū′klē-ŭs) Central point about which matter is gathered; controlling portion of a cell regulating metabolism and reproduction of the cell.

nulligravida (nŭl-ĭ-grăv′ĭ-dà) woman who has never been pregnant.

nullipara (nŭl-ĭp′à-rà) Woman who has never given birth to an infant of 500 g or more.

nurture (ner′cher) To feed, rear, foster, care for; nourishment, care, and training of growing children or things.

nystagmus (nĭs-tăg′mŭs) Constant, involuntary movement of the eyeballs.

oblique (ō-blēk′) Slanting; inclined.

obturator (ŏb′tū-rā″tŏr) Small, curved rod with an olive-shaped tip that fits inside a tracheostomy tube to aid in its insertion.

occiput (ŏk′sĭ-pŭt) Occipital bone or back part of the skull.

occlude (ŏ-klūd′) To close or plug.

occluded (ŏ-klūd′ĕd) Closed up; obstructed.

occult (ŏ-kŭlt′) Obscure, hidden.

oliguria (ŏl-ĭ-gū′rē-à) Diminished amount of urine production with subsequent scanty urination.

omphalocele (ŏm′făl-ō-sēl) Absence of the normal abdominal wall in the region of the umbilicus creating defects of varying sizes.

opaque (ō-pāk′) Lacking transparency.

ophthalmia neonatorum (ŏf-thăl′mē-à nē-ō-nā-tōr′-ŭm) Inflammation of the eyes of the newborn infant, particularly that caused by gonorrheal organisms.

opisthotonos (ŏ-pĭs-thŏt′ō-nŏs) Involuntary arching of the back because of irritation of the brain or spinal cord.

orchiopexy (or″kē-ō-pĕk′sē) Surgical fixation of a testis or testicle in the scrotum to correct undescent.

orthopnea (ŏr-thŏp-nē′à) Condition in which breathing is difficult except when the patient is in a standing or sitting position.

orthostatic (ŏr-thō-stăt′ĭk) Concerning an erect position or related to a standing position.

osmosis (ŏs-mō′sĭs) Passage of a liquid (solvent), usually water, through a semipermeable partition separating solutions of different concentrations to equalize the concentration of any substance dissolved in the solutions.

ossification (ŏs-ĭ-fĭ-kā′shŭn) Process of bone formation.

osteomalacia (ŏs″tē-ō-mà-lā′shē-à) Adult rickets or softening of the bone.

osteomyelitis (ŏs″tē-ō-mī-ĕ-lī′tĭs) Inflammation of the bone marrow and surrounding cells.

osteoporosis (ŏs″tē-ō-po-rō′sĭs) Deossification with decrease in bone tissue resulting in structural weakness.

otitis media (ō-tī′tĭs mē′dē-à) Middle ear infection.

ovary (ō′và-rē) Paired, almond-shaped gland that produces female hormones and female sex cells, or ova.

oviduct (ō′vĭ-dŭkt) Fallopian, or uterine, tube.

ovulation (ŏ-vŭ-lā′shŭn) Rupture of an ovarian follicle and the explusion of the ovum.

oxytocic (ŏk-sē-tō′sĭk) Medication that stimulates the uterus to contract.

palliative (păl′ē-à-tĭv) Alleviates without curing.

palpation (păl-pā′shŭn) Examination by touch or feel.

papule (păp′ū!) Small, solid elevation on the skin; the typical early stage of a pimple.

papulovesiculopustular (păp-ū-lō-vĕ-sĭk″ū-lō-pŭs′tū-lar) Papule or pimple with both vesicles and pustules.

paracentesis (păr-à-sĕn-tē′sĭs) Artificial withdrawal of fluid by puncture of a body cavity, especially the abdominal cavity.

paralytic (păr-à-lĭt′ĭk) Describes person suffering from loss of the ability to move a part or parts of his body.

parametrium (păr″à-mē′trē-ŭm) Outermost covering of the uterus formed in part by a portion of the peritoneum.

paraplegia (păr′-à-plē″-jà) Paralysis of legs and lower part of the body; both motion and sensation are affected.

parenchyma (pà-reng′kĭ-mà) Functioning portion of an organ as distinguished from supportive cells forming its framework.

parenteral (pà-rĕn′ter-àl) Pertaining to methods of drug or food administration other than through the use of the gastrointestinal tract (e.g., intravenous or subcutaneous routes).

paresis (pà-rē′sĭs) Organic mental illness; partial or incomplete paralysis.

paroxysmal (păr″ŏk-sĭz′măl) Of the nature of a sudden attack.

parturient (păr-tū′rē-ĕnt) Laboring or newly delivered mother.

parturition (păr-tū-rĭsh′ŭn) Childbirth; delivery.

patency (pā′tĕn-sē) State of being freely open.

pathogen (păth′ō-jĕn) Microorganism or substance capable of producing a disease.

pathologic (păth′à-lŏj′ĭ-kàl) Caused by or involving disease; concerning disease.

pediculosis (pĕ-dik-ū-lō′sĭs) Infestation of an individual by head, body, or pubic lice.

pelvimeter (pĕl-vĭm′ĕ-ter) Device used to measure the pelvis.

pendulous (pĕn′dū-lŭs) Hanging; lacking proper support.

percussion (per-kush′ŭn) Tapping the body lightly but sharply for diagnosis or therapy.

perinatal (pĕr-ĭ-nāt′àl) Associated with the period before or after birth.

perineum (per-ĭ-nē′ŭm) Area of the external genitalia in both male and female; specifically, the area between the vagina and the anus or the scrotum and the anus.

periorbital (pĕr′ē-or′bĭt′àl) Periosteum or outermost tissues covering the bone within the orbit of the eye.

periosteum (pĕr-ĭ-ŏs′tē-ŭm) Fibrous membrane that forms the covering of bones except at their articular surfaces.

peripheral (per-ĭf′er-àl) Located at the surface or away from the center of the body.

peristalsis (pĕr-ĭs-tăl′sĭs) Progressive, wavelike movement that occurs involuntarily in hollow tubes of the body, especially the alimentary canal.

peritoneum (pĕr″ĭt-o-nē′ŭm) Serous membrane lining the interior of the abdominal cavity and surrounding the contained internal organs.

peritonitis (pĕr-ĭ-tō-nī′tĭs) Inflammation of the peritoneum.

permeable (pur′mē-à-bàl) Capable of being penetrated.

per se (per sā) Essentially; by itself; of itself.

pertussis (per-tŭs′ĭs) Whooping cough.

petechiae (pà-tē′kē-ī) Small, bluish purple dots on the skin resulting from capillary hemorrhages.

petrification (pĕt″rĭ-fĭ-kā′shŭn) Process of turning into stone.

phagocytosis (făg″ō-sī-tō′sĭs) Ingestion and digestion of bacteria and microscopic particles by phagocytes, certain white blood cells.

pharynx (făr′ĭnks) Musculomembranous passageway at the back of the nose and mouth partially shared by both the respiratory and digestive systems.

phlebitis (flĕ-bī′tĭs) Inflammation of a vein.

phlebotomy (flĕ-bŏt′ō-mē) Purposeful opening of a vein, usually to let out a considerable amount of blood for therapy.

photophobia (fō-tō-fō′bē-à) Unusual intolerance to light.

pica (pī′kà) Abnormal craving for substances not meant for consumption.

pigmentation (pĭg-mĕn-tā′shŭn) Coloration resulting from the deposit of certain substances in the skin.

pipette (pī-pĕt′) Narrow calibrated glass tube with both ends open, used to measure and transfer liquids from one container to another by application of oral suction.

pituitary gland (pī-tū′ĭ-tăr-ē) Endocrine gland located at the base of the brain involved in many body functions; the "master gland."

placenta (plà-sĕn′tà) Flattened, circular mass of spongy vascular tissue attached to the inside of the uterine wall that serves as the metabolic link between the fetus and the mother; from its surface protrudes the umbilical cord that carries food and oxygen to the fetus and waste away from the fetus; also serves as a point of attachment for the bag of waters that encloses the fetus.

placentae abruptio (See abruptio placentae.)

placenta previa (prē′vēà) Low implantation of the placenta near or over the cervix within the uterine cavity causing hemorrhage late in pregnancy.

plantar (plăn′tăr) Concerning the sole of the foot.

platelet (plā′lĕt) (blood platelet) Thrombocyte, a necessary element for blood clot formation.

platypelloid (plăt″ē-pĕl′oyd) Abnormal type of female pelvis, flattened from front to back.

pneumatocele (nŭ-mă′ō-sēl) Herniation of lung tissue; a sac or tumor containing gas.

pneumomediastinum (nŭ″mō-mē-dē-ăs-tī′nŭm) Air or gas in the mediastinal tissues located between the lungs.

pneumonia (nŭ-mō′nē-à) Inflammation of the lung tissue.

pneumothorax (nŭ-mō-thō′răks) Collection of air or gas in the pleural cavity (the potential space between the two coverings of the lungs).

polyarthritis (pŏl″ē-är-thrī′tĭs) Inflammation that involves more than one joint, often migratory in character.

polycystic (pŏl-ē-sĭs′tĭk) Composed of many cysts, that is, little sacs usually containing fluid.

polycythemia (pŏl″ē-sī-thē′mē-à) Abnormal condition characterized by an excess of red blood cells.

polydactylism (pŏl-ē-dăk′tĭl-ĭzm) Presence of extra fingers or toes.

polydipsia (pŏl-ē-dĭp′sē-à) Excessive thirst and fluid intake.

polyhydramnios (pŏl″ē-hī-drăm′nē-ōs) Excessive volume of amniotic fluid.

polymorphonuclear (pŏl″ē-mor-fō-nü′klē-er) Leukocyte having a lobated or segmented nucleus.

polyphagia (pŏl-ē-fā′jē-à) Excessive appetite.

polyuria (pŏl-ē-ū′rē-à) Excessive urinary output.

portal of entry Avenue by which an infectious agent gains entrance into the body.

precipitate (prē-sĭp′ĭ-tāt) *delivery* Birth that occurs with such rapidity that proper preparation and medical supervision are lacking.

preeclampsia (prē-ĕk-lamp′sē⁺a) Toxemia of pregnancy uncomplicated by convulsion or coma; pregnancy-induced hypertension (see eclampsia).

prehension (prē-hĕn′shŭn) Use of the hands to pick up small objects; grasping.

prepuce (prē′pŭs) Foreskin of the penis or hood of the clitoris.

presentation In obstetrics, relationship of the length of the fetus to the length of the uterus.

presenting part Part of the baby that comes through or attempts to come through the pelvic canal first; often synonymous with "obstetric presentation."

primigravida (prī-mĭ-grăv′ĭ-dà) Woman who is having or has had one pregnancy.

primipara (prī-mĭp′à-rà) Strictly speaking, a woman who has given birth to one infant over 500 g; however, in the delivery room, a woman in the process of labor with her first viable child is often called a primipara.

progesterone (prō-jĕs′tĕr-ōn) Female sex hormone manufactured by the corpus luteum of the ovary and, during pregnancy, by the placenta; aids in preparing the lining of the uterus for pregnancy and maintaining a pregnancy once established.

progestin (prō-jĕs′ tĭn) Any progestational hormone; a synonym for progesterone.

prognosis (prog-nō′sĭs) Prediction regarding the course of a disease and the likelihood of recovery.

prolapse (prō-lăps′) Falling out of place (e.g., a rectocele).

prophylactic (prō-fĭ-lăk′tĭk) That which prevents disease.

prophylaxis (prō-fĭ-lăk′sĭs) Preventive treatment.

proptosis (prăp-tō′sĭs) Forward displacement.

prostaglandin (prŏs″tă-glănd-ĭn) Group of fatty acid derivatives present in many tissues, including prostate, involved in regulating many body processes.

prostate (prŏs′tāt) Exocrine gland found at the base of the male bladder that secretes an alkaline fluid stimulating sperm motility.

prosthesis (prō-thē′sĭs) Artifical body part.

proteinuria (prō-tē-ĭn-ū′rē-à) Finding of protein usually albumin, in the urine.

prothrombin (prō-thrŏm'bĭn) Chemical substance found in the blood, necessary to coagulation.

protozoa (prō-tō-zō'á) (sing. protozoon) Simple microscopic animals, usually single celled.

protrusion (prō-trü'zhŭn) State or condition of being forward or projecting.

protuberant (prō·tōō'bàr-ànt) Bulging.

pruritus (prü-rī'tŭs) Itching.

pseudohermaphroditism (sū"dō-hĕr-măf'rō-dīt-ĭzm) Condition in which an individual possesses external genitalia resembling those of one sex and the internal sex organs, or gonads, of the opposite sex.

psychosis (sī-kō-'sĭs) Serious mental disturbance involving personality disintegration and loss of contact with reality.

psychosocial (sī"kō-sō'shàl) Involving both psychological and social factors.

ptyalism (tī'á-lĭzm) Excessive salivation.

puberty (pū'ber-tē) Period in life when one becomes capable of reproduction.

puerperium (pū-er-pīr'ē-ŭm) Six-week period following childbirth.

purpura (pur'pū-rà) Purple discoloration that occurs as a result of spontaneous bleeding into the skin or mucous membranes.

pustule (pŭs'tūl) Pus-filled papule; a superficial cutaneous abscess.

pyelogram (pī'ĕl-ō-grăm) Radiograph of the ureters and renal pelves.

pyelonephritis (pī"ĕl-ō-nĕf-rī'tĭs) Infection of the renal pelvis and the working units of the kidney, the nephrons.

pyogenic (pī-ō-jĕn'ĭk) Producing pus.

pyrosis (pī-rō'sĭs) Heartburn.

quarantine (kwär'ăn-tēn) Confinement of a person or group of persons who have been exposed to a contagious disease to a specific place without outside contacts for the duration of the longest usual incubation period of the disease in question.

quickening (kwĭk'ĕn-ĭng) Maternal identification of fetal motion; felt by multiparas at about the sixteenth week of pregnancy and by primiparas 2 weeks later.

radiograph (rā'dĭ-ō-grăf) X-ray film.

rationale (răsh-ŭn-ăl') Logical reason for a course of action or procedure.

rectocele (rĕk'tō-sēl) Prolapse or displacement of the rectum because of weakening of the rectovaginal wall.

reduction (rē-dŭk'shŭn) In orthopedics, refers to realignment of a broken bone or the correct placement of a dislocation.

reflux (rē'flŭks) Return or backward flow (e.g., regurgitation of urine from the bladder into the ureter).

regurgitation (rē-gŭr-jĭ-tā'shŭn) Return of solids or fluids to the mouth from the stomach; any abnormal backflow of fluid within the body.

remission (rē-mĭsh'un) Lessening of severity or abatement of symptoms.

resorption (rē-sōrp'shŭn) Disappearance of all or part of a process, tissue, or exudate by biochemical reactions.

reservoir (rĕz'er-vwàr) Chamber or receptacle for holding fluid; store; reserve.

retinoblastoma (rĕt-ĭn-ō-blăs-tō'mà) Malignant tumor of the eye.

retinopathy (rĕt"ĭn-ŏp'a-thē) Any disorder of the retina.

retraction (rĕ-trăk'shŭn) State of being drawn back.

retroflexion (rĕt-rō-flĕk'shŭn) Bending or flexing backward; an abnormal position of the uterus bent backward toward the rectum, forming an angle between the cervix and the body of the organ.

retrograde (rĕt'rō-grād) Moving backward; degenerating from better to worse.

retrolental fibroplasia (rĕ"tro-lĕn'tàl fĭ"brō-plā'zē-à) Oxygen-induced separation of the retina of the eye behind the lens; characteristic of premature infants.

retroversion (rĕt-rō-ver'-shŭn) Turning or state of being turned back; backward displacement of the body of the uterus so that the cervix points toward the symphysis pubis instead of toward the sacrum.

Rh blood factor Blood protein found in approximately 85% of the American population; those persons who possess it are termed Rh positive.

rheumatism (rü' mà-tĭzm) Any of numerous conditions characterized by inflammation or pain in muscles, joints, or fibrous tissue.

rhinitis (rī-nī'tĭs) Inflammation of the nasal mucosa.

rickets (rĭk'ĕts) Disturbance in skeletal development because of poor nutritional intake or absorption of vitamin D and/or calcium or phosphorus; characterized by abnormal softening of the bones.

rubella (rü-bĕl'à) German, or 3-day, measles.

rubeola (rü-bē'ō-là) Red, or 2-week, measles.

sacrum (sā'krŭm) Fused bone that with the coccyx forms the lower portion of the spine and posterior surface of the pelvis.

salmonellosis (săl"mō-nĕl-ō'sĭs) Infection (including typhoid) caused by ingesting foods containing species of the genus *Salmonella*.

sarcoma (sär-kō'mà) Malignant tumor originating in connective tissue.

scabies (skā'bēz) Infestation of the skin by the itch mite *Sarcoptes scabiei*; "7-year itch."

sclera (sklĕ'rà) (pl. sclerae) White outercoating of the eyeball extending from the optic nerve to include the cornea.

scoliosis (skō-lĭ-ō′sĭs) Abnormal lateral spinal curvature.

scrotum (skrō′tŭm) Pouch forming part of the male external genitalia containing the testicles and part of the spermatic cord.

scultetus (skŭl-tē′tŭs) *binder* Many-tailed abdominal binder.

seborrhea (sĕb-ōr-ē′à) Functional disorder of the sebaceous (oil) glands of the skin and/or scalp causing crusting and scaling; on the scalp it may be called dandruff, milk crust, or cradle cap, depending on the location and density of the scaling.

sedative (sĕd′à-tĭv) Medication that quiets and reduces tension.

semen (sē′mĕn) Fluid discharge from the male reproductive organs that contains the sperm destined to fertilize the female ovum.

sensitization (sĕn-sĭ-tĭ-zā′shŭn) Process of making a person reactive to a substance such as a drug, plant, fiber, or serum.

sepsis (sĕp′sĭs) Presence or state of contamination, putrefaction, or infection.

septic (*adj.*, sepsis)

septicemia (sĕp-tĭ-sē′mē-à) Disease condition resulting from the absorption of pathogenic microorganisms and/or the poisons resulting from infectious processes into the blood.

sequela(e) (sē-kwē′là) Condition following and resulting from a disease.

sequestrum (sē-kwĕs′trŭm) (pl. sequestra) Fragment of a diseased, decaying bone that has become separated from surrounding tissue.

serology (ser-ŏl′ō-jĭ) Study of blood serum.

serosanguineous (sē″rō-săn-gwĭn′ē-ŭs) Containing both serum and blood.

show In obstetrics, the blood-tinged mucoid vaginal discharge that becomes more pronounced and red as cervical dilatation increases during labor.

shunt (shŭnt) To turn away from; to divert; a normal or artificially constructed passage that diverts a flow from one main route to another.

sibling (sĭb′lĭng) One of two or more children of the same parents.

smegma (smĕg′mà) Cheesy secretion of the sebaceous glands found in the area of the labia minora and the clitoris of the female or the prepuce in the male.

spastic (spăs′tĭk) Type of muscular action characterized by stiff, uncoordinated movement.

spasticity (spăs-tĭs′ĭ-tē) Stiff, awkward, uncoordinated movements caused by hypertension of the muscles, usually caused by brain damage.

sperm Male sex cell, spermatozoon, carrying the male hereditary potential.

spermatozoon (sper″ma-tō-zō-′on) (pl. spermatozoa) Male sex cell.

spermicide (sper′mĭ-sīd) Agent that kills spermatozoa.

sphincter (sfĭngk′ter) Circular muscle constricting or closing an opening.

spore (spōr) Protective form assumed by some bacilli (usage in bacteriology).

stasis (stā′sĭs) Cessation of flow in blood or other body fluids.

station (stā′shŭn) Depth of the presenting part in the pelvic canal as measured by the relationship of the presenting part to the ischial spines of the pelvis.

status asthmaticus (stăt′ŭs ăz-măt′ĭ-kŭs) Severe asthmatic condition that does not respond to usual treatment with epinephrine.

steatorrhea (stē-ăt-ōr-rē′à) Presence of excessive fat in the stool.

stenosis (stĕn-ō′sĭs) Abnormal narrowing of a passage or opening.

sterile (stĕr′ĭl) Free of living microorganisms, including spore forms.

stoma (stō′mà) Mouth or opening of a pore; a body opening, natural or artificial; term usually applied to a colostomy, ileostomy, or ileobladder opening.

strabismus (strà-bĭz′mŭs) Crossed or crooked eyes; squint.

streptococcus (strĕp-tō-kŏk′ŭs) (pl. streptococci) Spherical microorganism that forms a pattern like beads on a string.

striae (strī′ē) Stretch marks often seen on the skin of pregnant women.

stridor (strī′dōr) Harsh-sounding respirations.

subcostal (sŭb-kŏs′tàl) Lying beneath a rib or ribs or just below the last rib adjacent to the abdomen.

subinvolution (sub-ĭn-vō-lū′shŭn) Incomplete return of a part to its normal position or dimensions; term usually applied to an abnormal, incomplete return of the uterus to its prepregnant state after childbirth.

subluxation (sŭb″lŭk-sā′shŭn) Incomplete dislocation of a bone.

supine (sü-pīn′) Positioned on the back or palm up.

suprapubic (sü″prà-pū′bĭk) Above the pubis.

suprasternal (sü″prà-stur′nàl) Above the sternum, adjacent to the neck.

syndactylism (sĭn-dăk′tĭl-ĭzm) Fusion or webbing of two or more fingers or toes.

syndrome (sĭn′drōm) Complete picture of a disease; all the symptoms of a disease considered as a whole.

synthetic (sĭn-thĕt′ĭk) Artificially prepared.

systolic (sĭs-tŏl′ĭk) *pressure* Pertaining to systole; blood pressure at the time of greatest cardiac contraction.

tachycardia (tăk″ē-kär′dē-à) Excessive rapidity of the heart's action.

tachypnea (tăk″ĭp-nē′à) Rapid rate of breathing.

talipes (tăl′ĭ-pēz) Any of a number of deformities of the ankle or foot, usually congenital; clubfoot.

talipes valgus (văl′gŭs) The toes are turned out.

talipes varus (văr′rŭs) The toes are turned in.

telangiectasia (tel-ăn″jē-ĕk-tā′zē-ȧ) Small reddened areas often found on the eyelids, midforehead, and nape of the neck on newborn infants, caused by superficial dilatation of capillaries.

tendon (tĕn′dŭn) Fibrous tissue that connects muscle to bone or other structures.

teratogenic (tĕr″ȧ-tō-gĕn′ĭk) Capable of causing congenital malformation.

testis (tĕs′tĭs) (pl. testes) Paired, oval, male sex gland that produces a male sex hormone and spermatozoa.

testosterone (tĕs-tŏs′tĕr-ōn) Male hormone produced by the testes.

tetanus (tĕt′ȧ-nŭs) Lockjaw; a state of sustained muscular contraction.

tetany (tĕt′a-nē) Nervous disorder characterized by intermittent tonic spasms of the muscles that may be caused by inadequate calcium levels in the bloodstream.

therapeutic (thĕr′-ȧ-pū′tĭk) Having medicinal or healing properties; a healing agent.

thermal (ther′măl) Pertaining to heat.

thoracentesis (thō-răs-ĕn-tē′sĭs) Removal of fluids through the chest wall by the insertion of a special needle.

thrombocyte (thrŏm′bō-sīt) Blood platelet necessary to coagulation.

thrombocytopenia (thrŏm″bō-sī″tō-pēn′ĭ-a′) An abnormal decrease in the number of platelets in the blood.

thrombophlebitis (thrŏm″bō-flē-bī′tĭs) Inflammation of a vein in conjunction with the development of a blood clot.

thrombosis (thrŏm′-bō′sĭs) Formation of a blood clot.

thrombus (thrŏm′bŭs) Blood clot formed in a blood vessel or cavity of the heart.

thrush (thrŭsh) Fungous infection caused by *Candida albicans* in the mouth or throat, especially in infants; characterized by white patches that adhere to the mucous membranes.

tincture (tĭngk′tūr) Substance that, in solution, is diluted with alcohol.

tinea capitis (tĭn′ē-ȧ kăp′ĭ-tĭs) Ringworm of the scalp.

tinea corporis (kōr′por-ĭs) Any fungous skin disease, especially ringworm of the body.

tinea pedis (pĕd′ĭs) Fungous skin disease or ringworm of the foot; commonly called athlete's foot.

torsion (tōr′shŭn) Act of or condition of being twisted.

torticollis (tōr-tĭ-kŏl′ĭs) Wryneck or tilting of the head caused by the abnormal shortening of either sternocleidomastoid muscle.

toxemia (tŏk-sē′mē-ȧ) Presence of poisonous products in the blood and body; disease of unknown mechanism suffered by some pregnant women, characterized by high blood pressure, albumin in the urine, and edema (see eclampsia and preeclampsia [pregnancy-induced hypertension]).

toxoid (tŏks′oyd) Preparation that contains a toxin or poison produced by pathogenic organisms capable of producing active immunity against a disease but too weak to produce the disease itself.

tracheostomy (trā-kē-ŏst′ō-mē) Surgical opening of the trachea through the neck to help assure an airway; a planned intervention usually of some duration or permanence.

traction (trăk′shŭn) Process of pulling.

transcutaneous (trăns″kyōō-tā′nē-ŭs) Performed through the skin.

transilluminated (trăns-ĭl-lū mĭ-nā′tĕd) Inspection of cavity or organ by passing light through its walls.

translocation (trănz″lō-kā′shŭn) Displacement of part or all of one chromosome onto another.

transverse (trăns-vĕrs′) Lying at right angles to the long axis of the body; crosswise.

transverse presentation Presentation in which the fetus lies crosswise in the pelvis and cannot be delivered vaginally unless turned.

trauma (trăw′mȧ) Injury or wound; a painful emotional experience.

treponemal (trĕp″ō-nē′măl) Pertaining to a genus of spiral organisms, parasitic to man, with undulating or rigid bodies.

trichomonas vaginitis (trĭ-kŏm′ō′nȧs vȧ-jĭ-nī′tĭs) Inflammation of the vagina caused by the parasitic protozoan *Trichomonas vaginalis* that results in itching and a profuse, bubbly, yellow discharge.

trigone (trī′gōn) Triangular space; triangular area in the urinary bladder formed by the urethral outlet and the two ureteral openings.

trimester (trī-mĕs′tĕr) Three-month period of time.

trisomy (trī′sō-mē) Occurrence of three of a given chromosome in a cell rather than the normal diploid number of two.

trophozoite (trŏf-ō-zō′ĭt) Animal spore during its developmental stage; motile form of the ameba.

turbidity (tûr-bĭd′ȧ-tē) Cloudy or dense state; like a fog.

turgor (tur′gur) Normal tension in living cells; distention or swelling.

ubiquitous (ū-bĭk′wĕt-ŭs) Existing or seeming to exist everywhere.

μg (See microgram.)

ulcer (ŭl′ser) Raw area often depressed or forming a cavity caused by loss of normal covering tissue.

ultrasonography (ŭl″trȧ-sō-nŏg′rȧ-fē) Pulse echo diagnosis or technique using high-frequency, inaudible sound waves.

umbilicus (ŭm-bĭl′ĭkŭs or ŭm-bĭ-lī′kŭs) Site of the umbilical cord attachment; the navel.

uremia (ū-rē′mē-ȧ) Toxic condition associated with renal insufficiency and the retention in the blood of nitrogenous substances normally excreted by the kidney.

ureter (ū-rē′tur/ūr′ē-ter) Long tubes conveying the urine from the kidneys to the urinary bladder.

ureterocele (ū-rē′ter-ō-sēl) Ballooning of the lower end of the ureter.

urethra (ū-rē′thra) Canal through which the urine is discharged.

urethroplasty (ū-rē′thrō-plăs-tē) Operation to correct hypospadias; surgical repair of the urethra.

urogram (ū′rō-gram) X-ray photograph of any part of the urinary tract.

urticaria (ur-tĭ-kā′rē-ȧ) Wheals; hives; large, slightly raised, reddened or blanched areas often accompanied by intense itching.

uterine inertia (ū′ter-ĭn ĭn-er′shȧ) Abnormal relaxation of the uterus either during labor, causing lack of obstetric progress, or after childbirth, causing uterine hemorrhage.

uterus (ū′ter-ŭs) Hollow, muscular organ that serves as a protector and nourisher of the developing fetus and aids in its expulsion from the body; the womb.

vaccine (văk′sēn) Preparation containing killed or weakened living microorganisms that, when introduced into the body, cause the formation of antibodies against that type of organism, thereby protecting the individual from the disease.

vaccinia (văk-sĭn′ē-ȧ) (generalized) Numerous vaccination sites resulting from the spread of the vaccine to open lesions after a smallpox vaccination.

vagina (vȧ-jī′nȧ) Canal opening between the urethra and anus in the female that extends back to the cervix of the uterus.

valgus (văl′gŭs) Term denoting position, meaning "turned outward" or "twisted"; applied to a clubfoot with the toes turned outward.

varicella (văr-ĭ-sĕl′ȧ) Chicken pox; acute contagious disease, commonly of childhood, characterized by a body rash seen simultaneously in all stages of development.

varicosity (văr-ĭ-kŏs′ĭ-tē) Abnormal swollen vein, the walls of which are thinned and weakened.

variola (vă-rī′ō-la) Smallpox; severe contagious disease characterized by the formation of a typical rash and pronounced prostration; may cause death.

varus (vā′rŭs) Term denoting position, meaning "turned inward"; applied to a clubfoot with the toes turned inward.

vas deferens (văs dĕf′er-ĕnz) Excretory duct of the testis.

vasodilator (văs-ō-dī-lā′tŏr) Drug that dilates the blood vessels.

vein (vān) Blood vessel that carries blood to the heart.

ventricle (vĕn′-trĭk-ŭl) Small cavity or chamber; one of two lower chambers of the heart; one of several cavities in the brain where cerebrospinal fluid is formed or drains.

ventriculogram (vĕn-trĭk′ū-lō-grăm) Diagnostic test in which air is introduced into the ventricles of the brain through surgical openings in the scalp.

vernix caseosa (vĕr′nĭks cāz-ē-ō′sȧ) Yellowish, creamy substance on the fetus caused by the secretion of the sebaceous glands of the skin.

version (ver′shŭn) In obstetrics, the changing of the fetal presentation by internal or external manual maneuvers.

vertigo (ver′tĭ-gō) Dizziness.

vesicle (vĕs′ĭ-kŭl) Elevation of the skin, obviously containing fluid; a blister.

vesicular (vĕs-ĭk′ū-lar) Blisterlike.

vestibule (vĕs′tĭ-būl) Triangular space between the labia minora in which the openings of the urethra, vagina, and Bartholin's glands are located.

viable (vī′ȧ-bŭl) Capable of life; capable of living outside the uterus; subject to legal definition.

virulent (vĭr′ū-lĕnt) Highly poisonous; infectious.

virus (vī′rŭs) Submicroscopic infective agent.

viscid (vĭs′ĭd) Sticky.

viscosity (vĭs-kŏs′ĭ-tē) State of being thick, gummy, or sticky.

VMA (abbreviation for vanillylmandelic acid) (văn″-ĭ-lĭl-măn-del′-ĭk) Metabolic end product of adrenal medullary hormones (noradrenaline and adrenaline) excreted in the urine.

vulnerable Susceptible to being wounded; in an unfavorable condition.

vulva (vŭl′vȧ) External female genitalia.

wheal (wēl) Large, slightly raised, reddened or blanched area, often accompanied by intense itching.

zygote (zī′gōt) Fertilized egg.

INDEX